DISSEMINATION AND IMPLEMENTATION RESEARCH IN HEALTH

SECOND EDITION

DISSEMINATION AND IMPLEMENTATION RESEARCH IN HEALTH

Translating Science to Practice

EDITED BY

ROSS C. BROWNSON

GRAHAM A. COLDITZ

ENOLA K. PROCTOR

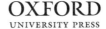

OXFORD
UNIVERSITY PRESS

OXFORD
UNIVERSITY PRESS

Oxford University Press is a department of the University of Oxford. It furthers
the University's objective of excellence in research, scholarship, and education
by publishing worldwide. Oxford is a registered trade mark of Oxford University
Press in the UK and certain other countries.

Published in the United States of America by Oxford University Press
198 Madison Avenue, New York, NY 10016, United States of America.

Library of Congress Cataloging-in-Publication Data
Names: Brownson, Ross C., editor. | Colditz, Graham A., editor. |
Proctor, Enola Knisley, editor.
Title: Dissemination and implementation research in health :
translating science to practice / edited by Ross C. Brownson,
Graham A. Colditz, Enola K. Proctor.
Description: Second edition. | Oxford ;
New York : Oxford University Press, [2018] |
Includes bibliographical references and index.
Identifiers: LCCN 2017029605 | ISBN 9780190683214 (pbk. : alk. paper)
Subjects: | MESH: Translational Medical Research—methods |
Information Dissemination
Classification: LCC R852 | NLM W 20.55.T7 |
DDC 610.72/4—dc23
LC record available at https://lccn.loc.gov/2017029605

1 3 5 7 9 8 6 4 2

Printed by Sheridan Books, Inc., United States of America

We dedicate this book to our spouses: Carol Brownson, Pat Cox, and Frank Proctor. We are grateful for their loving support, patience, and good humor.

CONTENTS

FOREWORD

Five years on down the road . . .

Perhaps the most frequently quoted statistic in dissemination and implementation (D&I) research is one that derives from Balas and Boren's seminal article in 2000: "It takes 17 years to turn 14 percent of original research to the benefit of patient care."[1] It is thus interesting to be writing this foreword 17 years after the publication of that article, and contemplating the second edition of this edited volume on D&I just 5 years removed from its inaugural version. By 2000 standards, we should still be some 12 years from the impact of the 2012 edition and yet it has been quite prominent in offering a comprehensive look at D&I research since its publication. And the field continues marching along.

Five years is the typical length of an NIH R01 grant, the standard for completion of a single definitive investigation of a set of research aims, and in the annals of D&I research history, it has been marked by a fair amount of progress made from the previous iteration. It is my intent in this foreword to provide a few reflections of where the field has gone, what D&I investigators have produced, both in terms of quality and quantity, and then to project into the next 5 years.

FIELD PROGRESS

Reflecting on the past few years, there has clearly been an increase in both the quality and quantity of dissemination and implementation research in health. The most recent versions of the trans-NIH program announcements (PARs) on D&I research were released in 2016, with another increase in representation of the components of the Agency, including Institutes, Centers, and Offices, which now number 18. The most recent versions highlight some of the areas in which D&I research is expanding, including greater focus on understanding adaptation of interventions in the context of implementation, sustainability of evidence-based practices (EBPs) over time, and even the de-implementation of ineffective or harmful practices still in use.[2-4] Over the past 5 years, tens of D&I research studies, including small grants, exploratory and developmental studies, and larger R01 grants, have been funded just through the PARs, and a number of additional NIH funding opportunity announcements have made the study of dissemination and implementation a core component of the scientific agenda moving forward.

We have also seen the contribution of other funders support advances in D&I research. The Patient Centered Outcomes Research Institute (PCORI) has identified communication and dissemination research as a key priority and has published several program announcements to stimulate more comparative effectiveness research in this area. The Agency for Healthcare Research and Quality has similarly articulated D&I research priorities for their extramural research program. In addition, the Veterans Administration's Quality Enhancement Research Initiative (QUERI) has continued support for D&I research since its inception in 1998, currently funding a series of centers targeting a variety of health care topics, including personalization of care, clinical care teams, and mobile health. Internationally, we have seen a complementary rise in solicitations of D&I research. The Canadian Institutes for Health Research and Canadian Cancer Society Research Institute, for example, have supported multiple grants in the D&I (or Knowledge Translation) space. The UK's Medical Research Council and the WHO have also supported D&I research (typically referred to as Implementation Science), and multiple foundations have also solicited work in this space.

D&I research has had a prominent role in a range of national conferences. The annual conferences on the science of dissemination and implementation have exceeded 1,100 participants annually, and the Society for Behavioral Medicine, American Society of Preventive Oncology, ASCO Quality Symposium, Society of Prevention Research, among others, have all featured D&I research as plenary sessions in recent years.

Training in Dissemination and Implementation Research has also continued at a frenzied pace. The NIH's Training Institute in Dissemination and Implementation Research in Health recently held trained its sixth cohort, and both MT-DIRC and IRI continue to bring in new investigators focusing on D&I research in cancer and mental health, respectively. Our neighbors to the North have continued the Knowledge Training Canada Summer Training Institutes as well, and additional academic courses, preconference workshops, certificate programs, and online training models have appeared to respond to the increased demand for D&I research knowledge.[5] In addition, a number of global implementation science training courses have emerged, including several partnerships between the National Institutes of Health, the World Cancer Congress, USAID, and many other international organizations.

More exciting to see has been the increase in the quality of D&I research conducted, much of which is referenced in this volume. The contributions of novel models and frameworks to explain dissemination and implementation processes continue to grow, beyond the previous published reviews[6-8] to better reflect the complexity and dynamism in the field. We've seen a number of new priority areas emerge—enhanced focus on sustainability, tailoring of interventions and implementation strategies to local contexts, scale-up across health systems, and the recognition of the need to study de-implementation.

We've seen more work to advance the research designs and available measures in our armamentarium. The former has included an expansion in the use of hybrid effectiveness-implementation designs,[9] the application of adaptive designs to implementation research questions,[10] as well as the full complement of research designs to apply both rigor and relevance to investigations.[11,12] The latter has seen much work to

operationalize D&I models, including the Society for Implementation Research Collaboration's Instrument Review Project and CFIR's measures database (CFIRguide.org), as well as the NCI's Grid-enabled Measures workspace for D&I research (https://cancercontrol.cancer.gov/brp/research/gem.html). And as referenced earlier, an increasing number of empirical studies of various approaches to improve adoption, implementation, adaptation, and sustainability of evidence-based health interventions.

SO WHERE IS D&I RESEARCH HEADING NEXT?

Pooling D&I Research Data

We have reached a new era of data sharing. Funding agencies have expanded the expectations for clinical trials, genomic studies, and a whole range of other research areas. As we have made progress in the development and validation of D&I construct measures, we will likely need to up our game in pooling common data elements across D&I studies. Both GEM and the SIRC instrument review projects have increased the democratization of measures, but we need to think about infrastructure needed to accept, compile, and analyze data across studies. This will be particularly important when we consider the potential contribution from analysis at the organization or system level, where any one study may be inadequate to generalize beyond the sample.

Mechanistic D&I Research

The field has not yet taken as much advantage of empirical investigations to capture a mechanistic understanding of what leads to successful D&I of EBPs. Many studies still focus more on answering whether dissemination or implementation strategies were successful rather than seeking to understand how and why these strategies led to differing levels of EBP adoption, implementation, and sustainment; what happened rather than how or why it happened. It is important for the next generation of studies to incorporate tests of hypothesized mechanisms of action so that no matter what the overall impact on D&I may be, we are advancing our understanding of what components of strategies we seek to target, whether they operate as designed, and how different mechanisms may work in concert to affect the overall implementation outcome.

Avoiding Silos Between D&I Research and D&I Practice

As the research community has embraced studies of D&I as a valid form of scientific activity, we have become aware that we may be creating a wedge between those advancing the science with those who work as D&I practitioners. The premise of D&I research was to break down the silos between research and practice, and the next generation of work in this area would be well served not to recreate a new set of barriers in the service of acceptability to biomedical research. We have also seen this to some degree in the ongoing discussions of similarities and differences between D&I research, quality improvement research, improvement science, and other areas of investigation. While some of these distinctions come from slightly different field histories, we should all be concerned that we are erecting even greater silos among investigators and between researchers and other key stakeholders. Chapter 11 in this volume focuses on participatory methods in D&I research, something that perhaps can help to address this issue by bringing all valuable perspectives to the table within specific studies.

Harnessing and Embracing All Evidence

On a related front, with processes of capturing data within front-line practice aided by technological savvy, an opportunity for the field to harness and embrace all available evidence to drive D&I decision-making seems within our reach. The more we increasingly see the health care community and public health systems as challenged by a dynamic world that is moving toward precision medicine, the more that D&I research can help us identify how best way to integrate research evidence, local knowledge, and stakeholder preferences, restoring the concept of evidence-based medicine to its 1995 definition.[14]

Return on Investment of D&I Research

Now that we see increased maturity in the D&I research field, we may finally be able to make more progress in being able to calculate the return on investments made to advance our science. We hypothesize that practicing high-value health care through provision of underutilized evidence-based practices may outstrip the benefit of discovering a new practice in an established area,[15] but we should seek to calculate how the results from D&I research contributes to improved value. Systems modeling may be useful in this endeavor, as may be synthesis of

the scientific products from discovery to delivery to see what bang for the buck D&I research generates.

If we are successful in moving these areas forward, I anticipate the fruits of our collective labors will be captured in subsequent editions of this book. The future is bright . . . .

David Chambers, DPhil
Deputy Director for Implementation Science
Division of Cancer Control and Population Sciences
National Cancer Institute
National Institutes of Health

REFERENCES

1. Balas EA, Boren SA. Managing clinical knowledge for health care improvement. In: Bemmel J, McCray AT, eds. *Yearbook of medical informatics.* Stuttgart: Schattauer; 2000: 65–70.
2. National Institute of Health (NIH). Dissemination and Implementation Research in health (R01). Available at: http://grants.nih.gov/grants/guide/pa-files/PAR-16-238.html. Accessed April 7, 2017.
3. National Institute of Health (NIH). Dissemination and Implementation Research in health (R03). Available at: http://grants.nih.gov/grants/guide/pa-files/PAR-16-237.html. Accessed April 7, 2017.
4. National Institute of Health (NIH). Dissemination and Implementation Research in health (R21). Available at: http://grants.nih.gov/grants/guide/pa-files/PAR-16-236.html. Accessed April 7, 2017.
5. Proctor EK, Chambers DA. Training in dissemination and implementation research: a field-wide perspective. *Transl Behav Med.* 2016 May 3. [Epub ahead of print]
6. Tabak RG, Khoong EC, Chambers DA, Brownson RC. Bridging research and practice: models for dissemination and implementation research. *Am J Prev Med.* 2012;43(3):337–350.
7. Mitchell SA, Fisher CA, Hastings CE, Silverman LB, Wallen GR. A thematic analysis of theoretical models for translational science in nursing: mapping the field. *Nurs Outlook.* 2010;58(6):287–300.
8. Nilsen P. Making sense of implementation theories, models and frameworks. *Implement Sci.* 2015;10:53.
9. Curran G.M, Bauer M, Mittman B, Pyne J.M., Stetler C. Effectiveness-implementation hybrid designs: combining elements of clinical effectiveness and implementation research to enhance public health impact. *Med Care.* 2012;50(3):217–226.
10. Kilbourne AM, Abraham KM, Goodrich DE, Bowersox NW, Almirall D, Lai Z, Nord KM. Cluster randomized adaptive implementation trial comparing a standard versus enhanced implementation intervention to improve uptake

of an effective re-engagement program for patients with serious mental illness. *Implement Science.* 2013;8:136.

11. Glasgow RE, Chambers D. Developing robust, sustainable, implementation systems using rigorous, rapid, and relevant science. *Clin Transl Sci.* 2012;5(1):48–55.

12. Brown CH, Curran G, Palinkas LA, Aarons GA, Wells KB, Jones L, Collins LM, Duan N, Mittman BS, Wallace A, Tabak RG, Ducharme L, Chambers DA, Neta G, Wiley T, Landsverk J, Cheung K, Cruden G. An overview of research and evaluation designs for dissemination and implementation. *Annu Rev Public Health.* 2017;38:1–22.

13. Minkler M, Salvatore A, Chang C. Participatory approaches for study design and analysis in dissemination and implementation research. In: Brownson R, Colditz G, Proctor E, eds. *Dissemination and implementation research in health: Translating science to practice.* 2nd ed. New York: Oxford University Press; 2018.

14. Sackett DL, Rosenberg WM, Gray JA, Haynes RB, Richardson WS. Evidence based medicine: what it is and what it isn't. *BMJ.* 1996;312(7023):71–72.

15. Woolf SH. The meaning of translational research and why it matters. *JAMA.* 2008;299(2):211–213.

PREFACE

Decades of support by governmental and private sources has produced a remarkable foundation of knowledge in all disciplines related to public health, mental health, and health care. The discovery of new knowledge should not occur in large measure to satisfy the curiosity of scientists; rather the goal must be to improve the human condition (lower morbidity and mortality, enhance quality of life). Yet the gap between care that *could be*, were health care informed by scientific knowledge, and the care *that is* in routine practice has been characterized as a "chasm" by the National Academy of Medicine. The lack of ability to apply research findings has sometimes been equated to a leaky or broken pipeline leading to a lag time of decades between discovery and application.

To understand and begin to fill these leaks, a new science has emerged. It goes by numerous titles, including: translational research, knowledge translation, knowledge exchange, technology transfer, and dissemination and implementation (D&I) research. Although the terminology can be cumbersome and changing existing practices complex, the underlying rationale is simple: too often, discovery of new knowledge begets more discovery (the next study) with little attention on how to apply research advances in real-world public health, social service, and health care settings. With early foundations in the work of Archie Cochrane in the 1970s showing that many medical treatments lacked scientific effectiveness, D&I research focuses on ways to increase the use of evidence-based interventions among practitioners. Research has shown that in efforts to disseminate practice guidelines using passive methods (e.g., publication of consensus statements, mass mailings), adoption has been relatively low, resulting in only small changes in the uptake of a new evidence-based practice. Thus, active approaches to D&I are needed, taking into account a wide array of contextual conditions.

A return on investment of the billions spent on basic and clinical research (discovery research) requires a marked increase in translational research, including the development of its tools and analytic approaches. These efforts have been receiving much greater attention in mainline medical and public health journals. There also is a small set of journals dedicated to D&I research, notably *Implementation Science* (begun in 2006) and *Translational Behavioral Medicine* (begun in 2011). Similarly, in multiple countries, federal agencies and foundations are beginning to support D&I research more fully. For example, recent funding announcements from the US National Institutes of Health (NIH) show the higher priority being placed on translational research. While NIH is placing renewed emphasis on T1 research from bench to bedside, we place emphasis on methods and research opportunities for moving from scientific discovery of efficacy to population-wide benefits.

There are tangible examples where the D&I gap has been shortened. This may be best illustrated over the 20th century in the United States where life expectancy rose from 49 years in 1900 to 77 years in 2000. In large part, this increasing longevity was due to the application of discoveries on a population level (e.g., vaccinations, cleaner air and water). Yet for every victory, there is a parallel example of progress yet to be realized. For example, effective treatment for tuberculosis has been available since the 1950s yet globally, tuberculosis still accounts for 2 million annual deaths with 2 billion people infected. In many ways, the chapters in this book draw on successes (e.g., what works in tobacco control) and remaining challenges (e.g., how to address translational research challenges in populations with health disparities).

What needs to happen to shorten the translational research gap?

- First, priorities need to shift. Of the US annual health expenditures, only about 0.1% is spent on health services research (where D&I research is nested). Shifting priorities toward health services research requires political will and a need for social change.
- Second, capacity for finding and implementing evidence-based practice needs to improve among numerous practitioners. For example, many individuals working in public health practice have no formal training in a public health discipline—which suggests the need for more and better on-the-job training. And for those with graduate training, keeping up with current research is a formidable—and sometimes impossible—challenge.
- Third, the science of D&I research needs further development. The range of research needs is vast and covered extensively in this volume.
- Fourth, capacity for conducting D&I research needs to be advanced through training. This training can occur in government agencies, academic institutions, and nongovernmental organizations (such as the World Health Organization).
- Fifth, provider capacity to implement change in health interventions and policies needs to be advanced. We need support for and successful models of training for implementation practice.
- And finally, to build this science and capacity, institutional support and incentives are needed. For example, academic institutions need to shift priorities for faculty to reward time spent in conducting D&I research.

As we began the 2nd edition of our book, we reflected on the significant progress in D&I science since the publication of the 1st edition. This led us to the need for several new or extensively revised chapters in this edition, including those on: ethics in D&I research, models and frameworks, systems science methods, implementation strategies, adaptation in D&I science, mixed-methods evaluation, worksite D&I, and working in lower resource countries. In the 2nd edition, 10 of 29 chapters are entirely new or extensively revised with mostly new material. In addition, all remaining chapters from the 1st edition have been updated.

We have organized the book in a format that covers the major concepts for D&I researchers and practitioners. It draws on the talents of some of the top D&I scholars in the world—crossing many disciplines, health topics, and intervention settings. Our book has four sections. The first section provides a rationale for the book, highlights core issues needing attention, and begins to develop the terminology for D&I research. In the second section, we highlight the historical development of D&I research and describe several key analytic tools and approaches. Some of the tools are well developed with a rich literature (e.g., economic evaluation, participatory approaches) and others are relatively new, developing fields (e.g., systems thinking). This section also emphasizes the need to better plan interventions for dissemination and think creatively about how lessons from business and marketing can be applied to health. The third section is devoted to design and analysis of D&I studies. It covers core principles of study design, measurement and outcomes, and evaluation. In addition, this section highlights the concepts of fidelity, adaptation, and external validity, which are fundamental to D&I science. The final section of the book focuses on settings and populations. Since D&I research occurs in places where people spend their lives (communities, schools, worksites) or receive care (health care, social service agencies), we devote chapters to specific settings. This section also recognizes the importance of policy influences on health, the science of addressing health disparities, and working in a global context. Our book concludes with a short chapter on future research directions.

The target audience for this text is broad and includes researchers and practitioners across many different disciplines including epidemiology, biostatistics, behavioral science, medicine, social work, psychology, and anthropology. It seeks to inform practitioners in health promotion, public health, health services, and health systems. We anticipate this book will be useful in academic institutions, state and local health agencies, federal agencies, and health care organizations. Although the book is intended primarily for a North American audience, there are authors and examples drawn from various parts of the world and we believe that much of the information covered will be applicable in both developed and developing countries. The challenges of moving research to practice and policy appear to be universal, so future progress calls for collaborative partnership and cross-country research.

Our book documents that in a time of substantial political changes resulting in increasing pressure on scientific and public resources, researchers must continue to meet the implied obligation to the public that the billions of dollars invested in basic science and etiologic research will yield specific and tangible benefits to their health. Taxpayers have paid for many new discoveries yet these are not being translated into better patient care, public policy, and public health programs. We believe that applying the principles in this volume will help to bridge the chasm between discovery and practice.

R. C. B.

G. A. C.

E. K. P.

ACKNOWLEDGMENTS

We are grateful to numerous individuals who contributed to the development of this book.

In particular, we are thankful to the outstanding team of authors who contributed chapters. Their exceptional knowledge and dedication is reflected in the chapters, providing an up-to-date snapshot of dissemination and implementation science. We also appreciate the assistance from Mary Adams, Matthew Brown, Lauren Carothers, Linda Dix, Maggie Padek, Mariah Robertson, and Cheryl Valko.

Development of this book was supported by the following awards: National Cancer Institute at the National Institutes of Health (5R01CA160327; 1R01CA124404-015; R25CA171994-02; P30 CA09184); National Institute for Mental Health at the National Institutes of Health (NIMH R25 MH080916); National Institute of Diabetes and Digestive and Kidney Diseases at the National Institutes of Health (1P30DK092950); and National Center for Advancing Translational Sciences at the National Institutes of Health (UL1 TR000448). The contents of this book are solely the responsibility of the authors and do not necessarily represent the official views of the National Institutes of Health.

We acknowledge the remarkable leadership of Washington University's Brown School of Social Work, Institute for Public Health, Alvin J. Siteman Cancer Center, Institute for Clinical and Translational Science, and Department of Surgery (Division of Public Health Sciences) for fostering an environment in which transdisciplinary and translational science are valued and encouraged. In particular, we are grateful to Tim Eberlein, Brad Evanoff, Eddie Lawlor, Mary McKay, Bill Powderly, and Mark Wrighton. Finally, we are indebted to Chad Zimmerman, Oxford University Press, who provided valuable advice and support throughout the production of this edition.

CONTRIBUTORS

Gregory A. Aarons, PhD
Department of Psychiatry, University of California San Diego, La Jolla, California and Child and Adolescent Services Research Center, San Diego, California

Danielle R. Adams, BA
School of Social Service Administration, University of Chicago, Chicago, Illinois

Jennifer D. Allen, ScD, MPH
Department of Community Health, Tufts School of Arts and Sciences, Medford, Massachussetts

Ana A. Baumann, PhD
Brown School of Social Work, Washington University in St. Louis, Missouri

LaShawnta Bell-Lewis, DrPH
VA Greater Los Angeles Healthcare System, Los Angeles, California

Jay M. Bernhardt, PhD, MPH
Moody College of Communication, University of Texas, Austin, Texas

Allan Best, PhD
InSource Research Group, British Columbia, Canada

C. Hendricks Brown, PhD
Department of Psychiatry and Behavioral Sciences, Northwestern University Feinberg School of Medicine, Chicago, Illinois

Leopoldo J. Cabassa, PhD
Brown School of Social Work, Washington University in St. Louis, Missouri

Christopher M. Casey, MPH
School of Public Health and Social Justice, Saint Louis University, St. Louis, Missouri

Patricia Chamberlain, PhD
Oregon Social Learning Center, Eugene, Oregon

David A. Chambers, DPhil
Division of Cancer Control and Population Sciences, National Cancer Institute, Bethesda, Maryland

Charlotte Chang, DrPH, MPH
Labor Occupational Health Program, School of Public Health, University of California, Berkeley, Berkeley, California

Todd B. Combs, PhD
Center for Public Health Systems Science, Brown School of Social Work, Washington University in St. Louis, St. Louis, Missouri

Brittany Rhoades Cooper, PhD
Department of Human Development, Washington State University, Pullman, Washington

Geoffrey M. Curran, PhD
Departments of Pharmacy Practice and Psychiatry, University of Arkansas for Medical Sciences and Central Arkansas Veterans Healthcare System, Little Rock, Arkansas

Sara Czaja, PhD
Departments of Psychiatry & Behavioral Science and Industrial Engineering, University of Miami, Coral Gables, Florida

James W. Dearing, PhD
Michigan State University, East Lansing, Michigan

Elizabeth A. Dodson, PhD, MPH
Prevention Research Center in St. Louis, Brown School of Social Work, Washington University in St. Louis, St. Louis, Missouri

James M. DuBois, DSc, PhD
Department of Medicine, Washington University
School of Medicine, St. Louis, Missouri

Elizabeth Eakin, PhD
The University of Queensland, Cancer Prevention
Research Centre, School of Public Health, Brisbane,
Australia

Mark G. Ehrhart, PhD
Department of Psychology, San Diego State University,
San Diego, California

Karen M. Emmons, PhD
Harvard T.H. Chan School of Public Health, Boston,
Massachusetts

Diane T. Finegood, PhD
Department of Biomedical Physiology & Kinesiology,
Simon Fraser University, British Columbia, Canada

Brianna Fjeldsoe, PhD
The University of Queensland, Cancer Prevention
Research Centre, School of Public Health, Brisbane,
Australia

Chandra L. Ford, PhD
Center for the Study of Racism, Social Justice and
Health, Department of Community Health Sciences,
Fielding School of Public Health, University of
California, Los Angeles

Bridget Gaglio, PhD
Clinical Effectiveness and Decision Science, Patient-
Centered Outcomes Research Institute (PCORI),
Washington, DC

Russell E. Glasgow, PhD
Department of Family Medicine and Dissemination
and Implementation Science Program of ACCORDS
(Adult and Child Consortium for Health Outcomes
Research and Delivery Science), University of
Colorado School of Medicine, Aurora, Colorado

Beth A. Glenn, PhD
UCLA Kaiser Permanente Center for Health Equity,
Department of Health Policy and Management,
Fielding School of Public Health and Center for
Cancer Prevention and Control Research, Jonsson
Comprehensive Cancer Center, University of
California, Los Angeles

Jeremy D. Goldhaber-Fiebert, PhD
Department of Medicine and Centers for Health Policy
and Primary Care and Outcomes Research, Stanford
University, Stanford, California

Ana Goode, PhD
The University of Queensland, Cancer Prevention
Research Centre, School of Public Health, Brisbane,
Australia

Steven Gortmaker, PhD
Department of Social and Behavioral Sciences,
Harvard T.H. Chan School of Public Health, Boston,
Massachusetts

Lawrence W. Green, DrPH
Department of Epidemiology and Biostatistics,
School of Medicine, University of California at San
Francisco

Alison B. Hamilton, PhD, MPH
VA HSR&D Center for the Study of Healthcare
Innovation, Implementation & Policy, US
Department of Veterans Affairs, Los Angeles,
California
Department of Psychiatry and Biobehavioral Sciences,
David Geffen School of Medicine, University of
California Los Angeles, Los Angeles California

Peggy A. Hannon, PhD, MPH
Health Promotion Research Center, Department of
Health Services, School of Public Health, University
of Washington, Seattle, Washington

Jeffrey R. Harris, MD, MPH, MBA
Department of Health Services, School of Public
Health, University of Washington, Seattle,
Washington

Genevieve Healy, PhD
The University of Queensland, Cancer Prevention
Research Centre, School of Public Health, Brisbane,
Australia

Bev Holmes, PhD
Michael Smith Foundation for Health Research, British
Columbia, Canada

Mary Hook, PhD, RN-BC
Center for Nursing Research and Practice, Aurora
Health Care, Milwaukee, Wisconsin

Sarah McCue Horwitz, PhD
Department of Child and Adolescent Psychiatry,
School of Medicine, New York University, New York,
New York

Kerk F. Kee, PhD
Chapman University, Orange, California

Jon F. Kerner, PhD
Strategy Division, Canadian Partnership Against
  Cancer, Toronto, ON Canada

JoAnn E. Kirchner, MD
VA Quality Enhancement Research Initiative (QUERI)
  for Team-Based Behavioral Health, Central Arkansas
  Veterans Healthcare System, North Little Rock,
  Arkansas
University of Arkansas for Medical Sciences, Little
  Rock, Arkansas

Mohammad Javad Koohsari, PhD
Waseda University, Tokyo, Japan

Matthew W. Kreuter, PhD, MPH
Health Communication Research Laboratory, Brown
  School of Social Work, Washington University in
  St. Louis, St Louis, Missouri

John Landsverk, PhD
Oregon Social Learning Center, Eugene, Oregon
  and Brown School of Social Work, Washington
  University in St. Louis, St Louis, Missouri

Rebekka Lee, ScD
Department of Social and Behavioral Sciences,
  Harvard T.H. Chan School of Public Health, Boston,
  Massachusetts

Cara C. Lewis, PhD
MacColl Center for Health Care Innovation, Kaiser
  Permanente Washington Health Research Institute,
  Seattle, Washington
Department of Psychiatry and Behavioral Sciences,
  University of Washington, Seattle, Washington
Department of Psychological and Brain Sciences,
  Indiana University, Bloomington, Indiana

Laura A. Linnan, ScD
Department of Health Behavior and Health Education,
  Gillings School of Global Public Health, University
  of North Carolina, Chapel Hill, North Carolina
Lineberger Comprehensive Cancer Center, Chapel Hill,
  North Carolina

Rebecca Lobb, ScD, MPH
Division of Public Health Sciences, Department of
  Surgery, Washington University School of Medicine,
  St. Louis, Missouri

Douglas A. Luke, PhD
Center for Public Health Systems Science, Brown
  School of Social Work, Washington University in St.
  Louis, St. Louis, Missouri

Jessie-Lee D. McIsaac, PhD
Healthy Populations Institute, Dalhousie University,
  Nova Scotia, Canada

Virginia R. McKay, PhD
Center for Public Health Systems Science, Brown
  School of Social Work, Washington University in
  St. Louis, St. Louis, Missouri

J. Curtis McMillen, PhD
School of Social Service Administration, University of
  Chicago, Chicago, Illinois

Meredith Minkler, DrPH, MPH
Community Health Sciences, School of Public
  Health, University of California, Berkeley, Berkeley,
  California

Brian S. Mittman, PhD
Kaiser Permanente Southern California Department of
  Research and Evaluation, Pasadena, California
VA HSR&D Center for the Study of Healthcare
  Innovation, Implementation & Policy,
  US Department of Veterans Affairs, Los Angeles
  California
Clinical and Translational Science Institute, University
  of California Los Angeles, Los Angeles, California

Alexandra B. Morshed, MSc
Center for Public Health Systems Science and
  Prevention Research Center in St. Louis, Brown
  School of Social Work, Washington University in
  St. Louis, St. Louis, Missouri

Joanna C. Moullin, PhD
Department of Psychiatry, University of California San
  Diego, La Jolla, California and Child and Adolescent
  Services Research Center, San Diego, California

Laura Murray, PhD
Department of Mental Health and International
  Health, Johns Hopkins Bloomberg School of Public
  Health, Baltimore, Maryland

Mona Nasser, DDS
Peninsula Dental School, Plymouth, UK

Mitsunori Ogihara, PhD
Department of Computer Science, University of Miami,
  Miami, Florida

Neville Owen, PhD
Swinburne University of Technology and the Baker
  Heart and Diabetes Institute, Melbourne, Australia

Lawrence A. Palinkas. PhD
Department of Children, Youth and Families, Suzanne Dworak-Peck School of Social Work, University of Southern California, Los Angeles, California

Tai-Quan Peng, PhD
Michigan State University, East Lansing, Michigan

Byron J. Powell, PhD
Department of Health Policy and Management, Gillings School of Global Public Health, University of North Carolina, Chapel Hill, North Carolina

Beth Prusaczyk, PhD, MSW
Department of Medicine, Vanderbilt University Medical Center, Nashville, Tennessee

Jonathan Purtle, DrPH, MSc
Department of Health Management & Policy, Drexel University Dornsife School of Public Health, Philadelphia, Pennsylvania

Borsika A. Rabin, PhD, MPH
Department of Family Medicine and Public Health, University of California, La Jolla, California

Ramesh Raghavan, MD, PhD
School of Social Work and School of Public Health, Institute for Health, Health Care Policy, and Aging Research, Rutgers University, New Brunswick, New Jersey

Shoba Ramanadhan, ScD, MPH
Center for Community-Based Research, Dana-Farber Cancer Institute, Boston, Massachusetts and Department of Social and Behavioral Sciences, Harvard T.H. Chan School of Public Health, Boston, Massachusetts

Barbara L. Riley, PhD
Propel Centre for Population Health Impact, Faculty of Applied Health Sciences, University of Waterloo, Ontario, Canada

Jennifer A. Rolls Reutz, MPH
Chadwick Center for Children and Families, Rady Childrens Hospital, San Diego, California

Lisa Saldana, PhD
Oregon Social Learning Center, Eugene, Oregon

Alicia L. Salvatore, DrPH, MPH
College of Public Health, University of Oklahoma Health Sciences Center, Oklahoma City, Oklahoma

Rachel C. Shelton, ScD, MPH
Department of Sociomedical Sciences, Columbia's Mailman School of Public Health, New York, New York

Jeffrey L. Smith, BS
VA Quality Enhancement Research Initiative (QUERI) for Team-Based Behavioral Health, Central Arkansas Veterans Healthcare System, North Little Rock, Arkansas

Justin D. Smith, PhD
Department of Psychiatry and Behavioral Sciences, Northwestern University Feinberg School of Medicine, Chicago, Illinois

Katherine A. Stamatakis, PhD, MPH
Department of Epidemiology, College for Public Health and Social Justice, Saint Louis University, St. Louis, Missouri

Joseph T. Steensma, EdD, MPH
Health Communication Research Laboratory, Brown School of Social Work, Washington University in St. Louis, St Louis, Missouri

Shannon Wiltsey Stirman, PhD
National Center for Posttraumatic Stress Disorder and Stanford University, Palo Alto, California

Takemi Sugiyama, PhD
Australian Catholic University, Melbourne, Australia

Rachel G. Tabak, PhD, RD
Prevention Research Center in St. Louis, Brown School of Social Work, Washington University in St. Louis, St Louis, Missouri

Wouter Vermeer, PhD
Department of Psychiatry and Behavioral Science, Northwestern University Feinberg School of Medicine, Chicago, Illinois

Cynthia A. Vinson, PhD, MPA
Division of Cancer Control and Population Sciences, National Cancer Institute, Bethesda, Maryland

Thomas J. Waltz, PhD, PhD
Eastern Michigan University, Ypsilanti, Michigan
HSR&D Center for Clinical Management Research, VA Ann Arbor Healthcare System, Ann Arbor, Michigan

Cameron D. Willis, PhD
Menzies Centre for Health Policy and the Australian
   Prevention Partnership Centre, University of Sydney,
   NSW, Australia

Antronette (Toni) Yancey, MD, MPH (deceased)
UCLA Kaiser Permanente Center for Health Equity,
   Department of Health Policy and Management,
   Fielding School of Public Health, Center for
   Cancer Prevention and Control Research, Jonsson
   Comprehensive Cancer Center, University of
   California, Los Angeles

1

The Promise and Challenges of Dissemination and Implementation Research

GRAHAM A. COLDITZ AND KAREN M. EMMONS

"To him who devotes his life to science, nothing can give more happiness than increasing the number of discoveries, but his cup of joy is full when the results of his studies immediately find practical applications."

—Louis Pasteur

"The ability of science to deliver on its promise of practical and timely solutions to the world's problems does not depend solely on research accomplishments but also on the receptivity of society to the implications of scientific discoveries."

—Agre and Leshner[1]

INTRODUCTION

Dissemination and implementation (D&I) of research findings into practice are necessary to achieve a return on investment in our research enterprise and to apply research findings to improve outcomes in the broader community. By not implementing prevention and treatment strategies equitably we incur avoidable morbidity and mortality.[2] At the level of molecular biology and pathogenesis of disease, the National Institutes of Health (NIH) Director, Francis Collins, seeks more rapid translation from discovery of receptors or pathways to first in-patient studies.[3] Whether we are focusing on genomic discovery or evidence that treatment of a condition improves outcomes, moving from scientific discovery to broader application brings society the full return on our collective investment in research. It is estimated that the biomedical research expenditures in the United States in 2012 exceeded $116 billion on health-related research.[4] Within this commitment, spending on health services research, models of care, and service innovations, "accounted for between 0.2% and 0.3% of national health expenditures between 2003 and 2011, an approximately 20-fold difference in comparison with total medical research funding,"[4(pp. 177–178)] Perhaps reflecting the low priority of research on implementation of scientifically proven approaches to care, in 2001, the Institute of Medicine noted a substantial gap between care that could be delivered if health care was informed by scientific knowledge and the care that is delivered in practice—defining this gap as a chasm.[5] It is precisely this gap that D&I is designed to address.

Implementation research is active and supports movement of evidence-based effective health care and prevention strategies or programs from the clinical or public health knowledge base into routine use (in some countries, the term "evidence-informed" is used).[6] The Centers for Disease Control and Prevention (CDC) has defined implementation research as "the systematic study of how a specific set of activities and designated strategies are used to successfully integrate an evidence-based public health intervention within specific settings" (RFA-CD-07-005).[7] The National Cancer Institute (NCI), in a request for proposals (RFP), has defined Implementation research as "the use of strategies to adopt and integrate evidence based health interventions and change practice patterns within specific settings." The Canadian Institutes of Health Research (http://www.cihr-irsc.gc.ca/ e/29418.html) use the following definition for knowledge translation: "a dynamic and iterative process that includes synthesis, dissemination, exchange and ethically-sound application of knowledge to improve the health of Canadians, provide more effective services and products and strengthen the health care system." Despite these definitions, a 2004 survey of readers in *Nature Medicine* showed little agreement and understanding of translational research.[8] Chapter 2 outlines terminology to help move to common understanding of terms in D&I.

While the translation of evidence-based interventions into practice to improve population health outcomes is a common theme of government agencies, the *process* for distribution of scientific findings, materials, and associated resources to support interventions is less developed. Dissemination is defined as "the targeted distribution of information and intervention materials to a specific public health or clinical practice audience."[9] Rabin et al. are more specific, calling for an active approach of spreading evidence-based interventions to the target audience via determined channels using planned strategies.[10] These definitions are similar to that of Lomas[11,12] but contrast to some extent with the approach of Curry,[13] who defines dissemination as a push–pull process. Those who adopt innovations must want them or be receptive (pull), while there is systematic effort to help adopters implement innovations (push). The intent of *dissemination research* is to spread knowledge and the associated interventions, building understanding of approaches to increased effectiveness of dissemination efforts. In understanding these approaches, numerous studies have shown that dissemination of evidence-based interventions using passive methods (e.g., publication of consensus statements in professional journals, mass mailings) has been ineffective, resulting in only small changes in the uptake of a new practice.[14] The intent of *implementation research* is to increase understanding of how to increase integration of evidence-based approaches into routine, real-world practices. Therefore, more targeted, active approaches to D&I are needed that take into account many factors, including the characteristics and needs of users, types of evidence needed, and organizational climate and culture. Greater stakeholder engagement across the D&I spectrum and systems approaches can increase the speed of change.[15] The definitions and other terms used in the field are described in more detail in chapter 2.

One useful model of translation of discovery to applications that will generate population health benefits comes from a thoughtful review by Bowen and colleagues. Reviewing the application of discovery to prevention of cancer, Bowen and colleagues note, "Our previous 30 years have taught us that dissemination does not just happen if we wait for it. New information is often needed to make it happen."[16(p. 483)] This call for research to improve understanding of methods for D&I remains true today. The challenges in D&I are broad and apply far beyond health and health care systems. In fact early examples, as we will see, come from other fields of learning. For example, much research in education has addressed the application of new knowledge to improve outcomes in children's learning.[17-19] The rapidly expanding field of D&I research has some common themes and lessons that this book will help bring together, so a more uniform understanding of the principles of D&I research methods and applications may help speed us to achieve the potential to improve population health. First, some key questions arise from the Bowen, et al. review that are applicable to the broader field of D&I research across health, education, and technology.

- How will we gather this information on effective interventions to form the evidence base?
- Will interventions be applicable to our setting?
- What methods should we use to decide what to disseminate or implement?
- Which strategies will give us the greatest impact on population health?
- What outcomes should be tracked to know if we are making progress?
- How long will it take to show progress, or when will it be observed?
- Will implementation be uneven across population subgroups leading to or exacerbating health disparities?

These are but a few of the questions raised by the call to action from Bowen and colleagues.[16] Other authors address specific questions in translation from clinical trials to policy and practice.[20,21] This book aims to lay out many options to help guide the field as it matures, thus speeding our progress toward improved health for all. This introductory chapter seeks to place D&I research in context, identify the challenges in moving forward, and the pressure to increase the emphasis on this aspect of knowledge translation and research utilization.

THE CHALLENGE IN TRANSLATING RESEARCH TO PRACTICE

There are a number of issues inherent in moving from discovery to application, which is essential if society is to fully benefit from our collective investment in research. Summarized below are some of the key issues that impact on our ability to translate evidence-based programs into real world practice.

Funding

Over the past 20 years, between 9% and 25% of the $30 billion NIH budget has been expended on prevention research[22,23]—that is, the direct and immediate application of effective intervention strategies to benefit the public's health.[24(p. 93)] Although this indicates a relatively low priority placed on prevention, the funding for D&I research is even lower. Farquhar has estimated that 10% or less of prevention research is focused on dissemination.[22] Across all funding sources through 2011—federal and foundations—spending on health services research, models of care, and service innovations, represented only 1/20th of biomedical research funding.[4] While Moses and colleagues use broad classification categories to assess trends in funding of pharmaceutical research over time (prehuman and preclinical; phase 1–3; phase 4; approval and regulatory; other and unclassified), D&I does not fall into any clear category for this or other analyses.[4] Rather, D&I research spans all areas from translating discoveries to bedside and broader clinical applications, to health services interventions to implement effective approaches to care. In global health it also spans from innovation in technology for extremely low-cost delivery systems to implementation in field settings.

Representation of D&I Science in the Scientific Literature

Another way to gauge the breadth of D&I research is to examine the types of articles appearing in the peer-reviewed literature. In a content analysis of 1,210 articles from 12 prominent public health journals, 89% of published studies were classified as basic research and development.[25] The authors classified another 5% of studies as innovation development, less than 1% as diffusion, and 5%

as institutionalization. Similarly, Sallis and colleagues conducted a content analysis of four journals and found that only 2% to 20% of articles fell in a phase defined as "Translate research to practice."[26] This is not terribly surprising, given the low level of funding for D&I science. In another review of three health promotion journals, dissemination research was poorly represented despite editorials calling for more D&I research.[27] This publication record follows funding priorities. Moreover, one-third of public health researchers themselves rate their dissemination efforts as poor.[28] In a cross-sectional study of researchers at universities, the NIH, and CDC, only 28% of researchers self-rated their efforts to disseminate research as "excellent/good" despite the overwhelming majority (87%) agreeing they have an obligation to disseminate their research findings.

Appropriate Outcomes

What are the outcomes for progress in D&I of discoveries? Appropriate outcomes can include more effective health services, better prevention, reduction in health disparities, or in nonhealth settings impact on the underlying root causes of population health—such as social services, better schooling for our children, or employment opportunities. There is growing interest in de-implementation (See NIH PAR-16-238) or reduction of the use of strategies and interventions that are not evidence based.[9] While the methods and issues may appear to differ across fields of study, in this book we set forth principles and methods that should be applicable across settings. Like statistics, which has a long history of development in agriculture (the leading industry of the time—Cochran wrote on meta-analysis of results from agriculture trial plots in 1937 and helped define modern approaches[29]), D&I research also grew from agriculture to guide thinking across many fields.[30] The history of D&I science is presented in more detail in chapter 3. With health care expenditures consuming an ever-increasing portion of national and state budgets in the developed world, methods to maximize our societal benefit must be refined and accessible to end users—and will likely be developed and refined most quickly in the context of health and wellness. In fact, data from the Organization for Economic Co-operation and Development (OECD) indicate that the average ratio of health expenditure to GDP has risen from 7.8% in 2000 to 9.0% in 2008, and is at 16.4% for the United States and 10.2% for Canada in 2013.[31] There is no shortage of academic research, but how do we sift through studies and draw inference to disseminate and implement effective programs and policies more broadly? A recurring question as we approach D&I research is "Will the evidence and intervention be applicable to the new setting?"

Acceptance of Delays in Adoption

Delay in adoption of scientific discoveries is not a new phenomenon. We can look at Bayesian methods used in statistics in the 1960s to evaluate the authorship of the Federalist papers.[32] In the process, described in detail by Fred Mosteller in his autobiography, an empirical test of the Bayesian approach gave new insight to manuscript classification.[33] Mosteller also presented on using Bayesian approaches to combine means (Lake Junaluska, North Carolina, 1946—see pages 186–187; also see On pooling data—JASA 1948).[34] These statistical methods have only much more recently been adapted to widespread use, with modern computer technology supporting this application. So advances in statistical methods development did not achieve widespread application for decades, perhaps in part due to the technical difficulty of implementing these approaches (lack of technology), but also reluctance on the part of investigators (intrapersonal factors). Both individual and structural barriers impeded implementation, reflecting a complex interplay of barriers to implementation of innovations.

How can the principles and methods we see presented in this book help us move more quickly to build on research findings and apply them to improve health? Do we need new ways of thinking, conducting, and reporting research, or can we take our existing approaches and through consensus apply what is known more rapidly? The challenge of implementation extends along the continuum from discovery of biologic phenomena to clinical application in research settings and the broader application in the population at large. While a range of approaches to describing this continuum has been developed, perhaps more pertinent from the D&I perspective is the perspective summarized by Green and colleagues as a leaky pipeline from research to practice.[35] Across these approaches to defining stages of translation and application, some common themes emerge; discovery on its own does not lead to use of knowledge; evidence of impact does not lead to uptake of new strategies; organizations often do not support the culture of evidence-based practice; and maintenance of change is

often overlooked, leading to regression of system level changes back to a prior state. The focus of an intervention for implementation, whether at the individual level or up through to system level changes or policies, determines in part the breadth of change toward improved population outcomes. The lag from discovery to application (implementation of effective programs and practices) may vary across disciplines. Examples from public health include the gap from perfecting the Papanicolaou test in 1943 to the establishment of screening programs in all US states in 1995, and the delay from the 1964 Surgeon General's report on smoking to effective statewide tobacco control programs and regulation of tobacco by the FDA in 2009.[36] Of course, early applications will typically be in place to varying degrees before full widespread programs are implemented and sustained. As Collins notes, many false starts or failures may be needed before successful translation of discoveries to human applications.[3] However, it is important to reduce the time lag from early adoption to comprehensive, widespread adoption, as this lag ultimately represents avoidable morbidity and mortality.

A frequently quoted statement about the total attrition in the funnel and the lapse between research and medical practice indicates that it takes 17 years to turn 14% of original research to the benefit of patient care, and is attributed to Balas & Boren.[37] The leakage or loss of medical-clinical research from the pipeline at each stage from completed research through submission, publication, indexing, and systematic reviews that produce guidelines and textbook recommendations for best practices, to the ultimate implementation of those practices in health care settings, all contribute to these estimates. Changing technologies and priorities of publishing, bibliographic data management, and systematic reviews and disseminating evidence-based guidelines will lead to different estimates over time and in different fields. Green and colleagues depict this flow of information as a leaky funnel. In it they identify many leakage points in the scientific process (Figure 1.1).[35]

Looked at from the other end of the funnel, identifying major advances in engineering that have improved quality of life in the 20th century, the National Academy of Engineering included electricity, electric motors, and imaging—each with a long line of scientific discovery and application before broader social impact was achieved.[38] Likewise the lag from

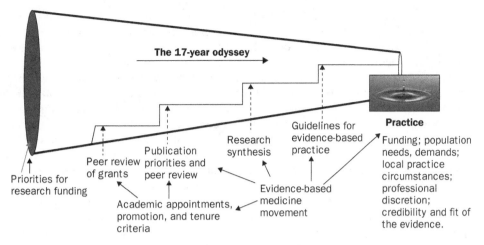

FIGURE 1.1 The funnel depicts loss in the pipeline from research to practice. (From Green et al [35])

original discovery to formal recognition with Nobel prizes grows exponentially.[39] A particular challenge in public health is that we are not producing a tangible product or commodity, as in the case with electricity and electric motors, but rather the intangible value of health, which may be even more challenging. That said, the path from scientific discovery to social benefit from broad implementation has common challenges across many scientific disciplines.

CASE STUDIES: FROM BENCH TO BEDSIDE TO POPULATIONS

Several case studies can help in illustrating the real-world challenges and successes in moving from research to practice. Of course, we learn from both successful translation of research to practice and also from failures.

Penicillin

Fleming discovered penicillin in 1928 (though others are attributed with noticing the effect of mold on bacteria in research laboratories). Use of penicillin was not implemented for more than 15 years, when an Australian Rhodes Scholar, Howard Florey, then in the Pathology Department at Oxford, evaluated penicillin in humans and with a team of scientists developed methods for mass production leading to widespread military use for infected soldiers.[40] Clearly the burden of infection reduced the military capability of the United Kingdom and allied forces in WWII, and increased the priority for effective antibiotics to

be available. Only after the War did civilian use become available, first in Australia and then more broadly. The time delay from discovery to clinical application is typical of the lag we still see today. Of course, war has a long history for development of new methods in trauma surgery, arterial limbs, and other areas of clinical medicine, but our focus in this book is broader application of scientific advances. This example not only includes several steps from discovery to clinical application during WWII and then broader community level application for effective health care, but also exemplifies how delays happen and how innovation is motivated by exceptional circumstances (unfortunately, all too often war leads to major innovations in technology for destruction and for sustaining lives). Systems for large-scale production were not available and the market forces did not support commercialization until after WWII.

Insulin

Insulin offers another extreme example we do not see replicated today. Pancreas extract was evaluated in dogs in physiology laboratories in numerous medical centers in the early 1900s. After only 6 or so months of experimentation, Banting and Best moved from their physiology laboratory and animal studies in the Medical Building at the University of Toronto to the delivery to humans at Toronto General Hospital.[41] The clinical condition favored rapid translation to practice, since patients routinely had a steady decline after onset of Type 1 or insulin-dependent diabetes, following standard therapies such as starvation and ultimately dying from metabolic imbalances.[42] Rapid physiologic evidence of response to pancreatic extract in terms of blood sugar and urinary ketones led to demand for pancreas extract outstripping supply. Few medical discoveries have had such a huge effect that they move so quickly from bench to bedside and broader application in clinics across North America. In fact, the will of the patients and their providers outpaced the slower development of approaches to large-scale production. Eli Lilly had a major interest from even before the discovery of the extraction methods in Toronto,[43] reinforcing the influence of market forces on implementation. More recent experience with HIV and the social forces brought to bear by AIDS activists, along with speeding of the drug approval process, and marketing show faster developments from identification of a new disease condition to effective treatment.[44] This time line spans from detection of AIDS cases in California and New York in 1981, to the viral cause identified in 1984, AZT as the first drug for treating AIDS in 1987, a US national education campaign in 1988, and combination antiretroviral therapy that is highly effective against HIV in 1996. Like diabetes, the political will generated by a patient population garnered support for scientific advances at exceptional speed with clear success, making efforts in cancer and other chronic disease management pale in comparison. AIDS research and systems delivery leave open research questions such as optimal scaling up strategies to bring effective prevention and treatment to all.

Smallpox

Smallpox epidemics raged in Boston in 1690 and 1702; inoculation was a folk remedy that was shown to be effective but political leaders forbade the use of inoculation as it was thought to spread the disease rather than prevent it. The 1721 epidemic had a major controversy as Reverend Cotton Mather and the Boston physician William Douglass disagreed as to the utility of inoculation. The Boston physician argued that inoculation spread the disease, while Reverend Mather had inoculated his son and was a vaccine advocate. Church leaders also debated the value of this medical intervention—Mather arguing that inoculation was a gift from God, while those opposed to inoculation claimed the epidemic afflicted people for divine reasons, and so did not want to interfere with the will of God.[45] Thus political will alone was not sufficient to implement a potentially major preventive strategy. Despite the

development of the Jenner vaccine in 1796, it was not until 1966 that the World Health Organization (WHO) established a goal to interrupt smallpox transmission throughout the world within a decade.[46] Because of a worldwide campaign to eradicate smallpox, the last known smallpox cases were observed near the 1976 goal—a case in Somalia in October 1977 and two laboratory infections in England in 1978.[47] The WHO certified that smallpox was eradicated from the world in December 1979. The enormous global public health commitment to achieve this goal of eradication was achieved after more than 150 years of less cohesive public health activity.

These examples of translating discovery to widespread application in varying time frames demonstrate the enormous variation in implementation and some of the social and political factors that may facilitate implementing effective programs and practices. We must balance timely implementation with the caution that pervades the scientific process. Too rapid implementation of ineffective or even harmful technologies will have deleterious consequences for population health. Tempering such caution is evidence from public health, where use of lead in petroleum (gasoline) was opposed by Alice Hamilton as early as 1925 because of the expected adverse health effects, almost 50 years before the US EPA began to restrict the lead content of gasoline in 1975, and 70 years before lead was phased out of gasoline entirely. Tobacco smoking continues to show just how slow we can be to implement effective prevention strategies when commercial interests oppose development of cohesive political will to advance population health. The authors contend, and the chapters in this book illustrate, that stronger methods for D&I research can help reduce this gap and bring us population benefits.

WHAT IS DISSEMINATION AND IMPLEMENTATION RESEARCH AND WHY DOES IT MATTER?

Given these historical examples, how do we conceptualize D&I research and classify it in relation to other systems or types of research? Growing emphasis on the pace of advances in medical systems leads to a number of approaches to classifying the continuum from discovery to delivery and the improvement of the health of the population. Classification of the research continuum from bench to bedside and use of population health metrics is now post hoc and continues to evolve.

Briefly, the language to describe these steps and procedures has evolved over the past decade (see chapter 2). Furthermore, the methods research to understand the limitations of research synthesis to gather information on effective interventions and inform next steps continues to provide caution in planning and evaluation of programs.[20,21] The Institute of Medicine has defined implementation research as an important component of the framework for clinical research, and Zerhouni called for reengineering the clinical research enterprise, but we are more broadly focused including clinical research, health systems, and prevention.[48] The NIH roadmap[49] defines T1 as moving from basic science to clinical applications (translation to humans); T2 as clinical research (up to phase 3 trials) moving to broader clinical practice (translation to patients); and T3 as D&I research following development of guidelines for practice moving research into health practice through diffusion, dissemination, and delivery research (translation to practice) (Figure 1.2). T4 research has now been added to evaluate real-world outcomes from applying discoveries and bringing them to practice (translation to population). No doubt further subdivisions will be proposed in coming years. Public health approaches may broadly be defined as practice based (though health departments and social marketing strategies for health promotion may be beyond most people's vision for practice-based research).[50] Accordingly, our methods must be robust and adaptive to the situation that they are applied in. In fact, the development and acceptance of a wide range of scientific methods as necessary for D&I research, beyond the randomized controlled trial, have helped to move the field significantly forward. These methods will be critical as new forms of discovery science proliferate, as some are anticipating with precision medicine. Both the NIH Precision Medicine Initiative and the NCI's Cancer Moonshot Initiative are seeking to accelerate the pace and impact of genetic and genomic research on health. Chambers et al. note the importance of implementation science as a mechanism for ensuring that precision medicine advances become integrated into health care delivery, which will ultimately be critical if the significant investment in these efforts is to be realized.[51]

A number of proposed models for D&I research are discussed in multiple chapters in this book. Some are "source-based" (i.e., they view D&I from the lens of researchers pushing out science) (see, e.g., chapter 11). Others are community centered, focusing on bringing research

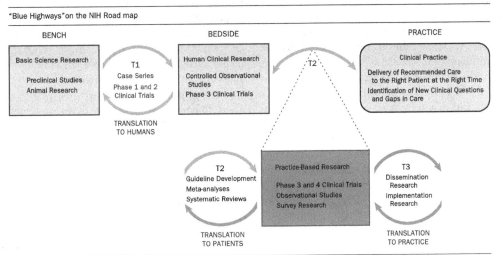

The current National Institutes of Health (NIH) Road map for Medical Research includes 2 major research laboratories (bench and bedside) and 2 translational steps (T1 and T2). Historically, moving new medical discoveries in to clinical practice (T2) has been haphazard, occurring largely through continuing medical education programs, pharmaceutical detailing, and guideline development. Proposed expansion of the NIH Roadmap (blue) includes an additional research laboratory (Practice-based Research) and translational step (T3) to improve incorporation of research discoveries in to day-to-day clinical care. The research roadmap is a continuum, with overlap between sites of research and translational steps. The figure includes examples of the types of research common in each research laboratory and translational step. This map is not exhaustive; other important types of research that might be included are community-based participatory research, public health research, and health policy analysis.

FIGURE 1.2 "Blue Highways" on the NIH Roadmap.

into practice settings. Systems approaches are also proposed to conceptualize the overall framework for D&I.[52] Underlying these approaches, the body of scientific evidence must be sufficient to justify moving from individual studies to broader practice (i.e., an evidence-based practice). How this is determined, through systematic synthesis, subgroup analysis, or other approaches continues to be debated. However, to move forward with an intervention one needs a strong scientific evidence base; political will to allocate resources to achieve the goal of implementation; and a social strategy that defines a plan of action to achieve the health goals.[53,54] As noted in examples earlier in the chapter, that lack of political will may hinder the uptake of effective public health interventions such as smallpox vaccination.

Scientific Evidence Base

In moving forward with D&I research, we can start with the first of these three dimensions: the scientific evidence base. Here we see confusion in the field over when we have a sufficient scientific evidence base ready for broader implementation.[55] In chapter 18, Green and Nasser highlight how the emphasis on internal validity in our research enterprise drives us to restricted populations and narrowly defined interventions. Do these interventions work? Will they work in a different setting? Will results from trials hold up with further evaluation?[21] The tension of priority on internal validity against external validity and the associated evidence to support broader applications of scientific findings continues within the scientific process.[56] Much of the evidence synthesis "industry" focuses on narrowing evidence to specific finite questions. In medicine and public health, this began by meta-analysis even excluding nonrandomized trials from study.[57] In an early application of research synthesis and meta-analysis to observational public health data, Berlin and Colditz evaluated quality of exposure measure and used regression methods to predict future health benefits from increases in physical activity.[58] Can stronger use of existing approaches to prediction (e.g., metaregression and network meta-analysis) help us understand when interventions will work and how large a benefit we might ultimately see? What range of benefits will fit within the distribution of findings to date?

The scope of synthesis has broadened over time—from consensus and review articles[59] to rigorous panel (systematic review) methods such as those used by the US and Canadian Preventive Services [60] and the CDC community guide. The GRADE system has been developed to more explicitly guide panel decision-making.[61-63] Despite these more formal approaches, a review of WHO Guidelines shows that they systematically omit guidance on active implementation strategies.[64]

While reporting standards have focused on the internal validity of clinical trials and observational studies [65] new approaches to make features of study design most relevant to effectiveness have been proposed (PRECIS and PRECIS-2).[66,67] By making explicit a number of dimensions such as flexibility of the comparison condition and experimental intervention; practitioner expertise; eligibility criteria participant compliance, and so forth, approaches such as metaregression[68] may be implemented to draw on these contextual factors to better understand if results can be applied in different settings. Furthermore, regression can then be used to predict what level of benefit may be seen in future applications (as has been done in the meta-analysis of BCG vaccine for prevention of tuberculosis).[69,70] While one often thinks of meta-analysis as driving for a common single answer to a clinical or public health problem, regression approaches and using meta-analysis to understand sources of heterogeneity highlight the many potentially untapped ways in which data can be synthesized to better inform policy and clinical decision making.[71] Importantly, Implementation Science should study how to translate findings to be contextually relevant— and while regression and synthesis offer traditional quantitative approaches, broader system and contextual measures are likely needed to fully capture translation to practice.[72]

Bero has studied the delay in implementation of clinical practices—guidelines are typically published and sit on a bookshelf.[14] Practice does not change. She reviews effectiveness for a range of approaches that are commonly used. Importantly, while the field of health care has moved substantially to accepting a role for research synthesis over the past quarter century, the study of how to implement the effective approaches to health and public health practice has been far less rigorous. Approaches to synthesis of strategies that work[73] could strengthen the field. In addition, Anderson and colleagues adapted some of the Bero factors as they apply to public health settings (Table 1.1).[74]

As in any field, a thorough review of evidence may provide a summary of where the field

TABLE 1.1 FACTORS INFLUENCING DISSEMINATION AMONG HEALTH ADMINISTRATORS, POLICY MAKERS, AND THE GENERAL PUBLIC

Category	Influential Factor
Information	• Sound scientific basis, including knowledge of causality • Source (e.g., professional organization, government, mass media, friends)
Clarity of contents	• Formatting and framing • Perceived validity • Perceived relevance • Cost of intervention • Strength of the message (i.e., vividness)
Perceived values, preferences, beliefs	• Role of the decision maker • Economic background • Previous education • Personal experience or involvement • Political affiliation • Willingness to adopt innovations • Willingness to accept uncertainty • Willingness to accept risk • Ethical aspect of the decision
Context	• Culture • Politics • Timing • Media attention • Financial, or political constraints

is or identify gaps that require further research.[75] Reviewing evidence in service organizations, Greenhalgh and colleagues[76] provide a model for diffusion of innovations in health service organizations, summarize methodology for review of evidence in this setting, and identify gaps to focus research on. They argue that research on diffusion of innovations should be theory driven; process rather than package oriented; ecological; collaborative; multidisciplinary; detailed; and participatory. They distinguish among "letting it happen," "helping it happen," and "making it happen" as related to diffusion and dissemination. Letting or helping it happen relies on the providers or consumers to work out how to use the science, in contrast with "making it happen," which places accountability for implementation on teams of individuals who may coach, support, or guide the implementation. Minkler et al. describe the value

of participatory research in speeding implementation of research findings (see chapter 11).

Policy and Politics (Political Will)

The framework of Kingdon[77] is useful in illustrating the policy making process and its impact on D&I research. Kingdon argues that policies move forward when elements of three "streams" come together. The first of these is the definition of the problem (e.g., a high cancer rate, or synthesis of the scientific knowledge base). The second is the development of potential policies to solve that problem (e.g., identification of policy measures to achieve an effective cancer control strategy). Finally, there is the role of politics, political will, and public opinion (e.g., interest groups supporting or opposing the policy). Policy change occurs when a "window of opportunity" opens and the three streams push policy change through.

But how do we summarize the stream of evidence to improve support to get resources allocated for implementation research or knowledge translation? Does the form of the evidence summary interact with the rate of uptake by end users, including policy makers? Lack of consistent approaches may again hinder the allocation of resources to these activities. Academic debate about the appropriateness of data, study populations, and the like, distracts from cohesion and a decision to move forward. The US Preventive Services Task Force separates the level of evidence from the magnitude of expected benefit when synthesizing data. They use a hierarchy of study designs to classify the source of evidence. This approach was expanded by the Institute of Medicine in their reports on vaccines[78] and health effects of Agent Orange[79] (see Mosteller and Colditz for descriptions).[75] It was adapted to a range of epidemiologic evidence on causes of cancer to guide risk assessment and prevention strategies.[80] Brownson and colleagues add to these design levels considerations of the research base contextual variables that inform implementation and adoption: individual, interpersonal, organizational, sociocultural, and political and economic.[81] Further research is needed to better understand the interplay of methods for research synthesis, presentation of summary data, and subsequent translation of research findings to policy and practice.

Prevention is lower on the priority list for public health funding at NIH and CDC than the discovery of new therapies, with emphasis on the research priority end of the Green pipeline and limited attention to practitioner needs and applications.[82] In contrast with best communication practices that include promotion with repeat messages, CDC rewards new approaches to prevention rather than sustaining effective programs, as exemplified by the contrast between the Australian Sun Smart program running for decades[83] and the CDC continuing to fund "novel" approaches to prevention of excess sun exposure. Quantifying improvements in population health contrasts with disease-focused treatment programs where individuals can self-identify demanding services and measurable outcomes. This identifiable benefactor (patient) contrasts with the beneficiaries of public health who are largely unknown.[82] Systems innovations to improve delivery of care equity and access to state of the art therapies all receive less support or are valued less by the population than services that are regarded as personal. The time frame for benefits of knowledge translation—D&I research—is in the future and runs counter to public policy and planning, conflicting with pressure to deliver services today.[82] In contrast with disease (e.g., breast cancer) and exposure advocacy groups (e.g., those focusing on environmental contaminants; or unions and related occupational exposures), prevention does not have a voice from those who benefit. Despite the apparent priority of tobacco control efforts since the 1964 Surgeon General's report, we have only halved the rate of smoking in the United States. While this reduction in smoking may have prevented more cancer deaths than all adult cancer therapy advances over the same time frame; it leaves us with an enormous lack of accomplishment when the full burden of smoking is summed up. Where are all those who quit smoking or never started and are not suffering or dying prematurely from lung cancer and many other chronic diseases? A lack of voice leads to limited political will and lack of resource allocation to achieve the benefits of translating research to practice. Sometimes governments do step in and do the right thing—as illustrated by the significant progress in tobacco control during the Obama presidency.[84] Based on the significant foundation of evidence about the health impacts of tobacco and strategies for effective tobacco control, the Obama administration implemented Food and Drug Administration regulation of tobacco (Family Smoking Prevention and Control Act enacted by Congress and signed by President Obama in 2009), improved coverage of tobacco cessation services by health plans via the 2010 Affordable Care Act, funded the first national media campaign designed to highlight the real human costs of smoking, expanded Medicare coverage for older smokers and expanded Medicaid coverage for pregnant smokers, and provided protection from exposure to second-hand tobacco smoke in public housing.

Social Strategy

In launching the first health goals for the nation, Richmond defined social strategy in the context of health—guiding both the landmark Healthy People 1980 and the first nutrition guidelines for the United States.[53] He proposed changes to promote health through health care providers, regulations, and community (individual and organizational changes). More recently, Koh and colleagues note the importance of integrating social determinants of health into Healthy People 2020.[84] The Healthy People initiative has represented an ambitious yet achievable health promotion and disease prevention agenda for over three decades, but only recently has this effort fully embraced a comprehensive social determinants perspective. Healthy People 2020 includes a new overarching goal to "create social and physical environments that promote good health for all" by accepting shared social responsibility for change.

Now we may expand this concept to incorporate the D&I elements—the innovation; the communication channel; the time; and the social system.[16] Proctor[85] proposes a model of Implementation research that defines the intervention (from the evidence base) and the implementation strategy (systems environment, organizational, group/learning, supervision, and individual providers/consumers) (Figure 1.3).

Here Proctor specifically defines the levels of change that an intervention is addressing: the larger system or environment, the organization, a group or team, or the individual. This is not unlike Richmond, who focused on policy level changes, provider level changes, and individual and community level changes to promote health.[53] One can ask, "Is there a parallel model for dissemination research addressing all these levels"?

WHAT IS MISSING— OUR SOCIAL CONTEXT FOR TRANSLATING RESEARCH INTO PRACTICE

To place the growing emphasis on D&I in the context of current funding, manpower needs,

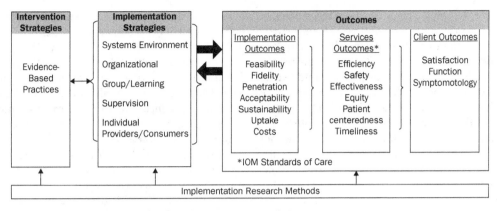

FIGURE 1.3 Proctor conceptual model of implementation research.[85]

and academic environments, we summarize a number of opportunities. We note the recent publication of reporting standards for implementation studies (StaRI)[86] and expect that the adoption of these standards over the coming years will further improve the quality of D&I research. Furthermore, topics such as scaling up and de-implementation are gaining greater attention and are briefly introduced.

Funding—NIH, CDC, AHRQ, and Canadian Priorities

Growing emphasis through funding adds credibility to the area of research implementation and evaluation. RFAs from NIH, CDC, and AHRQ (Agency for Healthcare Research and Quality) attest to the growing commitment of resources in the United States. The Canadian Institutes of Health Research have also increased emphasis on funding of D&I, or knowledge translation. Priority for methods development and application is included in these funding opportunities, and for many institutions provides the building block on which junior faculty members are themselves promoted (holding grants in addition to scientific productivity are often key components of promotion criteria). Many health care organizations are also beginning to recognize the importance of implementing evidence-based practices, which creates opportunities for research partnerships that can help to speed translation.

Education and Training

The need to align D&I training with career stage and goals for workforce development has been reviewed for North America.[87] Challenges to training identified by this review included core competencies versus specialization,[88] the rapid pace of

the developing field, and sustainability of training programs. Furthermore, for established schools of public health, identifying where this training fits in the methods and content areas covered across epidemiology, biostatistics, environmental health, health services research, and behavioral sciences remains challenging. Expanding shared resources of teaching materials and toolkits (see http://www.pcori.org/research-results/research-dissemination-and-implementation/dissemination-and-implementation) will help support these training endeavors. Several NIH-funded initiatives address skills development in specific areas of application including mental health implementation research;[89] cancer prevention and control;[88] and the training institute for D&I research in health, a collaboration with the Veterans Health Administration.[90]

Academic Rewards

Priority has historically been placed on novel contributions to science—that is, discovery. Even at the Nobel Prize level of recognition, debate was substantial regarding the role of Florey in moving from discovery of penicillin to the refinement of methods for mass production. From the point of view of impact it was clearly the application of methods leading to broad use that saved lives during WWII, not the discovery years earlier that lay dormant in a journal article. So how do we change our academic reward system to acknowledge that application of knowledge or translation to practice is an essential component of effective and affordable health and welfare services? Accountability, given the high levels of government funding for research in the United States and many other countries, does not on its own shift the reward system. In fact, Moses and Martin call for sweeping changes in the way we conduct research in academic medical centers and reward scientists to more efficiently translate research to practice.[91] We need models that are implemented and evaluated within our major academic centers to show that the translation of science to practice is an academic discipline with methods and outcomes that can be evaluated like any other discipline. However if junior investigators do not have options for a career path in these disciplines, then again the growth of this area will be limited. As an example, academic primary care has supported leading researchers at Dartmouth and Case Western to develop strategies for increased use of evidence-based preventive services, testing subsequent widespread implementation[92-95] and recognition at the level of membership in the Institute of Medicine in the National Academy. Broader recognition across health sciences disciplines will support methods development and applications to improve population health.

Innovation versus Replication (Delivery of Effective Programs)

Again, the criteria for funding of grants and the promotion of faculty often hinge on innovation and discovery. Moving a discovery from bench to clinical application or from one health department to a statewide intervention may not appear to be as innovative as a more focused basic science contribution. We might argue it is, however, far more complex and less likely to succeed! Can we refine metrics that will help us estimate lives saved or improvement in quality-adjusted life years to summarize the public health impact of D&I research? How should we quantify the contextual factors that moderate the effectiveness of implementation? As Titler asks,[96] can we become consistent in approaches to circumstances and setting in which implementation or translation to practice is effective, and define mechanisms for effective interventions?

Scaling Up

When we take evidence-based interventions to scale and deliver them to all population groups equitably, we achieve substantial population health benefits. A common and consistent definition of scaling up is not yet evident in the literature. Why aren't we studying large-scale implementation more routinely? How does scaling up differ from other implementation—if at all? Questions arise such as the strength of the evidence base—the ability to deliver the intervention

at low cost, the approaches to monitoring consistency or integrity of the intervention delivery, and outcomes across levels of health system (provider or heath department) and individuals. Will additional technical assistance be needed for broader implementation? How is this developed, delivered, and sustained? How flexible can and must the intervention be?[97] What are the measures of organizational success and of overall outcome? One design defined by Curran as effectiveness-implementation hybrid combines a dual focus on both clinical effectiveness and also implementation measures [98] This is described in detail for global mental health care, but could be a framework for other interventions that fall outside the responsive marketing and commercial sectors. How important is the original intervention design for delivery at scale? One guide for scaling up interventions sets out a step-by-step process.[99]

De-implementation

The need for research on de-implementation is highlighted in the PAR-16-238, which sees this as a means to move more quickly to effective and efficient delivery of evidence-based interventions. The PAR calls for "studies of the de-implementation of clinical and community practices that are not evidence-based, have been prematurely widely adopted, yield sub-optimal benefits for patients, or are harmful or wasteful." De-implementation is critically important because about 30% of all medical spending in the United States is unnecessary and doesn't add value. There has been a clinical focus on this over the last few years, largely as a result of the Choosing Wisely campaigns that targets reduction/elimination of low value care, but there has been relatively limited research emphasis in this area.

There are a wide range of terms that are used to describe de-implementation, including de-adoption, exnovation, and de-innovation.[100,101] Some authors use the term "misimplementation" to include both practices that are not evidence-based and should be stopped and practices that are evidence-based that should be implemented.[102] Regardless of the terminology, it is important to understand that this area actually represents three different types of problems: De-implementation is basically 3 different problems: (1) ending harmful practices, such as eliminating use of harmful drugs; (2) reducing use of ineffective practices, or those that offer no benefit over less invasive practices; and (3) reducing use of one practice while increasing the use of another.

Niven, et al.[100] recently completed the first knowledge synthesis in the area of de-implementation. They concluded that most de-implementation that occurs is the result of scientific evidence, is focused on market withdrawal of harmful drugs, and results from active interventions. It is also noted that de-implementation studies are largely observational, and little systematic or rigorous work in this area has been conducted.

There are many critical questions to be answered related to de-implementation, including whether the processes are similar across the three different types of de-implementation problems, and whether different people are needed to effectively address these different problems. There is also a real need to consider how to sustain de-implementation over time, especially when considering interventions other than drugs that are not driven by the market or regulatory factors.

There is also a critical need to understand the factors responsible for rapid and unplanned de-implementation, such as reduced use of hormone replacement therapy in the United States. Developing nimble mechanisms to allow for the study of population-level de-implementation as it is occurring may be particularly useful. For example, ongoing changes in practice such as elimination of PAP smears in Australia's national cervical screening program, from January 2017, and replacement with 5-year HPV testing, offer opportunities to consider the perspectives, facilitators, and barriers to de-implementation from the patient, provider, testing laboratory, and insurance perspectives. De-implementation will likely not be the inverse of implementation and dissemination uptakes.[103] Further, there are likely very different social factors at work in the implementation versus de-implementation context. For example, women have been told for decades that they must have yearly mammograms, and may have many friends who had breast cancer detected via routine mammography. Asking them now to have fewer mammograms, or at older ages to stop completely, may test their confidence in their provider and the health care system, and go against deeply rooted beliefs about taking care of themselves. Where to begin to remove inefficient or unnecessary practices remains an area of study to begin this process, as does identifying the characteristics of the people who will lead or resist de-implementation and how they may differ from those who lead implementation.[104] For example, the Choosing Wisely campaign launched in 2012 in the United States aims to encourage abandoning care that wastes resources or delivers no benefit in specific health areas, such as management of blood sugar and diabetes, and cancer screening. The approach to studying de-implementation mechanisms examines variation among systems, providers, patients, and the actual implementation strategies that may modify the success of the program.[105]

Systems to Quantify Benefits of Effective Programs (Outcomes)

How do we sum up the benefits of implementation and effective programs being delivered to broad sectors of the population? Ginexi and Hilton propose that focusing on evidence-based best practices may help bridge the gap from research to practice.[106] They argue that best and worst practice can inform practice improvement. How we quantify program fidelity and implementation remains at the core of the challenge. Proctor and colleagues[85] now propose a taxonomy of eight conceptually distinct implementation outcomes—acceptability, adoption, appropriateness, feasibility, fidelity, implementation cost, penetration, and sustainability—along with their nominal definitions. Further, they propose using a two-pronged agenda for research on implementation outcomes. Conceptualizing and measuring implementation outcomes (or process evaluation measures in the European framework) will advance understanding of implementation processes, enhance efficiency in implementation research, and pave the way for studies of the comparative effectiveness of implementation strategies. As noted in this book, several novel approaches are proposed but coming to agreement on when these measures are most helpful will require further study.

New methods are needed, and consistency across programs will add to the overall advance of the field. The magnitude of benefit, the proportion of the population reached, and the degree to which a program is sustained all impact the long-term population benefit. Proctor defines steps in the model of implementation, noting that conceptualizing and measuring implementation outcomes will advance understanding of implementation processes, enhance efficiency in implementation research, and pave the way for studies of the comparative effectiveness of implementation strategies.[85] Refinement to better incorporate ethical, legal, and social considerations through stakeholder engagement will further advance this model. The RE-AIM approach to evaluation is also summarized in chapter 19. Other approaches that apply across settings will make for a more robust area of inquiry.

SUMMARY

Given the growing emphasis on D&I as a means to increase the efficiency of the research enterprise, public policy, and the services with which we work, refining methods that will facilitate translation and implementation are imperative. Cultural changes within the academy and in linking researchers and practitioners will be necessary adjuncts to effective progress. Bringing the D&I research community to common understanding of answers to our over-arching questions will be a necessary step. Then we can more consistently answer the questions: How will we gather this information on effective interventions to form the evidence base? Will interventions be applicable to our setting? What methods should we use to decide what to disseminate or implement? Which strategies will give us the greatest impact on population health? What outcomes should be tracked to know if we are making progress? How long will it take to show progress, or when will it be observed? The methods outlined in this book will help us in answering these and other important questions.

SUGGESTED READINGS AND WEBSITES

Readings

Glasgow RE, Vinson C, Chambers D, Khoury MJ, Kaplan RM, Hunter C. National Institutes of Health approaches to dissemination and implementation science: current and future directions. *Am J Public Health*. 2012;102:1274–1281.
Addressing the gap between knowledge and practice, this paper reviews core values necessary to advance implementation science. These include rigor and relevance, efficiency, collaboration, improved collaboration, and cumulative knowledge.

Glasziou P, Chalmers I, Altman DG, et al. Taking healthcare interventions from trial to practice. *BMJ*. 2010;341:c3852.
Improved reporting of details of trials will enable use of results in practice. An example of this is illusrated and a call for increased reporting of intervention details to improve replication and use in practice.

Green LW, Ottoson JM, Garcia C, Hiatt RA. Diffusion theory and knowledge dissemination, utilization, and integration in public health. *Annu Rev Public Health*. 2009;30:151–174.

Rigrous review of public health implications of diffusion, dissemination, and implementation to improve public health practice and guide design of future research.

Ioannidis JP, Karassa FB. The need to consider the wider agenda in systematic reviews and meta-analyses: breadth, timing, and depth of the evidence. *BMJ*. 2010;341:c4875.
Thoughtful critique of limiations of meta-analysis of clinical interventions, the narrow scope of practice they cover, and the potential to draw misleading conclusions from systemaitc reviews and meta-analysis.

Lobb R, Colditz G. Implementation science and its application to population health. *Ann Rev Public Health* 2013:34:235–253.
Thoughtful review of the role that stakeholder engagement and more rigorous study of barriers to implementation can help identify how systems can implement effective innovations in health care delivery.

Proctor E, Silmere H, Raghavan R, et al. Outcomes for implementation research: conceptual distinctions, measurement challenges, and research agenda. *Adm Policy Ment Health*. 2011;38(2):65–76.
Groundbreaking summary of issues in design and evaluation of implementation research, setting out a model that defines steps in the process and discusses a model for quantfying benefits of program implementation.

Woolf SH. The meaning of translational research and why it matters. *JAMA*. 2008;299(2):211–213.
An important contribution defining stages of research and the importance of translation from bench to bedside and from reseach clinic to population wide applications. Also calls for research funding to be directed to inproving population health outcomes.

Selected Websites and Tools

Cancer Control P.L.A.N.E.T. http://cancercontrol-planet.cancer.gov/index.html
Cancer Control P.L.A.N.E.T. acts as a portal to provide access to data and resources for designing, implementing, and evaluating evidence-based cancer control programs. The site provides five steps (with links) for developing a comprehensive cancer control plan or program.

Dissemination and Implementation Research Core at the Institute for Clinical and Translational Science, Washington University in St. Louis, Enola Proctor, Director. http://icts.wustl.edu/icts-researchers/icts-cores/find-services/by-core-name/dissemination-implementation-research-core
The Dissemination and Implementation Research Core (DIRC) provides methodological expertise to advance translational (T3 and T4) research to inform and move efficacious health practices from clinical knowledge into routine, real-world use. The DIRC works with scientists to move forward scientific agenda and grant writing

related to dissemination and implementation (D&I) of health care discoveries. Furthermore, DIRC develops tools and methods for studying D&I.

Implementation Science exchange (IMPSCIX). https://impsci.tracs.unc.edu/
A public service of the North Carolina Translational and Clinical Sciences Institute (NC TRACS). UNC Chapel Hill. This free online resource offers help to design, get funded, and execute implementation science research projects.

Task Force on Community Preventive Services. http://www.thecommunityguide.org
The Community Guide provides a repository of the 200+ systematic reviews conducted by the Task Force, an independent, interdisciplinary group with staff support by the Centers for Disease Control and Prevention. Each review gives attention to the "applicability" of the conclusions beyond the study populations and settings in which the original studies were conducted.

Cochrane Collaboration. http://www.cochrane.org/
The Cochrane Collaboration prepares Cochrane Reviews and aims to update them regularly with the latest scientific evidence. Members of the organization (mostly volunteers) work together to assess evidence to help people make decisions about health care practices and policies. Some people read the health care literature to find reports of randomized controlled trials; others find such reports by searching electronic databases; others prepare and update Cochrane Reviews based on the evidence found in these trials; others work to improve the methods used in Cochrane Reviews; others provide a vitally important consumer perspective.

RE-AIM. http://www.RE-AIM.org
The acronym refers to Reach, Effectiveness, Adoption, Implementation, and Maintenance, all important dimensions in the consideration of D&I research and in the external validity or applicability of research results in original studies for the alternative settings and circumstances in which they might be applied. These were applied in the development of a set of guidelines for assessing and reporting external validity.

D-cubed. http://www.uq.edu.au/ evaluationstedi/Dissemination/?q=dissemination/
A review of dissemination strategies used by projects funded by the Australian Learning and Teaching Council) promotes dissemination strategies that have facilitated effective dissemination. A useful framework for dissemination and guide to use is provided.

REFERENCES

1. Agre P, Leshner AI. Bridging science and society. *Science.* 2010;327(5968):921.
2. Emmons KM, Colditz GA. Realizing the potential of cancer prevention—the role of implementation science. *N Engl J Med.* 2017;376(10):986–990.
3. Collins FS. Reengineering translational science: the time is right. *Sci Transl Med.* 2011;3(90):90cm17.
4. Moses H 3rd, Matheson DH, Cairns-Smith S, George BP, Palisch C, Dorsey ER. The anatomy of medical research: US and international comparisons. *JAMA.* 2015;313(2):174–189.
5. Institute of Medicine. *Crossing the quality chasm: A new health system for the 21st century.* Washington DC: National Academy Press; 2001.
6. Rubenstein LV, Pugh J. Strategies for promoting organizational and practice change by advancing implementation research. *J Gen Intern Med.* 2006;21 Suppl 2:S58–S64.
7. United States Department of Health and Human Services. Improving Public Health Practice through Translational Research. 2007; http://grants.nih.gov/grants/guide/rfa-files/rfa-cd-07-005.html. Accessed July 17, 2011.
8. Lost in clinical translation. *Nat Med.* 2004;10(9):879.
9. Department of Health and Human Services. Dissemination and Implementation Research in Health, PAR-16-238. 2016; PAR-16-238. Available at https://grants.nih.gov/grants/guide/pa-files/PAR-16-238.html. Accessed September 4, 2016.
10. Rabin BA, Brownson RC, Haire-Joshu D, Kreuter MW, Weaver NL. A glossary for dissemination and implementation research in health. *J Public Health Manag Pract.* 2008;14(2):117–123.
11. Lomas J. Diffusion, dissemination, and implementation: who should do what? *Ann N Y Acad Sci.* 1993;703:226–235; discussion 235–227.
12. Lomas J, Sisk JE, Stocking B. From evidence to practice in the United States, the United Kingdom, and Canada. *Milbank Q.* 1993;71(3):405–410.
13. Curry SJ. Organizational interventions to encourage guideline implementation. *Chest.* 2000;118(2 Suppl):40S–46S.
14. Bero L, Grillr R, Grimshaw J, Harvey E, Oxman AD, Thompson M. Closing the gap between research and practice: an overview of systematic reviews of interventions to promote the implementation of research findings. *BMJ.* 1998;317:465–468.
15. Lobb R, Colditz GA. Implementation science and its application to population health. *Annu Rev Public Health.* 2013;34:235–251.
16. Bowen DJ, Sorensen G, Weiner BJ, Campbell M, Emmons K, Melvin C. Dissemination research in cancer control: where are we and where should we go? *Cancer Causes Control.* 2009;20(4):473–485.
17. Crandall D. Implementation aspects of dissemination. *Sci Commun.* 1989;11(1):79–106.
18. Huberman M. Research utilization: the state of the art. *Knowledge, Technology & Policy.* 1991;7(4):13–33.

19. Huberman AM, Levinson NS, Havelock RG, Cox PL. Interorganizational arrangements. An approach to education practice improvement. *Knowledge: Creation, Diffusion, Utilization.* 1981;3(1):5–22.

20. Glasziou P, Chalmers I, Altman DG, et al. Taking healthcare interventions from trial to practice. *BMJ.* 2010;341:c3852.

21. Ioannidis JP, Karassa FB. The need to consider the wider agenda in systematic reviews and meta-analyses: breadth, timing, and depth of the evidence. *BMJ.* 2010;341:c4875.

22. Farquhar JW. The case for dissemination research in health promotion and disease prevention. *Can J Public Health.* 1996;87 Suppl 2:S44–S49.

23. Harlan WR. Prevention research at the National Institutes of Health. *Am J Prev Med.* 1998;14(4):302–307.

24. Institute of Medicine. *Linking research to public health practice. A review of the CDC's program of Centers for Research and Demonstration of Health Promotion and Disease Prevention.* Washington, DC: National Academy Press; 1997.

25. Oldenburg BF, Sallis JF, Ffrench ML, Owen N. Health promotion research and the diffusion and institutionalization of interventions. *Health Educ Res.* 1999;14(1):121–130.

26. Sallis JF, Owen N, Fotheringham MJ. Behavioral epidemiology: a systematic framework to classify phases of research on health promotion and disease prevention. *Ann Behav Med.* 2000;22(4):294–298.

27. Rychetnik L, Nutbeam D, Hawe P. Lessons from a review of publications in three health promotion journals from 1989 to 1994. *Health Educ Res.* 1997;12(4):491–504.

28. Tabak RG, Stamatakis KA, Jacobs JA, Brownson RC. What predicts dissemination efforts among public health researchers in the United States? *Public Health Rep.* 2014;129(4):361–368.

29. Cochran W. Problems arising in the analysis of a series of similar experiments. *J R Stat Soc Suppl.* 1937;4:102–118.

30. Rogers E. *Diffusion of innovations.* Third ed. London: The Free Press; 1993.

31. OECD. *Health at a Glance 2015.* 2015.

32. Mosteller F, Wallace D. *Inference and disputed authorship: The Federalist.* Reading, MA: Addison-Wesley Publishing Company; 1964.

33. Mosteller F. *The pleasures of statistics. The autobiography of Frederick Mosteller.* New York: Springer; 2010.

34. Mosteller F. On pooling data. *J Am Stat Assoc.* 1948;43:231–242.

35. Green LW, Ottoson JM, Garcia C, Hiatt RA. Diffusion theory and knowledge dissemination, utilization, and integration in public health. *Annu Rev Public Health.* 2009;30:151–174.

36. Brownson RC, Bright FS. Chronic disease control in public health practice: looking back and moving forward. *Public Health Rep.* 2004;119(3):230–238.

37. Balas EA, Boren SA. Managing clincal knowledge for health care improvement. In: Bemmel J, McCray A, eds. *Yearbook of medical informaticcs 2000: Patient-centered systems.* Stuttgart, Germany: Schattauer; 2000:65–70.

38. Goodwin I. Engineers proclaim top achievements of 20th century, but neglect attributing feats to roots in physics. *Physics Today.* 2000;53:48–49.

39. Fortunato S. Prizes: Growing time lag threatens Nobels. *Nature.* 2014;508(7495):186.

40. Bickel L. *Howard Florey: The man who made penicillin.* Melbourne: Melbourne University Press; 1972.

41. Banting FG, Best CH. The internal secretion of the pancreas. 1922. *Indian J Med Res.* 2007;125(3):251–266.

42. Banting FG, Best CH, Collip JB, Campbell WR, Fletcher AA. Pancreatic extracts in the treatment of diabetes mellitus. *Can Med Assoc J.* 1922;12(3):141–146.

43. Bliss M. *The discovery of insulin.* 25th Anniversary Edition. Chicago: University of Chicago Press; 2007.

44. U.S. Department of Health and Human Services. A Timeline of HIV/AIDS. 2017; https://www.aids.gov/hiv-aids-basics/hiv-aids-101/aids-timeline/ Accessed February 22, 2017, 2017.

45. Anonymous. The Boston Smallpox Epidemic, 1721. 2010; http://ocp.hul.harvard.edu/contagion/smallpox.html. Accessed December 5, 2010.

46. World Health Organizatio. *Handbook of resolutions and decisions of the World Health Assembly and the Executive Board.* Geneva: WHO; 1971.

47. Breslow L. The future of public health: prospects in the United States for the 1990s. *Annu Rev Public Health.* 1990;11:1–28.

48. Zerhouni E. Medicine. The NIH Roadmap. *Science.* 2003;302(5642):63–72.

49. Westfall JM, Mold J, Fagnan L. Practice-based research--"Blue Highways" on the NIH roadmap. *JAMA.* 2007;297(4):403–406.

50. Frieden TR. A framework for public health action: the health impact pyramid. *Am J Public Health.* 2010;100(4):590–595.

51. Chambers DA, Feero WG, Khoury MJ. Convergence of implementation science, precision medicine, and the learning health care system: a new model for biomedical research. *JAMA.* 2016;315(18):1941–1942.

52. Wandersman A, Duffy J, Flaspohler P, et al. Bridging the gap between prevention research and practice: the interactive systems framework for dissemination and implementation. *Am J Community Psychol*. 2008;41(3-4):171–181.

53. Richmond J, Kotelchuck M. Coordination and development of strategies and policy for public health promotion in the United States. In: Holland W, Detel R, Know G, eds. *Oxford textbook of public health*. Vol 1. Oxford: Oxford University Press; 1991.

54. Atwood K, Colditz GA, Kawachi I. From public health science to prevention policy: placing science in its social and political contexts. *Am J Public Health*. 1997;87(10):1603–1606.

55. Petticrew M, Tugwell P, Welch V, et al. Better evidence about wicked issues in tackling health inequities. *J Public Health*. 2009;31(3):453–456.

56. Lavis J, Davies H, Oxman A, Denis JL, Golden-Biddle K, Ferlie E. Towards systematic reviews that inform health care management and policy-making. *J Health Serv Res Policy*. 2005;10 Suppl 1:35–48.

57. Sacks H, Berrier J, Reitman D, Ancona-Berk V, Chalmers T. Meta-analysis of randomized controlled studies. *N Engl J Med*. 1987;316:450–455.

58. Berlin J, Colditz G. A meta-analysis of physical activity in the prevention of coronary heart disease. *Am J Epidemiol*. 1990;132:612–628.

59. Bastian H, Glasziou P, Chalmers I. Seventy-five trials and eleven systematic reviews a day: how will we ever keep up? *PLoS Med*. 2010;7(9):e1000326.

60. Preventive Services Task Force. *Guide to clinical preventive services*. 2nd ed. Baltimore: Williams and Wilkins; 1996.

61. Schunemann HJ, Oxman AD, Brozek J, et al. GRADE: assessing the quality of evidence for diagnostic recommendations. *Evid Based Med*. 2008;13(6):162–163.

62. Jaeschke R, Guyatt GH, Dellinger P, et al. Use of GRADE grid to reach decisions on clinical practice guidelines when consensus is elusive. *BMJ*. 2008;337:a744.

63. Guyatt GH, Oxman AD, Vist GE, et al. GRADE: an emerging consensus on rating quality of evidence and strength of recommendations. *BMJ*. 2008;336(7650):924–926.

64. Wang Z, Norris SL, Bero L. Implementation plans included in World Health Organisation guidelines. *Implement Sci*. 2016;11(1):76.

65. Moher D, Schulz KF, Altman DG. The CONSORT statement: revised recommendations for improving the quality of reports of parallel-group randomized trials. *Ann Intern Med*. 2001;134(8):657–662.

66. Thorpe KE, Zwarenstein M, Oxman AD, et al. A pragmatic-explanatory continuum indicator summary (PRECIS): a tool to help trial designers. *CMAJ*. 2009;180(10):E47–57.

67. Loudon K, Treweek S, Sullivan F, Donnan P, Thorpe KE, Zwarenstein M. The PRECIS-2 tool: designing trials that are fit for purpose. *BMJ*. 2015;350:h2147.

68. Berkey CS, Hoaglin D, Mosteller F, Colditz GA. A random-effects regression model for meta-analysis. *Statistics in Medicine*. 1995;14:395–411.

69. Colditz GA, Brewer TF, Berkey CS, et al. Efficacy of BCG vaccine in the prevention of tuberculosis. Meta-analysis of the published literature. *JAMA*. 1994;271(9):698–702.

70. Colditz GA, Berkey CS, Mosteller F, et al. The efficacy of bacillus Calmette-Guerin vaccination of newborns and infants in the prevention of tuberculosis: meta-analyses of the published literature. *Pediatrics*. 1995;96(1 Pt 1):29–35.

71. Colditz G, Burdick E, Mosteller F. Heterogeneity in meta-analysis of data from epidemiologic studies: A commentary. *Am J Epidemiol*. 1995;142:371–382.

72. Glasgow RE, Chambers D. Developing robust, sustainable, implementation systems using rigorous, rapid and relevant science. *Clin Transl Sci*. 2012;5(1):48–55.

73. Proctor EK, Landsverk J, Aarons G, Chambers D, Glisson C, Mittman B. Implementation research in mental health services: an emerging science with conceptual, methodological, and training challenges. *Adm Policy Ment Health*. 2009;36(1):24–34.

74. Anderson LM, Brownson RC, Fullilove MT, et al. Evidence-based public health policy and practice: promises and limits. *Am J Prev Med*. 2005;28(5 Suppl):226–230.

75. Mosteller F, Colditz G. Understanding research synthesis (meta-analysis). *Ann Rev Public Health*. 1996;17:1–32.

76. Greenhalgh T, Robert G, Macfarlane F, Bate P, Kyriakidou O. Diffusion of innovations in service organizations: systematic review and recommendations. *Milbank Q*. 2004;82(4):581–629.

77. Kingdon JW. *Agendas, alternatives, and public policies*. New York: Addison-Wesley Educational Publishers, Inc; 2003.

78. Institute of Medicine. *Adverse effects of pertussis and rubella vaccines*. Washington, DC: National Academy Press; 1991.

79. Institute of Medicine. *Veterans and agent orange. Health effects of herbicides used in Vietnam*. Washington, DC: National Academy Press; 1994.

80. Colditz GA, Atwood KA, Emmons K, et al. Harvard report on cancer prevention

volume 4: Harvard Cancer Risk Index. Risk Index Working Group, Harvard Center for Cancer Prevention. *Cancer Causes Control.* 2000;11(6):477–488.

81. Brownson RC, Fielding JE, Maylahn CM. Evidence-Based Public Health: A Fundamental Concept for Public Health Practice. *Annu Rev Public Health.* 2009;30:175–201.

82. Hemenway D. Why we don't spend enough on public health. *N Engl J Med.* 2010;362(18):1657–1658.

83. Dobbinson SJ, Wakefield MA, Jamsen KM, et al. Weekend sun protection and sunburn in Australia trends (1987-2002) and association with SunSmart television advertising. *Am J Prev Med.* 2008;34(2):94–101.

84. Koh HK, Piotrowski JJ, Kumanyika S, Fielding JE. Healthy people: a 2020 vision for the social determinants approach. *Health Educ Behav.* 2011;38(6):551–557.

85. Proctor E, Silmere H, Raghavan R, et al. Outcomes for implementation research: conceptual distinctions, measurement challenges, and research agenda. *Adm Policy Ment Health.* 2011;38(2):65–76.

86. Pinnock H, Barwick M, Carpenter CR, et al. Standards for Reporting Implementation Studies (StaRI): explanation and elaboration document. *BMJ Open.* 2017;7(4):e013318.

87. Chambers DA, Proctor EK, Brownson RC, Straus SE. Mapping training needs for dissemination and implementation research: lessons from a synthesis of existing D&I research training programs. *Transl Behav Med.* 2016. doi:10.1007/s13142-016-0399-3

88. Padek M, Colditz G, Dobbins M, et al. Developing educational competencies for dissemination and implementation research training programs: an exploratory analysis using card sorts. *Implement Sci.* 2015;10:114.

89. Proctor EK, Landsverk J, Baumann AA, et al. The implementation research institute: training mental health implementation researchers in the United States. *Implement Sci.* 2013;8:105.

90. Meissner HI, Glasgow RE, Vinson CA, et al. The U.S. training institute for dissemination and implementation research in health. *Implement Sci.* 2013;8:12.

91. Moses H, 3rd, Martin JB. Biomedical research and health advances. *N Engl J Med.* 2011;364(6):567–571.

92. Dietrich A, Carney P, Winchell C, et al. An office systems approach to cancer prevention in primary care. *Cancer Pract.* 1997;5:375–381.

93. Dietrich AJ, Tobin JN, Cassells A, et al. Telephone care management to improve cancer screening among low-income women: a randomized, controlled trial. *Ann Intern Med.* 2006;144(8):563–571.

94. Dietrich AJ, Tobin JN, Cassells A, et al. Translation of an efficacious cancer-screening intervention to women enrolled in a Medicaid managed care organization. *Ann Fam Med.* 2007;5(4):320–327.

95. Stewart EE, Nutting PA, Crabtree BF, Stange KC, Miller WL, Jaen CR. Implementing the patient-centered medical home: observation and description of the national demonstration project. *Ann Fam Med.* 2010;8 Suppl 1:S21–32; S92.

96. Titler MG. Translation science and context. *Res Theory Nurs Pract.* 2010;24(1):35–55.

97. Gopalan G, Franco LM, Dean-Assael K, McGuire-Schwartz M, Chacko A, McKay M. Statewide implementation of the 4 Rs and 2 Ss for strengthening families. *J Evid Based Soc Work.* 2014;11(1-2):84–96.

98. Curran GM, Bauer M, Mittman B, Pyne JM, Stetler C. Effectiveness-implementation hybrid designs: combining elements of clinical effectiveness and implementation research to enhance public health impact. *Med Care.* 2012;50(3):217–226.

99. Milat AJ, Newson R, King L, et al. A guide to scaling up population health interventions. *Public Health Res Pract.* 2016;26(1):e2611604.

100. Niven DJ, Mrklas KJ, Holodinsky JK, et al. Towards understanding the de-adoption of low-value clinical practices: a scoping review. *BMC Med.* 2015;13:255.

101. Gnjidic D, Elshaug AG. De-adoption and its 43 related terms: harmonizing low-value care terminology. *BMC Med.* 2015;13:273.

102. Brownson RC, Allen P, Jacob RR, et al. Understanding mis-implementation in public health practice. *Am J Prev Med.* 2015;48(5):543–551.

103. Davidoff F. On the undiffusion of established practices. *JAMA Intern Med.* 2015;175(5):809–811.

104. van Bodegom-Vos L, Davidoff F, Marang-van de Mheen PJ. Implementation and de-implementation: two sides of the same coin? *BMJ Qual Saf.* 2017;26(6):495–501.

105. Aron DC, Lowery J, Tseng CL, Conlin P, Kahwati L. De-implementation of inappropriately tight control (of hypoglycemia) for health: protocol with an example of a research grant application. *Implement Sci.* 2014;9:58.

106. Ginexi EM, Hilton TF. What's next for translation research? *Eval Health Prof.* 2006;29(3):334–347.

2

Terminology for Dissemination and Implementation Research

BORSIKA A. RABIN AND ROSS C. BROWNSON

INTRODUCTION

Dissemination and implementation (D&I) research is increasingly recognized as an important function of academia and is a growing priority for major health-related funding agencies (e.g., the National Institute of Health [NIH], the Centers for Disease Control and Prevention [CDC], the National Institute on Disability and Rehabilitation Research [NIDRR], the Canadian Institutes of Health Research [CIHR] and the World Health Organization [WHO]).[1-7] One challenging aspect of D&I research is the lack of standardized terminology.[8-13] As noted by Ciliska and colleagues: "closing the gap from knowledge generation to use in decision-making for practice and policy is conceptually and theoretically hampered by diverse terms and inconsistent definitions of terms."[14] A survey conducted by *Nature Medicine* on how their readers define the term "translational research" found substantial variation in interpretation by respondents. Some definitions were consistent with the NIH definition ("the process of applying ideas, insights and discoveries generated through basic scientific inquiry to the treatment or prevention of human disease"), others believed that only research that leads to direct clinical application should be defined as translational research, and only a small group emphasized the bidirectional nature of the process (i.e., bench to bedside and back).[15] This phenomenon can be partly explained by the relatively new appearance of D&I research on the health research agenda and by the great diversity of disciplines that made noteworthy contributions to the understanding of D&I research.[16-18] Some of the most important contributions originate from the nonhealth fields of agriculture, education, marketing, communication, and management.[19] The primary health-related areas presently contributing to D&I research include health

services research, HIV prevention, school health, mental health, nursing, cancer control, violence prevention, and disability and rehabilitation.[16,20-24] Further complexity is injected by the variation in terminology and classification of terms across countries. This book uses the term "dissemination and implementation research" to denote the newly emerging field in the United States; however, other countries and international organizations (e.g., the United Kingdom, Canada, the WHO) commonly use the terms "knowledge translation and integration," "population health intervention research," or "scaling up" to define this area of research.[7,25-27] Furthermore, Graham and colleagues identified 29 distinct terms referring to the some aspect of the D&I (or knowledge translation) process when they looked at the terminology used by 33 applied research funding agencies in nine countries.[27] A more recent review by McKibbon and colleagues identified 100 terms alone just to describe knowledge translation or KT research.[28]

Definitions presented in this chapter reflect the terminology used in the most frequently cited manuscripts, reports, websites, and databases on D&I research in health and in funding announcements of major federal funding agencies (e.g., NIH, CDC, NIDRR, CIHR). To identify terms and definitions, an initial search of the English language literature was conducted to identify peer-reviewed manuscripts and documents from governmental agencies (i.e., gray literature). Further papers and documents were identified from reference lists and expert recommendations using snowball sampling.[29] This chapter builds on a previously published article that used an expert discussion to select definitions to be included from a list of 106 definitions. Additional terms and their definitions were included based on recommendations from the authors and review of each chapter of this book. For each definition, the most relevant publications and chapters from this book were included so that readers may consult the literature for a more in-depth discussion of the term and its application.

To facilitate the thinking and discussion on D&I research, terms are presented using the three main sections proposed by Padek and colleagues to organize educational competencies for dissemination and implementation research.[30] The first section (**Definition, Background, and Rational**) provides definition for the most commonly used terms in D&I research as well as identifies stages of the research process continuum, their relationship to D&I-related activities, and defines varieties of Type 1 and 2 research. In section 2 (**Theories and Approaches**) the most commonly used models and frameworks that can inform planning and evaluation activities in D&I research are discussed along with concepts of designing for D&I and sustainability; adaptation and fidelity; D&I strategies; and factors associated with the success, speed, and extent of D&I. Finally, the third section (**Design and Analysis**) summarizes important concepts of study design and measurement that should be considered when evaluating D&I research. The list of terms and their organization is provided in Table 2.1.

SECTION 1: DEFINITION, BACKGROUND, AND RATIONALE

Innovation

The term "innovation" can refer to "an idea, practice, or object that is perceived as new by an individual or other unit of adoption."[19(p. 12)] Some authors use this term interchangeably with the term "evidence-based intervention."

A number of more specific terms denoting the subject of dissemination and implementation activities are commonly used in the context of health research and listed below.

Evidence-Based Intervention

The subjects of D&I activities are interventions with proven efficacy and effectiveness (i.e., evidence-based). Interventions within D&I research are defined broadly and may include programs, practices, processes, policies, and guidelines.[31] More comprehensive definitions of evidence-based interventions are available elsewhere.[32–36] In D&I research, we often encounter complex interventions (e.g., multilevel interventions using community-wide education) where the description of core intervention components and their relationships involve multiple

---

TABLE 2.1 DISSEMINATION AND IMPLEMENTATION
TERMS AND THEIR ORGANIZATION

SECTION 1: DEFINITION, BACKGROUND, AND RATIONALE	SECTION 2: THEORIES AND APPROACHES
Innovation	Stage Models
Evidence-based intervention	Theories and Frameworks
Empirically supported treatment	Diffusion of innovations
Evidence-informed practice	RE-AIM framework
Types of Evidence	Consolidated Framework for Implementation Research
Type 1 evidence	Designing for Dissemination, Implementation and Sustainability
Type 2 evidence	Audience Segmentation
Type 3 evidence	Fidelity and Adaptation
Processes for D&I	Fidelity
Diffusion	Adaptation
Dissemination	Core elements (components)
Implementation	Adaptome
Mis-implementation	Strategies for D&I
De-implementation	Dissemination strategy
Reach	Implementation strategy

TABLE 2.1 CONTINUED

Adoption	**Factors Associated with the Speed and Extent of D&I**
Sustainability/Sustainment	**Characteristics of the intervention**
Maintenance	Relative advantage
Institutionalization	Compatibility
Capacity building	Acceptability
Knowledge-for-Action terms	Appropriateness
Knowledge translation	Feasibility
Knowledge transfer	Implementation cost
Technology transfer	**Characteristics of the adopters**
Knowledge exchange	**Opinion leaders**
Knowledge integration	**Change agent**
Knowledge utilization	**Context**
Research utilization	Organizational culture
Knowledge brokering	Organizational climate
Knowledge broker	Readiness (organizational, practice, community)
Scale up and scaling up	
Evidence Synthesis Approaches	**SECTION 3: DESIGN AND ANALYSIS**
Scoping review	**Study Designs**
Realist review	**Pragmatic or practical clinical trial**
Types of Research	**Natural experiment**
Fundamental (or Basic) research	**Plausibility design**
Translational research	**Sequential, Multiple Assignment, Randomized Trial**
T1 research	**(SMART) design**
Efficacy research	**Stepped-wedge design**
T2 research	**Hybrid designs**
Effectiveness research	**Systems thinking**
Dissemination research	**Rapid, responsive, relevant research**
Implementation research	**Learning health care systems**
Mode I and II science	**Learning evaluation**
	Measurement considerations
Science-to-service gap	**Mixed methods**
Implementation gap	**Outcome variables**
Assimilation gap	Implementation outcomes
Population health intervention research	**Pragmatic measures**
Comparative Effectiveness Research to Accelerate	
Translation	**External validity**
Patient-centered outcomes research	**Standards for Reporting Implementation Studies**
Quality improvement	
Precision medicine	

settings, audiences, and approaches.[20,37] For a more detailed discussion of complex interventions, refer to Hawe et al.[37]

Empirically Supported Treatments

The term "empirically supported treatment" or EST is commonly used to describe psychological interventions that are proven to be efficacious. EST is different from the evidence-based intervention

or treatment terminology in that it requires that interventions are manualized and have at least two, independent, controlled experimental studies showing comparative effectiveness.[38–40]

Evidence-Informed Practice

The term "evidence-informed practice" expands the traditional evidence-based intervention terminology and intends to emphasize that health care and population health should always be context sensitive, and use a person- or client-focused (stakeholder) perspective and not be limited to the mere synthesis and application of scientific evidence.[41] In part, the "evidence-informed" framing seeks to emphasize that health-related decisions are not based only on research (particularly considering political and organizational factors).[42,43] This perspective highlights the importance of making health decisions using evidence-based methods (information based on the synthesis of scientific evidence) in conjunction with clinician and practitioner expertise and knowledge and information about the values, preferences, and circumstances of the target patient or population. Consequently, real-world experience suggests that the evidence should not be limited to quantitative evidence from highly controlled research trials but should also consider the use of many different levels and types of evidence including qualitative studies, case reports, and expert opinion.[44] Despite of the initial distinction in meaning between evidence-based and evidence-informed practice, the terms are commonly used interchangeably in the literature.

Additional terms denoting the subject of D&I activities include best practices, evidence-based processes, and evidence-based health care.[45,46]

Types of Evidence

The types of evidence available for decision making in health can be classified as Type 1, Type 2, and Type 3 evidence.[47] These evidence types differ in their characteristics, scope, and quality.

Type 1 Evidence

Type 1 evidence defines to the cause of a particular outcome (e.g., health condition). This type of evidence includes factors such as magnitude and severity of the outcome (i.e., number, incidence, prevalence) and the actionability of the cause (i.e., preventability or changeability) and often leads to the conclusion that "*something* should be done."[34,47]

Type 2 Evidence

Type 2 evidence focuses on the relative impact of a specific intervention to address a particular outcome (e.g., heath condition). This type of evidence includes information on the effectiveness or cost-effectiveness of a strategy compared to others and point to the conclusion that "*specifically, this should be done*."[34] Type 2 evidence (interventions) can be classified based on the source of the evidence (i.e., study design) as evidence-based, efficacious, promising, and emerging interventions.[47]

Type 3 Evidence

Type 3 evidence is concerned with the type of information that is needed for the adaptation and implementation of an evidence-based intervention.[32] This type of evidence includes information on how and under which contextual conditions interventions were implemented and how they were received and addresses the issue of "*how* something should be one." Type 3 is the type of evidence we have the least of and derives from the context of an intervention, particularly concepts of external validity.[47]

Processes for D&I

Diffusion

Diffusion is the passive, untargeted, unplanned, and uncontrolled spread of new interventions. Diffusion is part of the diffusion-dissemination-implementation continuum and it is the least focused and intense approach.[48,49]

Dissemination

Dissemination is an active approach of spreading evidence-based interventions to the target audience via determined channels using planned strategies.[48,49]

Implementation

Implementation is the process of putting to use or integrating evidence-based interventions within a setting.[50]

Mis-implementation

Mis-implementation involves one or both of two processes: the discontinuation of effective programs and the continuation of ineffective practices in the context of public health.[51] Mis-implementation is a broader term while de-implementation focuses on the discontinuation component of mis-implementation.

De-implementation

De-implementation is defined as stopping or abandoning practices that have not proved to be effective and are possibly harmful.[52] In medicine, the term "over use" is sometimes used to identified practices that should be ended. De-implementation gained increasing focus and support in health care and population health in many countries through initiatives like the Choosing Wisely campaign that encourages and supports practitioners to identify and abandon unproven or harmful practices.[53] De-implementation is believed to be an effective approach for improving patient outcomes and to achieve cost saving. Early evidence indicates that similar to dissemination and implementation efforts, de-implementation also requires active approaches and local champions for success. Factors associated with successful de-implementation efforts are still being studied, but they are believed to be similar to the factors relevant to determine the speed and extent of implementation and are multilevel and complex in nature.[54,55] Two main types of de-implementation include *substitution* (the replacement of the low value practice with a more promising alternative) and *disenchantment* (abandonment of practice due to information indicating its lack of effectiveness or cost-effectiveness).[54]

The terminology and strategies for de-implementation are still evolving and include terms such as termination, replacement, reversal, de-adoption, decrease use, disinvesting, and discontinue use.[55]

Reach

Reach refers to the ability of a program to engage its ultimate target audience, both in terms of quantity (number/percent of participant) and quality (representativeness of participants). The reach of a program can greatly influence the level of public health impact the program can achieve.[56]

Adoption

Adoption is the decision of an organization or community to commit to and initiate an evidence-based intervention.[19,57,58]

Sustainability

Sustainability describes the extent to which an evidence-based intervention can deliver its intended benefits over an extended period of time after external support from the donor agency is terminated.[59] A number of models and instruments are available to conceptualize and measure sustainability.[60] Most often sustainability is measured through the continued use of intervention components; however, Scheirer and Dearing suggest that measures for sustainability should also include considerations of maintained community- or organizational-level partnerships; maintenance of organizational or community practices, procedures, and policies that were initiated during the implementation of the intervention; sustained organizational or community attention to the issue that the intervention is designed to address; and efforts for program diffusion and replication in other sites.[61] As discussed in the following, three operational indicators of sustainability are: (1) **maintenance** of a program's initial health

benefits, (2) **institutionalization** of the program in a setting or community, and (3) **capacity building** in the recipient setting or community.[59]

Maintenance

Maintenance refers to the ability of the recipient setting or community to continuously deliver the health benefits achieved when the intervention was first implemented.[59]

Institutionalization

Institutionalization assesses the extent to which the evidence-based intervention is integrated within the culture of the recipient setting or community through policies and practice.[58,59,62] Three stages that determine the extent of institutionalization are: (1) *passage* (i.e., a single event that involves a significant change in the organization's structure or procedures such as transition from temporary to permanent funding), (2) *cycle or routine* (i.e., repetitive reinforcement of the importance of the evidence-based intervention through including it into organizational or community procedures and behaviors, such as the annual budget and evaluation criteria), and (3) *niche saturation* (the extent to which an evidence-based intervention is integrated into all subsystems of an organization).[59,63,64] Niche saturation is also referred to as *penetration* in the literature, as described by Lewis and colleagues in chapter 14.[65]

Capacity Building

This describes any activities (e.g., training, identification of alternative resources, building internal assets) that build durable resources and enable the recipient setting or community to continue the delivery of an evidence-based intervention after the external support from the donor agency is terminated.[59,63,66] Leeman and colleagues identified six strategies for capacity building: training, tools, technical assistance, assessment and feedback, peer networking, and incentives.[67]

Other terms that are commonly used in the literature to refer to program continuation include sustainment, incorporation, integration, local or community ownership, confirmation, durability, stabilization, and sustained use.[64]

Knowledge-for-Action Terms

The terms **knowledge translation, knowledge transfer, knowledge exchange, and knowledge integration** are commonly used especially outside of the United States to refer to the entire or some aspects of the D&I process. This chapter uses definitions coined by the CIHR and KT Canada, Graham and colleagues, Best and colleagues, and McKibbon and colleagues to define these terms.[5,27,28,68] As Best and colleagues suggested, these terms can be classified as linear (knowledge translation and transfer), relationship (knowledge exchange), or systems (knowledge integration) models of D&I.[68] Additional terms can be found on the WhatisKT wiki website: https://whatiskt.wikispaces.com/.

Knowledge Translation

Knowledge translation is the term used by the CIHR to denote "a dynamic and iterative process that includes synthesis, dissemination, exchange and ethically sound application of knowledge."[5] Knowledge translation occurs within a complex social system of interactions between researchers and knowledge users and with the purpose of improving population health, providing more effective health services and products, and strengthening the health care system.[5,27]

Knowledge Transfer

Knowledge transfer is a commonly used term both within and outside of the health care sector and is defined as the process of getting (research) knowledge from producers to potential users (i.e., stakeholders).[27,68] This term is often criticized for its linear (unidirectional) notion and its lack of concern with the implementation of transferred knowledge.[27]

Technology Transfer

Technology transfer is closely related to (some suggests it is a subset of) knowledge transfer and it refers to the process of sharing technological developments with potential users.[69,70] While knowledge transfer often refers to individuals as the recipient of the knowledge, technology transfer more often focuses on transfer to larger entities such as organizations, countries, or the public at large.[70] The object of technology transfer is often defined broadly as a process, product, know-how, or resource but its focus is still narrower than the focus of the more encompassing knowledge transfer.[70]

Knowledge Exchange

Knowledge exchange is the term used by the Canadian Health Services Research Foundation and describes the interactive and iterative process of imparting meaningful knowledge between knowledge users (i.e., stakeholders) and producers, such that knowledge users (i.e., stakeholders) receive relevant and easily usable information and producers receive information about users' research needs.[27,68] This term was introduced to, in contrast to the terms "knowledge translation" and "knowledge transfer," highlight the bi- or multidirectional nature of the knowledge transmission process (relationship model).[27,68,71]

Knowledge Integration

The term was introduced by Best and colleagues as the systems model for the knowledge transmission process and is defined as "the effective incorporation of knowledge into the decisions, practices and policies of organizations and systems."[68] The key assumptions around the knowledge integration process are that (1) it is tightly woven within priorities, culture, and context; (2) mediated by complex relationships; (3) needs to be understood from a systems perspective (i.e., in the context of organizational context and strategic processes); and (4) require the integration with the organization(s) and its systems.[68]

Knowledge Utilization

Knowledge utilization refers to the use of broadly defined knowledge including not only research evidence but also scholarly practice and programmatic interventions. It can be regarded as an overarching term that encompasses both research utilization and evidence-based practice.[72,73]

Research Utilization

Research utilization is a form of knowledge utilization; it has long traditions in the nursing literature and refers to "the process by which specific research-based knowledge (science) is implemented in practice."[73,74] Research utilization, similar to knowledge translation and knowledge transfer, follows a linear model and is primarily concerned with moving research knowledge into action.[27]

Knowledge Brokering

Knowledge brokering has emerged from the understanding that there is a belief, value, and practice gap between producers (i.e., researchers) and users (i.e., practitioners, policymakers) of knowledge and it involves the organization of the interactive process between these two groups to facilitate and drive the transfer and implementation of research evidence.[75-78] Specific tasks include synthesis and interpretation of relevant knowledge, facilitation of interaction and setting of shared agendas, building of new networks, and capacity building for knowledge use.[75,76] Knowledge brokering is described as a two-way process that not only aims at facilitating the uptake and use of evidence by practitioners and policymakers, but also focuses on prompting researchers to produce more practice-based evidence.[76]

Knowledge Broker

A knowledge broker is an intermediary (individual or organization) who facilitates and fosters the interactive process between producers (i.e., researchers) and users (i.e., practitioners, policymakers) of knowledge through a broad range of activities (see Knowledge Brokering).[75,79] More broadly, knowledge brokers assist in the organizational problem-solving process through drawing analogic links between solutions learned from resolving past problems, often in diverse domains, and demands of the current project. Knowledge brokers also help "make the right knowledge available to the right people at the right time."[79(p. 67)]

A more detailed discussion of knowledge brokering and knowledge brokers is provided by Hargadon.[79]

Scale Up and Scaling Up

The term is commonly used in the international health and development literature and refers to "deliberate efforts to increase the impact of health service innovations successfully tested in pilot or experimental projects so as to benefit more people and to foster policy and programme development on a lasting basis."[6,80,81] Scaling up most commonly refers to expanding the coverage of successful interventions; however, it can also be concerned with the financial, human, and capital resources necessary for the expansion.[6,82] It is suggested that sustainable scale up requires a combination of horizontal (e.g., replication and expansion) and vertical (institutional, policy, political, legal) scaling up efforts, which benefit from different D&I strategies (i.e., training, technical assistance hands-on support versus networking, policy dialogue, advocacy).[7] Furthermore, some researchers suggest that scale up has a broader reach and scope than D&I and expands to national and international levels.[83] The National Implementation Research Network uses the term "going to scale" when an evidence-based intervention reaches 60% of the target population that could benefit from it.[84]

Additional terms used to describe some aspect of the D&I process include knowledge cycle, knowledge management, knowledge mobilization, research transfer, research translation, expansion, linkage and exchange.[5,7]

Evidence Synthesis Approaches

In addition to more traditional evidence synthesis approaches of systematic reviews and meta-analysis, a number of more novel techniques are especially appropriate to use to summarize existing knowledge about D&I research and practice. These methods allow for a more relevant, real-world perspective on studies through a more inclusive, context-sensitive approach. For this chapter, two techniques were selected and are discussed here.

Scoping Review

Scoping reviews "aim to map rapidly the key concepts underpinning a research area and the main sources and types of evidence available"[(p. 194)] and can be efficiently used to explore complex areas or areas that have not been reviewed before.[85] The most important differences between a systematic review and a scoping review include level of specificity of the research question it is based on and the types of studies they draw upon. Systematic reviews generally start off with well-defined research questions and are most frequently based on a narrow range of quality-assessed studies. Scoping reviews intend to explore broader topics and include more diverse study designs, and are not concerned with quality assessment of included studies.[86] When undertaken as a stand-alone activity rather than in preparation of a systematic review, scoping reviews can be used to summarize and disseminate information about interventions to policymakers, practitioners, and consumers.[87]

Realist Review

Realist review is a method for reviewing and synthesizing information about complex, real-world interventions using an explanatory approach and focusing on "what works for whom, in what circumstances, in what respects and how."[89(p. S1:21)] Instead of determining if a certain intervention will work, realist reviews provide rich, contextual, and practical information regarding the mechanisms by which the intervention or program works under certain circumstances. This information can support implementation of programs at different levels. Realist review considers interventions as complex systems that function within systems and will be limited in terms of scope (how much can be looked at), the availability of information (the need for an array of primary sources for information), and the nature of effectiveness information (lack fast truth about effectiveness).[88,89]

Types of Research
Fundamental (or Basic) Research
Fundamental or basic research develops laboratory-based, etiologic models to provide theoretical explanation for generic or more specific phenomena of interest.[57]

Translational Research
T1 Research
T1 translational research uses discoveries generated through laboratory and/or preclinical research to develop and test treatment and prevention approaches. In other words, T1 clinical research moves science from "the bench" (fundamental research, methods development) to the patients' "bedside" (efficacy research).[57,90]

Efficacy Research
Efficacy research evaluates the initial impact of an intervention (whether it does more good than harm among the individuals in the target population) when it is delivered under optimal or laboratory conditions (or in an ideal setting). Efficacy trials typically use random allocation of participants and/or units and ensure highly controlled conditions for implementation. This type of study focuses on internal validity or on establishing a causal relationship between exposure to an intervention and an outcome.[57,91]

T2 Research
T2 translational research focuses on the enhancement of widespread use of efficacious interventions by the target audience. This type of research includes effectiveness research, dissemination research, and implementation research[57] and also referred to as "bedside to (clinical) practice (or trench)" translation.[90,92]

Effectiveness Research
Effectiveness research determines the impact of an intervention with demonstrated efficacy when

it is delivered under "real-world" conditions. As a result, effectiveness trials often must use methodological designs that are better suited for large and/or less controlled research environments with a major purpose to obtain more externally valid (generalizable) results.[57,91]

Dissemination Research
Dissemination research is the systematic study of processes and factors that lead to widespread use of an evidence-based intervention by the target population. Its focus is to identify the best methods that enhance the uptake and utilization of the intervention.[57,93]

Implementation Research
Implementation research seeks to understand the processes and factors that are associated with successful integration of evidence-based interventions within a particular setting (e.g., a worksite or school).[94] Implementation research assesses whether the core components of the original intervention were faithfully transported to the real-world setting (i.e., the degree of fidelity of the disseminated and implemented intervention with the original study) and also is concerned with the adaptation of the implemented intervention to local context.[94] Another, often overlooked but essential component of implementation research involves the enhancement of readiness through the creation of effective climate and culture in an organization or community.[20,95]

Finally, a broader interpretation of implementation research also includes the study of discontinuation of interventions and practices that do not work. See also **mis-implementation** and **de-implementation** in this chapter.[96]

More recently it was suggested that rather than two types (T1 and T2), four phases of translational research should be distinguished (T1 through T4).[90,97] According to this new classification: (1) T1 translational research is defined as translation of basic research into potential clinical application that leads to theoretical knowledge about a possible intervention; (2) T2 translational research involves efficacy studies and results in efficacy knowledge about interventions that work under optimal conditions; (3) T3 translational research involves effectiveness, dissemination, and implementation research and leads to applied knowledge about interventions that work in real-world settings; and (4) T4 translational research involves outcomes assessment at the population level and results in public health knowledge at the population level.[97,98]

Mode I and II Science

A similar model for the classification of research (knowledge production) established by Gibbons and colleagues was considered by the National Cancer Institute of Canada Working Group on Translational Research and Knowledge Transfer.[68,99] This model suggests the distinction of **Mode I** and **Mode II science**. **Mode I science** refers to traditional investigator-initiated scientific methods designed to produce discipline-based generalizable knowledge and is characterized by clear hypothesis, transparent methods, and replicability. **Mode II science** is defined as "*science in the context of its application*" and is described as context-driven, problem-focused research with the production of interdisciplinary knowledge.[68] Mode II science is concerned with contextual factors such as organizational structure, geography, attitudes, economics, and ethics.[68] Graham Harris introduces the concept of **Mode III science** that is not only done "in the context of its application but which also influences the context and application through engagement in a contextual and recursive debate." He further suggests that "to achieve this aspirational goal requires the establishment of a collaborative 'magic circle,' a creative collaboration linking the worlds of science, governance, industry, the media and the community."[100]

Science-to-Service Gap

Science-to-service gap refers to the phenomenon when the interventions that are adopted by individuals and organizations are not the ones that are known to be effective and hence most likely to benefit the target population.[84,101]

Implementation Gap

Implementation gap refers to the phenomenon when the interventions that are adopted by individuals and organization are not implemented with sufficient fidelity and consistency to produce optimal benefits.[84,101]

Assimilation Gap

Assimilation gap refers to the population-level (or public health) impact of interventions and describes the phenomenon when interventions that are adopted by individuals or organizations are not deployed widely (e.g., population level) and/or not sustained sufficiently at the individual or organizational level.[56,101,102]

Population Health Intervention Research

Population health intervention research (PHIR) emerged from the work of Hawe and colleagues and is supported by the CIHR through their Population Health Intervention Research Initiative for Canada.[103] PHIR uses scientific methods to produce knowledge on interventions operating either within or outside the health sector with potential to impact health at the population level.[25] Population health interventions include programs, policies, and resource-dsitribution processes and are often aimed at multiple systems, use multiple strategies, and are implemented both within and outside of the health sector into dynamic and complex systems.[103] PHIR integrates the components of evaluation research and community-based intervention research into traditional intervention research, and is concerned with multiple aspects of an intervention including efficacy and effectiveness, processes by which change is brought about, contextual factors that favor desirable outcomes, reach, differential uptake, dissemination, and sustainability.[104] PHIR considers both controlled and uncontrolled intervention designs and produces practice-relevant knowledge for real-world decision making.[104]

Comparative Effectiveness Research to Accelerate Translation (CER-T)

Comparative Effectiveness Research (CER) is defined as "the conduct and synthesis of research comparing the benefits and harms of different interventions and strategies to prevent, diagnose, treat and monitor health conditions in 'real-world' settings. The purpose of this research is to improve health outcomes by developing and disseminating evidence-based information to patients, clinicians, and other decision makers, responding to their expressed needs, about which interventions are most effective for which patients under specific circumstances."[89] **CER-T** refers to CER that is concerned with producing results that will disseminate and translate into population-level change.[105]

Patient-Centered Outcomes Research

Patient-centered outcomes research (PCOR) is a form of research that emphasizes the voice of various stakeholders but primarily patients in the process of evaluating health care options. PCOR is achieved through early and ongoing, meaningful engagement of stakeholders in all stages of the research process including: the identification of priority areas and questions for research, and dissemination and implementation of meaningful interventions. As defined by the Patient-Centered Outcomes Research Institute, "patient-centered outcomes research is the evaluation of questions and outcomes meaningful and important to patients and caregivers."[106(p. 1513)] The key premise is that patients have a unique perspective on their condition and through acknowledging this special perspective, PCOR will lead to better quality and stakeholder relevant responses and approaches to disease prevention, diagnosis, and treatment.[106,107] In this sense, PCOR is in line with the concept of designing for D&I and sustainability through the stakeholder-engaged development of interventions and the use of existing dissemination channels for the successful and active spread of effective interventions.

Quality Improvement

Quality improvement (QI) is defined as the concerted and ongoing activities that are undertaken systematically by diverse stakeholders to improve care. In the optimal case, this includes all relevant health care providers, organizational leaders, evaluators, patients, and their caregivers. QI efforts can address improving patient outcomes, health care services and system performance, and/or professional development (i.e., learning health care system) in the context of health care.[108-110] While QI and D&I science approach health care improvement from different paradigms and use different frameworks and methods, they share the ultimate goal of improving patient health outcomes. The main differences between QI and D&I science involve their scope, starting point, and speed of action. QI is generally initiated at the local level to address a specific issue for a clinic or health care system, while D&I science often starts with an evidence-based intervention or practice and explores how it can be spread and implemented at the health system or clinic level.[111] Usually QI efforts focus on or at least begin with very small "tests," even within a single health care team, using simple measures, often developed by local teams for rapid feedback (i.e., Plan-Do-Study-Act cycle). QI is also, by definition, iterative whereas D&I is usually seen as slower, larger in scope, and more likely to use explicit theoretical or conceptual models and well-validated measures. Recent reviews and thought pieces suggest that if we are to make

relevant, significant, and sustainable impact on health outcomes, D&I science should consider adopting some of the methods used by QI such as the iterative, rapid testing and adaptation of interventions and implementation strategies.[112] A proposal for the combination of QI and D&I science methods is described under **learning evaluation** in Section 3 of this chapter.[113]

Precision Medicine

Precision medicine merges information on genomic, biological, behavioral, environmental, and other data on individuals in order to identify factors that can support individualized treatment.[114,115] While to date most of the work in precision medicine has focused on the genomic and biological components, there is great need and opportunity in expanding our work to data elements related to the social and behavioral determinants of health, as well as patient values and preferences relevant for shared decision making. These latter factors are especially important when we consider the contextual and pragmatic issues involved in moving precision medicine activities from research into practice and policy. Chambers and colleagues suggested that the key potential of D&I science in precision medicine is to support the integration of various precision medicine interventions into learning health care systems.[114]

SECTION 2: THEORIES AND APPROACHES

Stage Models

Stage models propose that D&I of interventions occurs as a series of successive phases rather than as one event.[17,19,116,117] Although different stage models vary in the number and name of the identified stages,[17] all models suggest that D&I does not stop at the level of initial uptake; further steps are necessary to ensure the long-term utilization of an intervention.[118] This chapter identifies the stages as dissemination, adoption, implementation, and sustainability. Other commonly used models are the innovation-decision process (knowledge, persuasion, decision, implementation, and confirmation)[19] and the stages of the RE-AIM framework (reach, adoption, implementation, maintenance).[119] The different stages of the D&I process can be thought of as process variables or mediating factors (i.e., factors that lie in the causal pathway between an independent variable [e.g., the exposure to the intervention] and dependent variable [e.g., an outcome such as organizational change] and require different strategies and are influenced by different moderating variables).[120]

Theories and Frameworks

There are a number of theories, theoretical frameworks, and models that shape the way that we think about D&I research and guide our planning and evaluation activities.[12,93] Tabak and colleagues identified 63 distinct D&I models through their review,[121] which were further expanded with practice-relevant models by Rabin and colleagues to 87 models in their web-based interactive tool (http://dissemination-implementation.org). The most commonly used theories and frameworks include the Diffusion of Innovations theory,[19,118] theories of organizational change,[122] Social Marketing theory,[123] theories of communication,[124] individual and organizational decision making,[125] Community Organizing models,[126] the RE-AIM framework,[56] the Consolidated Framework for Implementation Research (CFIR),[127] the Precede-Proceed model,[128] the Interactive Systems Framework for D&I,[129] and the Practical, Robust Implementation and Sustainability model (PRISM),[130] the Knowledge-to-Action (KTA) model,[27] and the Promoting Action on Research Implementation in Health Services (PARiHS) framework.[131,132]

This chapter discusses one theory (Diffusion of Innovations), one framework (RE-AIM), and one metamodel (CFIR) that are commonly applied in D&I research in the field of health. More comprehensive discussion of diffusion and D&I theories is available in chapter 3 by Dearing and Kee.

Diffusion of Innovations

The diffusion of innovations theory was proposed by Rogers to explain the processes and factors influencing the spread and adoption of new innovations through certain channels over time.[19] Key components of the diffusion theory are: (1) perceived attributes of the innovation; (2) innovativeness of the adopter; (3) social system; (4) individual adoption process; and (5) diffusion system.[43] Some of these key components are discussed later in this chapter.

RE-AIM Framework

The RE-AIM framework developed by Glasgow and colleagues[56,91,133] provides a conceptual model to guide researchers and practitioners in the development of adequate multistage (reach, adoption, implementation, maintenance) and multilevel (individual, setting) indicators when evaluating D&I efforts.[119] A more comprehensive description of the RE-AIM framework and related tools can be found at: http://www.re-aim.org/.

Consolidated Framework for Implementation Research

The CFIR was developed by Damschroder and colleagues to provide "an overarching typology to promote implementation theory development and verification about what works where and why across multiple contexts."[127(p. 50)] CFIR is composed of five major domains (i.e., intervention characteristics, outer setting, inner setting, characteristics of the individuals involved, and the process of implementation) and each domain includes multiple constructs (e.g., evidence strength and quality, patient needs and resources, culture, evaluate).[127] A more detailed description of CFIR and related terminology and tools are available at: http://cfirguide.org/.

Designing for Dissemination, Implementation, and Sustainability

Designing for Dissemination, Implementation, and Sustainability (D4DIS) refers to a set of processes that are considered and activities that are undertaken throughout the planning, development, and evaluation of an intervention to increase its dissemination and implementation potential.

Some authors refer to the understanding and consideration of the user context (receiver "pull").[134] Others talk about the need to considering target users' needs, assets, and timeframes.[135] D4DIS builds on the premises that (1) effective dissemination of interventions requires an active, systematic, planned and controlled approach;[31] (2) planning for D&I and sustainability in the early stage of conceptualization and development of the intervention can increases the success of later D&I and sustainability efforts;[136] (3) early involvement of and partnership with target users in the conceptualization and development process can increase the likelihood of success for later dissemination and implementation efforts;[134] (4) close understanding of and building on the characteristics, beliefs, norms, and wants of target adopters can positively influence their perception of a new intervention and consequently will increase the likelihood of adoption, implementation, and sustained use of the intervention;[134] and (5) study designs and measures that generate practice-relevant evidence facilitate and inform later stage D&I and sustainability efforts.[137] Brownson and colleagues organized strategies for D4DIS into three broad categories of **systems changes** (e.g., shift in funder priorities and researcher incentives, developing measures, tools, and reporting standards), **processes** (e.g., early engagement of stakeholders, use of D&I models, identification of appropriate delivery methods) and **products** (e.g., identify appropriate message, develop user friendly summaries).[135]

Audience Segmentation

Audience segmentation is the process of distinguishing between different subgroups of users and creating targeted marketing and distribution strategies for each subgroup. Dearing and Kreuter suggest that "segmentation of intended audience members on the basis of demographic, psychographic, situational, and behavioral commonalities" allows for the design of products and messages that are perceived more relevant by the intended target audience.[134] A more detailed discussion about marketing approaches for D&I are described in chapter 12.

Fidelity and Adaptation

Understanding the nature and origin of changes made to the evidence-based interventions and implementation strategies during the implementation process and assessing how these modifications might have impacted outcomes, as well as using this information to inform future implementation efforts, is a critical topic for D&I research. This section defines terms related to fidelity, adaptations, and core components.

Fidelity

Fidelity measures the degree to which an intervention is implemented as it is prescribed in the original protocol.[17,57] Fidelity is commonly measured by comparing the original evidence-based intervention and the disseminated and implemented intervention in terms of: (1) adherence to the program protocol, (2) dose or amount of program delivered, (3) quality of program delivery, and (4) participant reaction and acceptance.[138]

In the case of complex interventions, the measurement of fidelity focuses more on the function and process of the intervention rather than the individual components.[37] A more comprehensive discussion of fidelity measurement of complex interventions is found in Hawe et al.[37]

Adaptation

For the success of D&I, interventions in most cases need to be adapted to fit the local context (i.e., needs and realities).[7] Adaptation is defined as the degree to which an evidence-based intervention is changed or modified by a user during adoption and implementation to suit the needs of the setting or to improve the fit to local conditions.[19] The need for adaptation and understanding of context has been called Type 3 evidence (i.e., the information needed to adapt and implement an evidence-based intervention in a particular setting or population) (see more on this under **Types of Evidence** earlier in this chapter).[32,47] Ideally, adaptation will lead to at least equal intervention effects as shown in the original efficacy or effectiveness trial. Furthermore, while modifications might facilitate implementation and sustainability by improving the fit between the intervention and the population or the facility, program fidelity and outcomes of interest may be affected. To reconcile the tension between fidelity and adaptation, the **core components** (or essential features) of an intervention (i.e., those responsible for its efficacy/effectiveness) must be identified and preserved during the adaptation process.[139] Frameworks like the Stirman adaptation and modification framework can support the systematic documentation of adaptations and modifications happening during implementation and can inform future implementation and scale-up efforts.[140] For a more comprehensive discussion of fidelity and adaptation see chapters 16 and 17 and a number of seminal papers on the topic.[139,141-144]

Although in this chapter it is defined differently, translation is another term commonly used in the literature to denote the adaptation of relevant research findings to make them useful for a variety of audiences.[145] Furthermore, "reinvention" is another term that also has been used as a synonym to adaptation.

Core Elements (or Components)

The terms core elements or components can refer to the intervention (core intervention elements or components) and is defined as the active ingredients of the intervention that are essential to achieving the desired outcomes of the intervention.[9] Some authors differentiate between core intervention elements or components and customizable components, which latter can be modified to local context without harming the effectiveness of the intervention.[61] While understanding of the core elements or components of an intervention or the implementation process can facilitate the adaptation and sustainability of the intervention in a new context (i.e., setting, audience),[61] the identification of these core elements is not always straightforward.[9] Identification can be facilitated by the use of theoretical frameworks during the development of the intervention and detailed description of the elements or components but as Fixsen and colleagues noted, "the eventual specification of the core intervention components for any evidence-based program or practice may depend upon careful research and well-evaluated experiential learning from a number of attempted replications."[9(p.26)]

Core elements or components can also refer to the implementation process (core implementation elements or components) and indicate of the drivers of the implementation process that are indispensable for the successful implementation of an intervention.[9]

An extensive discussion of core intervention and implementation components that can be used to successfully implement evidence-based interventions is provided in the report of Fixsen and colleagues.[9,146]

Adaptome

Adaptome was proposed by Chambers and Norton as a common data platform that would allow the systematic capturing and storing of data about adaptations happening during the delivery and implementation of evidence-based interventions across diverse settings and populations. This approach emphasizes the need for ongoing learning about optimal delivery strategies as fit between the intervention and setting and population is maximized. Furthermore, it highlights the need for a paradigm shift from the linear conceptualization of intervention development, testing, and dissemination and implementation to a more iterative, nonlinear approach where the permanence of evidence-base is not assumed.[147]

Strategies for D&I
Dissemination Strategy

Dissemination strategies describe mechanisms and approaches that are used to communicate and spread information about interventions to targeted users.[50] Dissemination strategies are concerned with the packaging of the information about the intervention and the communication channels that are used to reach potential adopters and target audience. Passive dissemination strategies include mass mailings, publication of information including practice guidelines, and untargeted presentations to heterogeneous groups.[31] Active dissemination strategies include hands-on technical assistance, replication guides, point-of-decision prompts for use, and mass media campaigns.[31] It is consistently stated in the literature that dissemination strategies are necessary but not sufficient to ensure widespread use of an intervention.[84,134]

Implementation Strategy

Implementation strategies refer to the systematic processes or methods, techniques, activities, and resources that support the adoption, integration, and sustainment of evidence-based interventions into usual settings.[148–150] Fixsen and colleagues refer to implementation strategies as core implementation components or implementation drivers and list staff selection, preservice and in-service training, ongoing consultation and coaching, staff and program evaluation, facilitative administrative support, and systems interventions as components.[9,84] Powell and colleagues differentiated discrete (i.e., individual implementation actions such as reminders, educational meetings), multifaceted (i.e., combination of two or more discrete strategies such as training with technical assistance), and blended (i.e., protocolized implementation strategies). They used a review and expert consensus approach to create a consolidated compilation of 73 discrete implementation strategies and respective definitions.[149,151] Chapter 15 discusses these strategies in more detail.

Factors Associated with the Speed and Extent of D&I

Several factors (i.e., moderators) influence the extent to which D&I of evidence-based interventions occur in various settings.[19] Moderators are factors that alter the causal effect of an independent variable on a dependent variable.[120] In this case, organizational capacity can moderate the effect of an intervention on a desired outcome. These factors can be classified as the characteristics of the intervention, characteristics of the adopter (organizational and individual), and contextual factors. Adoption rate will be influenced by the interaction among the attributes of the innovation, characteristics of the intended adopters, and the given context.[20]

Characteristics of the Intervention
Rogers identifies five perceived attributes of an innovation that are likely to influence the speed and extent of its adoption: (1) relative advantage (effectiveness and cost efficiency relative to alternatives); (2) compatibility (the fit of the innovation to the established ways of accomplishing the same goal); (3) observability (the extent to which the outcomes can be seen); (4) trialability (the extent to which the adopter must commit to full adoption); and (5) complexity (how simple the innovation is to understand).[19,141] Relative advantage and compatibility are particularly important in influencing adoption rates.[19]

Relative Advantage
Relative advantage refers to the degree to which the evidence-based intervention is perceived by potential adopters as better (e.g., more effective, less costly, takes less time, etc.) than the process or practice it replaces.[19]

Compatibility
Compatibility refers to the perceived fit of the evidence-based intervention with "existing values, past experiences, and needs of potential adopters"[19(p. 15)] as well as practices and processes in place at the adopting organization or setting (e.g., patient flow, community practices).[19]

Acceptability
Acceptability is related to the ideas of complexity and relative advantage; it refers to a specific intervention and describes whether the potential implementers, based on their knowledge of or direct experience with the intervention, perceive it as agreeable, palatable, or satisfactory.[65]

Appropriateness
Appropriateness is related to the idea of compatibility and is defined as the perceived fit and relevance of the intervention for a given context (i.e., setting, user group) and/or its perceived relevance and ability to address a particular issue.

Organizational culture and organizational climate might explain whether an intervention is perceived as appropriate by a potential group of implementers.[65]

The concepts of acceptability and appropriateness are related terms but not identical. While an intervention might be perceived as a good fit to address an issue in question (i.e., appropriate), it might not be perceived as acceptable due to its characteristics and vica versa.

Feasibility
Feasibility is closely related to the concepts of compatibility and trialability and refers to the actual fit, suitability, or practicability of an intervention in a specific setting. Perceived feasibility plays key role in the early adoption process.[65] A more detailed discussion of this concept is provided in chapter 14.

Implementation Cost
Implementation cost (or incremental cost) is defined as the cost impact of an implementation effort and depends on the costs of the particular intervention, the implementation strategy used, and the characteristics of the setting(s) where the intervention is being implemented. Understanding implementation cost can be especially important for comparative effectiveness research.[65]

A more detailed discussion of the concepts of acceptability, appropriateness, feasibility, and implementation cost is provided in chapter 14.

Characteristics of the Adopters
Characteristics of the adopters can be discussed at the individual and organizational/community level. Attributes of the organization/community include its size, formalization, perceived complexity, and readiness for the implementation of the innovation. The characteristics, attitudes, and behaviors of individuals within an adopting organization (e.g., position in the organization, education, individual concerns and motivations) may also determine the uptake and use of an innovation.[152] Rogers classifies the individual adopters according to their degree of innovativeness into five categories: (1) innovators, (2) early adopters, (3–4) early and late majority, and (5) laggards.[19,141]

Opinion Leader
Opinion leaders are members of a community or organization who have the ability to influence attitudes and behaviors of other members of the

organization or community. Opinion leadership is based on perceived competence, accessibility, and conformity to system norms and is not a function of formal position. Opinion leaders serve as models for other members of the organization or community for innovation decisions, hence they can facilitate or impede the dissemination and adoption process.[19]

Change Agent

Change agents are representatives of change agencies that are external to an organization or community and their goal is to influence the innovation decisions of members of the organization or community. Change agents often use opinion leaders from an organization or community to facilitate the dissemination and adoption process.[19]

Contextual Factors

Contextual factors may include the broader political, social, and organizational characteristics as well as the more immediate, local-level features for the implementation of the intervention.[31,153] Examples of contextual factors include social support, legislations and regulations, social networks and norms, culture, incentives, and processes. Understanding the delivery context for the intervention is essential for the success of the D&I and closely linked to the concepts of fidelity and adaptation.[154] When findings from D&I studies are considered with context taken into account, a greater understanding around the mechanisms leading to said results might emerge more readily.[155] Only less than half of the existing D&I theories and frameworks include some aspect of context as a construct.[156] Ones that are most useful conceptualize context at multiple levels and from the perspective of multiple stakeholders (e.g., CFIR, PRISM). Furthermore, while it is acknowledged as a critical area of influence for D&I, systematic documentation of context is still rarely reported on.[155] Context is best assessed using **mixed methods approaches,** which requires the collection of rich qualitative data in addition to more traditional quantitative data collection efforts (see chapter 20). Glasgow and colleagues propose a template for interviews and observations to collect contextual information that can be applied across settings and topic areas.[155] Recent efforts in the organizational change literature discussed context in terms of the inner (organizational) context including structural and cultural features, and system readiness and

the outer (interorganizational) context including interorganizational networks and collaborations.[20] They also identified several core aspects of context including leadership, infrastructure, and unit variability.[157]

A few more common contextual factors (organizational culture, organizational climate, and organizational readiness for change) are defined in this section.

Organizational Culture

Organizational culture is defined as the organizational norms and expectations regarding how people behave and how things are done in an organization.[158,159] This includes implicit norms, values, shared behavioral expectations, and assumptions that guide the behaviors of members of a work unit.[160] Organizational culture refers to the core values of an organization, its services or products as well as how individuals and groups within the organization treat and interact with each other. Schein defined it as "the pattern of shared basic assumptions that was learned by a group as it solved its problems of external adaptation and internal integration, and that has worked well enough to be considered valid and, therefore, to be taught to new members as the correct way to perceive, think, and feel in relation to those problems."[161(p. 17)]

Organizational Climate

Organizational climate refers to the employees' perceptions of and reaction to the characteristics of the work environment.[162–168]

Organizational Readiness for Change

Organizational readiness for change is defined as the extent to which organizational members are psychologically and behaviorally prepared to implement a new intervention. Organizational readiness is widely regarded as an essential antecedent to successful implementation of change in health care and social service organizations.[169–171]

Factors that are associated with organizational readiness for change include (1) change valence (i.e., the employees' perception of the personal benefit of implemented change), (2) change efficacy (i.e., the perception of their capability of implementing the change); (3) discrepancy (i.e., the employees' belief in the necessity of change to bridge the gap between the organization's current and desired state); and (4) principal support (i.e., the employees' perception of the commitment of the formal organizational leaders and opinion leaders to support successful implementation of change) and are discussed in more detail in chapter 8.

SECTION 3: DESIGN AND ANALYSIS

Study Designs

Traditional randomized controlled trials (RCTs) are not always desirable or feasible for the evaluation of dissemination and implementation programs. To achieve a greater understanding of external validity, a variety of study designs that take into count contextual factors should be considered for the evaluation of dissemination and implementation efforts, including quasi-experimental designs, interrupted times-series design, before–after designs, adequacy and plausibility designs, cluster (or group) randomized designs, participatory research methods, and pragmatic clinical trials.[172,173] This section provides definitions for a number of innovative design options relevant to D&I science. For a more detailed discussion of designs for D&I, see chapter 13 and work by Brown and colleagues.[174]

Pragmatic (or Practical) Clinical Trial

PCTs are clinical trials that are concerned with producing answers to questions faced by decision makers.[175] Tunis and colleagues define PCTs as studies that "(1) select clinically relevant alternative interventions to compare, (2) include a diverse population of study participants, (3) recruit participants from heterogeneous practice settings, and (4) collect data on a broad range of health outcomes."[175] PCTs that take into rather than "take out of" (i.e., control for) consideration the large number of mediators and moderators that influence the D&I process are more likely to produce practice-based evidence than their highly controlled counterparts.[172]

Natural Experiment

Natural experiment is a form of observational study design and is defined as "naturally occurring circumstances in which subsets of the population have different levels of exposure to a supposed causal factor, in a situation resembling an actual experiment where human subjects would be randomly allocated to groups."[120(p. 25)]

Plausibility Design

Plausibility design is used to document impact and rule out alternative explanations when an RCT approach is not feasible or acceptable (i.e., complexity of intervention, known efficacy or effectiveness in small scale, ethical concerns). Plausibility studies include comparison groups and also address potential confounders.[173]

Sequential Multiple Assignment Randomized Trial Design

Sequential, multiple assignment, randomized trials (SMARTs) can be used to develop adaptive interventions and adaptive implementation strategies and involve multiple intervention stages, each indicating a decision point in the development of the adaptive intervention. Adaptive interventions and adaptive implementation strategies allow for using individual (e.g., preference, severity of condition) or setting level (e.g., local processes and resources) variables to adapt an intervention or implementation strategy and individual (e.g., treatment response, adherence) or setting level (e.g., uptake by providers, screening rates at clinic) outcomes to further readapt or refine the intervention or implementation strategy during implementation. These modifications can be important to address changes in circumstances, to reduce burden and cost, and increase success as well as align with the more iterative approach to intervention and implementation strategy development, as suggested in the **adaptation** and **adaptome** sections of this chapter.[176,177]

Stepped-Wedge Design

Stepped-wedge design uses a sequential roll-out of the intervention to target sites or individuals in a manner that all sites or participants will receive the intervention by the end of the trial but the order in which they receive is determined randomly. Data collection happens at the end of each time segment or wedge. Stepped-wedge design is especially favorable to more traditional randomized trial designs when roll out of the intervention is not practical or feasible at once and when the intervention is believed to do more benefit than harm.[178] The use of the stepped-wedge design increased over the past decade and is especially suitable for multisite scale-up studies, as it aligns with the realities of real-world settings.[179]

Hybrid Designs

Hybrid study designs or effectiveness-implementation hybrid designs blend the design characteristics of effectiveness and implementation studies to generate more timely uptake of desirable interventions, more effective implementation strategies, and more relevant information for future scale up activities. Curran and colleagues identified three types of hybrid designs. Hybrid type 1 includes a primary focus on testing the effectiveness of an intervention while implementation-relevant data is also collected as a secondary outcome. Hybrid type 2 involves the parallel testing of intervention and implementation strategy effectiveness. Hybrid 3 primarily focusing on testing of the effectiveness of an implementation strategy while also gathering information on the intervention impact on relevant outcomes are secondary outcomes.[180]

Systems Thinking

Systems thinking is the process of understanding how things influence one another other within a whole. It is based on the premise that societal problems are complex and that the response to these complex problems is only possible by intervening at multiple levels and with the engagement of stakeholders and settings across the different levels, including the home, school, workplace, community, region, and country.[181,182] Systems thinking is not only concerned with applying multiple strategies at multiple levels but also focuses on the interrelationships within and across levels and how interventions need to take these relationships into account in their design and implementation.[181,182] Chapter 9 provides a detailed discussion on the concept of systems thinking for D&I.

System science approaches to study design include system dynamics method, agent-based modeling, social network analysis, system engineering, intelligent data analysis, and decision analysis with microsimulation modeling.

Learning Health Care Systems

Learning Healthcare System is defined by the Institute of Medicine as a system in which, "science, informatics, incentives, and culture are aligned for continuous improvement and innovation, with best practices seamlessly embedded in the delivery process and new knowledge captured as an integral by-product of the delivery experience."[183] As suggested by Chambers, Feero, and Khoury, D&I science has a critical role to play in creating and sustaining Learning Healthcare Systems through providing evidence-based strategies, frameworks, and measures to support ongoing learning and integration of evidence into practice.[114]

Rapid, Responsive, Relevant Research

The concept of rapid, responsive, relevant (R3) research was coined by Riley and colleagues to provide a framework and set of strategies for a rapid learning health research approach and to address limitations of traditional health research. Key criticisms of traditional health research include its slow pace, high cost and resource nature, and most importantly its lack of relevance to stakeholders that use the information for decision making. Proposed strategies to achieve R3 research include greater and more meaningful stakeholder engagement, use of innovative, rapid, and flexible designs, streamlining of the review process, and creation and better use of research infrastructure, rapid learning systems, and other health information technologies.[184]

Learning Evaluation

Learning evaluation is a multiorganization assessment approach that blends principles of quality improvement and D&I science. Balasubramanian and colleagues described the process as follows: "qualitative and quantitative data are collected to conduct real-time assessment of implementation processes while also assessing changes in context, facilitating quality improvement using run charts and audit and feedback, and generating transportable lessons."[113]

Measurement Considerations

In the context of measures of the D&I process, three main components should be considered: moderators (i.e., factors associated with the speed and extent of dissemination and implementation), mediators (i.e., process variables), and outcomes. Moderators and mediators are defined in a previous section of this chapter. The measurement of moderators and mediators can help to identify the factors and processes that lead to the success or failure of an evidence-based intervention to achieve certain outcomes. To reflect the complexity of interventions and diversity in the interest of potential stakeholders (i.e., policymakers, practitioners, clinicians), in D&I research we commonly measure multiple moderators, mediators, and outcomes and assess their relationship.[185]

Mixed Methods

Mixed methods designs involve the collection and analysis of multiple, both quantitative and qualitative data in a single study to answer research questions using a parallel (quantitative and qualitative data collected and analyzed concurrently), sequential (one type of data informs the collection of the other type), or converted (data is converted—qualitized or quantitized—and reanalyzed) approach. The mixed methods research design can generate rich data from multiple levels and a number of stakeholders and hence is appropriate to answer complex research questions (also see Systems Thinking).[186,187]

Outcome Variables

Outcome variables, the end results of evidence-based interventions, in D&I research are often different from those in traditional health research and have to be defined broadly, including short- and long-term outcomes, individual and organizational- or population-level outcomes, impacts on quality of life, adverse consequences, and economic evaluation.[31] Although, individual-level variables can also be important (e.g., behavior change variables such as smoking or physical activity), outcome measures in D&I research are typically measured at organizational, community, or policy level (e.g., organizational change, community readiness for change).

Implementation Outcomes

Implementation outcomes are distinct from system outcomes (e.g., organizational-level measures) and individual-level behavior and health outcomes, and are defined as "the effects of deliberate and purposive actions to implement new treatments, practices, and services."[65(p. 65)] Implementation outcomes are measures of implementation success, proximal indicators of implementation processes, and key intermediate outcomes of effectiveness and quality of care. The main value of implementation outcomes is to distinguish intervention failure (i.e., when an intervention is ineffective in a new context) from implementation failure (i.e., when the incorrect deployment of a good intervention causes lack of previously documented desirable outcomes).[65] Proctor and colleagues proposed the following implementation outcomes: acceptability, adoption, appropriateness, costs, feasibility, fidelity, penetration, and sustainability.[65]

Pragmatic Measures

Pragmatic measures were proposed by Glasgow and Riley as a set of criteria that should apply to instruments used in real-world studies including studies of D&I. In addition to the traditional criteria of validity and reliability, the key characteristics of an ideal pragmatic measure include: (1) measures outcomes important to a diverse set of stakeholders (i.e., practitioners, patients, researchers), (2) imposes a low burden from both data collection and analysis perspective (i.e., brief, user-friendly, low cost), (3) has a broad applicability (i.e., works across populations, settings, languages and cultures), (4) is sensitive to change (i.e., able to track change over time), (5) yields information that enhances patient engagement, (6) is actionable (i.e., based on information realistic action can be taken), (7) has public health relevance, and (8) does no harm (e.g., interferes with relationships, has unintended negative consequences).[188,189]

External Validity

External validity is the degree to which findings from a study (or set of studies) can be generalizable to and relevant for populations, settings, and times other than those in which the original studies were conducted.[190] Standardized and detailed reporting on factors that influence external validity (such as those recommended in the RE-AIM framework) can contribute to more successful D&I efforts.[56,137,191] In addition, Green and Glasgow have proposed rating criteria for external validity.[137] The concept of external validity is discussed in detail in chapter 18.

Standards for Reporting Implementation Studies

The Standards for Reporting Implementation Studies is a checklist compromised of 27 items and provides guidelines for implementation studies on reporting transparently, accurately, and consistently on various aspects of their work. The guidelines were developed using findings from a systematic review, a consensus-building e-Delphi exercise, and input from an international group of experts.[96]

SUMMARY

In order for a field to prosper and thrive, a common language is essential. As is often the case when many disciplines and numerous organizations converge in the development of a field, D&I research is still characterized by inconsistent terminology.

When compiling this chapter, we encountered a number of challenges. Our research was limited to English language documents, so we may have missed important information from non-English speaking countries. Another challenge was the lack of consensus on the overall classification of terms in the literature that may lead to apparent contradictions. For example, this chapter defines the different stages (dissemination, adoption, implementation, and sustainability) of the process under the umbrella term "D&I research." Other stage models may discuss adoption and sustainability as a distinct stage.[138] Finally, it is important to note that the three-section classification introduced in this chapter was not developed to impose a rigid structure, rather it is used as an organizing framework that allows us to discuss terms in the domain where they are most commonly applied. At the end of this book, the index provides an alphabetized list of terms with respective page numbers to facilitate the search for definitions and the fuller context for each term.

The lack of agreed-upon language for D&I research impedes the systematic analysis and summary of existing evidence in the field and the communication across different stakeholders (i.e., researchers, practitioners, policymakers).[11,192] The purpose of this chapter is not to advocate or argue the superiority of one term or classification scheme over another, but to facilitate communication by beginning to define commonly used terms in D&I research for researchers, practitioners, policymakers, and funding agencies. A common language should help accelerate the scientific progress in D&I research by facilitating comparison of methods and findings, as well as identifying gaps in dissemination knowledge.

Since the first edition of this chapter, a number of efforts were undertaken to create such ontology (i.e., agreed upon terms, definitions, and their interrelationships) and related data harmonization efforts. A few examples include: work by Padek and colleagues on identifying and organizing D&I research competencies;[30] Powell and colleagues on creating a consolidated compilation of implementation strategies;[150,151] Larsen and colleagues in suggesting ways to create an ontology for behavior change interventions;[193] Niven and colleagues' review of terminology for de-adoption;[55] the work described by Colquhoun and colleagues on developing a common terminology and overarching framework for KT interventions and related WhatisKT wiki page (https://whatiskt.wikispaces.com/);[13] the systematic review and organization of D&I models by Tabak and colleagues[121] and the related Dissemination and Implementation Models (www.dissemination-implementation.org) web-based tool created by Rabin and colleagues; the efforts undertaken by Lewis and colleagues to develop a shared repository of instruments for Implementation Science (https://societyforimplementationresearchcollaboration.org/sirc-instrument-project/);[194] and work by Rabin and colleagues to develop a D&I-focused workspace on NCI's Grid-enabled Measures Database (https://www.gem-beta.org/public/wsoverview.aspx?cat=8&wid=11&aid=0), a crowd-sourcing propelled wiki database of behavior health measures.[189]

While the "state-of-the-art" might still not be advanced enough to resolve all of the existing inconsistencies in terminology, this chapter represents the tremendous amount of development that happened over the past 5 years to create platforms and approaches for a more consistent, agreed upon language for D&I research across topic areas, stakeholder groups, and geographical areas. As the D&I field makes progress toward a shared terminology, we can expect to see higher quality D&I research and greater contribution of D&I science to improving public health and clinical practice.

ACKNOWLEDGEMENTS

The authors are thankful to Ms. Shannon Keating for her assistance with the preparation of the first edition of this chapter. We are also grateful to Melinda Davis, Jonathan Purtle, Shari Rogal, and Nicole Vaughn, who provided valuable input on the organizing structure and approaches used in this chapter, and to Russell Glasgow for reviewing and helping refine some of the definitions.

An earlier version of this chapter was published in the Journal of Public Health Management and Practice in 2008 and was coauthored by Drs. Debra Haire-Joshu, Matthew Kreuter, and Nancy Weaver. We appreciate the contributions from these coauthors.

SUGGESTED READINGS AND WEBSITES

Readings

Fixsen DL, Naoom SF, Blase KA, Friedman RM, Wallace F. *Implementation Research: A synthesis of the literature*. Tampa, Florida: National Implementation Research Network, University of South Florida; 2005.
A monograph that summarizes findings from the review of the research literature on implementation including findings from the domains of agriculture, business, child welfare, engineering, health, juvenile justice,

manufacturing, medicine, mental health, nursing and social services. The authors organize and synthesize critical lessons regarding implementation from these domains and provide definitions for constructs and processes.

Ottoson JM, Hawe P, eds. *Knowledge utilization, diffusion, implementation, transfer, and translation: Implications for evaluation.* Vol 124. San Francisco: Jossey-Bass and the American Evaluation Association; 2009.

A monograph on issues and terminology for knowledge utilization, diffusion, implementation, transfer, and translation. The authors recommend more consideration of background, contextual factors that may influence a policy or program, and how this impacts evaluation efforts.

Glasgow RE, Vogt TM, Boles SM. Evaluating the public health impact of health promotion interventions: the RE-AIM framework. *Am J Public Health.* 1999;89(9):1322–1327.

In this seminal article, Glasgow et al. evaluate public health interventions using the RE-AIM framework. The model's five dimensions (reach, efficacy, adoption, implementation, and maintenance) act together to determine a particular program's public health impact. The article also summarizes the model's strengths and limitations, and suggests that failure to evaluate on all five dimensions can result in wasted resources.

Feldstein AC, Glasgow RE. A practical, robust implementation and sustainability model (PRISM) for integrating research findings into practice. *Jt Comm J Qual Patient Saf.* 2008;34(4):228–243.

This article describes the Practical, Robust Implementation and Sustainability Model (PRISM), a comprehensive approach to implementation science. The model emphasizes the importance of considering worker perspectives, building partnerships, and providing for program sustainability.

Graham ID, Logan J, Harrsion MB, et al. Lost in knowledge translation: time for a map? *J Contin Educ Health Prof.* 2006;26:13–24.

This article reviews the terms used to describe the knowledge to action (KTA) process, and describe a framework for conceive of this process. The authors stress the importance of relationships to facilitate the knowledge to action process, as well as a common definition of how KTA works.

Colquhoun H, Leeman J, Michie S, Lokker C, Bragge P, Hempel S, McKibbon KA, Peters GJ, Stevens KR, Wilson MG, Grimshaw J. Towards a common terminology: a simplified framework of interventions to promote and integrate evidence into health practices, systems, and policies. *Implement Science.* 2014:1;9:51.

This paper describes an effort to create harmonized terminology and identify and overarching framework for KT using an expert workgroup approach.

Niven DJ, Mrklas KJ, Holodinsky JK, Straus SE, Hemmelgarn BR, Jeffs LP, et al. Towards understanding the de-adoption of low-value clinical practices: a scoping review. *BMC Med.* 2015;13:255.

This paper provides a systematic review of the literature on de-adoption, document current terminology and frameworks, map the literature to a proposed framework, identify gaps in our understanding of de-adoption, and identify opportunities for additional research.

Websites and Tools
What is KT wiki?
https://whatiskt.wikispaces.com/

This web-based resource provides an inventory of knowledge translation or KT terms, their definitions, and links to related resources. The What is KT wiki functions as a collaborative environment to define and compare terms and concepts used to describe getting research into practice across a variety of disciplines.

Dissemination and Implementation Models
http://dissemination-implementation.org/

This interactive website was designed to help researchers and practitioners to select the D&I Model that best fits their research question or practice problem, adapt the model to the study or practice context, fully integrate the model into the research or practice process, and find existing measurement instruments for the model constructs.

REFERENCES

1. National Cancer Institute. *The National Cancer Institue Startegic Plan for Leading the Nation.* 2006.
2. National Cancer Institute. Designing for Dissemination. n.d.; http://cancercontrol.cancer.gov/d4d/. Accessed Accessed on August 9, 2010.
3. National Institute for Occupational Safety and Health. Communication and Information Dissemination. n.d.; http://www.cdc.gov/niosh/programs/cid/. Accessed Accessed on August 9, 2010.
4. National Institute on Disability and Rehabilitation Research. NIDRR's Core Areas of Research. n.d.; https://www2.ed.gov/rschstat/research/pubs/programs.html. Accessed on July 28, 2017.
5. Canadian Institutes of Health Research. Knowledge Translation at CIHR. 2007; http://www.cihr-irsc.gc.ca/e/29418.html. Accessed on July 28, 2017.
6. Mangham LJ, Hanson K. Scaling up in international health: what are the key issues? *Health Policy and Planning.* 2010;25:85–96.
7. World Health Organization. *Practical guidance for scaling up health service innovations.*

Geneva: World Health Organization; 2009. http://apps.who.int/iris/bitstream/10665/44180/1/9789241598521_eng.pdf

8. National Center for the Dissemination of Disability Research. *A review of the literature on dissemination and knowledge utilization.* Austin, TX: Southwest Educational Development Laboratory, National Center for the Dissemination of Disability Research 1996. http://ktdrr.org/ktlibrary/articles_pubs/ncddrwork/NCDDR_lit_review_on_dissem.pdf

9. Fixsen DL, Naoom SF, Blase KA, Friedman RM, Wallace F. *Implementation Research: A synthesis of the literature.* Tampa, Florida: National Implementation Research Network, University of South Florida; 2005.

10. Kerner J, Rimer B, Emmons K. Introduction to the special section on dissemination: dissemination research and research dissemination: how can we close the gap? *Health Psychol.* 2005;24(5):443–446.

11. Glasgow RE, Marcus AC, Bull SS, Wilson KM. Disseminating effective cancer screening interventions. *Cancer.* 2004;101(5 Suppl):1239–1250.

12. Crosswaite C, Curtice L. Disseminating research results—the challenge of bridging the gap between health research and health action. *Health Promotion International.* 1994;9(4):289–296.

13. Colquhoun H, Leeman J, Michie S, et al. Towards a common terminology: a simplified framework of interventions to promote and integrate evidence into health practices, systems, and policies. *Implement Sci.* 2014;9:51.

14. Ciliska D, Robinson P, Armour T, et al. Diffusion and dissemination of evidence-based dietary strategies for the prevention of cancer. *Nutr J.* 2005;4(1):13.

15. Lost in clinical translation. *Nat Med.* 2004;10(9):879.

16. Dobbins M. *Is scientific research evidence being translated into new public health practice?* Toronto: Central East Health Information Partnership; 1999.

17. Mayer JP, Davidson WS. Dissemination of innovations. In: Rappaport J, Seidman E, eds. *Handbook of community psychology.* New York: Plenum Publishers; 2000:421–438.

18. Green LW, Johnson JL. Dissemination and utilization of health promotion and disease prevention knowledge: theory, research and experience. *Can J Public Health.* 1996;87 Suppl 2:S11–S17.

19. Rogers EM. *Diffusion of innovations.* 5th ed. New York: Free Press; 2003.

20. Greenhalgh T, Robert G, Macfarlane F, Bate P, Kyriakidou O. Diffusion of innovations in service organizations: systematic review and recommendations. *Milbank Q.* 2004;82(4):581–629.

21. Solomon J, Card JJ, Malow RM. Adapting efficacious interventions: advancing translational research in HIV prevention. *Eval Health Prof.* 2006;29(2):162–194.

22. Proctor EK, Landsverk J, Aarons G, Chambers D, Glisson C, Mittman B. Implementation research in mental health services: an emerging science with conceptual, methodological, and training challenges. *Adm Policy Ment Health.* 2009;36(1):24–34.

23. Saul J, Duffy J, Noonan R, et al. Bridging science and practice in violence prevention: addressing ten key challenges. *Am J Community Psychol.* 2008;41(3-4):197–205.

24. Bowen DJ, Sorensen G, Weiner BJ, Campbell M, Emmons K, Melvin C. Dissemination research in cancer control: where are we and where should we go? *Cancer Causes Control.* 2009;20(4):473–485.

25. Hawe P, Potvin L. What is population health intervention research? *Can J Public Health.* 2009;100(1):Suppl I8–14.

26. Tetroe J. *Knowledge Translation at the Canadian Institutes of Health Research: A Primer.* National Center for the Dissemination of Disability Research; 2007.

27. Graham ID, Logan J, Harrsion MB, et al. Lost in knowledge translation: time for a map? *J Contin Educ Health Prof.* 2006;26:13–24.

28. McKibbon KA, Lokker C, Wilczynski NL, et al. A cross-sectional study of the number and frequency of terms used to refer to knowledge translation in a body of health literature in 2006: a Tower of Babel? *Implement Sci.* 2010;5:16.

29. Balbach ED. *Using case studies to do program evaluation.* Sacramento, CA: California Department of Health Services; 1999.

30. Padek M, Colditz G, Dobbins M, et al. Developing educational competencies for dissemination and implementation research training programs: an exploratory analysis using card sorts. *Implement Sci.* 2015;10:114.

31. Rabin BA, Brownson RC, Kerner JF, Glasgow RE. Methodologic challenges in disseminating evidence-based interventions to promote physical activity. *Am J Prev Med.* 2006;31(4 Suppl):S24–S34.

32. Rychetnik L, Hawe P, Waters E, Barratt A, Frommer M. A glossary for evidence based public health. *J Epidemiol Community Health.* 2004;58(7):538–545.

33. Sackett DL, Rosenberg WM, Gray JA, Haynes RB, Richardson WS. Evidence based medicine: what it is and what it isn't. *BMJ.* 1996;312(7023):71–72.

34. Brownson RC, Baker EA, Leet TL, Gillespie KN. *Evidence-based public health.* New York: Oxford University Press; 2003.

35. Guyatt G, Rennie D, eds. *Users' guides to the medical literature. A manual for evidence-based clinical practice.* Chicago: American Medical Association Press; 2002.

36. Jenicek M. Epidemiology, evidenced-based medicine, and evidence-based public health. *J Epidemiol.* 1997;7(4):187–197.

37. Hawe P, Shiell A, Riley T. Complex interventions: how "out of control" can a randomised controlled trial be? *BMJ.* 2004;328(7455):1561–1563.

38. Chambless DL, Hollon SD. Defining empirically supported therapies. *J Consult Clin Psychol.* 1998;66(1):7–18.

39. Task Force on Promotion and Dissemination of Psychological Procedures. Training in and dissemination of empirically validated treatments: report and recommendations. *Clin Psychol.* 1995;48:3–23.

40. La Roche MJ, Christopher, M. S. Changing paradigms from empirically supported treatment to evidence-based practice: a cultural perspective. *Prof Psychol Res Pract.* 2009;40(4):396–402.

41. Miles A, Loughlin M. Models in the balance: evidence-based medicine versus evidence-informed individualized care. *J Eval Clin Pract.* 2011;17(4):531–536.

42. Armstrong R, Pettman TL, Waters E. Shifting sands—from descriptions to solutions. *Public Health.* 2014;128(6):525–532.

43. Yost J, Dobbins M, Traynor R, DeCorby K, Workentine S, Greco L. Tools to support evidence-informed public health decision making. *BMC Public Health.* 2014;14:728.

44. Woodbury MG, Kuhnke, J.L. Research 101: Evidence-based practice vs. evidence-informed practice: what's the difference? *Wound Care Canada* 2004;12(1):26–29.

45. Borkovec TD, Castonguay LG. What is the scientific meaning of empirically supported therapy? *J Consult Clin Psychol.* 1998;66(1):136–142.

46. Gambrill E. Evidence-based practice: Implications for knowledge development and use in social work. In: Rosen A, Proctor E, eds. *Developing practice guidelines for social work intervention.* New York: Columbia University Press; 2003:37–58.

47. Brownson RC, Fielding JE, Maylahn CM. Evidence-based public health: a fundamental concept for public health practice. *Ann Rev Public Health.* 2009;30:175–201.

48. Lomas J. Diffusion, dissemination, and implementation: who should do what? *Ann N Y Acad Sci.* 1993;703:226–235; discussion 235–227.

49. MacLean DR. Positioning dissemination in public health policy. *Can J Public Health.* 1996;87 Suppl 2:S40–S43.

50. National Institutes of Health. PA-10-038: Dissemination and Implementation Research in Health (R01). 2010.

51. Brownson RC, Allen P, Jacob RR, et al. Understanding mis-implementation in public health practice. *Am J Prev Med.* 2015;48(5):543–551.

52. Prasad V, Ioannidis JP. Evidence-based de-implementation for contradicted, unproven, and aspiring healthcare practices. *Implement Sci.* 2014;9:1.

53. Levinson W, Kallewaard M, Bhatia RS, et al. "Choosing Wisely": a growing international campaign. *BMJ Qual Saf.* 2015;24(2):167–174.

54. van Bodegom-Vos L, Davidoff F, Marang-van de Mheen PJ. Implementation and de-implementation: two sides of the same coin? *BMJ Qual Saf.* 2017;26(6):495–501.

55. Niven DJ, Mrklas KJ, Holodinsky JK, et al. Towards understanding the de-adoption of low-value clinical practices: a scoping review. *BMC Med.* 2015;13:255.

56. Glasgow RE, Vogt TM, Boles SM. Evaluating the public health impact of health promotion interventions: the RE-AIM framework. *Am J Public Health.* 1999;89(9):1322–1327.

57. Sussman S, Valente TW, Rohrbach LA, Skara S, Pentz MA. Translation in the health professions: converting science into action. *Eval Health Prof.* 2006;29(1):7–32.

58. Hoelscher DM, Kelder SH, Murray N, Cribb PW, Conroy J, Parcel GS. Dissemination and adoption of the Child and Adolescent Trial for Cardiovascular Health (CATCH): a case study in Texas. *J Public Health Manag Pract.* 2001;7(2):90–100.

59. Shediac-Rizkallah MC, Bone LR. Planning for the sustainability of community-based health programs: conceptual frameworks and future directions for research, practice and policy. *Health Educ Res.* 1998;13(1):87–108.

60. Luke DA, Calhoun A, Robichaux CB, Elliott MB, Moreland-Russell S. The Program Sustainability Assessment Tool: a new instrument for public health programs. *Prev Chronic Dis.* 2014;11:130184.

61. Scheirer MA, Dearing JW. Agenda for Research on the sustainability of public health programs. *Am J Public Health* 2011;101(11):2059–2067.

62. Goodman RM, Steckler A. A model for the institutionalization of health promotion programs. *Fam Community Health.* 1989;11(4):63–78.

63. Pluye P, Potvin L, Denis J. Making public health programs last: conceptualizing sustainability. *Eval Program Plann.* 2004;27:121–133.

64. Johnson K, Hays C, Center H, Daley C. Building capacity and sustainable prevention innovations: a sustainability planning model. *Eval Program Plann.* 2004;27:135–149.

65. Proctor E, Silmere H, Raghavan R, et al. Outcomes for implementation research: conceptual distinctions, measurement challenges, and research agenda. *Adm Policy Ment Health*. 2011;38:65–76.

66. Community Partnership for Healthy Children. Funding alternatives. *Spotlight (A Sierra Health Foundation Initiative)*. 2002;4(3):1–4.

67. Leeman J, Calancie L, Hartman MA, et al. What strategies are used to build practitioners' capacity to implement community-based interventions and are they effective?: a systematic review. *Implement Sci*. 2015;10:80.

68. Best A, Hiatt RA, Norman CD. Knowledge integration: conceptualizing communications in cancer control systems. *Patient Educ Couns*. 2008;71(3):319–327.

69. National Science Foundation. *Science and engineering indicators 2006*. 2006.

70. Oliver ML. The transfer process: Implications for evaluation. In: Ottoson SM, Hawe P, eds. *Knowledge utilization, diffusion, implementation, transfer, and translation: Implications for evaluation*. Vol 124. San Francisco: Jossey-Bass and the American Evaluation Association; 2009:61–73.

71. Mitton C, Adair CE, McKenzie E, Patten SB, Perry BW. Knowledge transfer and exchange: review and synthesis of the literature. *The Milbank Quarterly*. 2007;85(4):729–768.

72. Loomis ME. Knowledge utilization and research utilization in nursing. *Image J Nurs Sch*. 1985;17(2):35–39.

73. Estabrooks CA. The conceptual structure of research utilization. *Res Nurs Health*. 1999;22(3):203–216.

74. Estabrooks CA, Wallin L, Milner M. Measuring knowledge utilization in healthcare. *Int J Policy Eval Manag*. 2003;1:3–36.

75. Ward VL, House AO, Hamer S. Knowledge brokering: exploring the process of transferring knowledge into action. *BMC Health Serv Res*. 2009;9:12.

76. van Kammen J, de Savigny D, Sewankambo N. Using knowledge brokering to promote evidence-based policy-making: The need for support structures. *Bull World Health Organ*. 2006;84(8):608–612.

77. Lomas J. Using "linkage and exchange" to move research into policy at a Canadian foundation. *Health Aff (Millwood)*. 2000;19(3):236–240.

78. Caplan N. The two-communities theory and knowledge utilization. *American Behavioral Scientist*. 1979;22(3):459–470.

79. Hargadon AB. Brokering knowledge: linking learning and innovation. *Res Organ Behav*. 2002;24:41–85.

80. Simmons R, Fajans P, Ghiron L. Introduction. In: Simmons R, Fajans P, Ghiron L, eds. *Scaling up health service delivery: From pilot innovations to policies and programmes*. Geneva: World Health Organization; 2007:vii–xvii.

81. Johns B, Torres TT. Costs of scaling up health interventions: a systematic review. *Health Policy and Planning*. 2005;20(1):1–13.

82. Hanson K, Cleary S, Schneider H, Tantivess S, Gilson L. Scaling up health policies and services in low- and middle-income settings. *BMC Health Serv Res*. 2010;10(Suppl1):I1.

83. Norton WE, Mittman B. *Scaling-up health promotion/disease prevention programs in community settings: barriers, facilitators, and initial recommendations*. The Patrick and Catherine Weldon Donaghue Medical Research Foundation; 2010.

84. Blase KA, Fixsen DL, Duda MA, Metz AJ, Naoom SF, Van Dyke AK. Implementing and sustaining evidence-based programs: Have we got a sporting chance? Blueprints Conference; April 8, 2010; University of North Carolina, Chapel Hill.

85. Mays N, Roberts, E., Popay, J. Synthesising research evidence. In: Fulop N, Allen, P., Clarke A., Black, N., eds. *Studying the organisation and delivery of health services: Research methods* London: Routledge; 2001:188–219.

86. Arksey H, O'Malley, L. Scoping studies: towards a methodological framework. *Int J Soc Res Method: Theory & Practice*. 2005;8(1):19–32.

87. Dijkers M. What is a scoping review?. *KT Update*. 2015;4(1).

88. Pawson R. *Evidence-based policy. a realist perspective*. London: Sage; 2006.

89. Pawson R, Greenhalgh T, Harvey G, Walshe K. Realist review: a new method of systematic review designed for complex policy interventions. *J Health Serv Res Policy*. 2005;10:S21–S39.

90. Woolf SH. The meaning of translational research and why it matters. *JAMA*. 2008;299:211–213.

91. Glasgow RE, Lichtenstein E, Marcus AC. Why don't we see more translation of health promotion research to practice? Rethinking the efficacy-to-effectiveness transition. *Am J Public Health*. 2003;93(8):1261–1267.

92. National Institute of Health. *Roadmap for medical research*. 2002.

93. Johnson JL, Green LW, Frankish CJ, MacLean DR, Stachenko S. A dissemination research agenda to strengthen health promotion and disease prevention. *Can J Public Health*. 1996;87 Suppl 2:S5–S10.

94. National Institutes of Health. PA-10-040: Dissemination and Implementation Research in Health (R21). 2010.

95. Center for Mental Health in Schools at UCLA. *Systemic change and empirically-supported practices: The implementation problem*. Los Angeles: Author; 2006.

96. Pinnock H, Barwick M, Carpenter CR, et al. Standards for Reporting Implementation Studies (StaRI) statement. *BMJ*. 2017;356:i6795.

97. Szilagyi PG. Translational research in pediatrics. *Acad Pediatr*. 2009;9(2):71–80.

98. Khoury MJ, Gwinn M, Yoon PW, Dowling N, Moore C, Bradley C. The continuum of translation research in genomic medicine: how can we accelerate the appropriate integration of human genome discoveries into health care and disease prevention. *Genet Med*. 2007;9(10):665–674.

99. Gibbons M, Limoges C, Nowotny H, Schwartzman S, Scott P. *The new production of knowledge: The dynamics of science and research in contemporary societies*. London: Sage; 1994.

100. Harris G. Evidence, uncertainty and risk. In: *Seeking sustainability in an age of complexity*. Cambridge: Cambridge University Press; 2007.

101. Panzano P, Sweeney HA, Seffrin B, Massatti R, Knudsen KJ. The assimilation of evidence-based healthcare innovations: A management-based perspective. *The Journal Behavioral Health Services Research*. 2012;39(4):397–416.

102. Fichman RG, Kemerer CF. The illusory diffusion of innovation: an examination of assimilation gaps. *Information Systems Research*. 1999;10(3):255–275.

103. Canadian Institutes of Health Research. Population Health Intervention Research. 2007; http://www.cihr-irsc.gc.ca/e/38731.html.

104. Institute of Population and Public Health. *Population health intervention research. Spotlight on research*. Toronto: Author; 2007.

105. Glasgow RE, Steiner, J.F. Comparative effectiveness research to accelerate translation: Recommendations for an emerging field of science. In: Brownson RC, Proctor, E.K., Colditz, G.A., eds. *Dissemination and implementation research in health*. New York: Oxford; 2012:72–93.

106. Frank L, Basch E, Selby JV, Patient-Centered Outcomes Research Institute. The PCORI perspective on patient-centered outcomes research. *JAMA*. 2014;312(15):1513–1514.

107. Selby JV, Beal AC, Frank L. The Patient-Centered Outcomes Research Institute (PCORI) national priorities for research and initial research agenda. *JAMA*. 2012;307(15):1583–1584.

108. Batalden PB, Davidoff F. What is "quality improvement" and how can it transform healthcare? *Qual Saf Health Care*. 2007;16(1):2–3.

109. "Health Resources and Services Administration." Quality Improvement. *Quality Improvement Methodology*. https://www.hrsa.gov/quality/toolbox/methodology/qualityimprovement/index.html. Accessed March 15, 2017.

110. Kao LS. Implementation science and quality improvement. In: Dimick JB, Greenberg, C.C., eds. *Success in academic surgery: Health services research*. London: Springer; 2014:85–100.

111. Bauer MS, Damschroder L, Hagedorn H, Smith J, Kilbourne AM. An introduction to implementation science for the non-specialist. *BMC Psychol*. 2015;3:32.

112. Rosin R. Keynote Address: The Innovation Conundrum. Paper presented at: 9th Annual Conference on the Science of Dissemination and Implementation; December 14–15, 2016, 2016; Washington, DC.

113. Balasubramanian BA, Cohen DJ, Davis MM, et al. Learning evaluation: blending quality improvement and implementation research methods to study healthcare innovations. *Implement Sci*. 2015;10:31.

114. Chambers DA, Feero WG, Khoury MJ. Convergence of implementation science, precision medicine, and the learning health care system: a new model for biomedical research. *JAMA*. 2016;315(18):1941–1942.

115. National Cancer Institute. National Cancer Moonshot Initiative. http://www.cancer.gov/research/key-initiatives/biden-cancer-initiative. Accessed March 25, 2017.

116. Goodman RM, Tenney M, Smith DW, Steckler A. The adoption process for health curriculum innovations in schools: a case study. *J Health Educ*. 1992;23:215–220.

117. Brownson RC, Ballew P, Dieffenderfer B, et al. Evidence-based interventions to promote physical activity: what contributes to dissemination by state health departments? *Am J Prev Med*. 2007;33(1 Suppl):S66–S73; quiz S74–S68.

118. Oldenburg B, Glanz K. Diffusion of innovation. In: Glanz K, Rimer BK, Viswanath K, eds. *Health behavior and health education*. 4th ed. San Francisco, CA: John Wiley & Sons, Inc.; 2008:313–334.

119. Dzewaltowski DA, Estabrooks PA, Glasgow RE. The future of physical activity behavior change research: what is needed to improve translation of research into health promotion practice? *Exerc Sport Sci Rev*. 2004;32(2):57–63.

120. Last JM. *A dictionary of epidemiology*. 4th ed. New York: Oxford University Press; 2001.

121. Tabak RG, Khoong EC, Chambers DA, Brownson RC. Bridging research and practice: models for dissemination and implementation research. *Am J Prev Med*. 2012;43(3):337–350.

122. Butterfoss FD, Kegler MC, Francisco VT. Mobilizing organizations for health promotion: theories of organizational change In: Glanz K, Rimer BK, Viswanath K, eds.

Health behavior and health education. 4th ed. San Francisco, CA: John Wiley & Sons, Inc.; 2008:335–362.

123. Storey JD, Saffitz GB, Rimon JG. Social Marketing. In: Glanz K, Rimer BK, Viswanath K, eds. *Health behavior and health education.* 4th ed. San Francisco, CA: Wiley, John & Sons, Inc.; 2008:435–464.

124. Finnegan JRJ, Viswanath K. Communication theory and health behavior change: the media studies framework In: Glanz K, Rimer BK, Viswanath K, eds. *Health behavior and health education.* 4th ed: San Francisco, CA: John Wiley & Sons, Inc.; 2008:363–388.

125. Kegler MC, Glanz K. Perspectives on group, organization, and community interventions In: Glanz K, Rimer BK, Lewis FM, eds. *Health behavior and health education.* 4th ed: San Francisco, CA: John Wiley & Sons, Inc.; 2008:389–404.

126. Bracht NK, Rissel C. A five stage community organization model for health promotion: empowerment and partnership strategies. In: Bracht N, ed. *Health promotion at the community level: New advances.* Thousand Oaks, CA: Sage Publications; 1999:289–304.

127. Damschroder LJ, Aron DC, Keith RE, Kirsh SR, Alexander JA, Lowery JC. Fostering implementation of health services research findings into practice: a consolidated framework for advancing implementation science. *Implement Sci.* 2009;4:50.

128. Green LW, Kreuter M. *Health program planning: An educational and ecological approach.* 4th ed. New York: McGraw-Hill; 2005.

129. Wandersman A, Duffy J, Flaspohler P, et al. Bridging the gap between prevention research and practice: the interactive systems framework for dissemination and implementation. *Am J Community Psychol.* 2008;41(3-4):171–181.

130. Feldstein AC, Glasgow RE. A practical, robust implementation and sustainability model (PRISM) for integrating research findings into practice. *Jt Comm J Qual Patient Saf.* 2008;34(4):228–243.

131. Kitson A, Harvey G, McCormack B. Enabling the implementation of evidence based practice: a conceptual framework. *Qual Health Care.* 1998;7(3):149–158.

132. Rycroft-Malone J, Kitson A, Harvey G, et al. Ingredients for change: revisiting a conceptual framework. *Qual Saf Health Care.* 2002;11(2):174–180.

133. Glasgow RE, Klesges LM, Dzewaltowski DA, Bull SS, Estabrooks P. The future of health behavior change research: what is needed to improve translation of research into health promotion practice? *Ann Behav Med.* 2004;27(1):3–12.

134. Dearing JW, Kreuter MW. Designing for diffusion: how can we increase uptake of cancer communication innovations? *Patient Educ Couns.* 2010;81 Suppl:S100–S110.

135. Brownson RC, Jacobs JA, Tabak RG, Hoehner CM, Stamatakis KA. Designing for dissemination among public health researchers: findings from a national survey in the United States. *Am J Public Health.* 2013;103(9):1693–1699.

136. Kerner JF, Guirguis-Blake J, Hennessy KD, et al. Translating research into improved outcomes in comprehensive cancer control. *Cancer Causes Control.* 2005;16 Suppl 1:27–40.

137. Green LW, Glasgow RE. Evaluating the relevance, generalization, and applicability of research: issues in translation methodology. *Eval Health Prof.* 2006;29(1):126–153.

138. Rohrbach LA, Grana R, Sussman S, Valente TW. Type II translation: transporting prevention interventions from research to real-world settings. *Eval Health Prof.* 2006;29(3):302–333.

139. Castro FG, Barrera M, Jr., Martinez CR, Jr. The cultural adaptation of prevention interventions: resolving tensions between fidelity and fit. *Prev Sci.* 2004;5(1):41–45.

140. Stirman SW, Miller CJ, Toder K, Calloway A. Development of a framework and coding system for modifications and adaptations of evidence-based interventions. *Implement Sci.* 2013;8:65.

141. Dearing JW. Evolution of diffusion and dissemination theory. *J Public Health Manag Pract.* 2008;14(2):99–108.

142. Bopp M, Saunders RP, Lattimore D. The tug-of-war: fidelity versus adaptation throughout the health promotion program life cycle. *J Prim Prev.* 2013;34(3):193–207.

143. Carvalho ML, Honeycutt S, Escoffery C, Glanz K, Sabbs D, Kegler MC. Balancing fidelity and adaptation: implementing evidence-based chronic disease prevention programs. *J Public Health Manag Pract.* 2013;19(4):348–356.

144. Cohen DJ, Crabtree BF, Etz RS, et al. Fidelity versus flexibility: translating evidence-based research into practice. *Am J Prev Med.* 2008;35(5 Suppl):S381–S389.

145. Brownson RC, Kreuter MW, Arrington BA, True WR. Translating scientific discoveries into public health action: how can schools of public health move us forward? *Public Health Reports.* 2006;121:97–103.

146. Blase K, Fixsen, D. *Core intervention components: Identifying and operationalizing what makes programs work.* https://aspe.hhs.gov/report/core-intervention-components-identifying-and-operationalizing-what-makes-programs-work. Accessed on July 28, 2017.

147. Chambers DA, Norton WE. The Adaptome: advancing the science of intervention adaptation. *Am J Prev Med.* 2016;51(4 Suppl 2):S124–S131.

148. National Institutes of Health. PA-08-166: Dissemination, Implementation, and Operational Research for HIV Prevention Interventions (R01). 2009.

149. Powell BJ, McMillen JC, Proctor EK, et al. A compilation of strategies for implementing clinical innovations in health and mental health. *Med Care Res Rev.* 2012;69(2):123–157.

150. Proctor EK, Powell BJ, McMillen JC. Implementation strategies: recommendations for specifying and reporting. *Implement Sci.* 2013;8:139.

151. Powell BJ, Waltz TJ, Chinman MJ, et al. A refined compilation of implementation strategies: results from the Expert Recommendations for Implementing Change (ERIC) project. *Implement Sci.* 2015;10:21.

152. Elliott JS, O'Loughlin J, Robinson K, et al. Conceptualizing dissemination research and activity: the case of the Canadian Heart Health Initiative. *Health Education and Behavior.* 2003;30(3):267–282.

153. Waters E, Doyle J, Jackson N, Howes F, Brunton G, Oakley A. Evaluating the effectiveness of public health interventions: the role and activities of the Cochrane Collaboration. *J Epidemiol Community Health.* 2006;60(4):285–289.

154. Bauman LJ, Stein RE, Ireys HT. Reinventing fidelity: the transfer of social technology among settings. *Am J Community Psychol.* 1991;19(4):619–639.

155. Balasubramanian BA, Heurtin-Roberts S, Krasny S, et al. Contextual factors related to implementation and reach of a pragmatic multisite trial— The My Own Health Report (MOHR) Study. *J Am Board Fam Med.* 2017;30(3):337–349.

156. Dissemination and Implementation Models in Health. http://www.dissemination-implementation.org/. Accessed March 15, 2017.

157. Stetler CB, Ritchie J, Rycroft-Malone J, Schultz A, Charns M. Improving quality of care through routine, successful implementation of evidence-based practice at the bedside: an organizational case study protocol using the Pettigrew and Whipp model of strategic change. *Implement Sci.* 2007;2:3.

158. Gilson L, Schneider H. Managing scaling up: what are the key issues? *Health Policy and Planning.* 2010;25:97–98.

159. Verbeke W, Volgering M, Hessels M. Exploring the conceptual expansion within the field of organizational behaviour: organizational climate and organizational culture. *J Manage Stud.* 1998;35:303–330.

160. Cooke RA, Rousseau DM. Behavioral norms and expectations: a quantitative approach to the assessment of organizational culture. *Group Organ Stud.* 1988;13:245–273.

161. Schein E. *Organizational culture and leadership.* 3rd ed. San Francisco: Jossey-Bass; 2004.

162. Glisson C, James LR. The cross-level effects of culture and climate in human service teams. *J Organ Behav.* 2002;23:767–794.

163. James LR, Hater JJ, Gent MJ, Bruni JR. Psychological climate: implications from cognitive social learning theory and interactional psychology. *Pers Psychol.* 1978;31:783–813.

164. James LR, Sells SB. Psychological climate: theoretical perspectives and empirical research. In: Magnusson D, ed. *Toward a psychology of situations: An international perspective.* Hillsdale, NJ: Erlbaum; 1981:275–295.

165. Litwin G, Stringer R. *Motivation and organizational climate.* Cambridge, MA: Harvard University Press; 1968.

166. Hellriegel D, Slocum JWJ. Organizational climate: measures, research and contingencies. *Acad Manage J.* 1974;17:255–280.

167. Reichers A, Schneider B. Climate and culture: An evolution of constructs. In: Schneider B, ed. *Organizational climate and culture.* San Francisco: Jossey-Bass; 1990: 5–39.

168. Schneider B. Organizational climate: an essay. *Pers Psychol.* 1975;28(4):447–479.

169. Lehman WE, Greener JM, Simpson DD. Assessing organizational readiness for change. *J Subst Abuse Treat.* 2002;22(4):197–209.

170. Weiner BJ. A theory of organizational readiness for change. *Implement Sci.* 2009;4:67.

171. Weiner BJ, Amick H, Lee SY. Conceptualization and measurement of organizational readiness for change: a review of the literature in health services research and other fields. *Med Care Res Rev.* 2008;65(4):379–436.

172. Rabin BA, Glasgow RE, Kerner FJ, Klump MP, Brownson RC. Dissemination and implementation research on community-based cancer prevention: a systematic review. *Am J Prev Med.* 2010;38(4):443–456.

173. Victora C, Habicht J, Bryce J. Evidence-based public health: moving beyond randomized trials. *Am J Public Health.* 2004;94(3):400–406.

174. Brown H, Curran, G., Palinkas, L.A., Aarons, G.A. An overview of research and evaluation designs for dissemination and implementation. *Annu Rev Public Health.* 2017;38:1–22.

175. Tunis SR, Stryer DB, Clancy CM. Practical clinical trials: increasing the value of clinical research for decision making in clinical and health policy. *Jama.* 2003;290(12):1624–1632.

176. Lei H, Nahum-Shani I, Lynch K, Oslin D, Murphy SA. A "SMART" design for building individualized treatment sequences. *Annu Rev Clin Psychol.* 2012;8:21–48.

177. Kilbourne AM, Neumann MS, Pincus HA, Bauer MS, Stall R. Implementing evidence-based interventions in health care: application of the replicating effective programs framework. *Implement Sci.* 2007;2:42.

178. Brown CA, Lilford RJ. The stepped wedge trial design: a systematic review. *BMC Med Res Methodol.* 2006;6:54.

179. Beard E, Lewis JJ, Copas A, et al. Stepped wedge randomised controlled trials: systematic review of studies published between 2010 and 2014. *Trials.* 2015;16:353.

180. Curran GM, Bauer M, Mittman B, Pyne JM, Stetler C. Effectiveness-implementation hybrid designs: combining elements of clinical effectiveness and implementation research to enhance public health impact. *Med Care.* 2012;50(3):217–226.

181. Leischow SJ, Best A, Trochim WM, et al. Systems thinking to improve the public's health. *Am J Prev Med.* 2008;35(2 Suppl):S196–S203.

182. Trochim WM, Cabrera DA, Milstein B, Gallagher RS, Leischow SJ. Practical challenges of systems thinking and modeling in public health. *Am J Public Health.* 2006;96(3):538–546.

183. Institute of Medicine. *The learning healthcare system: Workshop summary.* Washington DC: National Academies Press; 2007.

184. Riley WT, Glasgow RE, Etheredge L, Abernethy AP. Rapid, responsive, relevant (R3) research: a call for a rapid learning health research enterprise. *Clin Transl Med.* 2013;2(1):10.

185. Glasgow RE. What outcomes are the most important in translational research?. Paper presented at: In Proceedings of "From clinical science to community: The science of translating diabetes and obesity research" conference 2004; Bethsada, Maryland.

186. Tashakkori A, Teddlie C. *Handbook of mixed methods in the social and behavioral research.* 2nd ed. Thousand Oaks, CA: SAGE Publications; 2010.

187. Johnson RB, Onwuegbuzie AJ. Mixed methods research: a research paradigm whose time has come. *Educ Researcher.* 2004;33(7):14–26.

188. Glasgow RE, Riley WT. Pragmatic measures: what they are and why we need them. *Am J Prev Med.* 2013;45(2):237–243.

189. Rabin BA, Purcell P, Naveed S, et al. Advancing the application, quality and harmonization of implementation science measures. *Implement Sci.* 2012;7:119.

190. Green LW, Ottoson JM, Garcia C, Hiatt RA. Diffusion theory and knowledge dissemination, utilization, and integration in public health. *Annu Rev Public Health.* 2009;30:151–174.

191. Rothwell PM. External validity of randomised controlled trials: "to whom do the results of this trial apply?". *Lancet.* 2005;365(9453):82–93.

192. Cunningham-Sabo L, Carpenter WR, Peterson JC, Anderson LA, Helfrich CD, Davis SM. Utilization of prevention research: searching for evidence. *Am J Prev Med.* 2007;33(1 Suppl):S9-S20.

193. Larsen KR, Michie S, Hekler EB, et al. Behavior change interventions: the potential of ontologies for advancing science and practice. *J Behav Med.* 2017;40(1):6–22.

194. Lewis CC, Stanick CF, Martinez RG, et al. The Society for Implementation Research Collaboration Instrument Review Project: a methodology to promote rigorous evaluation. *Implement Sci.* 2015;10:2.

3

Historical Roots of Dissemination and Implementation Science

JAMES W. DEARING, KERK F. KEE, AND TAI-QUAN PENG

INTRODUCTION

A worldwide science of dissemination and implementation (D&I) has emerged, driven by new media, the interests of philanthropies and the needs of government agencies, and the persistent and growing applied problems that have been addressed but not solved by the dominant research paradigms in disciplines such as psychology, sociology, and political science. Dissemination science is being shaped by researchers in the professional and applied fields of study, including public health, health services, communication, marketing, resource development, forestry and fisheries, education, criminal justice, and social work. A number of peer-reviewed journals[1–10] have since 2004 devoted special issues/sections to the topic of dissemination or implementation of evidence-based practices.

Research about D&I is a response to a general acknowledgment that successful, effective practices, programs, and policies resulting from clinical and community trials, demonstration projects, and community-based research as conducted by academicians very often do not affect the services that clinical staff, community service providers, and other practitioners fashion and provide to residents, clients, patients, and populations at risk. In any one societal sector (populated, for example, by planners for health care delivery, or city-level transportation and parkway planners), the state of the science (what researchers collectively know) and the state of the art (what practitioners collectively do) coexist more or less autonomously, each realm of activity having little effect on the other. In the United States, this situation has been referred to as a "quality chasm" by the US Institute of Medicine.[11]

Dissemination science is the study of how evidence-based practices, programs, and policies can best be communicated to an interorganizational societal sector of potential adopters and implementers to produce uptake and effective use, such as among clinics on behalf of patients or among elementary schools on behalf of children. This definition means that dissemination embeds the objectives of both *external validity*, the replication of positive effects across dissimilar settings and conditions, and *scale-up*, the replication of positive effects across settings and conditions.[12] A *potential adopter* is someone who is targeted by a change agency to make a decision about whether to try an *innovation*, an idea, practice, program, policy, or technology that is perceived to be new. In public health or health care delivery, the innovation may be an evidence-based intervention that shows the potential to improve the well-being of a segment of a population.

Implementation science is the study of what happens prior to, and after, adoption occurs, especially in organizational settings. Many studies of implementation focus on field-based tests of external validity to understand the extent to which an evidence-based program or practice will still be effective when subjected to realistic practice conditions. A smaller proportion of implementation research concerns post-adoption behavior among practitioners under actual practice conditions, when implementation and sustainability traditionally have gone unobserved. An *implementer* is someone who will actually change his or her behavior to use an innovation in practice. In organizations, the people who make the decision to adopt an innovation are often not the users of innovations. The extent and quality of implementation and client or constituent responses to it have become dependent variables of study just as important, and sometimes more important, than initial adoption. Implementation researchers have not much studied sustainability, which may be even more important than implementation, though this is beginning to change.[13] So dissemination science and implementation science merge the study and objectives of diffusion with those of organizational change. For example, public health researchers or practitioners can conduct combined D&I studies that target many county departments of public health with a new disease prevention program (a dissemination study objective) and then focus on understanding what is done with the program in a purposively derived sample of all adopting departments (an implementation study objective). The questions by public health researchers and practitioners about D&I can lead to rather different but perhaps equally fascinating projects, including questions such as:

- For a given public health program, does the change agency target types of organizations that are the most logical adopters serving the most needy clients or populations, or does the change agency simply target convenient or familiar organizations that they could easily contact because of a preexisting database?
- Does the change agency develop messages about the new program based on systematic formative evaluation?
- To what extent does the change agency strategically consider *when* to introduce the new program or do they just disseminate information as it becomes available?
- What is the competition for attention from the proponents of other similar programs and how does this change over time?
- What proportion of organizations targeted with dissemination messages respond by contacting the change agency for more information?
- How many try the new program (which might qualify them as adopters) of all those targeted (a measure of *reach*)?
- Was the program truly new conceptually to decision-makers in the adopting organizations, or were they already experimenting with similar programs?
- Do some organizations invest resources in adoption (taking the time to learn about the program, pay licensing fees, attend trainings, order booklets and train-the-trainer materials, become certified as coaches, etc.) but then never implement the program?

- What proportion of adopting organizations actually offer the program but then discontinue it?
- How many organizations stay in a holding pattern of adopting/not implementing/not discontinuing?
- What proportion of implementers offer the program as its designers intended with the same content, same number of modules, same behavior stimuli, same support, and checks on enrollee or client performance?
- What types of adaptations to the program are made by implementers? Do they offer all the program's core components? Are they true to the program's theory of behavior change? Do they drop some components, customize others, and/ or create their own to better suit their organization and their clients?
- Does the implementing organization change in ways unanticipated by the program designers? Does learning the one program serve as a trigger or precipitating event for organizational decision-makers to adopt other, consonant or complementary public health programs?
- Do implementers think they are offering the program as the designers intended but, in practice, do something quite different?
- What is the client or enrollee yield? How many individuals sign up? How many complete all modules or classes? How many people actually do the variety of behavior changes—wearing pedometers, meeting in groups, writing in diaries, coming to class, completing their workbook, monitoring their progress—as suggested (and tested in efficacy trials) by the program designers?
- Is the public health program sustained by the organization? Do clients or enrollees continue their participation, too? Is fidelity or adaptation a better predictor of sustainability?
- What are the individual outcomes (weight loss, muscle tone, etc.) and public health impacts (for example, proportion of obese people in intervention communities)?
- How can implementers identify opinion leaders who are looked to by others for advice and example for practice improvement?
- How can cutting-edge computational approaches help health researchers

understand public attention and emotion toward health issues?

Given this range of dissemination science and implementation science questions that can be studied, it can be argued that these foci represent a most important type of diffusion of innovations study. The key, we suggest, is the stimulation of or tapping into intrinsic motivation of the staff in public health, health care and other types of organizations and among their clients and program enrollees in communities. Certain innovations are met with enthusiasm, open arms, and eager learners who go on to champion new programs and advocate them to others. Innovations spread rapidly when people want them and can access them.

Where does the current emphasis on D&I science come from? How are new media altering the diffusion of new practices, programs, and beliefs? We turn to the diffusion of innovations paradigm to address these questions.

THE CLASSIC DIFFUSION PARADIGM

Diffusion is the process through which an innovation is communicated through certain channels over-time among the members of a social system.[14] For example, Barker[15] reports on three international development efforts in relation to diffusion concepts. In Haiti, a United States Agency for International Development (USAID) effort to conduct HIV prevention education in rural villages identified and recruited village voodoo practitioners, who are almost always considered credible and trusted sources of advice by Haiti villagers, to encourage villagers to participate in village meetings with USAID change agents. Meeting attendance exceeded campaign objectives by 124%. In Nepal, where vitamin A deficiency contributes to very high rates of infant and maternal mortality, the innovation of kitchen gardens was diffused among households through neighbor social modeling, resulting in heightened knowledge, positive attitudes, increased vegetable and fruit growing and consumption, and improvements in vitamin A nutrition. In Mali in 1999, a study of 500 Malian youth evaluated their information-seeking behavior and perceptions of source credibility concerning reproductive health. A lack of accurate knowledge among youth was attributed to their most trusted sources of information being friends and siblings; youth did not consider information

sources such as health agents and teachers to be accessible enough or trustworthy. In all three cases, the innovations of HIV prevention education, kitchen gardens, and reproductive health information are unlikely to impact Haitian villagers, Nepali infants and mothers, and Malian youths if the diffusion process is not stimulated by accessing trusted, informal opinion leaders.

Diffusion studies have demonstrated a mathematically consistent sigmoid pattern (the S-shaped curve) of over-time adoption for innovations that are perceived to be consequential by potential adopters, when the decisions to adopt are voluntary as opposed to them being compulsory, and with attendant logically related propositions, qualifying this literature as a theory of social change.[16] Many studies have shown a predictable over-time pattern when an innovation spreads, the now familiar S-shaped cumulative adoption curve. The "S" shape is due to the engagement of informal opinion leaders (as in Barker's study reported earlier) in talking about and modeling the innovation for others to hear about and see in action (Figure 3.1). For any given consequential innovation, the rate of adoption tends to begin slow, accelerate because of the activation of positive word of mouth communication and social modeling by the 5% to 8% of social system members who are sources of advice (i.e., opinion leaders) for subsequent other adopters, and then slow as system potential is approached. Box 3.1 provides a summary of the evolving opinion leader research for D&I interventions.

Key components of diffusion theory are:

1. The *innovation*, and especially potential adopter perceptions of its *attributes* of cost, effectiveness, compatibility, simplicity, observability, and trialability (see Table 3.1)
2. The *adopter*, especially each adopter's degree of *innovativeness* (earliness relative to others in adopting the innovation)
3. The *social system*, such as a geographic community, a distributed network of collaborators, a professional association, or a province or state, especially in terms of the *structure* of the system, its informal *opinion leaders*, and potential adopter perception of *social pressure* to adopt
4. The *individual adoption-process*, a stage-ordered model of awareness, persuasion, decision, implementation, and continuation[34]

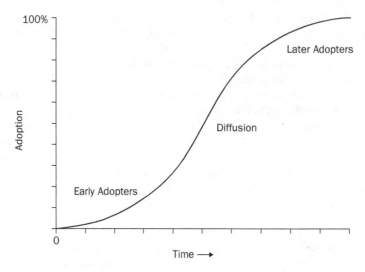

FIGURE 3.1 The generalized cumulative curve that describes the curvilinear process of the diffusion of innovation.

5. The *diffusion system*, especially an external *change agency* and its paid *change agents* who, if well trained, correctly seek out and intervene with the client system's opinion leaders and paraprofessional aides, and support the enthusiasm of unpaid emergent innovation champions

Diffusion occurs through a combination of (1) the need for individuals to reduce personal uncertainty when presented with information about an innovation and (2) the need for individuals to respond to their perceptions of what specific credible others are thinking and doing, and to generally felt social pressure to do as others have done. Uncertainty in response to an innovation typically leads to a search for information and, if the potential adopter believes the innovation to be interesting and with the potential for benefits, a search for evaluative judgments of trusted and respected others (informal opinion leaders). This advice-seeking behavior is a heuristic that allows the decision-maker to avoid comprehensive information-seeking, reflecting Herbert Simon's seminal insight about the importance of everyday constraints in "bounding" the rationality of our decision making.[35]

Needs or motivations differ among people according to their degree of innovativeness (earliness in adoption relative to others): The first 2.5% to adopt (*innovators*) tend to do so because of novelty and having little to lose; the next 13.5% to adopt (*early adopters*, including the subset of

about 5% to 7% informal opinion leaders) do so because of an appraisal of the innovation's attributes; the subsequent 34% of early majority adopters and 34% of late majority adopters do so because others have done so. They come to believe that adoption is the right thing to do (an imitative effect rather than a carefully reasoned rational judgment). The last 16% to adopt do so grudgingly with reservations. Their recalcitrance is sometimes later proved to be well-justified, since new programs can have undesirable consequences.

One's orientation to an innovation and time of adoption are related to and can be predicted by each adopter's structural position in the network of relations that tie together a social system such as a school, community, or even a far flung professional network. When viewed sociometrically (especially who-seeks-advice-from-whom within a social network) in two-dimensional space, the pattern of diffusion begins on the periphery of a network as the first to try the innovation experiment with it; central members of the network—informal opinion leaders who are a special subset of early adopters—then adopt if they judge the innovation to have important advantages over current practices; the many others then follow, who pay attention to what these sociometrically central and highly connected network members do and advise.[36] This outside-inside-outward progression of adoption, when graphed as the cumulative number of adoptions over time, reflects an S-shaped diffusion curve (see Figure 3.1).

BOX 3.1

EMPIRICAL IDENTIFICATION OF OPINION LEADERS

Opinion leaders are "individuals who exert an unequal amount of influence on the decisions of others"[17] within a social system. They can play important roles in the diffusion of creative ideas, innovative products, and new practices. Although the conceptualization of opinion leaders is rather clear, the empirical identification of opinion leaders has proved nontrivial.[18] In the past, self-reported individual attributes, such as education degree, social-economic status, and trust-worthiness, were employed to measure individuals' opinion leadership. However, such attribute-based measurement does not well capture the influence-susceptible relationship between opinion leaders and followers, which is central to Rogers and Cartano's conceptualization of opinion leaders.[19] Advances in network science can be combined with marketing approaches to help dissemination and implementation researchers identify and intervene with opinion leaders for health.[20]

Individual persons or groups in a social system are considered network nodes, which can be connected with one another via multiple types of links based on their similarities, social relations, interactions, or flows.[21] Such networks can be examined at the macro level to discover statistical regularities, at the meso level to reveal structural organizations, and at the micro level to uncover the positions occupied by individuals in a social system.[22] Micro-level analysis can allow research-ers or practitioners to identify who is better connected in a social system and who is less so. Individuals in better connected positions have greater influence than those in poorly connected positions,[23] as the latter are dependent on the former for valued resources (e.g., knowledge, eval-uation, and investment). Network science provides an array of centrality metrics to quantify the "better connected" positions, including degree centrality, closeness centrality, betweenness cen-trality, and eigenvector centrality.[24-26] More on network science is found in chapter 10.

These four metrics have been used separately or in combination to identify opinion leaders for various health issues (e.g., obesity, HIV/AIDS, and smoking) among the general public,[27,28] medical professionals,[29] and specific groups of patients.[30] Albalawi and Sixsmith[27] employed the degree centrality of Twitter users to identify which users have the potential to raise awareness of health issues and advocate for health in Saudi Arabia. They identified 100 accounts with the greatest potential to influence, including religious men/women, traditional media, commercial companies, sports-related accounts, politically related accounts, and health accounts. Holliday et al.[28] developed a peer support network among high school students in the United Kingdom and employed the degree, closeness, and betweenness centrality metrics to identify and engage opinion leaders.

In addition to these four centrality metrics, network scientists have developed more sophis-ticated algorithms to identify opinion leaders in social networks, such as the stability-sensitivity method,[31] the path counting method,[32] and VoteRank.[33] These metrics and algorithms can be applied in D&I science to help researchers and practitioners better understand, detect, and engage opinion leaders, which can facilitate the diffusion of ideas and practices among certain populations.

Forefathers of the Diffusion Model

The French judge cum sociologist Gabriel Tarde explained diffusion as a societal-level phenome-non of social change in his 1903 book, *The Laws of Imitation*, including the identification of an S-shaped curve in cumulative adoptions over time, the role of conversation in producing mimicry, and the importance of informal opinion leaders in jumpstarting the S-shaped curve. As a judge, Tarde had taken note of the way people coming before the bench used new slang and wore new clothing fashions as if on cue. In Germany at the same time, Georg Simmel, a political philosopher,

TABLE 3.1 DEFINITIONS AND APPLICATION OF INNOVATION ATTRIBUTES

Innovation Attributes	Definitions	Application to Public Health and Health Care Delivery
Cost	Perceived cost of adopting and implementing an innovation	How much time and effort are required to learn to use the innovation and routinze its use? How long does recouping of costs take?
Effectiveness	The extent to which the innovation works better than that which it will displace	Does a gain in performance outweigh the downsides of cost? Do different stakeholders agree on the superiority of the innovation?
Simplicity	How simple the innovation is to understand	How easy is an evidence-based program for adopters/implementers to understand and/or if it requires a steep learning and much training before actual implementation?
Compatibility	The fit of the innovation to established ways of accomplishing the same goal	How much/little would an evidence-based program disrupt the existing routine and/or workflow of the adopting/implementing organization?
Observability	The extent to which outcomes can be seen	How much and/or how quickly will the results of an evidence-based program become visible to an implementing organization, its clients, funders, and peer organizations?
Trialability	The extent to which the adopter must commit to full adoption	If an evidence-based program can be implemented as a pilot project without much investment and be abandoned without incurring much sunk cost?

was writing about how individual thought and action was structured by the set of interpersonal relations to which a person was subject. Tarde's perspective was the forerunner for the macro, social system perspective on diffusion as the means by which cultures and societies changed and progressed. Simmel's contribution, explicated in his book, *Conflict: The Web of Group Affiliations*, was the forerunner for understanding how social network position affects what individuals do in reaction to innovations, and when. Together, these perspectives provided an explanation for how system-level effects pressured the individual to adopt new things, and how individuals can affect change through their relationships in social networks.

Following Tarde and Simmel, European anthropologists seized on diffusion as a means to explain the continental drift of people, ideas, means of social organization, and primitive technologies. American anthropologists such as Alfred Kroeber in the 1920s also conducted historical studies but they confined their analyses— for the first time called *diffusion* study—to more

discrete innovations in smaller social systems such as a community or a region of the country. Anthropologists studying diffusion focused not only on spread of innovations but on how cultures in turn shaped those innovations[37] by giving them new purposes and by adapting them to suit local needs—the beginnings of what we now call implementation science. The studies of these early diffusion researchers encouraged sociologists to take up diffusion work in contemporary 1920s and 1930s society, focusing on informal communication in friendship or social support networks as an explanation for the city-to-rural spread of innovations, the importance of jurisdictions as barriers to diffusion, and the importance of proximity to the spread of ideas.[38] And diffusion was not only understood as a one-way process: The American sociologist Pitirim Sorokin saw diffusion as inherently recursive. More developed countries extract raw materials from developing countries and send back finished goods; classical music composers, for example, absorb ideas from folk tunes into the creation of symphonies.[36] Public health and health care can be interpreted recursively, too: Epidemiologic data about communities and practice-based research results are "diffused" to researchers, who develop new public health and health care interventions and seek to disseminate them back to those same practitioner systems and communities.[39]

A landmark event for diffusion science occurred in 1943 with a report on the diffusion of hybrid seed corn in two Iowa communities.[40] This seminal article set the paradigm for many hundreds of future diffusion studies by emphasizing individuals as the locus of decision, adoption as the key dependent variable, a centralized innovation change agency that employed change agents, and the importance of different communication channels for different purposes at different times in the individual innovation-decision process. The Ryan and Gross article propelled diffusion study to center stage among rural sociologists. It also made the application of diffusion concepts a key set of tools in the work of agricultural extension agents. Rural sociologists were closely wedded to the extension services for funding and for providing the distribution system by which diffusion study ideas could be tested. The academics were practice oriented. From 1954 to 1969, key faculty in the Iowa State University Department of Sociology gave an estimated 600 presentations about the diffusion process, many to extension service groups. In 1958 alone, there were 35 publications reporting diffusion data collected in the United States by rural sociologists. Six years later, rural sociology publications about diffusion in less developed countries reached a peak of 20.[41] Diffusion studies by rural sociologists began to wane in 1969, but by that time scholars in sociology, medical sociology, education, communication, and public health had begun diffusion research, such as Coleman, Katz and Menzel's classic study of physician's drug-prescribing behavior as a result of social network ties.[42]

Synthesizing the Diffusion Paradigm

The diffusion of innovations paradigm began to synthesize its approaches, central challenges, and lessons learned beginning in the 1960s. Internationally, an "invisible college" of rural sociologists had formed based in the American Midwest, drawn together both by intellectual questions and funding opportunities for research into a coauthorship, collaborative, and competitive network.[43] As these questions were answered by rural sociologists, diffusion research became fashionable to scholars in other disciplines and fields who conceptualized somewhat different problems, especially concerning policymakers as adopters and the conditions of innovation and spread in complex organizations. Yet diversification did not limit the centrality of diffusion scholarship as it importantly related to the growing paradigms of knowledge utilization and technology transfer studies and then to the evidence-based medicine movement.[44]

Everett M. Rogers, trained as a rural sociologist at Iowa State University, defended his dissertation in 1957 after growing up poor on an Iowa farm.[45,46] While the dissertation was ostensibly about the diffusion of 2-4-D weed spray among farmers, Rogers' real interest was in drawing generalizations that he believed were warranted on the basis of commonalities he had discovered by reading diffusion studies being published in different fields. The authors of the studies were not aware that other researchers were studying diffusion in fields different from theirs. Rogers expanded his chapter 2 literature review into the 1962 seminal book, *Diffusion of Innovations*, synthesizing what was known about diffusion in general terms. His modeling of diffusion as an over-time social process and, at the individual level, as a series of stages that a person passes through in relation to an innovation would soon come to be recognized across fields of study as the diffusion of innovations paradigm. Though Rogers[47] would remain for decades the single most recognizable name associated with the diffusion of innovations, many other scholars were studying diffusion. And many diffusion scholars took a slightly different approach than Rogers. Many of these scholars were former students and colleagues of his; their contributions continue to push the paradigm forward and outward. In particular, some working in the paradigm took a macro structural perspective on diffusion, especially those in population planning, demography, economics, and international relations. Anthropologists studying the spread of culture and linguists studying the spread of language also preferred a structural perspective on diffusion, which conceptualized waves of innovations washing over societies. To these structuralists, the study of diffusion was the study of social change writ large. For them, units of adoption are countries or cultures.

This macro orientation to diffusion was highly enticing to scholars because of its deductive and parsimonious potential based in a simple mathematical law of nature that describes a logistic (S-shaped or exponential) growth curve. Marketing scientists, epidemiologists, demographers, and political scientists instantly appreciated the predictive potential and eloquence of the population perspective on diffusion. Mathematical modeling formed the basis of this work, most of which continues today in fields such as family planning apart from more qualitatively informed micro-level studies of diffusion.[48]

So a major part of Rogers' contribution was in persuasively showing how macro-level processes of system change could be linked to micro-level behavior. These ideas harkened back to Simmel and Tarde, that individuals were influenced by system norms, and system structure and rules were the cumulative results of individual actions. Diffusion was one of the very few social theories that persuasively linked macro with micro-level phenomena.

KNOWLEDGE UTILIZATION AND TECHNOLOGY TRANSFER

The agricultural extension model, with its basis in the training of social change concepts to full-time staff who were experts in areas such as cherry blight, zebra mussel eradication, and pine beetle control, was critical to the popularity of the diffusion of innovations paradigm. It was also important in the genesis of two closely related bodies of research. *Knowledge utilization* has been a robust paradigm for 40 years; its central problem was not how a new practice came to be voluntarily adopted by many people, but rather how knowledge in the form of prior results of a social program (the effectiveness of school busing, or of curbside recycling, or of business enterprise zones in cities) affected the subsequent decisions of elected representatives and policy staff in government. This is another route to social change, one that relies more on policy action by formal authorities followed by the compulsory adoptions of others than the traditional diffusion attention to informal influence. Were ineffective programs phased out by policymakers while effective programs were replicated and expanded? Did the social and education programs that managed to spread across the American states deserve to spread? The key intellectual contributor to this paradigm was the education scholar, Carol H. Weiss.[49] Weiss' studies of policy decision-making showed that rational expectations between evidence and program continuation/expansion were not supported by

social science study. And beyond the expectation of a rational outcomes-to-funding relationship, Weiss and other knowledge utilization researchers of the policymaking process showed that any direct program evaluation-to-policy decision link was rare; rather, policymaking was inherently political.[50] Many more factors besides evidence of program effectiveness factored into decision-making.[51] When program evidence did affect subsequent decisions by policymakers, it did so through a circuitous cumulative learning by policymakers and staff as they became "enlightened" over time in terms of general programming lessons. In a gradual, accretionary way, indirect and partial knowledge diffusion did occur.

From the perspective of knowledge utilization, Blake and Ottoson[52] maintain that dissemination is the process of moving information from one source to another (as from program evaluators to policy makers), and the ultimate purpose of dissemination should be utilization by users. When utilization by users is achieved, information/knowledge has impact. This perspective has evolved with the field of knowledge utilization studies, through "waves" of research from the empirical studies in the 1940s by rural sociologists to studies of international development and family planning in the 1970s, to research in the 1990s about how research could improve human services in health and education.[53,54]

Researchers studying *technology transfer* identified a different problem. Beginning with Mansfield in the 1960s, scholars such as Leonard-Barton and von Hippel focused on the firm, especially complex organizations such as multinational corporations that partly by virtue of their size exhibited problems of coordination, knowledge sharing, and even knowing what was going on across its many divisions let alone having a managerial system for knowing which practices were more effective than others.[55] Whereas diffusion was about innovations that usually began with a single source and then spread broadly, technology transfer was one-to-one or "point-to-point." How can an innovative work-flow redesign or unit-based team approach to scheduling that produce huge productivity gains in Argentina be applied to improve the same company's productivity in Canada? What sorts of adaptation might be necessary?[56]

Contrary to the technology transfer label, Dunn, Holzener, and Zaltman[57(p. 120)] argued that, "Knowledge use is transactive. Although one may use the analogy of 'transfer,' knowledge is never truly marketed, transferred or exchanged. Knowledge is really negotiated between the parties involved." Similarly, Estabrooks and colleagues[58(p. 28)] clarify that the Canadian Institutes of Health Research defines knowledge translation as the "exchange, synthesis and ethically sound application of knowledge—within a complex system of interactions among researchers and users." In other words, the notions of transaction, negotiation, interactions, and synthesis are key to the conceptualization of transfer (and dissemination/diffusion) of information/knowledge from producers to users. In health research and organizational technology transfer, one needs to understand what is being transferred, by whom, to which targets, through what process, and with what outcomes.[59] So effective transfer has knowledge utilization at its core.[51]

EVIDENCE-BASED MEDICINE AND EVIDENCE-BASED PUBLIC HEALTH

Literatures about diffusion of innovations, knowledge utilization, and technology transfer have found new application and expansion in the fields of medicine and public health. *Evidence-based medicine* is the conscientious, explicit, and judicious use of current best evidence in making decisions about the care of individual patients. The practice of evidence-based medicine means integrating individual clinical expertise with the best available external clinical evidence from systematic research.[60]

Evidence-based medicine is an approach to medical practice that emphasizes the role of research literature (new information, latest knowledge), usually in the form of clinical practice or medical guidelines (increasingly based on comparative effectiveness research), over prior training and clinical experiences such that each becomes an input in decision-making about each particular patient's health. Although evidence-based medicine has been controversial among some medical professionals[61] and somewhat misunderstood as a movement to displace traditional practices in medicine, advocates[62] argue for augmentation rather than displacement. Clinical epidemiology, for example, has become infused with evidence-based knowledge generation, rapid critical appraisal of evidence, efficient storage and retrieval, and evidence synthesis.[63] When all four components are effectively practiced, the quality of patient care increases.

The desire for valid and generalizable evidence to inform decisions also has been applied to the domain of public health. Brownson and colleagues[64] proposed the following attributes as key to defining evidence-based public health: (1) Decisions are guided by best available peer-reviewed evidence and literature from a range of methodologies; (2) evidence-based public health approaches systematically make use of data and information systems; (3) its practice frameworks for program planning come from theories rooted in behavioral science; (4) the community of users are involved in processes of decision-making and assessment; (5) evidence-based public health approaches carry out sound evaluation of programs; and (6) lessons learned are shared with stakeholder groups and decision-makers. Simmons, Fajans, and Ghiron[65] additionally emphasize contextual factors as key in matching practice refinements to local conditions.

During the dissemination of evidence-based practices, we believe that it is useful to consider the interplay between the technical rationalities of knowledge producers or change agencies, and users' narrative rationalities, whether those users are patients and community members or health care providers and public health professionals. Technical rationalities are based on logics that are predictive, instructive, and technocratic, while narrative rationalities are stories of experiences that are interpretive, contextual, and dynamic.[66] Narratives can be illuminating to program planners as well as inform ongoing attempts to improve care and public health practice.[67,68] Collectively, these two perspectives represent the state of the science (what researchers collectively know) and the state of the art (what practitioners collectively do). New media and emerging technologies can facilitate the access to and use of both technical rationalities (guideline content) and narrative rationalities (for example, clinical practitioners' perspectives about how they have implemented such guidance given the realities of their practices).

NEW (AND NEWER) MEDIA

What are the effects of new information and communication technologies on dissemination activities by change agencies, the social diffusion processes that may result as potential adopters consider an innovation, and how implementation in organizations unfolds?

Collective knowledge of the diffusion of innovations paradigm has given way to a focus on those paradigmatic concepts that can be operationalized in purposive tests of how to best disseminate and implement evidence-based health practices, programs, and policies.[69] This has long been an objective in trying to spread effective innovations for improved global health as well as for domestic health care and public health.[70,71] New media, in the ways in which they affect the dissemination of information by change agencies, the subsequent diffusion process among targeted adopters, and the resultant critical stage of implementation of evidence-based practices in organizations, are iteratively changing how we work and how targeted adopters respond to change initiatives. D&I researchers and practitioners are well-advised to be agile.

The traditional notion of an innovation as predesigned by centralized change agents is increasingly inaccurate. Increasingly, innovations are malleable and coproduced by researchers, practitioners, and those persons who adopt them, whether the researchers in question have this intention or not. Such a perspective on change has the advantage of enabling learning from those persons who are best positioned to make insightful and applicable real-time improvements to an innovation: users themselves.[72] This shift in emphasis to utilization by users would wed source perspectives on change with those of innovation users-as-creators. Utilization properly involves both the logics of innovation producers with the experiential expertise of users who are sensitized to issues of context and compatibility.

Technologies can facilitate information access and knowledge creation in the context of dissemination. In terms of information access, it is clear that information technologies and certain new media accelerate our ability to disseminate information worldwide.[73] Do they also accelerate diffusion (that is, resultant decision-making) among those health care and public health practitioners whom we sometimes try to reach and affect?[74] Technologies increase the dissemination of knowledge about innovations and expand reach in terms of health promotion,[75] disease prevention,[76] health compliance, telehealth,[77,78] and cybermedicine.[79] Technologies allow easy access to new information and latest knowledge via specialized knowledge management systems (such as medical literature databases) that health care providers can use to inform their medical practice, and general knowledge management systems (such as public web-based search engines) to help patients make better health-related choices in life.[80]

Furthermore, technologies may intensify the diffusion process among connected adopters whom change agents may target for change,[81] including tapping their weak ties and strong ties,[82] and designing strategic messages to drive views, comments, and shares on social media.[83] Traditionally and still today, diffusion is facilitated by mass media and interpersonal networks among people. In today's wired societies and more specifically in our networked market segments that are organized by common interests and professions, new media create new online social communities that are critical to the facilitation of information knowledge dissemination beyond geographically/temporally bound communities of the past. Technologies intensify the dissemination process by elevating social media platforms and their amateur broadcasters as well as new networks among people who do not know each other except through online communities[84] to an emerging position of intermediary, thus giving information/knowledge another push for dissemination throughout social systems.[85]

In terms of knowledge creation, technologies are enabling new and expanded professional networks among health care providers and public health professionals, leading to interorganizational sharing and cross-fertilization of information and knowledge about common challenges.[86] New media make coproduction of knowledge between producers and users easier to achieve because of the low cost and high speed for feedback and ongoing communication.[87] Technologies support automatic and cumulative data acquisition (including electronic medical records in health care organizations and online data mining) for computations and analyses that, in turn, can produce more knowledge. In this way, the use of technologies demonstrates Sorokin's view that diffusion is inherently recursive. We surmise that if potential adopters of innovations feel that they have been involved in the creation of or refinement of an innovation, their adoption and implementation is more likely. If new media lead to the experience of broader participation in knowledge creation, then those media will stimulate not only dissemination but diffusion, too. Box 3.2 provides a summary of applications of computational social science to D&I research in health.

SUMMARY

This chapter has tried to show the evolution of diffusion of innovations theory, and how concepts from that paradigm as well as knowledge

BOX 3.2

COMPUTATIONAL SOCIAL SCIENCE AND PUBLIC HEALTH RESEARCH

Computational social science (CSS) has penetrated health research due to widely available, massive ("BIG") datasets and increasingly sophisticated computational methods.[88] The computational paradigm has triggered the creativity of researchers from different disciplines (e.g., computer science, physics, communication and epidemiology) to examine health phenomena at an unprecedented scale.

The most visible application of CSS in public health is the forecasting of disease outbreaks with search query data. Ginsberg et al.[89] tracked the search volumes of 45 influenza-related queries at Google and found that the searching trends of these queries could alert the general public to flu pandemics earlier than could government statistics from the Centers for Disease Control and Prevention in the United States. Although recent studies found that Google search trends would overestimate the epidemic degree of influenza in the United States,[90,91] this study has prompted scholars to apply query data to monitor the trends of various diseases, such as dengue,[92] stroke,[93] and tuberculosis.[94] Researchers were also inspired to employ data from other social media platforms (e.g., Twitter) for influenza surveillance.[95] Such surveillance and forecasting of specific diseases is of great significance for public health professionals who can send timely alerts to the public and prepare adequate resources to address outbreaks.

Another notable application of CSS in health is the mining of voluminous textual information on the Internet to understand and monitor how the public thinks about and feels toward health issues. By combining manual content analysis and automatic text mining algorithms, researchers analyzed information collected from various online sources (e.g., Twitter, blogs, and news) to understand public confidence toward vaccination,[96] discover major themes underlying public discussion about measles[97] and Zika,[98] and examine public sentiment toward depression and anxiety disorder.[99]

A third application of CSS in public health is to investigate how offline and online social connections among individuals may lead to the diffusion of health behaviors. By creatively utilizing several large-scale longitudinal datasets, Nicholas Christakis, James Fowler, and their colleagues[100–103] conducted a series of studies to investigate how a specific health phenomenon (e.g., obesity, smoking, alcohol consumption, drug use, and depression) can spread across network ties. Researchers have designed experiments on social media platforms (e.g., Facebook and Twitter) to examine how individuals' online connections may lead to changes in health behavior in various domains, such as fitness,[104,105] sexual health,[106] and smoking.[107]

With the increasing availability of datasets from more platforms and the rapid development of computational algorithms, the CSS paradigm will contribute more theoretical insights and methodological options for dissemination and implementation research in health.

---

utilization and technology transfer research have contributed to the evidence-based medicine and evidence-based public health emphases in D&I. The authors suggest that D&I researchers and practitioners will continue to find relevance and applicability in these former research traditions as they seek ways to study and apply new information and communication technologies to the challenges of dissemination activity by innovation proponents, diffusion responses by adopters, and then subsequent implementation and sustained use.

SUGGESTED READINGS

Readings

Dearing JW, Smith DK, Larson RS, Estabrooks CA. Designing for diffusion of a biomedical intervention. *Am J Prev Med.* 2013;44(1S2):70–76.
The authors suggest how diffusion concepts can be applied during strategic planning for the roll-out of an evidence-based intervention for HIV/AIDS prevention. The article emphasizes the importance of formative evaluation to understand and then appeal to the

motivations of potential adopters and implementers in community health centers.

Estabrooks C, Derksen L, Winther C, et al. The intellectual structure and substance of the knowledge utilization field: a longitudinal author co-citation analysis, 1945 to 2004. *Implement Sci.* 2008;3(1):49. *This article is a bibliographic analysis of the knowledge utilization field between World War II and the present and how it has evolved in that time. The authors cite the emergence of evidence-based medicine during this time period, a major advance with significant influences on models of evidence-based practice in other fields, including public health.*

Green LW, Ottoson JM, Garcia C, Hiatt RA. Diffusion theory and knowledge dissemination, utilization, and integration in public health. *Annu Rev Public Health.* 2009;30:151-174. *Green et al. provide a rigorous review of the public health implications of diffusion, dissemination, and implementation to improve public health practice and guide the design of future research. The article suggests a decentralized approach to D&I, as well as ways diffusion may be combined with other theories.*

Rogers EM. *Diffusion of innovations.* 5th ed. New York: Free Press; 2003. *Rogers's classic text on how ideas and opinions diffuse over time through various communication channels and networks. Because many new ideas involve taking a risk, people seek out others who have already adopted it. As a result, the new idea is spread through social networks over a period of weeks, months, or years.*

REFERENCES

1. *Health Psychol.* 2005;24(5).
2. *Acad Manage Exec.* 2005;19(2).
3. *J Health Commun.* 2004; 9 Suppl 1.
4. *Metro Univ.* 2006;17(4).
5. *Am J Pub Health.* 2006;96(2).
6. *Am J Prev Med.* 2006;31(4S).
7. *AIDS Educ Prev.* 2006;18 (Suppl A).
8. *J Pub Health Manag Pract.* 2008(14), 2.
9. *Res Soc Work Pract.* 2009;19(5).
10. *New Dir Eval.* 2009; Winter 2009(124).
11. Institute of Medicine. Crossing the quality chasm: A new health system for the 21st century. Washington, DC: Author; 2001.
12. Moffitt RA. Forecasting the effects of scaling up social programs: An economics perspective. In: Schneider B, McDonald S, editors. *Scale-up education.* Vol. 1. Lanham, MD: Rowman & Littlefield; 2007:173-186.
13. Scheirer MA, Dearing JW. An agenda for research on the sustainability of public health programs. *Am J Public Health.* 2011;101:2059-2067.
14. Rogers EM. *Diffusion of innovations.* 5th ed. New York: The Free Press; 2003.
15. Barker K. Diffusion of innovations: a world tour. *J Health Commun.* 2004;9:131-137.
16. Green LW, Gottlieb NH, Parcel GS. Diffusion theory extended and applied. *Adv Health Educ Promot.* 1991;3:91-117.
17. Rogers EM, Cartano DG. Methods of measuring opinion leadership. *Public Opin Quart.* 1962;26(3):435-441.
18. Kim DK, Dearing JW, eds. *Health communication research measures.* 2nd ed. New York: Peter Lang Inc.; 2016.
19. Flynn LR, Goldsmith RE, Eastman JK. Opinion leaders and opinion seekers: two new measurement scales. *J Acad Market Sci.* 1996;24(2):137.
20. Dearing JW. Social marketing and the diffusion of innovations. In: Stewart DW, editor. *Handbook of persuasion and social marketing.* New York: Praeger; 2014:35-66.
21. Borgatti SP, Mehra A, Brass DJ, Labianca G. Network analysis in the social sciences. *Science.* 2009;323(5916):892-895.
22. Lü L, Chen D, Ren X-L, Zhang Q-M, Zhang Y-C, Zhou T. Vital nodes identification in complex networks. *Physics Reports.* 2016;650:1-63.
23. Burt RS. The network structure of social capital. *Res Organ Behav.* 2000;22:345-423.
24. Bavelas A. Communication patterns in task-oriented groups. *J Acoust Soc Am.* 1950;22:725-730.
25. Bonacich P. Power and centrality: a family of measures. *Am J Sociol.* 1987;92(5):1170-1182.
26. Freeman LC. Centrality in social networks: conceptual clarification. *Soc Networks.* 1979;1(3):215-239.
27. Albalawi Y, Sixsmith J. Identifying Twitter influencer profiles for health promotion in Saudi Arabia. *Health Promot Intl.* 2017;32(3):456-463.
28. Holliday J, Audrey S, Campbell R, Moore L. Identifying well-connected opinion leaders for informal health promotion: the example of the ASSIST smoking prevention program. *Health Commun.* 2016;31(8):946-953.
29. Jonnalagadda S, Peeler R, Topham P. Discovering opinion leaders for medical topics using news articles. *J Biomed Semantics.* 2012;3:2-2.
30. Wang X, Shi J, Chen L, Peng T-Q. An examination of users' influence in online HIV/AIDS communities. *Cyberpsych Beh Soc N.* 2016;19(5):314-320.
31. Dangalchev C. Residual closeness in networks. *Physica A: Stat Mech Appl.* 2006;365(2):556-564.
32. Klemm K, Serrano MÁ, Eguíluz VM, Miguel MS. A measure of individual role in collective dynamics. *Sci Rep.* 2012;2:292.

33. Zhang J-X, Chen D-B, Dong Q, Zhao Z-D. Identifying a set of influential spreaders in complex networks. *Sci Rep.* 2016;6:27823.

34. Brownson RC, Ballew P, Brown KL et al. The effect of disseminating evidence-based interventions that promote physical activity to health departments. *Am J Public Health.* 2007;97(10):1900–1907.

35. Gigerenzer G, Reinhard S. *Bounded rationality: The adaptive toolbox.* Cambridge, MA: The MIT Press; 2001.

36. Kerckhoff AC, Back KW, Miller N. Sociometric patterns in hysterical contagion. *Sociometry* 1965;28(1):2–15.

37. Katz E. Theorizing diffusion: Tarde and Sorokin revisited. *The Ann Am Acad Politi SS.* 1999;566:144–155.

38. Katz E, Levin ML, Hamilton H. Traditions of research on the diffusion of innovation. *Am Sociol Rev.* 1963;28(2):237–252.

39. Orleans CT. Increasing the demand for and use of effective smoking-cessation treatments reaping the full health benefits of tobacco-control science and policy gains--in our lifetime. *Am J Prev Med.* 2007;33(6 Suppl):S340-S348.

40. Ryan B, Gross NC. The diffusion of hybrid seed corn in two Iowa communities. *Rural Sociol.* 1943;8(1):15–24.

41. Valente TW, Rogers EM. The origins and development of the diffusion of innovations paradigm as an example of scientific growth. *Sci Commun.* 1995;16(3):242–273.

42. Coleman JS, Katz E, Menzel H. The diffusion of an innovation among physicians. *Sociometry.* 1957;20:253–270.

43. Crane D. *Invisible colleges: Diffusion of knowledge in scientific communities.* Chicago: University of Chicago Press; 1972.

44. Estabrooks CA, Derksen L, Winther C et al. The intellectual structure and substance of the knowledge utilization field: a longitudinal author co-citation analysis, 1945 to 2004. *Implement Sci* 2008;3:49.

45. Rogers EM. A conceptual variable analysis of technological change. *PhD Dissertation* 1957; Ames, IA (Iowa State University).

46. Rogers EM. The fourteenth paw: growing up on an Iowa Farm in the 1930s. Singapore: *Asian Media Information and Communication Centre*; 2008.

47. Singhal A, Dearing JW. *Communication of innovations: A journey with Ev Rogers.* New Delhi: Sage Publications, Inc.; 2006.

48. Montgomery MR, Casterline JB. The diffusion of fertility control in Taiwan: evidence from pooled cross-section time-series models. *Pop Stud.* 1993;47(3):457–479.

49. Weiss CH, Bucuvalas MJ. *Social science research and decision-making.* New York: Columbia University Press; 1980.

50. Kingdon JW. *Agendas, alternatives, and public policies.* New York: Longman; 2003.

51. Anderson LM, Brownson RC, Fullilove MT et al. Evidence-based public health policy and practice: promises and limits. *Am J Prev Med* 2005;28(5 Suppl):226–230.

52. Blake SC, Ottoson JM. Knowledge utilization: implications of evaluation. *New Dir Eval.* 2009;124:21–34.

53. Backer TE. Knowledge utilization: the third wave. *Knowledge: Creation, Diffusion, Utilization.* 1991;12(3):225–240.

54. Green LW, Ottoson JM, Garcia C, Hiatt RA. Diffusion theory and knowledge dissemination, utilization, and integration in public health. *Annu Rev Public Health.* 2009;30:151–174.

55. O'Dell C, Grayson CJ. If only we knew what we know: identification and transfer of internal best practices. *Calif Manage Rev.* 1998;40(3):154–174.

56. Leonard-Barton D. Implementation as mutual adaptation of technology and organization. *Res Policy.* 1988;17(5):251–267.

57. Dunn W, Holzener B, Zaltman G. Knowledge utilization. In: Husen T, Postlethwaite TN, editors. *The international encyclopedia of education.* Vol. 1. New York: Pergamon Press; 1985.

58. Estabrooks CA, Thompson DS, Lovely JJE, Hofmeyer A. A guide to knowledge translation theory. *J Contin Educ Health Prof.* 2006;26(1):25–36.

59. Lavis JN, Robertson D, Woodside J, McLeod CB, Abelson J. How can research organizations more effectively transfer research kknowledge to decision makers. *Milbank Quart.* 2003;81(2):221–248.

60. Sackett DL, Rosenberg WMC, Gray JAM, Haynes RB, Richardson WS. Evidence based medicine: what it is and what it isn't. *Br Med J.* 1996;312:71–72.

61. Mykhalovskiy E, Weir L. The problem of evidence-based medicine: directions for social science. *Soc Sci Med.* 2004;59(5):1059–1069.

62. Haynes RB. What kind of evidence is it that evidence-based medicine advocates want health care providers and consumers to pay attention to? *BMC Health Serv Res.* 2002;2(1):3.

63. Sackett DL. Clinical epidemiology. what, who, and whither. *J Clin Epidemiol.* 2002;55(12):1161–1166.

64. Brownson RC, Fielding JE, Maylahn CM. Evidence-based public health: a fundamental concept for public health practice. *Annu Rev Public Health.* 2009;30:175–201.

65. Simmons, R., Fajans, P., & Ghiron L. (2007). *Scaling up health service delivery from pilot innovations to policies and programmes.* Geneva, Switzerland: Department of Reproductive Health and Research World Health Organization.

66. Browning LD. Lists and stories as organizational communication. *Commun Theory.* 1992;2:281–302.

67. Greene JD. Communication of results and utlization in participatory program evaluation. *Eval Program Plann.* 1988;11(4):341–351.

68. Doolin B. Narratives of change: discourse, technology and organization. *Organization.* 2003;10(4):751–770.

69. Dearing JW. Evolution of diffusion and dissemination theory. *J Public Health Manag.* 2008;14(2):99–108.

70. Rogers EM. *Communication strategies for family planning.* New York: Free Press; 1973.

71. Office of Behavioral and Social Sciences Research. *putting evidence into practice: The OBSSR Report of the Working Group on the Integration of Effective Behavioral Treatments into Clinical Care.* Washington, DC: Author; 1997.

72. von Hippel E. *Democratizing innovation.* Cambridge, MA: The MIT Press; 2005.

73. Edejer TT. Disseminating health information in developing countries: the role of the internet. *Br Med J.* 2000;321(7264):797–800.

74. Dearing JW, Maibach E, Buller DB. A convergent diffusion and social marketing approach for disseminating proven approaches to physical activity promotion. *Am J Prev Med.* 2006;1–13.

75. Korp P. Health on the Internet: Implications for health promotion. *Health Educ Res.* 2006;21(1):78–86.

76. Atherton H, Huckvale C, Car J. Communicating health promotion and disease prevention information to patients via email: a review. *J Telemed Telecare.* 2010;16(4):172–175.

77. Tuerk PW, Fortney J, Bosworth HB et al. Toward the development of national telehealth services: the role of Veterans Health Administration and future directions for research. *Telemed J E Health.* 2010;16(1):115–117.

78. Dellifraine JL, Dansky KH. Home-based telehealth: a review and meta-analysis. *J Telemed Telecare.* 2008;14(2):62–66.

79. Eysenbach G, Sa ER, Diepgen TL. Shopping around the Internet today and tomorrow: towards the millenium of cybermedicine. *Br Med J.* 1999;319(7220):1294.

80. Jadad AR, Haynes RB, Hunt D, Browman GP. The Internet and evidence-based decision-making: a needed synergy for efficient knowledge management in health care. *CMAJ.* 2000;162(3):362–365.

81. Dearing JW, Kreuter MW. Designing for diffusion: how can we increase uptake of cancer communication innovations? *Patient Educ Couns,* 2010; 81S:100–110.

82. Kee KF, Sparks L, Struppa DC et al. Information diffusion, Facebook clusters, and the simplicial model of social aggregation: a computational simulation of simplicial diffusers for community health interventions. *Health Commun.* 2016; 31(4): 385–399.

83. Liang YJ, Kee KF. Developing and validating the A-B-C framework of information diffusion on social media. *New Media Soc.* in press. doi: https://doi.org/10.1177/1461444816661552

84. Hawn C. Take two aspirin and tweet me in the morning: how Twitter, Facebook, and other social media are reshaping health care. *Health Aff (Millwood)W* 2009;28(2):361–368.

85. Shirky C. *Here comes everybody: The power of organizing without organizations.* New York: Penguin Press; 2009.

86. Eysenbach G. Medicine 2.0: social networking, collaboration, participation, apomediation, and openness. *J Med Internet Res.* 2008;10(3):e22.

87. Griffiths F, Lindenmeyer A, Powell J, Lowe P, Thorogood M. Why are health care interventions delivered over the internet? A systematic review of the published literature. *J Med Internet Res.* 2006;8(2):e10.

88. Lazer D, Pentland A, Adamic L, et al. Computational social science. *Science.* 2009;323(5915):721–723.

89. Ginsberg J, Mohebbi MH, Patel RS, Brammer L, Smolinski MS, Brilliant L. Detecting influenza epidemics using search engine query data. *Nature.* 2009;457(7232):1012–1014.

90. Butler D. When Google got flu wrong. *Nature.* 2013;494(7436):155–156.

91. Lazer D, Kennedy R, King G, Vespignani A. The parable of Google flu: traps in big data analysis. *Science.* 2014;343(6176):1203–1205.

92. Althouse BM, Ng YY, Cummings DAT. Prediction of Dengue incidence using search query surveillance. *Plos Neglected Tropical Diseases.* 2011;5(8):e1258.

93. Walcott BP, Nahed BV, Kahle KT, Redjal N, Coumans J-V. Determination of geographic variance in stroke prevalence using Internet search engine analytics. *Neurosurg Focus.* 2011;30(6):E19.

94. Zhou X, Ye J, Feng Y. Tuberculosis surveillance by analyzing Google trends. *IEEE T Bio-Med Eng.* 2011;58(8):2247–2254.

95. Broniatowski DA, Paul MJ, Dredze M. National and local influenza surveillance through Twitter: an analysis of the 2012-2013 influenza epidemic. *PLOS ONE.* 2013;8(12):e83672.

96. Larson HJ, Smith DMD, Paterson P, et al. Measuring vaccine confidence: analysis of data obtained by a media surveillance system used to analyse public concerns about vaccines. *Lancet Infect Dis.* 2013;13(7):606–613.

97. Mollema L, Harmsen IA, Broekhuizen E, et al. Disease detection or public opinion reflection? Content analysis of Tweets, other social media, and online newspapers during the measles outbreak in the Netherlands in 2013. *J Med Internet Res.* 2015;17(5):e128.

98. Fu K-W, Liang H, Saroha N, Tse ZTH, Ip P, Fung IC-H. How people react to Zika virus outbreaks on Twitter? A computational content analysis. *Am J Infect Control.* 2016;44(12):1700–1702.

99. Ji X, Chun SA, Wei Z, Geller J. Twitter sentiment classification for measuring public health concerns. *Soc Net Anal Mining.* 2015;5(1):13.

100. Christakis NA, Fowler JH. The spread of obesity in a large social network over 32 Years. *N Engl J M.* 2007;357(4):370–379.

101. Christakis NA, Fowler JH. The collective dynamics of smoking in a large social network. *NEngl J Med.* 2008;358(21):2249–2258.

102. Rosenquist JN, Fowler JH, Christakis NA. Social network determinants of depression. *Mol Psychiatry.* 2011;16(3):273–281.

103. Rosenquist JN, Murabito J, Fowler JH, Christakis NA. The spread of aocohol consumption behavior in a large social ntwork. *Ann Intern Med.* 2010;152(7):426-W141.

104. Centola D. An experimental study of homophily in the adoption of health behavior. *Science.* 2011;334(6060):1269.

105. Turner-McGrievy G, Tate D. Tweets, Apps, and Pods: results of the 6-month Mobile Pounds Off Digitally (Mobile POD) randomized weight-loss intervention among adults. *J Med Internet Res.* 2011;13(4):e120.

106. Bull SS, Levine DK, Black SR, Schmiege SJ, Santelli J. Social media–delivered sexual health intervention: a cluster randomized controlled trial. *Am J Prev Med.* 2012;43(5):467–474.

107. Graham AL, Cobb NK, Papandonatos GD, et al. A randomized trial of Internet and telephone treatment for smoking cessation. *Arch Intern Med.* 2011;171(1):46–53.

4

Ethical Issues in Dissemination and Implementation Research

JAMES M. DUBOIS AND BETH PRUSACZYK

INTRODUCTION

In contrast to theoretical ethics, which focuses on areas such as understanding the nature of ethical reasoning and ethical language, professional ethics are specific to a particular activity such as practicing medicine, investment banking, or doing research. Professional ethics are frequently a concoction of norms stemming from diverse sources including federal and state laws and regulations, the codes of professional associations, institutional policies, general ethical principles, scientific standards, and the decisions of oversight boards or stakeholder committees. Within the domain of research ethics, the content of these norms is also highly varied. In the broadest sense, the responsible conduct of research involves protection of human subjects as well as standards for ensuring data integrity, good mentoring, authorship, peer review, and the social value of research.[1] This chapter focuses primarily on the protection of human participants in D&I studies. It begins by reviewing the Belmont principles that undergird US research regulations and considering the ethical case for D&I research. It then proceeds to examine some ethical issues that might arise during the course of a public health, D&I research agenda in middle schools.

Moving beyond the content of the ethics of a profession, one may also focus on fostering ethical behavior. This can be accomplished not merely by teaching rules but also by increasing sensitivity to how ethical issues arise in specific contexts, fostering good ethical decision-making skills, creating an ethical climate in which leaders model good behavior and clearly state expectations, and by providing oversight.[2–4] After examining how D&I raises special challenges in determining which rules and regulations apply to a study (increasing ethical sensitivity), we consider a series of decision-making strategies that can guide behavior in challenging situations that arise in D&I research, for example, when disagreement exists regarding which rules apply to a study or stakeholders seek competing goals.

THE BELMONT PRINCIPLES

The Belmont Report: Ethical Principles and Guidelines for the Protection of Human Subjects of Research describes three general principles that are widely recognized in society and have implications for the ethical conduct of human subjects research.[5] The principle of *respect for persons* requires that insofar as human beings are capable of reasoning and self-determination, we should provide them with information about research studies and solicit their voluntary, informed consent. When human beings lack the cognitive capacity to provide informed consent (for example, due to young age or cognitive impairments) or when voluntariness might be compromised (for example, by being institutionalized or in a subordinate relationship to the researchers or sponsors of a project) then they are vulnerable and deserve additional protections. The *principle of beneficence* reminds us that research should pursue benefits that are proportionate to the risks involved, and that risks should be minimized and managed throughout studies. The *principle of justice* requires that, in general, those who are likely to benefit from a research study are the ones who should undertake the risks of research participation. Participants should not be recruited simply because it is convenient to access them (e.g., due to institutionalization).

When the Belmont Report was produced in the 1970s the emphasis was on avoiding the exploitation of vulnerable groups of individuals as occurred in Nazi experimentations on human subjects held in concentration camps and in the Public Health Service study of syphilis at

TABLE 4.1 BELMONT PRINCIPLES FOR THE PROTECTION OF HUMAN SUBJECTS APPLIED TO D&I RESEARCH

Belmont Principle	General Requirements	Application Questions in D&I Research
Respect for Persons	• Obtain informed consent • Provide additional protections when participants are incapable of providing informed consent	• Who needs to provide informed consent when implementation is studied? • How can the voluntariness of participation be ensured when participants are students or employees?
Beneficence	• Minimize risk of harms, establish appropriate protections • Ensure anticipated benefits justify risks	• Must implementation trials have equipoise? • When interventions are effective, how can benefits be provided to control groups?
Justice	• The populations that undertake risks in research should also be beneficiaries of research • Vulnerable populations should not be targeted due to convenience	• How can community partners be engaged to address concerns about social justice within D&I studies? • When is there an obligation to engage in D&I research in order to justify the investment in efficacy research?

Tuskegee. Today, we additionally recognize that justice requires that research serves people in need without regard to their sex, sexual preferences, or financial means. Ironically, the desire to protect vulnerable populations—for example, those living with often stigmatized diseases such as HIV or prisoners—may prevent them from benefiting from research participation and may slow advances in the treatment or prevention of diseases that disproportionately affect them.[6,7]

While the Belmont Report focused primarily on the treatment of research participants, which has led some to question their suitability for public health research,[8] each of its principles may be adapted to communities from which participants are drawn.[9] For example, while only individuals can provide informed consent in the traditional sense, community permission may be sought through a variety of means such as holding town hall meetings, surveying community members, establishing community advisory boards, or including community members as full research partners using action research or community-based participatory research designs.[8,10,11] Engaging communities may serve to increase transparency, provide researchers with valuable guidance, facilitate recruitment by fostering buy-in, and provide the permission of representatives

from the community.[11-14] Similarly, risks may be considered not only to individuals, but also to communities, including the risk of breaching trust or stigmatizing groups. Within some public health circles, the need to adapt general ethical principles to the special features of communities has led to recognition of a fourth principle, *respect for communities*.[15,16]

Table 4.1 presents the Belmont principles and illustrates how they relate to current questions about ethics in D&I research.

THE ETHICAL CASE FOR D&I RESEARCH

Many have argued that funders and researchers have an ethical duty to disseminate and implement knowledge and evidence from efficacy trials so their full benefits can be realized.[17-19] Only through implementation science can "our nation's investment in research in the life sciences yield the pay-off that patients and the public deserve."[19] The Public Health Leadership Society published *Principles of the Ethical Practice of Public Health*, which includes principles on the dissemination and implementation of information, policies, and programs.[18] One of the underlying values and beliefs of the principles states that information is not gathered for "idle interest" but that "Public health should seek to translate available information into timely action." The Society continues by saying that people have a *responsibility* to act on the basis of what they know.

Mann offers several reasons why researchers have an ethical obligation to disseminate research findings, including the need for providing social value, facilitating production of credible and relevant systematic reviews and meta-analyses, honoring the altruistic motivation of study participants and participants' right to know the results of studies they were enrolled in, and complying with codes of ethical conduct that require sharing new knowledge with colleagues and the public.[20] Mann believes it is the responsibility of research ethics committees (such as Institutional Review Boards [IRBs] in the United States) to ensure dissemination occurs; we believe the responsibility is shared with investigators as well.

As described in numerous chapters in this book, we know that some strategies for D&I are significantly more effective in achieving the goals of knowledge transfer, research utilization or adoption, and diffusion within communities, including utilizing audit and feedback, learning collaboratives, facilitation, and local needs assessments.[21–25] Thus, there is an imperative not only to engage in D&I, but also in research on D&I aimed at making D&I more effective in achieving their goals.

COMMON ETHICAL CHALLENGES IN D&I RESEARCH

Several authors have argued that that researchers and review boards must think about the ethical challenges of clinical efficacy studies differently from those of D&I research, a point that has also been made by others.[19,26–30] This chapter considers four questions that arise in D&I research more frequently than in common research activities such as drug trials:

1. Is it human subjects research?
2. Who are your research participants, and who should provide informed consent?
3. Is equipoise necessary?
4. How can scientific rigor be protected in real-world settings (e.g., when participation cannot be blinded or participants are not interested in D&I research)?

A Focal Case

In order to illustrate how these questions arise when conducting D&I research, we will build upon a case presented in chapter 24 on "Health Dissemination and Implementation within Schools." Lee and Gortmaker describe Planet Health, an obesity prevention program in middle schools. The Planet Health program aims to prevent obesity by "increasing physical activity, decreasing television viewing, improving diet through increased fruit and vegetable intake, and moderating fat intake."[31(p. 468)] The program is built around self-assessment and lessons delivered by social studies, language arts, math, and science teachers and micro units delivered by physical educators. The Planet Health field trial not only aimed to study the efficacy of the program, but also how the program was implemented and disseminated within the real-world context of schools. The project used a group- or cluster-randomized trial design. Initially, 10 schools that were matched on key characteristics were randomized to receive the Planet Health intervention or nothing (until the end of the project period).

In what follows, we consider diverse projects related to the Planet Health project—both real and fictitious—as well as ethical challenges and potential ethical solutions—again, both real and fictitious.

Is It Human Subjects Research?

US federal regulations define research as "a systematic investigation, including research development, testing and evaluation, designed to develop or contribute to generalizable knowledge" (45CFR46.102(d)).

Dissemination and implementation are systematic activities. As defined in chapter 2, dissemination involves spreading evidence-based practices to a target group using planned strategies. Implementation involves using evidence-based practices within a real-world setting. Understood in this manner, D&I activities do not contribute to generalizable knowledge and do not constitute research. Accordingly, many aspects of research ethics such as review by an IRB, informed consent of participants, and privacy protections may not pertain to D&I activities.

In contrast to dissemination activities, D&I research aim to study the effects of interventions and diverse variables on outcomes such as uptake of evidence-based practices. Chapter 23 by Hamilton and Mittman, describes eleven different research activities commonly performed across the life of an implementation research program, ranging from preimplementation studies through four phases of implementation studies.

Whether human subjects protections and review by an IRB are required is primarily determined by the purpose of a study and whether human subjects or identifiable information about individuals are involved. If the purpose of an implementation project is strictly to improve outcomes at a hospital or the health of children at a school, then the activity may be treated as a quality improvement project. However, even when federal regulations do not apply to quality improvement projects, institutions or community organizations may nevertheless require some level of review and oversight.[32] Similarly, if a study does not examine outcomes at the level of individuals, but only at the level of clusters or groups, it may not meet the definition of human subjects research and may not be addressed by research regulations. However, if determining the outcomes of a group involves examining identifiable, individual information, the regulations and IRB review do apply.[15]

Who Are Your Research Participants? Who Should Provide Consent?

D&I studies can be complicated because they may collect data on diverse outcomes, particularly in hybrid effectiveness-implementation designs.[33] For example, in the Planet Health study, investigators may be concerned with effectiveness— whether middle-school children who receive the intervention have lower rates of obesity than children who do not receive the intervention. If the effectiveness outcome involves gathering data through interaction with the children or in some other manner that involves the collection of individually identifiable data, then the children are research subjects. Depending on the risk level of the intervention and the feasibility of obtaining consent, an IRB might (a) waive elements of consent (e.g., permit an opt-out approach); (b) require written, signed parental permission; and (c) require the verbal or written signed assent of the children. In several studies by the Planet Health principal investigator, the authors state that they obtained both the written consent (permission) of parents and the consent (assent) of the children.[34,35] Requiring consent to establish the effectiveness of a hybrid D&I intervention can present a significant burden in school settings; it may mean excluding from participation students

who might benefit from the program, and it might be finding alternative classroom space and meaningful activities for nonparticipating children. In other cases, however, a participating school may have the authority to make participation in a project's educational activities required or at least routine, and consent and assent are sought only for the collection of individual data.[34]

In other legs of the Planet Health project, the outcomes were all related to implementation, rather than effectiveness: "dose, acceptability, feasibility, and intent to continue use." All of these outcomes could be measured by engaging teachers as subjects; student participation was not necessary.[31] A common challenge investigators face when conducting D&I research relates to the collection of data from employees or providers in organizations whose supervisors or administrative leaders may have access to or request access to the data. Employees or providers may worry that their participation in the study or their feedback on the intervention or implementation strategies could impact their job security or standing in the organization. Investigators should anticipate this prior to beginning the study and map out strategies to ensure the privacy of employees or providers is protected.

Is Equipoise Necessary?

Within the world of efficacy trials such as randomized, controlled trials of pharmaceuticals, it is common to speak of clinical equipoise as a requirement[36] (though even in this domain the concept is somewhat controversial and the term is not used in the Common Rule, 45CFR46).[37] Clinical equipoise is "a state of genuine uncertainty on the part of the clinical investigator regarding the comparative therapeutic merits of each arm in a trial."[36(p. 141)] For example, in a study with three arms that compares a new drug to a standard of care drug and to placebo, equipoise would require uncertainty about the comparative merits of each arm. If one embraces clinical equipoise as an ethical requirement for clinical trials, then the use of placebo cannot always be justified. For example, if a serious medical condition urgently requires some form of treatment (e.g., lung cancer), then a placebo must be administered alongside a known effective treatment. However, if all available medications have serious side effects (while placebo rarely does) and a positive placebo effect has been observed in a clinical population (as is often the case in patients with depression), then the use of placebo might be justified.[38]

Implementation trials rarely occur in the absence of prior trials demonstrating efficacy. However, the point of implementation trials such as Planet Health is to establish effectiveness in real-world settings (as well as to examine factors that affect implementation outcomes) (see chapter 24). That is to say, the fact that a strategy for preventing obesity in children has been proven efficacious in a controlled setting does not mean it will be effective in the real-world setting of a middle school, which requires effective training of teachers, buy-in from administrators and teachers, and resources to sustain the program on a larger scale. So, uncertainty does exist regarding the comparative merits of being in the intervention arm versus a control arm.

Moreover, it is unclear whether the notion of equipoise—which arose from within the patient–physician relationship, in which patients present with health needs in the context of a fiduciary relationship[39]—should be extrapolated to public health settings. Some argue that the notion could be grounded in the relationship of trust that exists between the state and research subjects (or by analogy, a school and its students), and it remains useful as IRBs evaluate studies.[40] However, The Ottawa Statement on the Ethical Design and Conduct of Cluster Randomized Trials states that:

> Researchers must adequately justify the choice of the control condition. When the control arm is usual practice or no treatment, individuals in the control arm must not be deprived of effective care or programs *to which they would have access, were there no trial.* (p. 7)[15] [emphasis added]

That is, in a nontherapeutic trial—a trial in which no patient–physician relationship preexists to treat or prevent an illness or disease—one should focus on not harming, but there is no strict obligation to provide benefits to which one ordinarily would not have access. Nevertheless, when prior trials lead study teams and community members to believe an intervention will improve the lives of participants, the question of justice cannot be avoided. Community input may be particularly important when it is not feasible (e.g., due to limited funding) to provide everyone with a known effective intervention.[41] However, when it is feasible—except for reasons of scientific design (specifically the need for a control group)—then it is possible to provide control groups with the intervention following

the conclusion of the study, if the intervention proves effective.[34] This approach is often defensible because until the conclusion of the implementation study, genuine uncertainty exists whether it will have its intended effect in a real-world setting. In fact this approach is possible in D&I through the increasing use of the stepped-wedge research design, in which the intervention is rolled out to all participants over time.[42] This design is adaptive and as the intervention and strategies are rolled out, data are collected and analyzed, then used to adapt the roll-out for the next group of participants. This ongoing data collection and adaptation does present potential challenges with IRBs who may request ongoing review and approval in tandem with the ongoing study procedures.

How Can Scientific Rigor Be Protected in Real-World Settings?

Emanuel, Wendler, and Grady reviewed international codes of research ethics to answer the question, "what makes research with human subjects ethical?"[43] *Scientific validity* was among the seven requirements that they identified. Research that lacks scientific merit exposes participants to risks for no purpose and wastes scarce research resources.

Threats to scientific validity in real-world settings are manifold. First, in real-world settings, it is difficult to identify all the factors that might mediate, moderate, or confound effects of interventions. Randomization may help establish that an intervention was effective; but implementation science aims to understand why and when it is effective in complex settings such as hospitals and schools. This may require not only statistical expertise, but very large sample sizes, which in turn requires tremendous resources and buy-in from stakeholder groups.

In 2007, the research team that implemented the Planet Health and other health promotion programs in public schools published a "lessons learned" paper. Although the paper discusses few specific challenges that arose within these studies, focusing rather on positive lessons (above all, the need for early and ongoing stakeholder engagement, liaisons between research teams and schools, and project champions), it offers the following general observation:

> Creating public health partnerships with schools is challenging for many reasons, including the numerous academic and non-academic demands placed on schools. In

addition, school programs often lack sufficient funds, are subject to political vicissitudes, exist in complex bureaucracies that foster fragmentation, and vary across localities.[44(p. 2)]

The authors of a paper on the importance of community engagement for ensuring the ethical design and conduct of research added caveats throughout. In particular, they offered two observations. First, communities are never fully engaged; they may lack organization, leaders, or spokespeople; they may be heterogeneous and speak with competing voices rather than one voice; and individuals may not want to engage researchers. Second, while community engagement may improve the conduct of research in many ways, it can also compromise scientific rigor when done poorly or when goals are not shared.[11]

How can one protect the rigor of a research study when problems arise, for example, when gatekeepers or IRBs resist the use of a control group, when parental consent is required and parents are not heavily engaged in their children's school activities, or when a commitment to co-design of a study[27] requires that the design be adaptive to emerging stakeholder concerns? The following sections offers strategies for addressing these and other concerns that may arise in D&I research.

STRATEGIES FOR ETHICAL DECISION-MAKING

A recent root cause analysis of why researchers were referred for remediation of research compliance and integrity violations found that researchers are at risk when they are overextended, rules and expectations are ambiguous (e.g., when moving into new areas of research or working in an unfamiliar culture), or relationships or communication are poor.[45] Engaging stakeholders well is time consuming (though often time saving in the long run), which is challenging for busy researchers; each institution has its own culture; and communication is difficult in studies that involve multiple sites or that gather data at several levels (e.g., schools, teachers, and students). Rules are often ambiguous in implementation trials because they include elements that do not exist in the standard clinical trials that IRBs routinely review. Relationships can be strained when diverse stakeholders have competing goals for a project.

What follows offers a series of evidence-informed professional decision-making strategies that can serve researchers well as they navigate

the challenges that may arise in D&I research.[46,47] As observed repeatedly throughout this chapter, stakeholder engagement is often key to navigating ethical and scientific issues in D&I research.[16,27,44] Each of these strategies can be applied by individual investigators, or adapted for application by research teams.

Seek Help

Uncertainty can arise at all stages of research regarding logistical, scientific, ethical or regulatory matters. Seeking help—the input of stakeholders, compliance officers, research ethicists, or more experienced colleagues—may provide new information, identify new options, or establish new relationships that can enable projects to move forward positively. Given the novelty of many D&I designs or interventions, seeking help from investigators who have previously conducted D&I research on the ethical issues they encountered and how they solved them may prove especially beneficial.

Manage Emotions

As research moves from experimental settings to real-world settings, projects become more politically charged, a greater number of competing voices must be heard, and accordingly, tensions can run high.[11,44] Managing emotions is a key component to successful professional decision-making and relationship development.[48,49] Strategies for managing emotions can include reappraising a situation, engaging in stress management practices such as relaxation or mindfulness, or simply taking a time out.[48,50,51]

Anticipate Consequences

In research and many other endeavors, we often focus on information that confirms what we expect.[52,53] Yet, deliberations about risks, benefits, fair outcomes, and protection of the trust of stakeholder groups, requires consideration of possible short-term and long-term, and positive and negative consequences of a project for different stakeholders.[54] Anticipating consequences is often best done in conjunction with many of the other strategies listed here, including seeking help, managing emotions, and testing assumptions.

Recognize Rules and Context

Recognizing rules sounds like a straightforward task. However, D&I research frequently spans the worlds of academic institutions and service organizations (e.g., hospitals, public health agencies, schools), which may have different rules and procedures. Moreover, research regulations require interpretation as they are applied to specific research protocols; for better or worse, the interpretation of rules offered by IRBs carries more authority than the interpretation of investigators. Additionally, community organizations may have unwritten rules that guide their interactions with researchers, rules that must be satisfied before partnership agreements can be established or executed successfully. Again, other strategies may assist in the execution of this strategy—particularly seeking help (e.g., calling the IRB or engaging communities through focus groups) and testing assumptions. Last, as with all human subjects research, there may be additional rules and regulations surrounding D&I research with some communities and populations such as prisoners, American Indians or Alaskan Natives, or pregnant women.

Test Assumptions and Motives

Researchers make a lot of assumptions, for example, assumptions about the value of a project, the needs of communities, the best design to test a hypothesis, the feasibility of recruiting participants, and the risks of a study to individuals or communities. Problems can arise when these assumptions are either mistaken or are not shared by other stakeholders. Good communication with others is an excellent way of testing assumptions. Sharing our thought processes with others enables correction of bias and reappraisal of situations, which in turn may reduce anxiety and facilitate constructive problem-solving.[55]

Researchers may also assume that IRBs have all the information they need to make effective decisions. However, particularly with complex and unfamiliar study designs, this may not be the case. D&I researchers may benefit significantly from serving on IRBs or writing protocols with detailed engagement of ethical issues.

SUMMARY

While these strategies may be beneficial to all researchers, the authors believe they are of particular value to D&I researchers because the nature of their work—context specific, complex, and unfamiliar to many peers, collaborators, and reviewers—means they will deal with uncertainty and conflict on a regular basis, and solutions to the problems they face will rarely be found through simple reference principles, rules, or regulations.

SUGGESTED READINGS AND WEBSITES

Readings

Macklin R. Ethical challenges in implementation research. *Pub Health Ethics*. 2014;7(1):86–93.

A good overview of ethical issues that arise in implementation research by a leading ethicist.

Gopichandran V, Luyckx VA, Biller-Andorno N, et al. Developing the ethics of implementation research in health. *Implement Sci*. 2016;11(1):161.

A very recent and comprehensive overview of ethical issues in implementation research with case studies.

Weijer C, Grimshaw JM, Eccles MP, et al. The Ottawa Statement on the Ethical Design and Conduct of Cluster Randomized Trials. *PLoS Med*. 2012;9(11):e1001346.

A thoughtful consensus statement on the ethical design of cluster randomized trials, a study design commonly used in clinical effectiveness research. This resource may be particularly useful in engaging institutional research ethics committees or institutional review boards.

DuBois JM, Bailey-Burch B, Bustillos D, et al. Ethical issues in mental health research: the case for community engagement. *Curr Opin Psychiatry*. 2011;24(3):208–214.

This article makes the case for community engagement in research and illustrates diverse approaches to community engagement suitable for a wide range of study designs. This paper tries to move beyond the all-or-nothing (or community-based participatory research-or-nothing) approach to community engagement in research.

Selected Websites and Tools

The Belmont Report. https://www.hhs.gov/ohrp/regulations-and-policy/belmont-report/

This website provides the full text of the Belmont Report, which describes the principles of respect for persons, beneficence, and justice, and applies them to the context of human research. This framework has been particularly influential in the United States, where specific rules and regulations are supposed to be based upon these principles.

Public Health Ethics Resources hosted by the Centers for Disease Control and Prevention. https://www.cdc.gov/od/science/integrity/phethics/resources.htm

This website collects a variety of useful materials in the area of public health ethics, many of which are open access.

Public Health Ethics Training Materials from the Centers for Disease Control and Prevention. https://www.cdc.gov/od/science/integrity/phethics/trainingmaterials.htm

This website provides access to training materials developed by the CDC, as well as other open access training materials in the area of public health ethics.

REFERENCES

1. Shamoo AE, Resnik DB. *Responsible conduct of research*. 3rd ed. New York: Oxford University Press; 2015.
2. Antes AL, DuBois JM. Aligning objectives and assessment in responsible conduct of research instruction. *J Microbiol Biol Educ*. 2014;15(2).
3. Rest JR, Narvez D, Bebeau MJ, Thoma SJ. *Postconventional moral thinking: A Neo-Kohlbergian approach*. Mahwah, NJ: Lawrence Erlbaum Associates, Inc.; 1999.
4. Mulhearn TJ, Steele LM, Watts LL, Medeiros KE, Mumford MD, Connelly S. Review of instructional approaches in ethics education. *Sci Eng Ethics*. 2017;23(3):883–912.
5. National Commission. *The Belmont report: Ethical principles and guidelines for the protection of human subjects of research*. Washington, DC: Department of Health, Education, and Welfare. National Commission, for the Protection of Human Subjects of Biomedical and Behavioral Research; 1979.
6. King PA. Justice beyond Belmont. In: Childress JF, Meslin EM, Shapiro HT, eds. *Belmont revisited. Ethical principles for research with human subjects*. Washington, DC: Georgetown University Press; 2005:136–147.
7. DuBois JM, Beskow L, Campbell J, et al. Restoring balance: a consensus statement on the protection of vulnerable research participants. *Am J Public Health*. 2012;102(12):2220–2225.
8. Quinn S. Ethics in public health research: Protecting human subjects: the role of community advisory boards. *Am J Public Health*. 2004;94(6):918–922.
9. Gostin L. Ethical principles for the conduct of human subject research: population-based research and ethics. *Law Med Health Care*. 1991;19(3-4):191–201.
10. Ross LF, Loup A, Nelson RM, et al. The challenges of collaboration for academic and community partners in a research partnership: points to consider. *J Empir Res Hum Res Ethics*. 2010;5(1):19–31.
11. DuBois JM, Bailey-Burch B, Bustillos D, et al. Ethical issues in mental health research: the case for community engagement. *Curr Opin Psychiatry*. 2011;24(3):208–214.
12. Frerichs L, Kim M, Dave G, et al. Stakeholder Perspectives on Creating and Maintaining Trust in Community-Academic Research Partnerships. *Health Education & Behavior: The Official Publication Of The Society For Public Health Education*. 2016.
13. Ross LF, Loup A, Nelson RM, et al. Human subjects protections in community-engaged research: a research ethics framework. *J Empir Res Hum Res Ethics*. 2010;5(1):5–17.
14. Ross LF, Loup A, Nelson RM, et al. Nine key functions for a human subjects protection program for community-engaged research: points to consider. *J Empir Res Hum Res Ethics*. 2010;5(1):33–47.
15. Weijer C, Grimshaw JM, Eccles MP, et al. The Ottawa Statement on the Ethical Design and Conduct of Cluster Randomized Trials. *PLoS Med*. 2012;9(11):e1001346.
16. Weijer C. Protecting communities in research: philosophical and pragmatic challenges. *Cam Q Healthc Ethics*. 1999;8(4):501–513.
17. Woolf SH. The meaning of translational research and why it matters. *JAMA*. 2008;299(2):211–213.
18. Public Health Leadership Society from http://www.apha.org/~/media/files/pdf/member-groups/ethics_brochure.ashx.
19. Solomon MZ. The ethical urgency of advancing implementation science. *Am J Bioeth*. 2010;10(8):31–32.
20. Mann H. Research ethics committees and public dissemination of clinical trial results. *Lancet*. 2002;360(9330):406–408.
21. Brownson RC, Colditz GA, Proctor E, eds. *Dissemination and implementation research in health. Translating science into practice*. New York: Oxford University Press; 2012.
22. Grol R, Grimshaw J. From best evience to best practice: effective implementation of change in patients' care. *Lancet*. 2003;2015(362): 1225–1230. http://ac.els-cdn.com/S0140673603145461/1-s2.0-S0140673603145461-main.pdf?_tid=db5a546a-f809-11e4-bce5-00000aacb35e&   acdnat=1431368374_458f913b23b8d c6e1279aff647619a10.
23. Squires JE, Estabrooks CA, Gustavsson P, Wallin L. Individual determinants of research utilization by nurses: a systematic review update. *Implement Sci*. 2011;6:1.
24. Eccles MP, Grimshaw JM, Johnston M, et al. Applying psychological theories to evidence-based clinical practice: identifying factors predictive of managing upper respiratory tract infections without antibiotics. *Implement Sci*. 2007;2:26.
25. Powell BJ, Waltz TJ, Chinman MJ, et al. A refined compilation of implementation strategies: results from the Expert Recommendations for Implementing Change (ERIC) project. *Implement Sci*. 2015;10(1):21.
26. Eccles MP, Weijer C, Mittman B. Requirements for ethics committee review for studies submitted to Implementation Science. *Implement Sci*. 2011;6(32):1–4.
27. Goodyear-Smith F, Jackson C, Greenhalgh T. Co-design and implementation research: challenges

and solutions for ethics committees. *BMC Med Ethics*. 2015;16:78.

28. Gopichandran V, Luyckx VA, Biller-Andorno N, et al. Developing the ethics of implementation research in health. *Implement Sci*. 2016;11(1):161.

29. Hutton JL, Eccles MP, Grimshaw JM. Ethical issues in implementation research: a discussion of the problems in achieving informed consent. *Implement Sci*. 2008;3:52.

30. Macklin R. Ethical challenges in implementation research. *Pub Health Ethics*. 2014;7(1):86–93.

31. Wiecha JL, El Ayadi AM, Fuemmeler BF, et al. Diffusion of an integrated health education program in an urban school system: Planet Health. *J Pediatr Psychol*. 2004;29(6):467–474.

32. Bellin E, Dubler NN. The quality improvement-research divide and the need for external oversight. *Am J Public Health*. 2001;91(9):1512–1517.

33. Curran GM, Bauer M, Mittman B, Pyne J, Stetler C. Effectiveness-implementation hybrid designs: combining elements of clinical effectiveness and implementation research to enhance pubic health impact. *Annals of HSR*. 2012;50(3):217–226.

34. Gortmaker SL, Cheung LW, Peterson KE, et al. Impact of a school-based interdisciplinary intervention on diet and physical activity among urban primary school children: eat well and keep moving. *Arch Pediatr Adolesc Med*. 1999;153.

35. Gortmaker SL, Lee RM, Mozaffarian RS, et al. Effect of an after-school intervention on increases in children's physical activity. *Med Sci Sports Exerc*. 2012;44.

36. Freedman B. Equipoise and the ethics of clinical research. *N Engl JMed*. 1987;317(3):141–145.

37. Castro M. Placebo versus best-available-therapy control group in clinical trials for pharmacologic therapies: which is better? *Proc Am Thorac Soc*. 2007;4(7):570–573.

38. Khan A, Warner HA, Brown WA. Symptom reduction and suicide risk in patients treated with placebo in antidepressant clinical trials: an analysis of the Food and Drug Administration database. *Arch Gen Psychiatry*. 2000;57(4):311–317.

39. Miller PB, Weijer C. Rehabilitating equipoise. *Kennedy Inst Ethics J*. 2003;13(2):93–118.

40. Binik A, Weijer C, McRae AD, et al. Does clinical equipoise apply to cluster randomized trials in health research? *Trials*. 2011;12:118–118.

41. Valdiserri RO, Tama GM, Ho M. The role of community advisory committees in clinical trials of anti-HIV agents. *IRB: Ethics Hum Res*. 1988;10(4):5–7.

42. Brown CA, Lilford RJ. The stepped wedge trial design: a systematic review. *BMC Med Res Methodol*. 2006;6(1):54.

43. Emanuel EJ, Wendler D, Grady C. What makes clinical research ethical? *JAMA*. 2000;283(20):2701–2711.

44. Franks A, Kelder S, Dino G, et al. School-based programs: lessons learned from CATCH, Planet Health, and Not-On-Tobacco. *Prev Chronic Dis*. 2007;4(2):1–9.

45. DuBois JM, Chibnall JT, Tait RC, Vander Wal JS. Lessons from researcher rehab. *Nature*. 2016;534:173–175.

46. DuBois JC, Chibnall JT, Tait RC, Vander Wal JS, Baldwin KA, Antes AL, Mumford MD. Professional decision-making in research (PDR): the validity of a new measure. *Sci Eng Ethics*. 2016;22(2):391–416.

47. Mecca JT, Medeiros KE, Giorgini V, et al. The influence of compensatory strategies on ethical decision making. *Ethics & Behavior*. 2014;24(1):73–89.

48. Thiel CE, Connelly S, Griffith JA. Leadership and emotion management for complex tasks: different emotions, different strategies. *Leadership Quart*. 2012;23(3):517–533.

49. Angie AD, Connelly S, Waples EP, Kligyte V. The influence of discrete emotions on judgement and decision-making: a meta-analytic review. *Cognition Emotion*. 2011;25(8):1393–1422.

50. Barrett LF, Gross J, Christensen TC, Benvenuto M. Knowing what you're feeling and knowing what to do about it: mapping the relation between emotion differentiation and emotion regulation. *Cognition Emotion*. 2001;15(6):713–724.

51. Roche M, Haar JM, Luthans F. The role of mindfulness and psychological capital on the well-being of leaders. *J Occup Health Psychol*. 2014;19(4):476–489.

52. Bazerman MH, Moore DA. *Judgment in managerial decision making*. 8th ed. New York: Wiley; 2013.

53. Nickerson RS. Confirmation bias: A ubiquitous phenomenon in many guises. *Rev Gen Psychol*. 1998;2(2):175–220.

54. Stenmark CK, Antes AL, Thiel CE, Caughron JJ, Wang XQ, Mumford MD. Consequences identification in forecasting and ethical decision-making. *J Empir Res Hum Res Ethics*. 2011;6(1):25–32.

55. DuBois JM, Kraus E, Mikulec A, Cruz S, Bakanas E. A humble task: restoring virtue in medicine in an age of conflicted interests. *Acad Med*. 2013;88(7):924–928.

5

The Conceptual Basis for Dissemination and Implementation Research

Lessons from Existing Models and Frameworks

RACHEL G. TABAK, DAVID A. CHAMBERS, MARY HOOK,
AND ROSS C. BROWNSON

INTRODUCTION

Dissemination and implementation (D&I) research can be dynamic and complex. Studies lacking adequate underpinning from a model may miss key information related to system-wide processes, organizational factors, and measures required for D&I.[1] Evidence from other fields, such as public health, have found that interventions using health behavior theories are more effective than those lacking a basis in theory, as the model can provide a way to focus the intervention on the process of behavior change.[2,3] Similarly, as D&I science advances, evidence is building to show that the interpretability of study findings is improved by use of models because the study can be better organized and strategies can more successfully intervene on and measure the components essential to a successful D&I outcome.[3–5]

There are a number of ways in which a model can improve a D&I study. Models provide a systematic structure for the development, management, and evaluation of D&I efforts, linking study aims, design, measures, and analytic strategies.[6] D&I models can help narrow the scope of a study, by assisting with the focus of the research question and guiding the selection of constructs to measure. Framing a study within a D&I model can also help explain why an evidence-based intervention (EBI) or D&I strategy works or does not work. Empirical findings from model-based studies provide evidence to support understanding the mechanisms for D&I strategies and moves D&I science forward. In this way, models can help on the front end to organize and understand phenomenon and on the back end to understand

why/how D&I strategies succeed or fail. This is particularly true if the field is to progress to precision implementation, which recognizes that models in D&I need to account for a different combination of factors affecting local implementation, and in this way, precision implementation can help to better specify/tailor implementation strategies to an individual setting. This is especially important as there are a number of pathways through which a D&I strategy can succeed or fail.

The purposes of this chapter are to introduce models to inform D&I research and to provide advice and examples on model selection, adaptation, and application.

TERMINOLOGY

In explaining the conceptual underpinnings of a field, we recognize the use of various terms, including theories, frameworks, and models. Theories and frameworks are distinct concepts, as defined in the following text and in chapter 2. A theory is generally considered to provide a systematic way of understanding events or behaviors by indicating relationships between constructs and concepts. Frameworks guide researchers to consider constructs in systematic efforts to develop and evaluate interventions.

- Theory: a set of interrelated concepts, definitions, and propositions that present a systematic view of events or situations by specifying relations among variables, in order to explain and predict events or situations.[7(p. 26)]

- Conceptual Framework: A type of intermediate theory that attempts to connect to all aspects of inquiry; can act like maps that give coherence to empirical inquiry.[8]

To avoid further complicating the already complex language of D&I science, and for simplicity and consistency, this chapter collectively describes theories and frameworks as models.

- Model: A description of analogy used to help visualize something that cannot be directly observed.[9]

Outside of the health field, there has been an evolution of models for D&I of innovations. For example, in the field of business/management, this thinking incorporated a number of different ways to think about change, including change as rational action;[10,11] and change as adaptation to environment, which included theories such as Contingency Theory,[12-14] Ecology theory,[15] and Institutional Theory.[16] A theory familiar to many D&I in health researchers, Rogers Diffusion of Innovation,[17] became part of this literature as change was conceptualized as innovation; a further conceptualization was cultural change.[18,19] The science of D&I in health has learned a great deal from fields beyond health about the value of models, and can continue to look to these fields (e.g., business, engineering, political science) to develop and adapt new model applications and build new theories.[20]

SELECTING AND ADAPTING A MODEL

Given the importance of models in guiding research and their availability in the literature, researchers embarking on D&I research may wonder: how do I select an appropriate model to guide my work? Several efforts to collect, organize, and synthesize the many models available to guide D&I science are available, and can be used in combination. In one review, models were organized based on three continua: construct flexibility, dissemination and/or implementation (D/I), and the levels of the socioecological framework (SEF).[6] At one end of the construct flexibility spectrum are broad models, those with more loosely defined or outlined constructs; at the other end, operational models offer more detailed step-by-step actions for organizing a D&I study. Because of the greater flexibility afforded by broad models, more responsibility is placed on the researchers

to operationalize, implement, and use the model; however, operational models, because of their specificity, tend to be more clearly defined for a particular context and activity. D/I refers to whether the model is focused on using active approaches to spread EBIs to the target audience via determined channels using planned strategies (dissemination) or has more of a focus on integrating an EBI within a setting (implementation); definitions for D&I have been provided in chapter 2. The SEF includes the levels: individual, organization, community, system, and describes that a model can operate at one or more of these; models can also include a policy component. In a review of 61 models, at least four fell into each of the five categories for the construct flexibility and D/I scales. Models were spread across the socioecological framework levels, and every model operated at more than one level. The majority of models included community and/or organizational levels. Only eight models touched on policy. Additional information about these models is also provided, including the field in which the model was developed as well as citations with examples where the model was used (where available).

A sample of the most highly cited, representative models from this review are displayed in Table 5.1, to demonstrate how these pieces of information about each model might be used. Within this sample are models representing all categories in terms of dissemination to implementation and construct flexibility, as well as all levels of the SEF. From the table it is possible to narrow down the list of available models to those that might best fit the intended study. To provide an additional tool to identify models and narrow the search, the models collected and organized in this review, as well as 25 models from another review with a greater focus on practitioners and clinicians,[3] have been included in a searchable website (http://dissemination-implementation.org/index.aspx).

Nilsen developed a strategy to categorize models and assist researchers in model selection based on study aim;[88] this, and the resource just mentioned, can be used in combination to help narrow the list of models and find the best fit. Nilsen's review identified five categories of models and associated each with one of three common aims for implementation science research. The first category, process models, includes models that focus on describing and/or guiding the process of translating research into practice. Process models incorporate the temporal sequence of implementation as well as the importance of

TABLE 5.1 SELECTED MODELS AND THEIR CATEGORIZATIONS

Model	Dissemination and / or Implementation	Construct Flexibility: Broad to Operational	SEF Level					Field of Origin	Studies that Use the Model	Number of Times the Model Has Been Cited*	Citation(s)
			System	Community	Organization	Individual	Policy				
Diffusion of Innovation	D only	1		x	x	x		Agriculture	21-28	79,570+	17
Streams of Policy Process	D only	2	x	x	x		x	Political Science	29-31	16,204‡	32,33
A Conceptual Model for the Diffusion of Innovations in Service Organizations	D > I	4		x	x			Health Services	34,35	3,789	36
Research Knowledge Infrastructure	D > I	4		x	x	x	x	Knowledge Transfer in Health and Economic/ Social Research Organizations	37	283, 881¶	38-41
Framework for Dissemination of Evidence-Based Policy	D > I	5		x	x	x	x	Public Health	42	10	43
Real-World Dissemination	D = I	1		x	x			Health Care	—	1234	44,45
Interactive Systems Framework	D = I	2	x	x	x	x		Violence Prevention	46-50	599	51
The RE-AIM Framework	D = I	4		x	x	x		Public Health	52-55	2020	56
The Precede-Proceed Model	D = I	5		x	x	x		Health	57-60	1088	61
CDC DHAP's Research-to-Practice Framework	I > D	4		x	x			HIV/AIDS Prevention	—	176, 63**	62-67
Active Implementation Framework	I only	3		x	x	x		Any Domain	68,69	3165	70,71
Implementation Effectiveness Model	I only	3		x	x	x		Management	72-77	2205	78,79

(continued)

TABLE 5.1 CONTINUED

Model	Dissemination and / or Implementation	Construct Flexibility: Broad to Operational	SEF Level					Field of Origin	Studies that Use the Model	Number of Times the Model Has Been Cited[*]	Citation(s)
			System	Community	Organization	Individual	Policy				
Sticky Knowledge	I only	3		x	x	x		Strategic Management and Medicine	80	61, 8696[‡‡]	81,82
Consolidated Framework for Implementation Research	I only	4		x	x	x		Health Services	83–86	1,615	87

[*] As of January 12, 2017

[†] For 2010 edition, as this is the first edition that appears in google scholar.

[‡] This citation number is provided for the 2003 edition (the 2nd edition).

[§] These are the citation numbers for Lavis[80] (283 citations) and Lavis[41] (881 citations) articles.

[**] These are the citation numbers for the 2006 Collins[62] (176 citations) and 2000 Neumann[64] (63 citations) articles. These were selected because the authors felt these articles best explained the model.

[‡‡] Citation numbers for both the Elwyn[81] (61 citations) and Szulanski[82] (8,696 citations) references are provided. Both were included because the authors felt the references were sufficiently different that the citation numbers for both would be useful.

barriers and facilitators to D&I efforts, but do not aim to identify or systematically structure what makes D&I efforts successful. Models in the categories of determinant frameworks, classic theories, and implementation theories are used to guide research aimed at understanding and/or explaining the factors that influence the outcomes of D&I efforts. Determinant frameworks describe five common determinants including the implementation object, the users/adopters, the context, the implementation strategy, and the outcome(s). Framework determinants may be based on theory, but limited in scope. Theory from implementation science or other fields is needed for research aimed at enhancing the understanding of relationships, change mechanisms, or to predict outcomes. The last category, evaluation frameworks, can guide D&I research by identifying specific aspects of the D&I effort to evaluate in order to determine success.

It is important to consider this variety of models available for use in D&I research, and to recognize the benefits of selecting an existing model from those already available, which include an opportunity to advance the field by providing empirical evidence for a model. Applying an existing model can be a source of innovation for a study, especially if it is a model not previously used in the field. However, there is no comprehensive model that will perfectly fit every study. It will likely be necessary to adapt a model and/or to combine multiple models in order to inform a study. Case study 1 outlines an example of adapting a model. While there are a number of models available, not all are well operationalized, and it may therefore require more effort to apply them in a study. The decision to attempt to develop a new model should be taken with extreme caution, as this is a large undertaking, and there are many models with similar and overlapping constructs that currently exist in the literature. Chambers has laid out a set of questions that can be asked about a D&I effort to inform the choice of a model, which have been adapted and summarized in Table 5.2.[89]

Case Study 1: Process for Selecting and Adapting a Framework for Evidence-Based Policy Research
Background
Evidence-based practice (EBP) is a core competency for professional nurses.[94] Little progress, however, has been made in closing the research-to-practice gap and supporting nurses who work

in acute care settings to consistently use EBP to achieve best outcomes.[95–100] Health care organizations utilize varied strategies to increase the uptake of EBP including embedding best practices into policies[5,101] and/or the content and clinical decision support tools in their electronic health record.[102] Although policy/technology based tools are increasingly utilized in health care to support the uptake of EBP, the impact of these strategies has not been empirically tested.

Context
This case study describes the selection and adaptation of a theory-based framework used to guide research evaluating the impact of an evidence-based policy innovation within the context of a health care organization.[42] The innovation was designed to support nurses to know and use best practices in caring for patients during hospitalization. A theory-based approach was needed to ensure that essential concepts and processes were captured in the study design and used to support the interpretation of the findings.

Methods: The Selection and Adaptation of the Framework
The selection and adaption of the framework was guided by the process described by Tabak et al.[6] The research team reviewed the inventory of commonly cited models (N = 61) to select one best suited for the proposed study. The Dissemination of Evidence-Based Policy (DEBP) framework[43] (see Figure 26-1 in chapter 26) was selected because it described the process for using a policy-based innovation to achieve desired outcomes using both passive and active dissemination strategies, utilized an operational (step-by-step) construct, and incorporated a multi-socioecological level evaluation. The DEBP describes the policy process and illustrates how passive and active dissemination activities can be targeted to key audiences and carried out in phases to achieve policy outcomes. The framework was adapted to accommodate the aims, setting, and outcomes for the proposed study with a detailed description of the adaptation process.

First, the DEBP framework was designed for health policy research conducted at the "big P" level, referring to the formal laws, rules, and regulations enacted by elected officials.[91] To adapt the framework for organization-level ("little p") policy research the researchers had to address several key issues. Health care organizations create and maintain written policy to guide decisions

TABLE 5.2 QUESTIONS TO CONSIDER WHEN SELECTING A MODEL[*]

Question	Considerations
What is/are the research question(s) I'm seeking to answer?	1. Reviewing D&I literature to identify and utilize essential concepts and established definitions[90] will enhance the overall generalizability of the effort. 2. Articulating a research question and aims can narrow the scope of which models might fit the study well. 3. Beginning with a research question allows the researcher to determine what evidence is needed to answer that question.
What is the scope of the study?	1. Explanatory investigations certainly benefit from models. 2. Earlier stage research such as measurement development or pilot work may not need to fully flesh the study out in terms of a model and might instead frame the study under the idea of a model.
What is the purpose of the model in the context of the study?[88]	Nilsen proposed[88] five categories within three aims a model can have in guiding a study to help guide selection: 1. Process models "describe and/or guide the process of translating research into practice." 2. Determinant frameworks help explain/understand influences on implementation outcomes by specifying determinants (barriers and facilitators). 3. Classic theories, which emerge from fields such as organizational theory, psychology, and sociology, can be applied to explain/understand implementation efforts. 4. Implementation theories, developed by implementation researchers, help understand/explain implementation. 5. Evaluation frameworks "specify aspects of implementation that could be evaluated to determine implementation success."
What socioecological level(s) of change am I seeking to explain?	1. Specifying the socioecological level in which the change will occur allows for selection of a model that corresponds to the types of change under investigation (e.g., individual, organizational, community, system). 2. When thinking about policy, it is important to consider that policy exists at two levels: "big P" policy (formal laws, rules, regulations enacted by elected officials) and "small p" policy (organizational guidelines, internal agency decisions/memoranda, social norms).[43]
What characteristics of context are relevant to the research questions?	1. Identifying aspects of the context that may be important to the D&I outcome are important steps.
What is the timeframe?	1. There is variability between models in terms of how many phases of the D&I process are included (e.g., exploration of an EBI to be adopted, EBI implementation, and sustainment of the practice). 2. A study may focus on some or all phases of the D&I process depending on the research question and the scope of the study. 3. For studies covering multiple phases, multistage stage models Reach Effectiveness Adoption Implementation Maintenance (RE-AIM)[91] and Exploration, Preparation, Implementation, and Sustainment (EPIS) framework[92] can help organize these in addition to providing context specific for those stages. 4. Other models may focus on a specific phase of the D&I process.
Are measures available?	1. Measures are one of the important ways in which a model and its constructs are operationalized and are a way to tie the model to the research question. 2. Resources to help researchers identify measures for the constructs in their selected models, including the availability/absence of psychometric properties for the measures, are available,[93] but considerable work is still needed.

TABLE 5.2 CONTINUED

Question	Considerations
Does the study need to be related to a single model, and how strict does the use of the model need to be?	1. Given the complexity of D&I research, it is possible that a single model may be inadequate or underspecified to fully inform a research study. 2. Models may be combined to complement their purpose (e.g., those laid out by Nilsen such as process models, implementation theories, or evaluation frameworks),[88] based on the level of context, and/or based on the phase of the D&I process under study.
Does the model need to be adapted to fit the goal, setting, population, or other context?[6]	1. Models often need to be adapted to fit the study; theoretical and/or empirical adaptations can contribute to advancing D&I science. 2. Caution must be taken when adapting a model to provide evidence that supports the change without compromising the core elements.[6]

*Adapted from Chambers 2016[89]

and activities related to governance, management, care, treatment, and services.[103] In this setting, policy decision-making often takes place at the level of the organization where "policy content" is produced based on three key inputs: "big P" policy requirements, published evidence, and practice-based evidence. To accurately reflect the differences associated with organizational use, the "policy process" concept was relocated to the upper left corner to represent that policy creation occurs at the level of the organization with the addition of the key inputs (Figure 5.1). The active dissemination process is focused solely on disseminating policy with accepted benefits,

complexity, and costs to organizational audiences (e.g., departments/units) who are responsible for implementing and maintaining it over time.

Second, the DEBP framework illustrates how passive and active strategies could be used to disseminate health policy. The framework featured a full range of strategies including passive (e.g., innovation development and awareness) and active strategies commonly used to support implementation within a setting (e.g., adoption, implementation, and maintenance).[90] To enhance conceptual clarity, the two D&I concepts were adjusted from "passive dissemination" and "active dissemination" to "dissemination" (passive

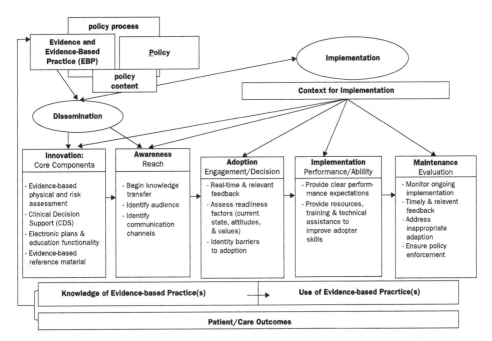

FIGURE 5.1 Framework for disseminating and implementing evidence-based policy.

and active) and "implementation." The framework title was adapted to the "Dissemination and Implementation of Evidence-based Policy" (DIEBP) framework to recognize the inclusion of the full range of interventions on a dissemination-to-implementation spectrum.

Beyond the policy process, the DEBP framework describes two factors that influence the outcomes associated with active dissemination—specifically the audience and the conditions that support the implementation of the approved policy. These attributes are commonly referred to as "context"—the "conditions or surroundings in which something exists or occurs, typically referring to an analytical unit higher than the phenomena directly under investigation."[88] The context includes characteristics of the adopters (e.g., individuals/unit) and the factors that influence EBP implementation (e.g., leadership, culture, interactions, staffing, skill mix, turnover, etc.).[104]

Last, the outcome component of the framework was refined with the addition of two intermediate outcomes with a feedback loop to depict the mechanisms used to provide practice and outcome-based evidence to update policies. The intermediate outcomes, clinician knowledge and use of best practices, are not commonly measured but are seemingly important for achieving the identified outcomes and for interpreting the findings of the study.

Lessons Learned

The policy dissemination process is one avenue for "hardwiring" best practices to promote the consistent use of EBP for patient care, but writing and disseminating policy does not ensure a practice change. The DIEBP framework was adapted to support the study aims, population, and setting. The adaptations made the process explicit and supported the research team to evaluate the strategies and measure the factors that may be impacting EBP policy implementation and outcomes.

The adapted framework draws attention to the policy process, the potential impact of health system (big P) and organizational (little p) policy, and the options leaders have for deploying EBP policy to impact outcomes. Passive dissemination may be efficient and cost-effective but it may not be sufficient to change practice. Implementation may cost more, but may result in better uptake with fewer resources used for quality improvement and service recovery. The use of implementation requires that the consistent use of best practice is a priority and that unit leaders have the knowledge, skills, and overall capacity for overseeing and maintaining practice changes. Further use and testing is needed to promote growth in this important area of D&I science.

APPLYING THE SELECTED MODEL

The next two case studies demonstrate the application of a model to a research question. Case Study 2 applies the Consolidated Framework for Implementation Research (CFIR)[87] to retrospectively explore an implementation effort related to healthy weight promotion. Case Study 3 applies the Interactive Systems Framework (ISF)[51] prospectively to an effort to increase the capacity for community organizations to address teen pregnancy prevention using science-based approaches.

Case Study 2: Consolidated Framework for Implementation Research
Background

Obesity has increased dramatically in the United States and many other countries over the past few decades,[105] and this has led to an increase in associated chronic diseases and substantial health care costs.[106,107] To address these, there has been an increase in program offerings from employers and insurers with a range of intensity.[108,109] Interventions delivered through the Internet have great potential for scalability.[110] While randomized controlled trials have demonstrated the benefit of these interventions for increasing physical activity, less attention has been paid to deploying Internet-based interventions into a broad population.[111]

Context

A large US insurance company began offering a wellness program, delivered via the Internet, to all employees with obesity in 2010. This program offered employees who did not meet certain health metrics the opportunity to join the wellness program, in order to be eligible for enhanced benefits. The multicomponent, automated, web-based lifestyle change intervention included the Walkingspree program (including an uploading pedometer, guided step-count goal setting, and web-based feedback), an online community, motivational and informational messaging, and diet tracking.[111]

The CFIR was developed based on multiple implementation theories and reviews of constructs important to effective implementation.[87] The CFIR is composed of five major domains: Intervention Characteristics, Outer Setting, Inner Setting, Characteristics of Individuals, and Process. Each domain contains several constructs, providing a "menu" for implementation scientists. For example, the Inner Setting domain includes constructs such as: Structural Characteristics, Networks & Communications, Culture, Implementation Climate, and Readiness for Implementation.

The research team conducted semistructured interviews with those critical to implementation of the program, in order to understand factors influencing implementation. The interview guide was developed based on the CFIR. As an example, the interview guide addressed the Outer Setting, including prompts related to the impact of relevant local, state, or national policies, regulations, or guidelines; the importance of member needs; and the influence of competitors implementing similar programs on program implementation efforts. The program evaluation also included assessments of program acceptance, adherence, and impact. The CFIR-based analysis identified factors in a number of domains, which were related to program implementation. In the Outer Setting, factors included federal policies (e.g., US Department of Labor Health Insurance Portability and Accountability Act guidelines) and rising costs associated with obesity. In the Inner Setting, organizational culture and support from leadership were influential as were Intervention Characteristics such as program design and the flexibility of the vendor that provided Walkginspree. The wellness program was implemented with a formal implementation Process, though in a short time frame.

Lessons Learned

The impact of interventions to modify health behaviors will be limited if they cannot be implemented on a large scale. The program evaluation was able to explore implementation through the CFIR. An appendix in the original publication provides a mapping of quotes from interview respondents on to relevant constructs,[111] which helps to deconstruct aspects of the intervention and its implementation that are critical to inform future efforts. This detailed evaluation, as well as the assessment of acceptance, adherence, and impact, was able to demonstrate the promise of a wellness program delivered through the Internet to promote physical activity among workers with obesity as well as important information regarding implementation. The implementation effort evaluated in this study engaged a large number of employees, many of whom adhered to the intervention and demonstrated sustained levels of physical activity above the program's initial goal despite modifications to the program, which were necessary to allow for large scale implementation.

Case Study 3: Interactive Systems Framework
Background

The Promoting Science-based Approaches to Teen Pregnancy Prevention project (PSBA) program is a multisite, capacity-building effort whose goal is to assist local prevention partners in the use of science-based approaches to prevent teen pregnancy.[48] While previous work had shown that coalitions were important partners in prevention, the model of building and strengthening teen pregnancy prevention coalitions to improve community level capacity to plan and implement effective and sustainable teen pregnancy prevention programming had limited success.[112] However, this work suggested the need for a focus on building the capacity of existing local coalitions or other types of community organizations that provide prevention programming directly to youth (i.e., focus more on capacity building of existing, youth-serving organizations than on building new community level infrastructures such as coalitions) to improve local prevention practice.

Context

The ISF[51] was adopted to allow for more specific and strategic planning about what capacities were needed at the local level and to develop a framework for systematically building these capacities.

The ISF was originally developed to be used by different types of stakeholders (e.g., funders, practitioners, researchers).[51] The ISF aims to help these diverse stakeholders see prevention through the lens of their own needs and perspectives as well as helping these stakeholders to better understand the needs of other stakeholders and systems. This framework identifies three systems: (1) the Prevention Synthesis and Translation System (which distills information about innovations and translates it into user-friendly formats); (2) the Prevention Support System (which provides training, technical assistance or other support to users in the field in order to build their capacity); and (3) the Prevention Delivery System (which implements innovations in the world of practice), each of which are necessary for the movement of innovations into widespread prevention practice at the community level.[51]

ISF informed the measures and evaluation for this PSBA project, including development of questions to document and evaluate the process and outcomes. This evaluation included a focus on how well the ISF-inspired capacity-building model was able to improve prevention practice among selected local partners. The ISF also guided how barriers identified in previous prevention efforts were addressed in the current project.

Lessons Learned

PSBA uses all three systems of the ISF to facilitate practice improvements and offers valuable research opportunities to investigate factors related to D&I processes across these systems. (I) In an effort to synthesize the elements needed to promote science-based approaches and increase the capacity of local providers, the PSBA project created an accessible and comprehensive manual called Promoting Science-based Approaches to Teen Pregnancy Prevention using Getting To Outcomes (PSBA-GTO).[48] (II) CDC's national, regional, and state partners have worked to: (1) strengthen their own general organizational capacity, (2) build science-based approaches-specific capacity to provide training and technical assistance using the PSBA-GTO process, and (3) through training and technical assistance, assist local partners in applying PSBA-GTO in their work. (III) In the PSBA project, the Prevention Delivery System includes all those local prevention partners who were invited to and have agreed to receive intensive technical assistance from state and regional grantees. Over the life of the project, each state and regional grantee was expected to have selected a convenience sample of 5 to 10 local partners and worked intensively with these partners to build their capacity to use science-based approaches to prevent teen pregnancy.

FUTURE DIRECTIONS

Given the plethora of models to guide D&I efforts and the importance of a theory-based approach to support these efforts, it is essential to consider how to make this available to D&I scientists and how to facilitate the selection process. While several options for categorization of existing models have been described,[6,88] further categorizing

models by (1) type of intervention, (2) type of provider, (3) type of setting, and (4) study aim, as well as utility for implementing multiple interventions simultaneously, could be beneficial to those selecting a model. There is much to be gained from employing models, including contributions to empirical testing and mechanistic D&I, which can be facilitated by enabling more researchers to select from existing models. As described, there are many models that have never been tested,[6,88] so empirical use of models has great potential to advance the field. Aside from models existing within D&I science and health, models for D&I may be adapted from fields outside of health such as education, business, and engineering. There is room for additional efforts in specialty topics of D&I science (e.g., adaptation, sustainment, and de-implementation) to describe how the models are used. While efforts to sort models have been described, further synthesis of existing models, including exploring the many common constructs across models could help extend the existing models to address key questions in D&I. A better connection between models and the measures to assess the model constructs is required for continuing to advance D&I science.[93] This highlights the importance of using a model in all stages of research, from designing the study to interpreting the findings.

SUMMARY

There are tangible benefits to the use of models to inform D&I research. However D&I scientists may find it difficult to select, adapt, and apply a model to their work. Guidance is provided on how to select a model, as answering several questions (e.g., the research question, scope of the study) can aid a research team in selecting a model. A case study example of adapting a model is also included, as for nearly all studies the selected model will need adaptation. Given the large number of models available and the amount of work required to develop a new model, a D&I researcher likely does not need to create a new model. There is a need to look outside the field of health research to identify other models that might inform D&I research, as reviews have identified gaps in availability of models for certain types of D&I research (e.g., policy research). The use and ongoing testing of theory-based approaches will increase our ability to ensure that essential concepts are considered, enhance interpretability, support the evaluation of outcome variations, and move the science forward.

SUGGESTED READINGS AND WEBSITES

Readings

Mitchell SA, Fisher CA, Hastings CE, Silverman LB, Wallen GR. A thematic analysis of theoretical models for translational science in nursing: mapping the field. *Nurs Outlook*. 2010;58(6):287–300.

This resource includes a literature search in which the 47 models identified are categorized into four thematic areas, which emerged from the review: (1) evidence-based practice and knowledge transformation processes, (2) strategic change to promote adoption of new knowledge, (3) knowledge exchange and synthesis for application and inquiry, and (4) designing and interpreting dissemination research to help aid model selection to guide D&I.

Tabak RG, Khoong EC, Chambers DA, Brownson RC. Bridging research and practice: models for dissemination and implementation research. *Am J Prevent Med*. 2012;43(3):337–50.

This narrative review identified 61 models used in D&I research and organized them according to several continua (construct flexibility, dissemination and/or implementation (D/I), and the levels of the socioecological framework) in order to assist with model selection. Additional information about each model including the field in which it originated, examples of studies (where available) that use the model, and the number of times the model was cited. Case studies demonstrating model use are also included.

Sales A, Smith J, Curran G, Kochevar L. Models, strategies, and tools. Theory in implementing evidence-based findings into health care practice. *J Gen Intern Med*. 2006;21 Suppl 2:S43–9.

This paper describes how efforts to implement evidence-based practices in clinical settings can be improved by using a theoretical foundation for the design and planning of intervention strategies and tool selection. The resource argues that a failure to truly link the theory, models, strategy, and tools in intervention design, when planning a change effort can result in suboptimal outcomes. The theories discussed in this resource are those most appropriate to clinical settings, often complex organizations.

Nilsen P. Making sense of implementation theories, models and frameworks. *Implement Sci*. 2015;10:53.

In this paper, Nilsen presents a strategy to categorize models to assist in model selection based on study aim. This review identified five categories of models and associated each with one of three common aims for implementation science research (describing and/or guiding the process of translating research into practice, understanding and/or explaining what influences implementation outcomes, and evaluating implementation): process models, determinant frameworks, classic theories, implementation theories, and evaluation frameworks.

Chambers DA. Guiding theory for dissemination and implementation research: A reflection on models used in research and practice. In: Beidas RS, Kendall PC, eds. *Dissemination and Implementation of evidence-based practices in child and adolescent mental health*. New York, NY: Oxford University Press; 2016:3.

This chapter offers guidance to researchers on using theories, models, and conceptual framework in support of D&I research. This includes examples of several prominent models in D&I research as well as guidance for application of models to practice and policy in addition to research. Also included in this chapter is information on model selection.

Wilson PM, Petticrew M, Calnan MW, Nazareth I. Disseminating research findings: what should researchers do? A systematic scoping review of conceptual frameworks. *Implement Science*. 2010, 5:91

This scoping review aimed to identify and describe conceptual/organizing frameworks, which could be of use to guide dissemination efforts by researchers. The review identified 33 frameworks, and among these, 20 were designed to help researchers in dissemination. Of the 33 frameworks identified, 28 were underpinned in some way by persuasive communication, diffusion of innovations theory, and social marketing. The frameworks are described in terms of their dissemination elements, theoretical foundations, and framework description.

Rycroft-Malone J, Bucknall T. (Eds.). *Model and frameworks for implementing evidence-based practice: Linking evidence to action*. Oxford, UK: Wiley-Blackwell, 2010.

This book aims to assist researchers in selecting and applying an appropriate model by providing considerable information and analysis about the included models. Model chapters are written by the model developer and include background, suitable applications, underlying theory, examples of use, strengths and weaknesses, and barriers and facilitators for use. Models included in this book were selected if they have wide recognition, evaluation and testing, transfer across different settings, and apply across disciplines.

Selected Websites and Tools

http://dissemination-implementation.org/index.aspx
This website provides a searchable database of models included in the review papers published by Mitchell et al. and Tabak et al. Search categories include dissemination to implementation, levels of the SEF, and

included constructs. The database includes information about each model's categorization as well as citations for the model, and where possible, examples of its use. Resources on adapting and integrating the model are also provided.

CFIR Technical Assistance Website: http://www.cfir-guide.org/
This website has considerable information for those interested in the Consolidated Framework for Implementation Research (CFIR). This includes an overview of the framework, its domains and constructs, and library of citations using CFIR. Other features of the site are tools and templates for data collection and analysis, including an interview guide tool, which is designed to help researchers build interview guides based on CFIR.

http://re-aim.org/
The RE-AIM website provides a number of resources related to the RE-AIM framework and external validity. Information on the overall framework and its application is provided, as well as is information on RE-AIM's components: Reach, Effectiveness, Adoption, Implementation, and Maintenance with examples of use. The website also includes many resources and tools including guides on how to calculate the components of RE-AIM as well as checklists and tools for intervention planning and assessing RE-AIM application.

REFERENCES

1. Stetler CB, Legro MW, Wallace CM, et al. The role of formative evaluation in implementation research and the QUERI experience. *J Gen Intern Med.* 2006;21 Suppl 2:S1–S8.
2. Glanz K, Bishop DB. The role of behavioral science theory in development and implementation of public health interventions. *Annu Rev Public Health.* 2010;31:399–418.
3. Mitchell SA, Fisher CA, Hastings CE, Silverman LB, Wallen GR. A thematic analysis of theoretical models for translational science in nursing: mapping the field. *Nurs Outlook.* 2010;58(6):287–300.
4. Sales A, Smith J, Curran G, Kochevar L. Models, strategies, and tools. Theory in implementing evidence-based findings into health care practice. *J Gen Intern Med.* 2006;21 Suppl 2:S43–S49.
5. Van Achterberg T, Schoonhoven L, Grol R. Nursing implementation science: how evidence based nursing requires evidence based implementation. *J Nurs Scholarsh.* 2008;40(4):302–310.
6. Tabak RG, Khoong EC, Chambers DA, Brownson RC. Bridging research and practice: models for dissemination and implementation research. *Am J Prev Med.* 2012;43(3):337–350.
7. Glanz K, Rimer BK, Viswanath K. Theory, research, and practice in health behavior. In: Glanz K, Rimer BK, Viswanath K, eds. *Health behavior and health education: Theory, research, and practice.* 5th ed. San Francisco: Jossey-Bass; 2015:23.
8. Wikipedia. Conceptual Framework. 2013; http://en.wikipedia.org/wiki/Conceptual_framework.
9. In Merriam-Webster online. Model & Theory. 2013; Retrieved from http://www.merriam-webster.coms.
10. Friedmann J, Hudson B. Knowledge and action: a guide to planning theory. *J. Am Inst Plann.* 1974;40(1):2–16.
11. Delbecq AL, Van de Ven AH. A group process model for problem identification and program planning. *J Appl Behav Sci.* 1971;7(4):466–492.
12. Hage J, Aiken M. Program change and organizational properties a comparative analysis. *Am J Sociol.* 1967:503–519.
13. Hage J, Aiken M. Routine technology, social structure, and organization goals. *Adm Sci Q.* 1969:366–376.
14. Hage J, Aiken M. *Social change in complex organizations.* Vol 43. New York: Random House; 1970.
15. Hannan MT, Freeman J. Structural inertia and organizational change. *Am Sociol. Rev.* 1984;49(2):149–164.
16. Dimaggio P, Powell W. The iron cage revisited: Institutional isomorphism and collective rationality in organizational fields. *Am Sociol Rev.* 1983;48(2):147–160.
17. Rogers EM. *Diffusion of innovations.* 5th ed. New York: Free Press; 2003.
18. Schein E. *Organizational culture and leadership: A dynamic view.* 1st ed. San Francisco: Jossey-Bass; 1985.
19. Lewin K. *Field theory in social science: Selected theoretical papers* (Dorwin Cartwright, ed). 1st ed. New York: Harper; 1951.
20. Wacker JG. A definition of theory: research guidelines for different theory-building research methods in operations management. *J Oper Manag.* 1998;16(4):361–385.
21. Dingfelder HE, Mandell DS. Bridging the research-to-practice gap in autism intervention: an application of diffusion of innovation theory. *J Autism Dev Disord.* 2011;41(5):597–609.
22. Glanz K, Steffen A, Elliott T, O'Riordan D. Diffusion of an effective skin cancer prevention program: design, theoretical foundations, and first-year implementation. *Health Psychol.* 2005;24(5):477–487.
23. Ball K. Compliance with surgical smoke evacuation guidelines: implications for practice. *AORN J.* 2010;92(2):142–149.
24. Ball K. Surgical smoke evacuation guidelines: compliance among perioperative nurses. *AORN J.* 2010;92(2):e1–e23.
25. Shively M, Riegel B, Waterhouse D, Burns D, Templin K, Thomason T. Testing a community

level research utilization intervention. *Appl Nurs Res.* 1997;10(3):121–127.

26. Wiecha JL, El Ayadi AM, Fuemmeler BF, et al. Diffusion of an integrated health education program in an urban school system: planet health. *J Pediatr Psychol.* 2004;29(6):467–474.

27. Al-Ghaith WA, Sanzogni L, Sandhu K. Factors influencing the adoption and usage of online services in Saudi Arabia. *EJISDC.* 2010;40(1):1–32.

28. Nanney MS, Haire-Joshu D, Brownson RC, Kostelc J, Stephen M, Elliott M. Awareness and adoption of a nationally disseminated dietary curriculum. *Am J Health Behav.* 2007;31(1):64–73.

29. Bugeja L, McClure RJ, Ozanne-Smith J, Ibrahim JE. The public policy approach to injury prevention. *Inj Prev.* 2011;17(1):63–65.

30. Craig RL, Felix HC, Walker JF, Phillips MM. Public health professionals as policy entrepreneurs: Arkansas's childhood obesity policy experience. *Am J Public Health.* 2010;100(11):2047–2052.

31. D'Abbs P. Alignment of the policy planets: behind the implementation of the Northern Territory (Australia) Living With Alcohol programme. *Drug Alcohol Rev* 2004;23(1):55–66.

32. Kingdon JW. *Agendas, alternatives, and public policies.* Boston: Little, Brown; 1984.

33. Kingdon JW. *Agendas, alternatives, and public policies.* Updated 2nd ed. Boston: Longman; 2010.

34. Deschesnes M, Trudeau F, Kebe M. Factors influencing the adoption of a Health Promoting School approach in the province of Quebec, Canada. *Health Educ Res.* 2010;25(3):438–450.

35. Hanbury A, Thompson C, Wilson PM, et al. Translating research into practice in Leeds and Bradford (TRiPLaB): a protocol for a programme of research. *Implement Sci.* 2010;5:37.

36. Greenhalgh T, Robert G, Macfarlane F, Bate P, Kyriakidou O. Diffusion of innovations in service organizations: systematic review and recommendations. *Milbank Q.* 2004;82(4):581–629.

37. Cordero C, Delino R, Jeyaseelan L, et al. Funding agencies in low-and middle-income countries: support for knowledge translation. *Bull World Health Organ.* 2008;86(7):524–534.

38. Ellen ME, Lavis JN, Ouimet M, Grimshaw J, Bedard PO. Determining research knowledge infrastructure for healthcare systems: a qualitative study. *Implement Sci.* 2011;6(1):60.

39. IWH. Institute for Work and Health—Knowledge Transfer & Exchange Guides. 2006; http://www.iwh.on.ca/kte-guides. Accessed October 15, 2011.

40. Lavis JN, Lomas J, Hamid M, Sewankambo NK. Assessing country-level efforts to link research to action. *Bull World Health Organ.* 2006;84(8):620–628.

41. Lavis JN, Robertson D, Woodside JM, McLeod CB, Abelson J. How can research organizations more effectively transfer research knowledge to decision makers? *Milbank Q.* 2003;81(2):221–248, 171–222.

42. Hook ML. Using Implementation Theory to Evaluate the Impact of Technology on Nurses' Knowledge and Use of Best Practices in Acute Care. Presentation at the 9th Annual Conference of the Science of Dissemination and Implementation, co-hosted by the National Institutes of Health and AcademyHealth; December 2016; Washington, DC.

43. Dodson E, Brownson R, Weiss S. Policy dissemination research. In: Brownson R, Colditz G, Proctor E, eds. *Dissemination and implementation research in health: Translating science to practice.* New York: Oxford University Press; 2012:437–458.

44. Adapted by Chambers D, Raingeisen H, Hoagwood K, Patel V. Leading clinical practice change. In: Dopson S, Mark A, eds. *Leading health care organizations.* Houndmills, UK: Palgrave Macmillan; 2003.

45. Pettigrew AM, Ferlie E, McKee L. *Shaping strategic change: making change in large organizations: The case of the National Health Service.* Thousand Oaks, CA: Sage; 1992.

46. Emshoff JG. Researchers, practitioners, and funders: using the framework to get us on the same page. *Am J Community Psychol.* 2008;41(3):393–403.

47. Lee SJ, Altschul I, Mowbray CT. Using planned adaptation to implement evidence-based programs with new populations. *Am J Community Psychol.* 2008;41(3-4):290–303.

48. Lesesne CA, Lewis KM, White CP, Green DC, Duffy JL, Wandersman A. Promoting science-based approaches to teen pregnancy prevention: proactively engaging the three systems of the interactive systems framework. *Am J Community Psychol.* J2008;41(3-4):379–392.

49. Ozer EJ, Cantor JP, Cruz GW, Fox B, Hubbard E, Moret L. The diffusion of youth-led participatory research in urban schools: the role of the prevention support system in implementation and sustainability. *Am J Community Psychol.* 2008;41(3):278–289.

50. Rolleri LA, Wilson MM, Paluzzi PA, Sedivy VJ. Building capacity of state adolescent pregnancy prevention coalitions to implement science-based approaches. *Am J Community Psychol.* 2008;41(3):225–234.

51. Wandersman A, Duffy J, Flaspohler P, et al. Bridging the gap between prevention research and practice: the interactive systems framework

for dissemination and implementation. *Am J. Community Psychol.* 2008;41(3-4):171–181.

52. Aittasalo M, Miilunpalo S, Ståhl T, Kukkonen-Harjula K. From innovation to practice: initiation, implementation and evaluation of a physician-based physical activity promotion programme in Finland. *Health Promot Int.* 2007;22(1):19.

53. De Meij JSB, Chinapaw MJM, Kremers SPJ, Van der Wal MF, Jurg ME, Van Mechelen W. Promoting physical activity in children: the stepwise development of the primary school-based JUMP-in intervention applying the RE-AIM evaluation framework. *Br J Sports Med.* 2010;44(12):879–887.

54. Glasgow RE, Nelson CC, Strycker LA, King DK. Using RE-AIM metrics to evaluate diabetes self-management support interventions. *Am J Prev Med.* 2006;30(1):67–73.

55. Van Acker R, De Bourdeaudhuij I, De Cocker K, Klesges L, Cardon G. The impact of disseminating the whole-community project '10,000 Steps': a RE-AIM analysis. *BMC Public Health.* 2011;11(1):3.

56. Glasgow RE, Vogt TM, Boles SM. Evaluating the public health impact of health promotion interventions: the RE-AIM framework. *Am J Public Health.* 1999;89(9):1322–1327.

57. Curran GM, Mukherjee S, Allee E, Owen RR. A process for developing an implementation intervention: QUERI Series. *Implement Sci.* 2008;3(1):17.

58. Gary TL, Bone LR, Hill MN, et al. Randomized controlled trial of the effects of nurse case manager and community health worker interventions on risk factors for diabetes-related complications in urban African Americans. *Prev Med.* 2003;37(1):23–32.

59. Guidotti TL, Ford L, Wheeler M. The Fort McMurray demonstration project in social marketing: Theory, design, and evaluation. *Am J Prev Med.* 2000;18(2):163–169.

60. Ottoson JM, Green LW. Community outreach: from measuring the difference to making a difference with health information. *J Med Libr Assoc.* 2005;93(4 Suppl):S49.

61. Green LW, Kreuter MW. *Health program planning: An educational and ecological approach.* 4th ed. New York: McGraw-Hill; 2005.

62. Collins C, Harshbarger C, Sawyer R, Hamdallah M. The diffusion of effective behavioral interventions project: development, implementation, and lessons learned. *AIDS Educ Prev.* 2006;18(4 Suppl A):5–20.

63. Collins CB, Jr., Johnson WD, Lyles CM. Linking research and practice: evidence-based HIV prevention. *Focus.* 2007;22(7):1–5.

64. Neumann MS, Sogolow ED. Replicating effective programs: HIV/AIDS prevention technology transfer. *AIDS Educ Prev.* 2000;12(5 Suppl):35–48.

65. Sogolow E, Peersman G, Semaan S, Strouse D, Lyles CM. The HIV/AIDS Prevention Research Synthesis Project: scope, methods, and study classification results. *J Acquir Immune Defic Syndr.* 2002;30 Suppl 1:S15–S29.

66. Sogolow ED, Kay LS, Doll LS, et al. Strengthening HIV prevention: application of a research-to-practice framework. *AIDS Educ Prev.* 2000;12(5 Suppl):21–32.

67. CDC-DHAP. HIV/AIDS Prevention Research Synthesis Project. 2011; https://www.cdc.gov/hiv/dhap/prb/prs/index.html.

68. Casado BL, Quijano LM, Stanley MA, Cully JA, Steinberg EH, Wilson NL. Healthy IDEAS: Implementation of a depression program through community-based case management. *Gerontologist.* 2008;48(6):828.

69. Graff CA, Springer P, Bitar GW, Gee R, Arredondo R. A purveyor team's experience: lessons learned from implementing a behavioral health care program in primary care settings. *Fam Syst Health.* 2010;28(4):356.

70. Fixsen DL, Mental LPF, Florida UoS. *Implementation research: A synthesis of the literature.* Chapel Hill, NC: National Implementation Research Network; 2005.

71. Institute FCD. National Implementation Research Network. 2008; http://nirn.fpg.unc.edu/learn-implementation/implementation-defined. Accessed October 15, 2011.

72. Dong L, Neufeld DJ, Higgins C. Testing Klein and Sorra's innovation implementation model: an empirical examination. *J Eng Technol Manage.* 2008;25(4):237–255.

73. Holahan PJ, Aronson ZH, Jurkat MP, Schoorman FD. Implementing computer technology: a multiorganizational test of Klein and Sorra's model. *J Eng Technol Manage.* 2004;21(1-2):31–50.

74. Osei-Bryson KM, Dong L, Ngwenyama O. Exploring managerial factors affecting ERP implementation: an investigation of the Klein-Sorra model using regression splines. *Inform Syst J.* 2008;18(5):499–527.

75. Robertson J, Sorbello T, Unsworth K. Innovation implementation: the role of technology diffusion agencies. *J Technol Manage Innovat.* 2008;3(3):1–10.

76. Sawang S. Innovation implementation effectiveness: a multiorganizational test of Klein Conn and Sorra's model. 2008.

77. Sheldon MR. Evidence-based practice in occupational health: description and application of an implementation effectiveness model. *Work.* 2007;29(2):137–143.

78. Klein KJ, Conn AB, Sorra JS. Implementing computerized technology: an organizational analysis. *J Appl Psychol*. 2001;86(5):811.

79. Klein KJ, Sorra JS. The challenge of innovation implementation. *Acad Manage Rev*. 1996;21(4):1055–1080.

80. Szulanski G. The process of knowledge transfer: A diachronic analysis of stickiness. *Organ Behav Hum Decis Process*. 2000;82(1):9–27.

81. Elwyn G, Taubert M, Kowalczuk J. Sticky knowledge: a possible model for investigating implementation in healthcare contexts. *Implement Sci*. 2007;2:44.

82. Szulanski G. Exploring internal stickiness: impediments to the transfer of best practice within the firm. *Strategic Manage J*. 1996;17:27–43.

83. Lash SJ, Timko C, Curran GM, McKay JR, Burden JL. Implementation of evidence-based substance use disorder continuing care interventions. *Psychol Addict Behav*. 2011;25(2):238–251.

84. Hartzler B, Lash SJ, Roll JM. Contingency management in substance abuse treatment: a structured review of the evidence for its transportability. *Drug Alcohol Depend*. 2012 Apr 1;122(1-2):1–10.

85. Sorensen JL, Kosten T. Developing the tools of implementation science in substance use disorders treatment: applications of the consolidated framework for implementation research. *Psychol Addict Behav*. 2011;25(2):262.

86. Williams EC, Johnson ML, Lapham GT, et al. Strategies to implement alcohol screening and brief intervention in primary care settings: a structured literature review. *Psychol Addict Behav*. 2011;25(2):206–214.

87. Damschroder LJ, Aron DC, Keith RE, Kirsh SR, Alexander JA, Lowery JC. Fostering implementation of health services research findings into practice: a consolidated framework for advancing implementation science. *Implement Sci*. 2009;4:50.

88. Nilsen P. Making sense of implementation theories, models and frameworks. *Implement Sci*. 2015;10:53.

89. Chambers DA. Guiding theory for dissemination and implementation research: A relection on models used in research and practice. In: Beidas RS, Kendall PC, eds. *Dissemination and implementation of evidence-based practices in child and adolescent mental health*. New York, NY: Oxford University Press; 2016:3.

90. Rabin BA, Brownson RC. Terminology for dissemination and implementation research. In: Brownson R, Colditz G, Proctor E, eds. *Dissemination and implementation research in health: Translating science to practice*. 2nd Edition. New York: Oxford University Press.

91. Glasgow RE, McKay HG, Piette JD, Reynolds KD. The RE-AIM framework for evaluating interventions: what can it tell us about approaches to chronic illness management? *Patient Educ Couns*. 2001;44(2):119–127.

92. Aarons GA, Hurlburt M, Horwitz SM. Advancing a conceptual model of evidence-based practice implementation in public service sectors. *Adm Policy Ment Health*. 2011;38(1):4–23.

93. Rabin BA, Lewis CC, Norton WE, et al. Measurement resources for dissemination and implementation research in health. *Implement Sci*. 22 2016;11:42.

94. American Nurses Association. *Nursing: Scope and standards of practice*. 3rd ed. Silver Spring, MD: ANA; 2015.

95. Pravikoff DS, Pierce ST, Tanner A. Evidence-based practice readiness study supported by academy nursing informatics expert panel. *Nurs. Outlook*. 2005;53(1):49–50.

96. Saunders H, Vehvilainen-Julkunen K. The state of readiness for evidence-based practice among nurses: An integrative review. *Int J Nurs Stud*. 2016;56:128–140.

97. Duffy JR, Culp S, Yarberry C, Stroupe L, Sand-Jecklin K, Coburn AS. Nurses' research capacity and use of evidence in acute care: baseline findings from a partnership study. *J Nurs Adm*. 2015;45(3):158–164.

98. Melnyk BM, Fineout-Overholt E, Gallagher-Ford L, Kaplan L. The state of evidence-based practice in US nurses: critical implications for nurse leaders and educators. *J Nurs Adm*. 2012;42(9):410–417.

99. Yoder LH, Kirkley D, McFall DC, Kirksey KM, StalBaum AL, Sellers D. CE: Original Research: staff nurses' use of research to facilitate evidence-based practice. *Am J Nurs*. 2014;114(9):26–37.

100. Yost J, Ganann R, Thompson D, et al. The effectiveness of knowledge translation interventions for promoting evidence-informed decision-making among nurses in tertiary care: a systematic review and meta-analysis. *Implement Sci*. Jul 14 2015;10:98.

101. Oman KS, Duran C, Fink R. Evidence-based policy and procedures: an algorithm for success. *J Nurs Adm*. 2008;38(1):47–51.

102. Hook ML, Burke LJ, Murphy J. An IT innovation for individualizing care: success with clinicians leading the way. *Stud Health Technol Inform*. 2009;146:493–497.

103. Joint Commission Resources I. *Environment of care: Essentials for health care*. Oakbrook IL: Joint Commission Resources; 2012.

104. Estabrooks CA, Squires JE, Hutchinson AM, et al. Assessment of variation in the Alberta

Context Tool: the contribution of unit level contextual factors and specialty in Canadian pediatric acute care settings. *BMC Health Serv Res.* 2011;11:251.

105. Finucane MM, Stevens GA, Cowan MJ, et al. National, regional, and global trends in body-mass index since 1980: systematic analysis of health examination surveys and epidemiological studies with 960 country-years and 9.1 million participants. *Lancet.* 2011;377(9765):557–567.

106. Sullivan PW, Ghushchyan V, Ben-Joseph RH. The effect of obesity and cardiometabolic risk factors on expenditures and productivity in the United States. *Obesity (Silver Spring).* 2008;16(9):2155–2162.

107. Finkelstein EA, Fiebelkorn IC, Wang G. State-level estimates of annual medical expenditures attributable to obesity. *Obes Res.* 2004;12(1):18–24.

108. Pelletier KR. A review and analysis of the clinical and cost-effectiveness studies of comprehensive health promotion and disease management programs at the worksite: update VII 2004-2008. *J Occup Environ Med.* 2009;51(7):822–837.

109. Baicker K, Cutler D, Song Z. Workplace wellness programs can generate savings. *Health Aff (Millwood).* 2010;29(2):304–311.

110. Strecher V. Internet methods for delivering behavioral and health-related interventions (eHealth). *Annu Rev Clin Psychol.* 2007;3:53–76.

111. Zulman DM, Damschroder LJ, Smith RG, et al. Implementation and evaluation of an incentivized Internet-mediated walking program for obese adults. *Transl Behav Med.* 2013;3(4):357–369.

112. Chervin DD, Philliber S, Brindis CD, et al. Community capacity building in CDC's Community Coalition Partnership Programs for the Prevention of Teen Pregnancy. *J Adolesc Health.* 2005;37(3 Suppl):S11–S19.

6

The Role of Economic Evaluation in Dissemination and Implementation Research

RAMESH RAGHAVAN

INTRODUCTION

Over the past several decades, many new and highly efficacious interventions have been developed in health and public health settings thanks to considerable investments in intervention research. Unfortunately, these advances in the development of interventions have not been accompanied by their spread to real-world, community settings. Bridging this gap between science and practice is a principal goal of dissemination and implementation (D&I) research, the former being concerned with increasing the use of evidence-based interventions widely by a target population, and the latter being concerned with the integration of evidence-based interventions within particular service settings such as schools or worksites (please see the chapter 2 for more formal definitions of these terms). Much of D&I research focuses on processes or strategies— or *activities*—by and through which interventions can be spread to, or adopted by, target audiences. In the field of implementation science, where the study of these activities is more developed, there are several distinct implementation strategies, which are designed to systematize the uptake of an intervention in a provider setting.

The challenge for the target audience of D&I research, whether a population of practitioners, or a provider organization, is that many of these activities are highly complex endeavors and, consequently, are likely to be very expensive to deploy within practice settings. Authors of a recent study costing the implementation of a chronic care model reported that the dominant human resources costs identified in the study were due to the 15 individuals charged with implementing the model,[1] suggesting that ignoring implementation costs can have serious consequences to an organization's bottom line. Most health and public health service delivery environments in the community do not have access to research funds, nor the personnel required to execute these activities within their settings. And current reimbursement mechanisms do not cover the entirety of the costs of disseminating and implementing interventions. Hence, organizations that want to deliver new interventions have to think carefully about the affordability of implementing that intervention.

To help support such a decision, an economic analysis of D&I processes and strategies is required, one which systematically examines what outcomes a strategy—or a set of competing strategies—achieves, and the costs of achieving those outcomes. This type of analysis can often be accomplished via a partnership between academic researchers and providers. Once a provider organization knows how much it will cost them to implement an intervention, for example, and what the returns are likely to be of spending those dollars, it can then take an informed decision regarding whether or not to participate in such an implementation. In essence, this argument is an extension and application to the field of implementation science of the theory and practice of economic evaluations of interventions. Just as economic evaluations can provide one particular perspective in assessing the benefit of interventions, economic evaluations also can be of use to D&I researchers. A very expensive implementation strategy that produces small improvements in outcomes is likely to be less attractive than another implementation strategy that produces the same improvement but at a fraction of the cost. Conducting economic evaluations of competing implementation strategies is one way in which D&I researchers can justify scaling up the use of their implementation strategy, and pave the way for comparative cost-effectiveness studies of intervention strategies.

This chapter presents an overview of how D&I research can be evaluated from an economic point of view. We do not, in this chapter, discuss or evaluate any intervention which may be disseminated and implemented; we assume the effectiveness of that intervention. Because implementation science has better developed strategies whose costs can be assessed, this chapter accentuates implementation strategies and illustrates costing one particular implementation strategy as a case example. This approach, however, also can be extended to quantifying the costs of dissemination processes. D&I researchers are interested in both proximal outcomes—such as fidelity (an implementation outcome), or timeliness of care (a service outcome)—as well as distal outcomes, such as improvements in client health and well-being.[2] Each of these types of outcomes can be subject to an economic evaluation. As a first step, for example, researchers might quantify the relative costs of different implementation strategies and compare changes in an intermediate outcome, such as fidelity, resulting from the use of those strategies. This type of analysis provides a researcher with the incremental costs of improving the fidelity to an intervention. The next step might be to examine if these improvements in fidelity have resulted in improvements in a distal outcome, such as improved client health. This type of a sequenced analysis provides information on whether the costs of implementation are a good value for a provider organization attempting to deploy a given evidence-based intervention.

The chapter begins by providing a brief review of economic concepts, and in the next section discusses cost and outcome estimation from a D&I perspective. Using the Breakthrough Series Collaborative as a case study, a suggested approach is outlined to costing this implementation strategy and comparing its costs versus a "usual" implementation. Finally, observations are provided regarding the implications of economic evaluations for the field of D&I research in particular, and for policy in general.

BRIEF REVIEW OF ECONOMIC EVALUATIONS

Economic evaluations use a formal methodology to quantify whether or not the money that is spent on the purchase of health care goods and services represents the best use of that money.[3] This kind of information is one among many other factors (such as availability of a good or service, or practitioner familiarity with an intervention, for example) that drive decision-making. This information is important not only for policymakers but also for administrators, executive directors, and budget managers within hospitals and health care facilities, who each day face decisions regarding whether their organizational expenditures are producing the biggest "bang for the buck."

More formally, economic evaluations have been defined as the ". . . comparative analysis of alternative courses of action in terms of both their costs and consequences."[3] Why is such an analysis necessary? In health, as in several other areas of human activity, many decisions have to be made under conditions of scarcity. If a decision is taken to invest some resources into approach A, then those same resources cannot be used to support some other approach B. Because approach B now cannot be supported, any potential benefits that might have accrued if it had been supported are foregone. These foregone potential benefits of approach B are referred to as *opportunity costs*. The purpose of economic analysis is to ask the question—is the support of A the best possible use of available resources given its opportunity costs? The answer to this question is arrived at by comparing and quantifying the next-best use of available resources (supporting B), and comparing those costs and outcomes to A. Economic evaluations are also central to the estimation of *value*, one definition of which is ". . . the health outcomes achieved per dollar spent."[4] As such, economic evaluations are key to constructing a health system designed around improving outcomes, instead of one focused solely on delivering products and services.

The aforementioned definition suggests that economic evaluations are characterized by two features. First, they are *comparative*, requiring a choice between two proposed alternatives. Second, this comparison between the two proposed alternatives is based on the analysis of the *costs* and *consequences* (or outcomes) of each alternative. Comparing approach A against approach B is what makes economic evaluations *incremental*, in that it is the relative difference in costs and consequences between the two alternatives that is used to drive decision-making.

A common type of economic evaluation used in the health care literature is the *cost-effectiveness analysis*, which examines the relative costs of different interventions designed to affect a health outcome. A cost-effectiveness analysis expresses its results in the form of a ratio:

Incremental cost-effectiveness ratio

$$= \frac{\text{Cost}_{\text{Intervention A}} - \text{Cost}_{\text{Intervention B}}}{\text{Outcome}_{\text{Intervention A}} - \text{Outcome}_{\text{Intervention B}}}$$

where the denominator reflects the gain in a health outcome resulting from Intervention A measured in, say, years of life gained, or reductions in the value of an abnormally high laboratory test result. The numerator reflects the increased costs required to procure that gain.[5] This ratio is called the Incremental Cost Effectiveness Ratio, commonly abbreviated as ICER. An ICER is most interpretable as dollars per unit outcome gained. For example, assume that we are evaluating two competing cancer drugs that have different costs, and our outcome is the number of years of cancer-free survival. If we find an ICER of $50,000, we would say that an expenditure of $50,000 more would be expected to produce one additional year of survival free from cancer. Cost-effectiveness ratios also can be constructed, not against a next-best option, but against doing nothing or a placebo condition; in that case, they are referred to as Average Cost-Effectiveness Ratios.

The task for decision-makers is easiest if Intervention A is cheaper, and produces better outcomes, than Intervention B; in this case Intervention A is the obvious choice from a cost-effectiveness perspective. If Intervention A is costlier than Intervention B but produces better outcomes, then administrators have to decide whether those increased outcomes are worth the added cost. Or, given that Intervention B produces worse outcomes than the more expensive Intervention A, administrators will have to decide if they and their patients can afford to live with the poorer outcomes given the lowered costs of Intervention B. In this example, is $50,000 too much or too little? And who gets to decide whether a year of added life is "worth" $50,000? And can we really afford to spend $50,000 on purchasing an additional year of life given the other things that we could do with that money? It is perhaps obvious that these are not economic but ethical questions,[6] and policymakers have to consider noneconomic elements that go into the making of a decision regarding adopting a given strategy.

A related type of economic evaluation is the *cost–utility analysis,* where the goal is to measure costs associated with changes in client-level or patient-level health-related quality of life (which incorporates preferences with regard to a health outcome instead of using the health outcome per se). These preferences are operationalized and expressed in changes in quality-adjusted life years (QALYs), which form the denominator in these types of studies.[7] Another type of economic evaluation, *cost–benefit analysis,* examines only those outcomes (benefits) that can be quantified in dollar terms. Unlike cost-effectiveness analyses and cost–utility analyses that allow the determination of cost-per-unit-outcome, cost–benefit analyses place dollar values on the outcome and compare whether or not the monetary benefits of an intervention are greater than its costs.[8]

Not all analyses consider costs as well as consequences. Studies frequently deal with either comparisons of costs, or comparisons of consequences, but not both of these. Others do not examine any comparisons at all, confining themselves to quantifying costs associated with a particular approach; this is a necessary precursor to comparison studies. Other studies examine *cost offsets,* for example, examining if costs of treating depression can be partially recouped by reductions in utilization of general medical services by patients suffering from depression.[9] These various types of studies are not considered in this chapter; the discussion is confined to economic evaluations that compare both costs and consequences between two or more competing approaches.

This has necessarily been a cursory overview of the area; further details on how to perform economic evaluations in health care are available elsewhere.[5,10–12] For a study team wishing to perform an economic evaluation as part of a D&I study, it is important to not only consult these sources but to enlist the assistance of a health services researcher with expertise in economic evaluations.

Examples from the Literature

In the field of health care, much of the focus of economic evaluations has been on analyzing *interventions,* a term that we use to encompass activities that are preventative as well as curative in purpose. For example, cost-effectiveness studies have been performed on the use of vaccine to prevent cervical cancer caused by the human papilloma virus (HPV),[13] on screening for maternal depression following childbirth,[14] and on the use of exercise-based treatments in various diseases,[15] among several others. These analyses are designed to provide guidance to health care administrators and payers—to continue these examples—on whether or not to deploy an inoculation program using the HPV vaccine, whether or not to screen for maternal depression following childbirth, or whether or not to add an exercise treatment to extant treatment for individuals suffering from various diseases. In other words, they are all designed to provide an answer to the question, "What intervention makes the most economic sense to deploy?"

ECONOMIC EVALUATIONS IN DISSEMINATION AND IMPLEMENTATION RESEARCH

Dissemination and implementation research, however, requires the answer to a slightly different question—"What are the costs of a particular dissemination approach?" or "Which implementation strategy makes the most economic sense to deploy?" D&I researchers who develop implementation strategies, and organizations considering using an implementation strategy to deploy a desired intervention, both want to know whether the money used to deploy that implementation strategy represents the best use of organizational dollars. Is it really necessary to spend the money on a lengthy process to train, evaluate, and supervise practitioners in delivering an intervention? Or will a weekend seminar suffice? Even more cheaply, why not simply give them a treatment manual and have them deliver the treatment to their clients? Is the added cost of deploying that implementation strategy really that much better than the seminar when it comes to, say, how well practitioners learn to use that intervention (an intermediate outcome), or how well their clients get (the final outcome)?

The answer to this question requires an adaptation to D&I research of the economic evaluation approach described in the previous section. In other words, the purpose of conducting a cost-effectiveness analysis of an implementation strategy, for example, is to quantify the following ratio:

Implementation cost-effectiveness ratio

$$= \frac{\text{Cost}_{\text{ImplementationStrategy}} - \text{Cost}_{\text{"Usual" implementation}}}{\text{Outcome}_{\text{ImplementationStrategy}} - \text{Outcome}_{\text{"Usual" implementation}}}$$

Here, the denominator quantifies the gains in an intermediate or final, clinical outcome; the numerator compares the costs required to achieve those gains. A "usual" implementation is—to continue the example—the weekend seminar, and the candidate implementation strategy is being compared with it on measures of its costs and ability to produce outcomes. As in the intervention example in the prior section, the choice for administrators depends on their valuation of the relative costs and outcomes of one implementation strategy over another. This ratio, which has a similar interpretation as the ICER discussed in the prior section, we will call an incremental implementation cost-effectiveness ratio.

There are several named or "branded" implementation strategies, including leadership facilitation; community development teams;[16] the Breakthrough Series Collaborative;[17] the Translating Initiatives for Depression into Effective Solutions model;[18] the Network for the Improvement of Addiction Treatment model;[19] Cascading Diffusion; Research Practice Partnership; Quality Enhancement Research Initiative;[20] the Availability, Responsiveness, Continuity model;[21] Replicating Effective Programs;[22] the IDEAL model;[23] and several others.[24] The (usually) highly structured nature of these strategies allows them to be subject to an economic evaluation. In contrast, models of diffusion[25] present greater challenges to economic evaluators because each of their elements need to be operationalized before costs can be attached to them. The overall goal of economic evaluations of D&I approaches is to quantify their incremental costs associated with producing change in intermediate or final outcomes.

Perspective

What costs to capture usually depends on whose perspective is adopted. The cost of a single day of hospital care, for example, is either the amount of money paid to the hospital by the health plan (health plan perspective); the total expenditure undertaken by the hospital on that patient that day, including labor costs, medicines, and overhead (organizational perspective); out-of-pocket payments made to the hospital (patient perspective); or *all* costs associated with the hospital stay, irrespective of who incurs them, including the opportunity costs of all resources donated to the hospital (societal perspective).[11] Economic evaluations of interventions usually take a variety of perspectives, including those of the social planner (societal perspective) as well of the entity making the decision whether or not to adopt the intervention being evaluated (i.e., the payer). The latter perspective is important because the payer is making the decision of whether or not to adopt the intervention; the reason the societal perspective is also important is because the payer may vary by intervention and disease, so results using the societal perspective provide a common metric for comparing all treatments across all disorders across all patient populations.

Implementation studies largely seem to adopt the organizational (or program) perspective, which is likely appropriate given that organizations bear the costs of implementing interventions, and that third-party payers do not as yet explicitly resource the costs of implementation in their rate-setting decisions. Dissemination studies, by corollary, should likely take the perspective of the organization disseminating the information—a not-for-profit entity, a professional society, or some other knowledge purveyor.

Cost Estimations

In this chapter, costs are classified into direct labor, indirect labor, and nonlabor costs.[26] *Direct labor costs* are the costs associated with client contact, for example, the cost of delivering an intervention by a practitioner, and measured by the time cost for the practitioner to deliver that intervention. *Indirect labor costs* are also associated with client contact, but occur outside of an examination or intervention room, for example, the time cost of scoring a rating instrument. *Nonlabor costs* are overhead, and include costs associated with clients (e.g., the actual cost to obtain that rating instrument), as well as costs that cannot be assigned to a particular client (e.g., the cost of utilities, administrative support, and building space that are necessary to deliver interventions). The costs of treatment (i.e., service costs), therefore, are the sum of direct labor costs, indirect labor costs, and nonlabor costs associated with delivering that intervention. The costs of disseminating and implementing that intervention are the sum of indirect labor costs and nonlabor costs associated with all implementation activities. Examples of the indirect labor costs of implementation include the cost of practitioner time spent in training and supervision, foregone clinical revenues due to the loss of these practitioners' billable hours, and the time cost of the supervisor assisting the practitioners in delivering the intervention. Examples of nonlabor

costs include the costs of tuition and manuals, and the costs of travel, if necessary (please see Table 6.1 for an example of these costs as applied to implementation).

Outcomes

As in economic evaluations of interventions, economic evaluations of D&I are also concerned with the achievement of client-level health outcomes. However, clinical outcomes are but one type of outcome of interest to dissemination and implementation scientists.[27] Proctor and colleagues define implementation outcomes as "... the effects of deliberate and purposive actions to implement new treatments, practices, and services").[2] These outcomes not only encompass distal clinical outcomes, but also more proximal implementation and service outcomes (Figure 6.1). Hence, cost-effectiveness analyses can be conducted on the costs of achieving gains on a measure of practitioner fidelity to an intervention (an implementation outcome), or on the costs of achieving gains on a measure of timeliness of care (a service outcome), or both.

Some implementation scientists may want to compare implementation strategies on gains in patient quality-adjusted life years or QALYs (cost–utility analysis). Scientists interested in capturing practitioner preferences across competing implementation strategies can use an instrument like the Evidence-Based Practice Attitude Scale.[28] Such studies examining gains in practitioner preference across competing implementation strategies may be useful to implementation scholars seeking an alternative way to examine implementation outcomes such as practitioner acceptability of an intervention. Practitioner-level outcomes also can be measured directly. In mental health, for example, practitioner fidelity to an intervention is an important metric. (Fidelity is the extent to which an intervention as implemented resembles the original protocol of the investigators who developed the intervention.[29,30]) Using fidelity as a practitioner-level outcome, implementation strategies can be compared with respect to the congruence between the deployed intervention and original protocol, and the costs that are necessary to achieve such congruence.

The field of operationalizing D&I outcomes is relatively new, and more development needs to occur before these can be used in economic evaluations. Conceptually, however, implementation outcomes perhaps are of more relevance to D&I scholars than are clinical outcomes, and future

TABLE 6.1 IMPLEMENTATION COSTS FOR THE BREAKTHROUGH SERIES COLLABORATIVE

	Time in hours (a)	Hourly wage (inclusive of fringe benefits) (b)	Cost (a)×(b) = (c.)
Indirect Labor Costs			
Prework			
Practitioner (e.g., *clinician, public health educator*)			
Online training course			
Familiarization with training methodology			
Readiness assessment			
Initial skills-based training			
Administrator			
Familiarization with training methodology			
Readiness assessment			
Manager/Supervisor			
Familiarization with training methodology			
Readiness assessment			
Learning Session			
Practitioner			
Time cost of training			
Administration of instruments			
Scoring of instruments			
Administrator			
Time cost of participation			
Quality assurance			
Manager/Supervisor			
Time cost of participation			
Quality assurance			
Action Period			
Practitioner			
Time cost of participation in case conference			
Nonlabor Costs			
Prework			
Tuition costs			
Cost of curiculum (manual and materials)			
Audiotapes, DVDs, and other recording materials			
Travel costs			
Airfare			
Hotel stay			
Meals and other expenses			
Learning Session			
Costs of supervision/case consultation			

	Time in hours (a)	Hourly wage (inclusive of fringe benefits) (b)	Cost (a)×(b) = (c.)

TABLE 6.1 CONTINUED

Telephone charges
Travel costs
Airfare
Hotel stay
Meals and other expenses
Action Period
Costs of supervision/case
consultation
Telephone charges
   Costs of audiovisual
   materials (DVDs, etc.)
Mailing charges

work that conducts economic evaluations using these consequences is necessary.

Time Horizon

A time horizon (or analytic horizon) is a period of time within which all costs and consequences can be expected to occur. Intervention researchers sometimes use long time horizons because client outcomes following an intervention can take decades (survival after chemotherapy for a malignancy, for example). If D&I researchers are also examining clinical (patient) outcomes, then the issue of specifying an appropriate time horizon is critical. If, however, D&I researchers are only studying dissemination or implementation or service outcomes, and if these outcomes are coterminus with D&I costs, then the issue of specifying a long time horizon is less critical.

Discounting

Discounting is a way to downwardly adjust future costs and consequences in order to derive their present value. Costs are discounted because the value of receiving $1 today is more than the value of receiving $1 ten years from now. An individual can invest that $1 today, and reinvest any interest earnings and obtain in 10 years a sum of money greater than $1. Health outcomes are

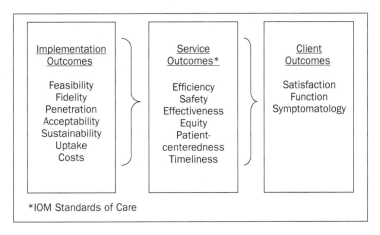

FIGURE 6.1 Implementation outcomes.

(From Proctor and colleagues.[2])

also discounted because most people would rather enjoy better health now than better health 10 years from now.[31] If D&I researchers focus on dissemination and implementation costs, and on implementation and service outcomes, all occurring within a short time horizon, then discounting is of lesser relevance. D&I researchers studying distal client outcomes will need to identify and incorporate appropriate cost and health outcome discounting approaches.

Examples from the Literature

The bulk of the literature on economic analyses of D&I seems to have focused on the implementation of clinical practice guidelines (also known as practice parameters or clinical protocols). Economic evaluations of selected preventive interventions recommended by the Task Force on Community Preventive Services have also been conducted.[32]

A systematic review of guideline implementation studies by Grimshaw and colleagues[33] revealed that 63 of 235 studies (approximately a quarter) provided information on costs of implementation. Strategies to implement these clinical guidelines varied and included dissemination of educational materials, educational meetings, audit and feedback, and the use of clinical reminders, deployed either singly or in combination. Over half of these 63 studies were cost–outcome studies that did not compare alternative implementation strategies, some were cost descriptions, and 11 were cost-effectiveness studies. Many guideline implementation studies since the date of publication of that review seem to focus on cost analyses,[34,35] although cost-effectiveness and cost–benefit studies offer support for patient-focused educational strategies in the implementation of practice guidelines in diabetic care[36] and in asthma care.[37]

Researchers publishing in other disciplines have also conducted economic analyses of D&I within their own disciplines. In the field of infectious diseases, for example, researchers have conducted cost descriptions of competing strategies to ensure infection control,[38] and of widespread versus focused spraying strategies for vector control as a preventive strategy for malaria,[39] have compared competing vaccination strategies with respect to costs and consequences,[40] and have reported cost analyses of alternative strategies to perform screening for a variety of communicable diseases.[41] Researchers have also performed cost descriptions of a community-directed

intervention strategy to implement treatments to reduce roundworm infestation,[42] and of a community health worker-based implementation strategy to deploy interventions to reduce malaria.[43] In the field of health care management, scholars have conducted studies on the costs associated with electronic health record implementation.[44] In the field of pharmaceutical services research, scholars have conducted cost analyses of a strategy to optimize use of a certain high-risk class of medications,[45] and a review reported on equivocal results of cost studies designed to implement strategies to reduce prescribing of acid-suppressive medications.[46] Reviews of studies examining implementation of clinical pathways (which are structured intervention protocols also called care protocols or care pathways) for a variety of illnesses have also reported modest, though highly heterogeneous and variable, reductions in hospital costs.[47]

Since the last edition of this book, there have been a few studies that have examined the outcomes associated with these differential costs. For example, one study examining the costs of developing and implementing 16 disease management programs, and their effects on outcomes for 1,322 patients over the course of a year later found modest outcomes—and consequently wide variations in incremental cost-effectiveness ratios—for these programs.[48] Economic evaluations are occurring across the D&I intellectual landscape. Study protocols on the evaluation of competing implementation strategies to address low back pain[49] and cost analysis of an implementation of Dutch national guidelines designed to reduce vaginal breech deliveries[50] are examples of future studies that can provide valuable information once they are completed.

Two principal challenges seem to characterize this burgeoning literature on the economics of implementation. First, there is variation in the literature regarding which activities should have costs attached to them when it comes to implementation. For example, in a study of guideline implementation, should the cost of developing the guideline be counted, as some authorities suggest?[51] It is not entirely clear that it should be. In mental health, for example, there is considerable information on the costs of treatment;[52–56] to include all of these costs within the costs of implementation would comingle an economic evaluation of treatment with an economic evaluation of its implementation. One study valued the time spent by teachers, parents, school administrators, and project staff associated with implementing a behavioral intervention for children at risk for conduct problems.[57] While time costs are a critical element of the costs of implementation, equating time costs with the costs of implementation can underestimate the true cost of implementing interventions when there are (expensive) manuals and other nonlabor costs associated with implementing the intervention. Another study of service costs included the costs of quality assurance—a category that included "clinical case review, clinical supervisions, team meetings, and case staffing"[26]—in addition to case management and the costs of treatment, but did not include added costs associated with implementation. Other studies that have examined cognitive behavioral therapy implementation have calculated the time taken to train the practitioners, as well as the costs of ongoing supervision, but not nonlabor costs associated with implementation,[58-60] while other studies have excluded costs of supervision from the costs of implementation.[61] Clearly, some unifying framework for cost estimations is necessary in the field of implementation research. It also seems necessary to distinguish between one-time (fixed) costs, such as the costs of initial training; regularly scheduled but fixed costs, such as the costs of ongoing group or peer supervision; and variable costs that increase incrementally with, say, providing client services, such as the costs of rating instruments and their administration.

Second, many studies examine heterogeneous implementation outcomes. Some focus on clinical (patient) outcomes only,[42] a justifiable outcome given that the ultimate goal of implementation is to improve client or patient well-being. Others examine provider behavior,[46] while others study various other aspects of the implementation enterprise. In order to standardize the economic evaluation of implementation, some agreement on the appropriate outcomes for implementation is also necessary.

CASE STUDY—COSTING THE BREAKTHROUGH SERIES COLLABORATIVE IMPLEMENTATION STRATEGY

With the aforementioned caveats, one suggested approach to assessing the costs of D&I within a short time horizon from an organizational perspective is described here; this approach is an example of an activity-based costing strategy[62]

and has its origins in the field of accounting. The basic premise of an activity-based strategy is that it is *activities* performed by various individuals that primarily consume resources, and that it is these activities that are also responsible for producing outcomes. Consequently, understanding the resources consumed by these various activities can be used to allocate costs associated with these activities, and serve as a basis for evaluating the outcomes that result from such activities. Activity-based costing is not the only way to account for costs; traditional accounting strategies such as Relative Value Units develop costs based on procedures, and are far more widely used in health care. But because dissemination and implementation are fundamentally activities in which implementers, providers, administrators, and (to a slightly lesser degree) clients are engaged, and since goods or products are a relatively minor driver of dissemination and implementation costs, this chapter uses activity-based costing instead of a more traditional accounting approach.

Table 6.1 displays a worksheet listing the various elements of a typical Breakthrough Series Collaborative (BSC) strategy, which has been primarily used to implement interventions, but which could be adapted to the use of diffusion researchers. Learning collaboratives—of which the BSC is a "flavor"—are an understudied implementation strategy, although one recent study suggested greater provider engagement and program completion with learning collaboratives compared with on-site training.[63] Table 6.2 displays elements of a weekend seminar (the "usual" dissemination or implementation approach); costs can be attached to each of the elements listed in the tables. The difference in costs between the BSC and "usual" implementation forms the numerator of a cost-effectiveness analysis for the BSC implementation strategy. Tables 6.1 and 6.2 are largely based on the idea that one way to capturing costs associated with D&I is to adapt methods of service costing[10,64] to a D&I approach. This approach assumes that the same intervention can have varying D&I costs depending on whether it is implemented using a weekend seminar or a multimonth implementation strategy. These added costs make one implementation strategy more expensive than another.

Costing a D&I strategy requires a close familiarity with the strategy. A full description of the BSC model is beyond the scope of this chapter, and the reader is referred to overviews of this

TABLE 6.2 IMPLEMENTATION COSTS FOR A WEEKEND SEMINAR
("USUAL" IMPLEMENTATION)

	Time in hours (a)	Hourly wage (inclusive of fringe benefits) (b)	Cost (a)×(b) = (c).
Indirect Labor Costs			
Prework			
Practitioner			
Reading intervention materials			
At the Seminar			
Practitioner			
Time cost of training			
Nonlabor Costs			
Prework			
Tuition costs			
Cost of curriculum (manual and materials)			
Audiotapes, DVDs, and other recording materials			
Travel costs			
Airfare			
Hotel stay			
Meals and other expenses			
At the Seminar			
Telephone charges			
Travel costs			
Airfare			
Hotel stay			
Meals and other expenses			

strategy.[17] *Indirect labor costs* of the BSC model are generated by practitioners, administrators, and supervisors. During the *prework* phase, much of the time of practitioners, administrators, and supervisors is spent in familiarization with the BSC training model (the Institute of Healthcare Improvement requires the formation of three-member teams comprising practitioners as well as administrative staff). This stage also requires an organizational assessment, which must be completed prior to participation in the model. All of these indirect labor costs can be quantified by using the same approach as used for service costs—they represent time costs of participating in these activities. If the time taken in these tasks by practitioners and other personnel is quantified, this time can be multiplied by wage and fringe information, resulting in the cost of participation.

These three sets of personnel also incur opportunity costs during the *learning session* phase, where teams gather in person to discuss the results of their implementation, establish new goals for treatment, and strategize about ways to overcome observed challenges. These learning sessions lead to *action periods*, where practitioners actually deploy the strategies elicited during the learning session. Implementation costs are incurred by practitioners, supervisors, and administrators during these action periods. The BSC model is cyclical, iterative, and cumulative, with learning sessions leading to action periods, which in turn lead to new learning sessions. Hence, organizations have to be prepared to invest in several iterations of this process in order to successfully achieve implementation.

The BSC model is also associated with *nonlabor costs*. In the *prework* phase, these include the costs of procuring training in the intervention using the BSC model (tuition, and other materials) as well as travel expenses for (minimally) one practitioner, an administrator, and a supervisor. Costs of tuition involve two types of costs—the costs of learning about the intervention (which are charged by its developers) and the costs of learning how to implement it using the particular implementation strategy (e.g., the costs of training in the BSC methodology, which are charged by the Institute of Healthcare Improvement). Although organizations bear the costs of learning about the intervention (which is a part of treatment cost), it is best to count the costs of implementation alone here. This is because it may be difficult to disaggregate costs of an implementation strategy from the costs of the treatment that will be deployed using it. In other words, there may be no way to teach the "how" of an intervention without also teaching the "what" of an intervention. (It is, however, possible to do the reverse—teach the "what" of an intervention without teaching the "how" of it.) If researchers find themselves in this quandary, a sensitivity analysis that clearly distinguishes the costs of treatment from the costs of its implementation should be shown.

Implementation costs of the BSC approach during the learning sessions and action periods are largely time costs associated with case consultation, and the material costs associated with developing audiovisual materials of sessions undertaken by trainee psychotherapists (DVDs or videotapes), and then mailing them to trainers. To the extent that some learning sessions occur in person rather than over the telephone, travel costs need to be factored into the indirect nonlabor costs. The estimation of these costs is done in the same manner as for nonlabor costs for the service (treatment). All of these costs unfold over time (since the BSC approach may spill over into a succeeding fiscal year), and with stage of the implementation process (as different elements of the implementation process manifest and recede with implementation). Organizations undertaking their cost estimations will need to be cognizant of these time horizons, and use appropriate discounting for complicated, multiyear implementation endeavors.

These cost domains can be easily generalized to other implementation strategies so long as all these strategies require time for learning, ongoing supervision, case consultation, curricula and other materials, and travel. Some types of generic training will require the resourcing of idiosyncratic costs, and provider organizations will need to identify and quantify these idiosyncratic costs

in order to accurately capture their overall cost of implementing a treatment.

The denominator of an economic evaluation depends on whether investigators are interested in clinical outcomes, or in a particular intermediate outcome. In the latter instance, to some extent, the denominator also depends on the intervention that is being implemented. Researchers wishing to study client improvement across several mental health interventions can use a generic instrument such as the Child Behavior Check List,[65,66] and examine improvements in this measure across the BSC and "usual" implementation conditions. Researchers wishing to study a particular implementation outcome such as fidelity will need to use a fidelity scale developed for a specific intervention—if the intervention is trauma-focused cognitive-behavioral therapy,[67,68] then investigators will need to use the fidelity scale developed for this intervention.[69] The difference in fidelity measures between practitioners participating in the BSC implementation strategy and those participating in the weekend seminar, then, forms the denominator in the cost-effectiveness intervention.

IMPROVING THE STATE OF THE ART IN THE ECONOMICS OF DISSEMINATION AND IMPLEMENTATION

The relative paucity of studies reporting on economic evaluations of D&I suggests that researchers are currently focused on developing and refining D&I strategies rather than on evaluating them from an economic perspective. This section outlines some overarching themes emerging from this review.

First, the bearers of the costs of D&I efforts are likely to emerge as its key stakeholders. Provider organizations currently bear much of the costs of implementation, and information purveyors and health communicators bear much of the costs of dissemination. These organizations will need to be cognizant of the added costs imposed as a result of the use of D&I strategies, and clearly distinguish them from intervention costs. As discussed earlier, much of the variations in D&I costs likely result from the complexity of the D&I strategy, and approaches that require a large number of stakeholders and change agents interacting with various individuals within an organization over prolonged periods of time, or approaches that use highly expensive communicative media like television, likely will be very expensive with respect to D&I costs. In contrast, leaner approaches involving fewer personnel who do much of their work using videoconferencing, telephone consultations, and remote viewing of trainee's sessions will incur fewer implementation costs. Provider organizations that do not possess many resources will need to carefully consider their financial ability to implement treatments using expensive D&I approaches, and D&I scholars developing new approaches should provide data on the long-term advantages of their approaches to these various stakeholders.

Second, because D&I approaches have associated costs, this cost information can be used to develop a future research agenda on the comparative cost-effectiveness of D&I strategies. Currently, there are few studies directly comparing one implementation strategy against another on their relative ability to achieve implementation, service, or clinical outcomes. Incorporating costs into the mix will permit researchers to not only ask if a particular implementation strategy works, but whether its outcomes are worth the money. Those strategies that produce greatest change in outcomes at lowest cost are likely to be the ones that are most practicable in everyday use. Much like for service costs, the costs of D&I are a function of price (the expense of various elements that go into a given approach) and quantity (how long it takes to disseminate or implement a treatment using this strategy, and with what intensity), aggregated over all resources required for the D&I effort. Thus, the most cost-efficient implementation strategies are likely to be the ones that reduce the complexity of the D&I process, the various resources necessary for the strategy, and the total duration of D&I while still producing desirable outcomes.[27]

Third, the field of D&I needs widespread use of costing toolkits, something that is simple enough to be used by practitioners and implementation scientists, that unifies a common set of costing methodologies suited for D&I, that standardizes procedures for capturing costs, that is flexible enough to be applicable across varied D&I strategies, that is robust across the varied organizations and service settings within which D&I work is being conducted, and that serves as a common platform for training and development of economic evaluations in the field. In the area of intervention science, for example, the World Health Organization, as part of its **Cho**osing Interventions that are Cost Effective (CHOICE)

program, has spent the past two decades developing what is perhaps the most comprehensive costing toolkit available.[70,71] Similar efforts have been underway within D&I—examples include an approach developed for implementation of sex offender treatment,[72] or the Cost of Implementing New Strategies approach,[73] and an adaptation of a cost calculator based on child protection practices in Britain.[74] A common framework for economic evaluations within D&I that builds upon these efforts is now necessary because the growth of the field requires that implementation scientists evaluate the same things in much the same way.

Fourth, the rate-limiting step in the economics of D&I research is the cottage industry of D&I strategies, many of which are developed in highly resourced research settings with seemingly little attention being paid to their deployment in lower resource environments, are highly particularistic, appear to be unnecessarily complex and overconceptualized, appear to be indistinguishable from other strategies in terms of focus or intent, and are too poorly described to promote understanding of what implementers actually are supposed to do and what they are supposed to achieve. Activity-based costing—the approach in this chapter—requires that the activities are clear so that costs can be attached to them; also, the outcomes need to be well operationalized so that the incremental effects of these strategies can be captured. At the present time, reviews of implementation strategies implore the field to name and define these strategies,[75] and the prolix and turgid terminology of the field is referred to as a "Tower of Babel."[76] If it is unclear what an implementation strategy actually is, it is impossible to conduct any rigorous economic evaluation of it. Economic evaluators, therefore, may need to confine themselves to the best operationalized and measured implementation strategies. They might also consider advocating for the culling of several marginal strategies, so that those that remain can be subject to appropriate analysis.

Fifth, an important contribution of economic evaluations of implementation strategies will be in the ascertainment of value, which needs a more central space within the firmament of implementation research. Conceptual frameworks exist to help decision-makers decide how best to allocate resources between interventions, their implementation, and research—all to maximize a desired goal.[77] In an elaboration of a value framework for implementation, Walker and colleagues derived constructs from a payer perspective.[78]

The *expected value of perfect implementation* represents the highest possible outcome that can be achieved when implementation is "perfect." The *expected value of actual implementation* represents the outcome that would occur under more naturalistic circumstances. The more cost-effective an intervention is, and the more widely applicable it is, the higher is its expected value of actual implementation.[79] This is what a payer would be willing to pay in order to secure some desirable health outcome (so, for example, payers should be willing to make considerable investments in implementation strategies that increase the percentage of children vaccinated, based on this model). The *value of the implementation activity*, then, is the difference between the expected value of actual implementation and its actual implementation cost. If the cost of implementing an intervention is small, and the effects of the implementation strategy result in highly desirable outcomes, then this is a high-value implementation strategy that needs to be supported. Empirical investigations using these frameworks have yielded intriguing findings, such as declining returns to implementation as natural diffusion occurs,[79] suggesting that investments in implementation should be early, intensive, and time limited.

Delivering a treatment, especially one that comes with expensive D&I costs, is very expensive; high-fidelity implementation requires considerable investment of organizational resources. Because multiprovider organizations are more likely to possess the kinds of resources and the economies of scale required to undertake successful implementation, it is likely that much of the traction in the economics of implementation will occur within large organizations. It also seems apparent that an organization's returns on investment in a treatment are greatest when most of the organization's clients are those who require that particular treatment. To train all clinicians in all treatments is likely to be cost prohibitive. For this reason, the economics of implementation also suggest greater organization and specialization in the health care enterprise.

From a policy perspective, the principal challenge is how to pay for implementation, and this is another area where a focus on value can help decision-makers.[80] In health care, there are efforts focused around twin approaches of *value-based purchasing* [81] (assisting health care purchasers to contract with plans that offer greater value rather than merely lower cost) and *pay-for-performance*,[82] which involve tying fiscal and nonfiscal rewards and punishments to a variety of performance outcomes, such as health outcomes, patient satisfaction, scores on quality scorecards, screening rates, prescribing practices, adherence to clinical guidelines, and investments in information technology, among others. More recently, pay-for-performance approaches have also been proposed for population-level health outcomes such as health inequalities.[83] Scholars have proposed methods for determining the policy cost-effectiveness of implementation, which attempts to provide guidance to policymakers on the relative costs and outcomes of implementation strategies, and is expressed as a function of the cost-effectiveness of treatment, and cost-effectiveness of the practice (organization).[84] But in many disciplines, such as in mental health, the data necessary to determine these cost-effectiveness ratios are not extant. Paying for implementation, then, is an alternative to paying for outcomes in such cases where outcomes are very difficult to pay for given problems in assessing risk.[85] If efficacious treatments are identified, then the task for policymakers is to help resource the delivery of these treatments by paying for their implementation.

SUMMARY

D&I imposes costs upon knowledge purveyors, provider organizations, public health organizations, and payers (including governments). However, whether these added costs will result in improved service delivery and, perhaps more importantly, client outcomes and improvements in population health remains an open question. If emerging studies reveal that defined implementation strategies are more cost effective than "usual" implementation, then policymakers and service providers will need to resource these added costs of implementation in order to assure the success and sustainability of high-quality health services over the long term.

SUGGESTED READINGS AND WEBSITES

Readings

Drummond MF, Sculpher MJ, Torrance GW, O'Brien BJ, Stoddart GL. *Methods for the economic evaluation of health care programmes.* 3rd ed. Oxford: Oxford University Press; 2005.

Gold MR, Siegel JE, Russell LB, Weinstein MC. *Cost-effectiveness in health and medicine.* New York: Oxford University Press; 1996.

These are two of the standard texts on conducting economic evaluations in the health sciences.

Kilo CM. A framework for collaborative improvement: lessons from the Institute for Healthcare Improvement's Breakthrough Series. *Qual Manage Health Care.* 1998;6(4):1–13.
This article was used to motivate the Breakthrough Series case.

Fixsen DL, Naoom SF, Blase KA, Friedman RM, Wallace F. *Implementation research: A synthesis of the literature.* Tampa, FL: University of South Florida, Louis de la Parte Florida Mental Health Institute, The National Implementation Research Network; 2005.

Proctor EK, Landsverk J, Aarons G, Chambers D, Glisson C, Mittman B. Implementation research in mental health services: an emerging science with conceptual, methodological, and training challenges. *Adm Policy Ment Health.* 2009;36(1):24–34.
These are two good overviews of the field of implementation research.

Weinstein MC, Siegel JE, Gold MR, Kamlet MS, Russell LB, for the Panel on Cost-Effectiveness in Health and Medicine. Recommendations of the panel on cost-effectiveness in health and medicine. *JAMA.* 1996;276:1253–1258.
A consensus statement that outlines appropriate methodology for the use of cost-effectiveness analyses in health.

Selected Websites and Tools

The following Internet resources are focused around economic evaluations of interventions, either curative or preventative. The general approach described in these resources, however, can be applied to evaluations of D&I activities.

Chronic Disease Cost Calculator Version 2, Centers for Disease Control and Prevention. http://www.cdc.gov/chronicdisease/calculator/index.html.
This tool provides state-level estimates of the cost of several chronic diseases in the Umited States. Cost is measured as medical expenditures and absenteeism costs. Diseases covered are arthritis, asthma, cancer, cardiovascular diseases, depression, and diabetes.

Cost-Effectiveness Analysis Registry, Center for the Evaluation of Value and Risk in Health, Institute for Clinical Research and Health Policy Studies, Tufts Medical Center. http://healtheconomics.tuftsmedicalcenter.org/cear4/Home.aspx.
Originally based on the articles by Tengs et al.,86,87 this website includes a detailed database of cost-effectiveness analyses, cost-effectiveness ratios, and QALY weights.

Guide to Clinical Preventive Services, Third Edition. http://www.ahrq.gov/clinic/uspstfix.htm.
The U.S. Preventive Services Task Force developed and updates this guide, intended for primary care clinicians, other allied health professionals, and students. It provides recommendations for clinical preventive interventions— screening tests, counseling interventions, immunizations, and chemoprophylactic regimens—for more than eighty target conditions. Systematic reviews form the basis for the recommendations. The Guide is provided through the web site of the Agency for Healthcare Research and Quality.

Task Force on Community Preventive Services. Economic Reviews. http://www.thecommunityguide.org/about/economics.html.
The Community Guide provides a repository of the 200+ systematic reviews conducted by the Task Force, an independent, interdisciplinary group with staff support by the Centers for Disease Control and Prevention. This link is for their economic reviews section, which reviews the applications of cost-effectiveness analyses to interventions analyzed by the Community Guide.

REFERENCES

1. Panattoni L, Dillon EC, Hurlimann L, Durbin M, Tai-Seale M. Human resource costs of implementing a tiered team care model for chronically ill patients according to lean management principles. *JPCRR.* 2016;3(3):186.
2. Proctor E, Silmere H, Raghavan R, et al. Outcomes for implementation research: conceptual distinctions, measurement challenges, and research agenda. *Adm Policy Ment Health Ment Health Serv Res.* 2011;38(2):65–76.
3. Drummond MF, Sculpher MJ, Torrance GW, O'Brien BJ, Stoddart GL. *Methods for the economic evaluation of health care programmes.* 3rd ed. Oxford; New York: Oxford University Press; 2005.
4. Porter ME. What is value in health care? *N Engl J Med.* 2010;363(26):2477–2481.
5. Gold MR, Siegel JE, Russell LB, Weinstein MC. *Cost-effectiveness in health and medicine.* New York: Oxford University Press; 1996.
6. Brock D. Ethical issues in the use of cost effectiveness analysis for the prioritization of health resources. In: Khushf G, ed. *Handbook of bioethics: Taking stock of the field from a philosophical perspective.* Dordrecht: Springer Netherlands; 2004:353–380.
7. Dasbach EJ, Teutsch SM. Cost-Utility Analysis. In: Haddix AC, Teutsch SM, Shaffer PA, Dunet DO, eds. *Prevention effectiveness: A guide to decision analysis and economic evaluation.* New York: Oxford University Press; 1996:130–142.

8. Clemmer B, Haddix AC. Cost-Benefit Analysis. In: Haddix AC, Teutsch SM, Shaffer PA, Dunet DO, eds. *Prevention effectiveness: A guide to decision analysis and economic evaluation.* New York: Oxford University Press; 1996:85–102.

9. Simon GE, Katzelnick DJ. Depression, use of medical services and cost-offset effects. *J Psychosomat Res.* 1997;42(4):333–344.

10. Drummond MF, McGuire A. *Economic evaluation in health care: Merging theory with practice.* New York: Oxford University Press; 2001.

11. Petitti DB. *Meta-analysis, decision analysis, and cost-effectiveness analysis: Methods for quantitative synthesis in medicine.* 2nd ed. New York: Oxford University Press; 2000.

12. Warner KE, Luce BR. *Cost-benefit and cost-effectiveness analysis in health care: Principles, practice, and potential.* Ann Arbor, MI: Health Administration Press; 1982.

13. Armstrong EP. Prophylaxis of cervical cancer and related cervical disease: a review of the cost-effectiveness of vaccination against oncogenic HPV types. *J Manag Care Pharm.* 2010;16(3):217–230.

14. Paulden M, Palmer S, Hewitt C, Gilbody S. Screening for postnatal depression in primary care: cost effectiveness analysis. *BMJ.* 2009;339:b5203.

15. Roine E, Roine RP, Rasanen P, Vuori I, Sintonen H, Saarto T. Cost-effectiveness of interventions based on physical exercise in the treatment of various diseases: a systematic literature review. *Int J Technol Assess Health Care.* 2009;25(4):427–454.

16. Evans SW, Green AL, Serpell ZN. Community participation in the treatment development process using community development teams. *J Clin Child Adolesc Psychol.* 2005;34(4):765–771.

17. Kilo CM. A framework for collaborative improvement: lessons from the Institute for Healthcare Improvement's Breakthrough Series. *Qual Manage Health Care.* 1998;6(4):1–13.

18. Luck J, Hagigi F, Parker L, Yano E, Rubenstein L, Kirchner J. A social marketing approach to implementing evidence-based practice in VHA QUERI: the TIDES depression collaborative care model. *Implement Sci.* 2009;4(1):64.

19. McCarty D, Gustafson DH, Wisdom JP, et al. The Network for the Improvement of Addiction Treatment (NIATx): enhancing access and retention. *Drug Alcohol Depend.* 2007;88(2-3):138–145.

20. Rubenstein LV, Mittman BS, Yano EM, Mulrow CD. From understanding health care provider behavior to improving health care: the QUERI framework for quality improvement. *Med Care.* 2000;38(6,Suppl1):I129–I141.

21. Glisson C, Schoenwald SK. The ARC organizational and community intervention strategy for implementing evidence-based children's mental health treatments. *Ment Health Serv Res.* 2005;7(4):243–259.

22. Kilbourne AM, Neumann MS, Pincus HA, Bauer MS, Stall R. Implementing evidence-based interventions in health care: application of the replicating effective programs framework. *Implement science.* 2007;2:42.

23. Solberg LI, Reger LA, Pearson TL, et al. Using continuous quality improvement to improve diabetes care in populations: the IDEAL model. Improving care for Diabetics through Empowerment Active collaboration and Leadership. *Jt Comm J Qual Improv.* 1997;23(11):581–592.

24. McLaughlin CP, Kaluzny AD. *Continuous quality improvement in health care: theory, implementations, and applications.* 3rd ed. Sudbury, MA: Jones and Bartlett; 2006.

25. Lawrence RS. Diffusion of the U.S. Preventive Services Task Force recommendations into practice. *J Gen Intern Med.* 1990;5:S99-S103.

26. Zarkin GA, Dunlap LJ, Homsi G. The substance abuse services cost analysis program (SASCAP): a new method for estimating drug treatment services costs. *Eval Prog Plann.* 2004;27(1):35–43.

27. Proctor EK, Landsverk J, Aarons G, Chambers D, Glisson C, Mittman B. Implementation research in mental health services: an emerging science with conceptual, methodological, and training challenges. *Adm Policy Ment Health.* 2009;36(1):24–34.

28. Aarons GA. Mental health provider attitudes toward adoption of evidence-based practice: the Evidence-Based Practice Attitude Scale (EBPAS). *Ment Health Serv Rese.* 2004;6(2):61–74.

29. Rabin BA, Brownson RC, Haire-Joshu D, Kreuter MW, Weaver NL. A glossary for dissemination and implementation research in health. *J Public Health Manag Pract.* 2008;14(2):117–123.

30. Fixsen DL, Naoom SF, Blase KA, Friedman RM, Wallace F. *Implementation research: A synthesis of the literature.* Tampa, FL: University of South Florida, Louis de la Parte Florida Mental Health Institute, The National Implementation Research Network; 2005.

31. Brouwer WB, Niessen LW, Postma MJ, Rutten FF. Need for differential discounting of costs and health effects in cost effectiveness analyses. *BMJ.* 2005;331:446–448.

32. Task Force on Community Preventive Services. Economic Reviews. n.d.; http://www.thecommunityguide.org/about/economics.html. Accessed 1/10/11.

33. Grimshaw JM, Thomas RE, MacLennan G, et al. Effectiveness and efficiency of guideline dissemination and implementation strategies. *Health Technol Assess*. 2004;8(6):iii-iv, 1–72.

34. Koskinen H, Rautakorpi UM, Sintonen H, et al. Cost-effectiveness of implementing national guidelines in the treatment of acute otitis media in children. *Int J Technol Assess Health Care*. 2006;22(4):454–459.

35. Hoeijenbos M, Bekkering T, Lamers L, Hendriks E, van Tulder M, Koopmanschap M. Cost-effectiveness of an active implementation strategy for the Dutch physiotherapy guideline for low back pain. *Health Policy*. 2005;75(1):85–98.

36. Dijkstra RF, Niessen LW, Braspenning JCC, Adang E, Grol RTPM. Patient-centred and professional-directed implementation strategies for diabetes guidelines: a cluster-randomized trial-based cost-effectiveness analysis. *Diabet Med*. 2006;23(2):164–170.

37. Tschopp JM, Frey JG, Janssens JP, et al. Asthma outpatient education by multiple implementation strategy. outcome of a programme using a personal notebook. *Respir Med*. 2005;99(3):355–362.

38. Mubayi A, Zaleta CK, Martcheva M, Castillo-Chavez C. A cost-based comparison of quarantine strategies for new emerging diseases. *Math Biosci Eng*. 2010;7(3):687–717.

39. Dambach P, Schleicher M, Stahl H-C, et al. Routine implementation costs of larviciding with Bacillus thuringiensis israelensis against malaria vectors in a district in rural Burkina Faso. *Malaria J*. 2016;15(1):380.

40. Coudeville L, Van Rie A, Getsios D, Caro JJ, Crepey P, Nguyen VH. Adult vaccination strategies for the control of pertussis in the United States: an economic evaluation including the dynamic population effects. *PloS One*. 2009;4(7):e6284.

41. Kania D, Sangare L, Sakande J, et al. A new strategy to improve the cost-effectiveness of human immunodeficiency virus, hepatitis B virus, hepatitis C virus, and syphilis testing of blood donations in sub-Saharan Africa: a pilot study in Burkina Faso. *Transfusion*. 2009;49(10):2237–2240.

42. CDI Study Group. Community-directed interventions for priority health problems in Africa: results of a multicountry study. *Bull World Health Organ*. 2010;88(7):509–518.

43. Onwujekwe O, Uzochukwu B, Ojukwu J, Dike N, Shu E. Feasibility of a community health worker strategy for providing near and appropriate treatment of malaria in southeast Nigeria: an analysis of activities, costs and outcomes. *Acta Tropica*. 2007;101(2):95–105.

44. Slight SP, Quinn C, Avery AJ, Bates DW, Sheikh A. A qualitative study identifying the cost categories associated with electronic health record implementation in the UK. *J Am Med Inform Assoc*. 2014;21(e2):e226–e231.

45. Burns TL, Ferry BA, Malesker MA, Morrow LE, Bruckner AL, Lee DL. Improvement in appropriate utilization of recombinant human erythropoietin pre- and post-implementation of a required order form. *Ann Pharmacother*. 2010;44(5):832–837.

46. Smeets H, Hoes A, de Wit N. Effectiveness and costs of implementation strategies to reduce acid suppressive drug prescriptions: a systematic review. *BMC Health Serv Res*. 2007;7(1):177.

47. Rotter T, Kugler J, Koch R, et al. A systematic review and meta-analysis of the effects of clinical pathways on length of stay, hospital costs and patient outcomes. *BMC Health Serv Res*. 2008;8(1):265.

48. Tsiachristas A, Cramm JM, Nieboer AP, Rutten-van Mölken MP. Changes in costs and effects after the implementation of disease management programs in the Netherlands: variability and determinants. *Cost Eff Resour Alloc*. 2014;12(1):1.

49. Jensen CE, Riis A, Pedersen KM, Jensen MB, Petersen KD. Study protocol of an economic evaluation of an extended implementation strategy for the treatment of low back pain in general practice: a cluster randomised controlled trial. *Implement Sci*. 2014;9(1):1.

50. Vlemmix F, Rosman A, Fleuren M, et al. Implementation of the external cephalic version in breech delivery. Dutch national implementation study of external cephalic version. *BMC Pregnancy Childbirth*.10(1):20.

51. McIntosh E. Economic evaluation of guideline implementation studies. In: Makela M, Thorsen T, eds. *Changing professional practice. Theory and practice of clinical guidelines implementation*. Copenhagen: Danish Institute for Health Services Research and Development; 1999:77–98.

52. Anderson DW, Bowland BJ, Cartwright WS, Bassin G. Service-level costing of drug abuse treatment. *J Subst Abuse Treat*. 1998;15(3):201–211.

53. Foster EM, Connor T. Public costs of better mental health services for children and adolescents. *Psychiatr Serv*. 2005;56(1):50–55.

54. Nabors LA, Leff SS, Mettrick JE. Assessing the costs of school-based mental health services. *J School Health*. 2001;71(5):199–200.

55. Cuffel BJ, Jeste DV, Halpain M, Pratt C, Tarke H, Patterson TL. Treatment costs and use of community mental health services for schizophrenia by age cohorts. *Am J Psychiatry*. 1996;153(7):870–876.

56. Foster EM, Summerfelt WT, Saunders RC. The costs of mental health services under the Fort Bragg Demonstration. *J Ment Health Adm*. 1996;23(1):92–106.

57. Foster E, Johnson-Shelton D, Taylor T. Measuring time costs in interventions designed to reduce behavior problems among children and youth. *Am J Communi Psychol.* 2007;40(1/2):64–81.

58. McCrone P, Knapp M, Kennedy T, et al. Cost-effectiveness of cognitive behaviour therapy in addition to mebeverine for irritable bowel syndrome. *Eur J Gastroenterol Hepatol.* 2008;20(4):255–263.

59. Scheeres K, Wensing M, Bleijenberg G, Severens JL. Implementing cognitive behavior therapy for chronic fatigue syndrome in mental health care: a costs and outcomes analysis. *BMC Health Serv Res.* 2008;8:175.

60. Foster EM, Olchowski AE, Webster-Stratton CH. Is stacking intervention components cost-effective? An analysis of the Incredible Years program. *J Am Acad Child Adolesc Psychiatry.* 2007;46(11):1414–1424.

61. Byford S, Barrett B, Roberts C, et al. Cost-effectiveness of selective serotonin reuptake inhibitors and routine specialist care with and without cognitive behavioural therapy in adolescents with major depression. *B J Psychiatry.* 2007;191(6):521–527.

62. Baker JJ. *Activity-based costing and activity-based management for health care.* Gaithersburg, MD: Aspen; 1998.

63. Nadeem E, Weiss D, Olin SS, Hoagwood KE, Horwitz SM. Using a Theory-Guided Learning Collaborative Model to Improve Implementation of EBPs in a State Children's Mental Health System: A Pilot Study. *Adm Policy Ment Health Ment Health Serv Res.* 2016:1–13.

64. Drummond MF. *Methods for the economic evaluation of health care programmes.* 2nd ed. Oxford: Oxford University Press; 1997.

65. Achenbach TM. *Manual for the child behavior checklist/4-18 and 1991 profile.* Burlington, VT: University of Vermont Department of Psychiatry; 1991.

66. Achenbach TM. *Manual for the child behavior checklist/2-3 and 1992 profile.* Burlington, VT: Department of Psychiatry; 1992.

67. Cohen JA, Mannarino AP, Deblinger E. *Treating trauma and traumatic grief in children and adolescents.* New York: Guilford Press; 2006.

68. Cohen JA, Mannarino AP, Deblinger E. *Child and parent trauma-focused cognitive behavioral therapy treatment manual.* Philadelphia: Drexel University College of Medicine; 2006.

69. Child Sexual Abuse Task Force and Research & Practice Core National Child Traumatic Stress Network. How to Implement Trauma-Focused Cognitive Behavioral Therapy. 2004; http://www.nctsnet.org/nctsn_assets/pdfs/TF-CBT_Implementation_Manual.pdf. Accessed 1/10/11.

70. Johns B, Baltussen R, Hutubessy R. Programme costs in the economic evaluation of health interventions. *Cost Eff Resour Alloc.* 2003;1(1):1.

71. Edejer T-T, Baltussen R, Adam T, et al. *WHO guide to cost-effectiveness analysis.* Geneva: World Health Organization; 2003.

72. Jennings WG, Zgoba KM. An application of an innovative cost-benefit analysis tool for determining the implementation costs and public safety benefits of SORNA with educational implications for criminology and criminal justice. *J Crim Just Educ.* 2015;26(2):147–162.

73. Saldana L, Chamberlain P, Bradford WD, Campbell M, Landsverk J. The Cost of Implementing New Strategies (COINS): a method for mapping implementation resources using the Stages of Implementation Completion. *Child Youth Serv Rev.* 2014;39:177–182.

74. Holmes L, Landsverk J, Ward H, et al. Cost calculator methods for estimating casework time in child welfare services: a promising approach for use in implementation of evidence-based practices and other service innovations. *Child Youth Serv Rev.* 2014;39:169–176.

75. Proctor EK, Powell BJ, McMillen JC. Implementation strategies: recommendations for specifying and reporting. *Implement Sci.* 2013;8(1):1.

76. McKibbon KA, Lokker C, Wilczynski NL, et al. A cross-sectional study of the number and frequency of terms used to refer to knowledge translation in a body of health literature in 2006: a Tower of Babel? *Implement Sci.* 2010;5(1):16.

77. Fenwick E, Claxton K, Sculpher M. The value of implementation and the value of information: combined and uneven development. *Med Decis Making.* 2008;28(1):21–32.

78. Walker S, Faria R, Whyte S, et al. Getting cost-effective technologies into practice: the value of implementation. Report on framework for valuing implementation initiatives. *Policy Research Unit in Economic Evaluation in Health and Care Interventions.* 2014; http://www.eepru.org.uk/Valueofimplementation-framework-024.pdf. Accessed 12/25/16.

79. Whyte S, Dixon S, Faria R, et al. Estimating the cost-effectiveness of implementation: is sufficient evidence available? *ValueHealth.* 2016;19(2):138–144.

80. Proctor EK, Knudsen KJ, Fedorovicius N, Hovmand P, Rosen A, Perron B. Implementation of evidence-based practice in community behavioral health: agency director perspectives. *Adm Policy Ment Health.* 2007;34(5):479–488.

81. Deas TM, Jr. Health care value-based purchasing. *Gastrointest Endosc Clin North Am.* 2006;16(4):643–656.

82. Rosenthal MB, Dudley RA. Pay-for-performance: will the latest payment trend improve care? *JAMA*. 2007;297(7):740–744.

83. Asada Y. A summary measure of health inequalities for a pay-for-population health performance system. *Prev Chronic Dis*. 2010; http://www.cdc.gov/pcd/issues/2010/jul/09_0250.htm. Accessed 1/11/11.

84. Mason J, Freemantle N, Nazareth I, Eccles M, Haines A, Drummond M. When is it cost-effective to change the behavior of health professionals? *JAMA*. 2001;286(23):2988–2992.

85. Raghavan R. Using risk adjustment approaches in child welfare performance measurement: applications and insights from health and mental health settings. *Child Youth Serv Rev*. 2010;32(1):103–112.

86. Tengs TO, Wallace A. One thousand health-related quality-of-life estimates. *Med Care*. 2000:583–637.

87. Tengs TO, Adams ME, Pliskin JS, et al. Five-hundred life-saving interventions and their cost-effectiveness. *Risk Anal*. 1995;15(3):369–390.

7

Designing for Dissemination in Chronic Disease Prevention and Management

NEVILLE OWEN, ANA GOODE, TAKEMI SUGIYAMA, MOHAMMAD JAVAD KOOHSARI, GENEVIEVE HEALY, BRIANNA FJELDSOE, AND ELIZABETH EAKIN

INTRODUCTION

Epidemiological, behavioral, and public health research continue to generate findings with great potential to inform the prevention and management of major chronic diseases—type 2 diabetes, cardiovascular disease, and breast and colon cancer in particular. There have been significant research advances across several evidence domains: on understanding relationships of behavior with health outcomes; on developing measurement methods for use in public health research; on identifying the individual, social and environmental determinants of health behaviors; and on a wide range of behavior-change interventions that have been developed and tested systematically.[1,2]

However, the actual translation of this broad array of knowledge into effective policies and programs has been limited.[3] Research findings may be promulgated, but their uptake will not happen automatically. Designing explicitly for dissemination is required. Such evidence-to-practice translation gaps have been characterized in several ways, for example:

The metaphor of the "leaky pipeline" is compelling. [4] Much that is important in maintaining the rigor and integrity of prevention efforts can leak away, as that knowledge moves from the research evidence base through the mechanisms of translation into the broadness of policy and the constraints of practical application.

The "push-pull" metaphor[5] characterizes many of the relevant challenges in designing for dissemination: efforts at dissemination by researchers (the "push" element) can be limited in their momentum, or the initial momentum can rapidly decay; furthermore, the motivations and capacities of practitioners, policymakers, and others (the "pull" element) to translate, adopt, and implement can be held back by the multiple limitations of systems for funding, administration, staffing, communication, and implementation of programs.

Such conceptions point broadly to the need for an increased emphasis on *designing for dissemination*.[6,7] In practice, such concepts and models can help to guide initiatives through the relevant networks and partnerships required for successful dissemination.[8] However, designing for dissemination in practice remains a somewhat marginal priority for many researchers and can thus limited in its scope.

The approach to designing for dissemination in this chapter is flavored by Geoffrey Rose's[9,10] perspective on the balancing of population and high-risk approaches—addressing both the *prevention* and *management* of chronic disease. While these are chronic disease examples, the principles apply to a wide range of health-related topics. These two approaches are complementary, reflecting Rose's perspective on the *strategy of preventive medicine*: that overall health is improved by both population-wide and high-risk approaches.

THERE REMAINS MUCH SCOPE FOR IMPROVING THE PRACTICE OF DESIGNING FOR DISSEMINATION

For both public health and clinical settings (the population and the high-risk contexts), there are unmet needs to pursue systematically the dissemination of evidence-based practices acts as a constraint on potential benefits that would flow from new discoveries.

For example Brownson and colleagues[11] identified a large sample of researchers in the United States, surveying them to identify gaps in practice among researchers and areas where there is potential for improvement in designing for dissemination. They surveyed authors of relevant papers in public health and the recipients of government-sponsored research support. Over three quarters declared that they spent less than 10% of their time on dissemination-related research and activities. A little over half identified having an individual or group in their research program dedicated to dissemination. Less than 20% stated that they used a framework or theory as a conceptual guide to dissemination activities. Only one-third sated that they "always" or "usually" involved stakeholders in the conduct of their research.

There thus remains considerable room for improvement in designing for dissemination. Reflecting on the findings of their survey, Brownson and colleagues[11] concluded that:

1. Dissemination generally does not occur spontaneously and naturally.
2. Passive approaches to dissemination are largely ineffective.
3. Single-source prevention messages are generally less effective than comprehensive, multilevel approaches.
4. Stakeholder involvement in the research or evaluation process is likely to enhance dissemination (so-called practice-based research).
5. Theory and frameworks for dissemination are beneficial.
6. The process of dissemination needs to be tailored to specific audiences.

Table 7.1, which builds on the framework developed by Brownson and colleagues,[11] outlines the key complexities and many of the major practicalities of designing for dissemination, classified in terms of the relevant system changes, processes, and products that can be involved. Many of the elements to consider in designing for dissemination are closely related to concepts of external validity (see chapter 18).

The need to understand these limitations and opportunities has a broader relevance for the practice of designing for dissemination, not only in the United States where influential guiding models have been developed. For example,

through a survey of researchers from Brazil, the United Kingdom, and the United States, Tabak and colleagues[12] have identified attributes of how the dissemination process is pursued. They explored further details of practices in designing for dissemination, and researchers' perceptions of the factors that they believed to be associated with successful dissemination. The significance of dissemination to nonresearcher audiences was widely recognized across all three countries; however, the communication outlets identified for putting forward dissemination-related research findings could only be classified as being "traditional academic venues."

Across the respondents from all three countries, self-rated dissemination effort was found to be related to several predictive factors (including the availability of resources to support dissemination efforts to distinctly). However, the factors related to these dissemination efforts had quite low prevalence in this three-country sample. Among all of the researchers surveyed, less than one-third rated their level of effort for the dissemination as being excellent. Overwhelmingly, the constraints identified were limited support and resources to properly support researchers who might want to disseminate their findings.

These self-ratings very likely reflect best-case scenarios. Even when researchers' stated intentions strongly endorse the importance of dissemination, researchers generally identified that they lacked the supports to increase dissemination efforts. Additional resources and training in designing for dissemination along with improved partnerships could help bridge the research-practice gap.[13-15]

Against the background of these concerns and conceptual models to guide designing for dissemination, examining the particulars of dissemination initiatives can be informative. This chapter first considers some particulars of designing for dissemination, taking two case examples from physical activity and sedentary behavior as primary-prevention concerns. It then considers a further case example from a high-risk group: disease-management among middle-aged and older adults living with diabetes. These case studies illustrate many of the principles in Table 7.1. While other health behaviors or issues are not discussed here, implications for other prevention and management concerns should be apparent to the reader.

TABLE 7.1 PRINCIPLES FOR DESIGNING FOR DISSEMINATION[11]

Domain	Subdomain	Sample Actions
System changes	Shift research funder priorities and processes.	• Make dissemination (e.g., a dissemination plan) a scoreable part of funding announcements. • Include stakeholders in the grant review process. • Provide rapid funding for practice-based research with high dissemination potential. • Provide supplemental funding for dissemination.
	Shift researcher incentives and opportunities.	• Provide academic incentives and credit, including impacts on promotion and tenure decisions (provide prototype promotion/tenure policies). • Hire faculty with practice experience. • Provide opportunities for faculty to spend time in practice settings. • Conduct training to improve dissemination, implementation, evaluation, and translation.
	Develop new measures and tools.	• Identify measures for evaluating dissemination efforts. • Maintain systems for tracking the measures. • Develop tools for designing for dissemination.
	Develop new reporting standards.	• Develop standards for reporting research that focus more fully on dissemination. • Promote new dissemination and implementation reporting standards.
	Identify infrastructure requirements.	• Identify people required for dissemination and evaluation. • Identify system requirements (information technology, media).
Processes	Involve stakeholders as early in the process as possible.	• Engage as advisors and collaborators. • Engage in the research process.
	Engage key stakeholders (receptors) for research through audience research.	• Identify gaps in research, relevance of methods, messages. • Ensure stakeholders represent potential adopter organizations. • Identify opinion leaders for uptake. • Identify barriers to dissemination. • Identify success and failure stories.
	Identify models for dissemination efforts.	• Review existing frameworks for applicable constructs. • Pilot test measures for assessing model constructs among key stakeholders. • Develop models for dissemination actions that are context relevant.
	Identify the appropriate means of delivering the message.	• Identify the optimal disseminator [usually *not* the researcher]. • Link the researcher, practice, and policy specialists with the disseminator. • Identify channels for dissemination/mode of knowledge transfer.

(continued)

TABLE 7.1 CONTINUED

Domain	Subdomain	Sample Actions
Products	Identify the appropriate message.	• For interventions, document evidence of effectiveness, cost of implementation, and cost effectiveness. • For etiologic research, address risk communication. • Document evidence of disseminability/ease of use.
	Develop summaries of research in user friendly, nonacademic formats (audience tailoring).	• Develop issue briefs, policy briefs, case studies. • Identify potential roles for social media (e.g., Twitter, Facebook). • Deliver presentations to stakeholders.

DESIGNING FOR DISSEMINATION THROUGH ENVIRONMENTAL INITIATIVES: ACTIVE TRANSPORT

Environmentally focused initiatives have the potential to be wide reaching, available broadly across the social spectrum, and sustainable, illustrating key elements of designing for dissemination in Rose's population-wide prevention context. Here, the broad aim is to make healthy choices more realistic choices within the context of people's everyday lives. There have been impressive successes in the dissemination of environmental approaches, particularly in the field of tobacco control in countries like the United States and Australia, in reducing road traffic accidents, and in changing public practices in relation to alcohol use. As was the case during the early stages of tobacco control (e.g., stop smoking groups, self-help books), the first organized approaches to increasing participation in physical activity focused on factors operating at the individual level (e.g., promoting motivation, goal setting, confidence, incentives for change).[16] However, widespread and sustainable physical activity changes are only likely to be achieved by initiatives designed to make participation an attractive default choice, through the identification and implementation of the relevant environmental changes.[16,17]

For such approaches to inform designing for dissemination, contextual and behavioral specificity[18,19] should be taken into account, with a focus on "behavior settings" for physical activity dissemination.[20,21] A behavior setting involves the combination of physical and social environments, in which certain behaviors may be observed or expected. For example, exercise for fitness or health purposes, carried out in health club facilities or community gymnasia may be determined by distinct individual, social, and environmental factors that dissemination will need to address. Designing for dissemination in the physical activity context will require multiple strategies, because each domain embodies different behavior settings, the relevant behaviors are influenced by different factors, and the engagement of different partners will be required to design for dissemination.

Daily travel or transport within a city is a particular "behavior setting" within which there remain significant implementation challenges to increasing participation in physical activity.[22] Active transport such as walking and cycling contributes to health because these alternatives to automobile use involve physically active options. However, automobile use is the most common transport mode and will result in longer sitting time, which is now known to have detrimental effects on weight gain, metabolic health outcomes, and risk of major chronic diseases, in addition to other risks associated with lack of physical activity.[23] The rapidly increasing body of evidence in the population-health benefits of active transport, combined with advocacy for environmental initiatives to promote walking and biking, has engaged multiple sectors beyond health, such as urban design, planning, and transportation sectors.[24-27] However, the systematic use of dissemination-relevant research evidence in this relatively new field lags behind the enthusiasm and the imperatives for doing so. For evidence to influence transport mode choice, designing for dissemination needs to build transport and urban designers/planners' understanding of the changes that will yield health benefits through increasing activity.

Neighborhood walkability, a composite construct typically consisting of residential density, land use, mix and street connectivity, has been demonstrated through a range of studies to be associated with health-related physical activity.[17,18,22,28] Such evidence is important for engaging the requisite "processes" in designing for dissemination (see Table 7.1) via the involvement and contributions of policymakers and the other "gatekeepers" of dissemination in the urban design planning, transportation, and geography fields. For these "gatekeeper" constituencies— who have practical concerns and obligations to do what will make a difference in ways that will be justifiable and defensible—a set of explanations is required about how the attributes of neighborhoods can increase physical activity.[29] Such explanations need to be supported conceptually (see italicized terms following) and also be practical in their focus. To this end, the context and benefits of addressing a neighborhood walkability may be explained as follows:

- The presence of destinations such as retail outlets and other facilities (service, recreational) in the local neighborhood, and the attributes of the routes by which they may be accessed can provide *instrumental cues* (relating to the feasibility and efficiency of walking or biking).
- Aesthetic attributes can provide *evaluative and affective cues* that may make active behavioral choices more or less attractive (in a negative way, poor neighborhood aesthetic attributes might foster residents' staying indoors to watch television, or driving an automobile rather than spending time outdoors or walking or biking to destinations).
- Built-environment attributes can provide *normative cues* about behavioral choices that are expected of people (large parking lots and the absence of sidewalks around shopping centres, seeing few other people in the local neighborhood walking or using bicycles).
- Built-environment attributes may prompt people to anticipate the likely *positive or negative outcomes* of such choices. Such outcomes might include a greater variety of pleasant social interactions, or prolonged

waiting to cross busy roads and exposure to exhaust fumes.

Urban design and public health practitioners and policymakers who are the gatekeepers for designing for dissemination in the active transport context are more likely to be engaged if the aforementioned constructs can be put forward in more simple, operational terms. Further, user-friendly monitoring tools can support dissemination. Walkability has been a tool for researchers due to its reliance on spatial data and geographical technologies, but there are newly emerging potentials for broader adoption of simplified neighbourhood walkability using Space Syntax methods, which only requires readily available street data to calculate walkability.[30,31] There are now also user-friendly and publicly available tools for assessing neighbourhood walkability.[32] For example, Walk Score® is a free, web-based tool that evaluates how a particular location is supportive of residents' active behaviors.[33]

Attributes of Research to Support Designing for the Dissemination of Active Transport Initiatives in Multiple Countries

Informing designing for dissemination through fostering interactions at the local and international level between researchers and practitioner constituencies has considerable potential.[34] The Council on the Environment and Physical Activity (CEPA) of the International Society for Physical Activity and Health has been established. The purpose of CEPA is to build strong evidence-based links from the research that is being supported through the International Physical Activity and the Environment Network (IPEN) study. IPEN investigators from multiple disciplines in multiple countries are conducting rigorous research on physical activity and the environment, with the explicit purpose of promoting internationally and locally relevant designing for dissemination initiatives (*www. ipenproject.org*) through pursuit of the following objectives:

1. To stimulate and support interdisciplinary research on physical activity and the environment
2. To build capacity for using the best available methods, and encourage the use of common protocols and measures

3. To increase communication and collaboration among researchers in developing new measures, adapting measures for local contexts, and organizing networks focusing on specific population subgroups, geographic regions, and research question
4. To communicate with policymakers in ways that are outside the usual academic methods (i.e., academic articles, academic meetings)
5. To encourage formation of interdisciplinary teams to conduct research that provides the evidence-base for dissemination
6. To encourage teams from different countries to carry out joint and pooled analyses, with the aim of identifying unique environmental and cultural determinants of physical activity that may be more broadly disseminated
7. To support physical activity/built environment researchers to become more effective advocates for disseminating evidence-based approaches to environmental and policy change (for example, through opportunities with these key constituencies through the Active Living Research organization [http://activelivingresearch.org/] and associated conferences)

These seven objectives of CEPA illustrate the logic of how designing for dissemination through the interactions of settings-focused research, policy, and practice may be pursued in the field of physically active transport.

DESIGNING FOR THE DISSEMINATION OF A WORKPLACE SITTING-REDUCTION INITIATIVE

Too much sitting is now recognised as a serious public health concern that is in addition to an established focus on physical inactivity. On average, sedentary time (sitting, reclining, or lying awake with low energy expenditure) occupies more than half of an adults' waking hours, with this proportion expected to continue to escalate. Notably, there is increasing evidence that frequently breaking up sitting with even light intensity activities, including standing, and slow walking, may provide cardiometabolic health benefits.[35] Underpinned by this research, new preventive messages, interventions, and policies to reduce prolonged sitting are now emerging.

There is a plethora of new findings from epidemiological, experimental, and intervention studies (at this stage, primarily efficacy studies), demonstrating that significant health benefits are highly likely to accrue from reducing and breaking up prolonged periods of time spent sitting.[36] Sedentary behavior is a thus a new element of the established physical activity agenda in chronic disease prevention and disease management.

Compared with promoting physical activity, addressing sedentary behavior illustrates the different challenges for designing for dissemination, within which the "pull" elements[5] are compelling. Sitting has been characterized as the "new smoking"—in broadcast and online media, blogs, and commentaries. In this context, where there has been rapid uptake of the idea that *too much sitting* is bad for health, there is also recognition that it is an issue that should be considered and addressed in a careful and systematic fashion, with reference to the state of the relevant evidence. This is now evident in many areas of business and industry where "active working" options are being introduced.

Sitting time can be highly contextually driven and is often dictated by the "behavior settings" in which it occurs.[2] This is illustrated in the neighbourhood activity-environments examples described earlier and applies similarly to the office-workplace environment.[37] For office workers, the majority of their daily sitting time is accrued in the workplace, with office workers spending on average 70% to 80% of their working day sitting. Further, much of this sitting time is accrued in prolonged, unbroken bouts of 30 minutes or longer;[38] a pattern potentially placing them at increased risk for poor cardiometabolic and musculoskeletal health.[39] Considering that sitting is a norm in most office-based workplaces, there is thus a "designing for dissemination" imperative in this field.

The *Stand Up Australia* Research and Dissemination Initiative

Within this context, the *Stand Up Australia* collaborative research program on understanding the benefits of reducing prolonged sitting time in the workplace was initiated with the explicit intention of designing for dissemination. The *Stand Up Australia* program comprises pragmatic, research-led intervention trials that evaluate the effectiveness of different activity-promoting strategies (organizational, environmental, individual;

alone or in combination) to enable adults to stand up, sit less, and move more in the workplace, with a particular focus on the desk-based workplace. This program of research has demonstrated that it is feasible and acceptable to introduce activity-promoting strategies within the desk-based workplace to create a dynamic work environment (i.e., a working environment that encourages more movement, more often), and that such strategies can lead to substantial (e.g., more than 1.5 hours reduction in sitting per 8-hour workday[40]) and sustained[41] reductions in workplace sitting time.

There is now strong demand from workplaces for advice, assistance, and support in implementing such activity-permissive strategies into their policy and practice (the "pull" element in designing for dissemination[5]). The *BeUpstanding Champion Toolkit*[42] was designed to address this need, based on evidence from *Stand Up Australia* and the broader sedentary behavior field. The key adaptations from the research protocol were the transfer of program implementation and evaluation from the research team to a workplace champion, with the champion guided by multimedia resources provided in an online, website-based format.[42] The "train the champion" approach was used in recognition that workplace champions, as role models and drivers of the program, are critical for successful workplace change.[43]

The *BeUpstanding* program is designed to be implemented at the level of the work team (broadly defined as a colocated group, employed by one organization, and having the same workplace policies) over 3 months. Increased activity and decreased sitting are primarily targeted through organizational and environmental level approaches (e.g., standing meetings, centralized bins), with the strategies chosen by each work team. In line with best practice and existing frameworks for program delivery, the program is underpinned by: a participative and collaborative approach; tailoring of strategies to the organization; visible organizational support for the program; a strong evaluation framework; and communication of program outcomes. The dissemination toolkit resides on a dedicated website and includes the following features:

- A website "landing page" to provide the rationale and business case for program participation
- Embedded evaluation via automated tracking of program delivery through Google analytics and smart features, and an inbuilt, customised online data collection and feedback module
- Dedicated *BeUpstanding* social media channels (Facebook, Twitter, Instagram) to connect champions with other champions, facilitating the sharing of ideas and progress and creating a support community for change
- An "evidence portal" (e.g., email/ social media tool/blog) to update the champions and staff on the latest research evidence.

Understanding the successes or otherwise of designing for the dissemination of such approaches will require detailed but pragmatic evaluations. In this context, it is possible to gather data independent of researcher input using such tools as website analytics, online workplace audits, and online surveys for staff and champions. It is also important to identify predicted outcomes of the dissemination process, which can include:

- *Uptake:* The documentation of number of work teams registered for the program and the characteristics of participating work teams.
- *Implementation*: Documenting the completion by participants and participating organizations of program components; and, documenting barriers and facilitators to implementation.
- *Effectiveness:* Changes in workplace sitting time, workplace time spent in more physical activities, related attitudes and knowledge, and perceptions of workplace culture to prolonged sitting.
- *Costs*: The economic outcomes of the program dissemination may be considered in terms of costs and benefits to employers and employees.

Embedding evaluation into the dissemination design ensures the generation of practice-based evidence: a key element for supporting the wide-scale integration of the *BeUpstanding Champion Toolkit* into workplace policy and practice.

DESIGNING FOR DISSEMINATION TO A HIGH-RISK GROUP

The Logan Healthy Living Program

The Logan Healthy Living Program (LHLP) was a cluster-randomized trial evaluating a 12-month telephone-delivered physical activity and dietary behavior intervention, targeting Australian primary care patients with type 2 diabetes or hypertension from a low-income community.[44] The LHLP trial was a pragmatic trial[45–47] designed explicitly to inform subsequent dissemination. In addition to documenting the primary behavioral outcomes of the trial,[44] key elements of the evidence base needed to inform dissemination were also examined. These included:

- Cost-effectiveness analysis[48]
- Data on intervention implementation were systematically collected, allowing for evaluation of dose-response outcomes.[49]
- Maintenance data 6 months following the end of the intervention[50]

In brief, the original LHLP trial, in which the primary outcomes were self-reported physical activity and dietary behavior, resulted in significant between-group improvements favoring the intervention group. This was the case for all dietary outcomes, including energy from total fat and saturated fat, vegetable intake, fruit intake, and grams of fiber; and, a significant within-group improvement was observed for both treatment and usual care groups for moderate-to-vigorous physical activity.[44] Results were maintained at an 18-month follow-up, 6 months following the end of intervention.[50] The intervention was also shown to be cost effective, and a higher dose of intervention, particularly during the latter part of the intervention, was shown to be related to behavior-change outcomes.[51]

As described in the following, the evidence generated in the LHLP trial, along with a systematic review of telephone delivered interventions,[47] played a significant role in informing the dissemination of the LHLP intervention into community-based practice. To highlight the opportunities, practicalities, and compromises involved in the dissemination of the LHLP, an account of the adaptations and supportive factors that were necessary to facilitate adoption and implementation in a community setting is provided.[52]

Funding and Broader Contextual Opportunity

Resources for dissemination are crucial, particularly those related to the infrastructure and staffing necessary for program delivery. The ability to conduct the LHLP dissemination study was influenced in large part by the availability of dedicated state government funding to enable the implementation of locally relevant solutions to better manage and prevent chronic disease. One of the sites to receive funding was the Logan area in which the LHLP trial was conducted. As mandated by the initiative, this presented an opportunity to consider the dissemination of local, evidence-based programs targeted at the primary and secondary prevention of chronic disease within the Logan community.

Strong Credibility and Community Partnerships

The conduct of the LHLP research trial in the Logan community involved the development of a partnership with the Greater Metro South Brisbane Medicare Local, a state-funded organization providing administrative, technical, and professional development support to local area primary care practices. This core partnership and other strong relationships in the Logan community were important to enhancing local trust in the trial, aiding recruitment and ultimately influencing dissemination: its successful translation from research to practice. At the same time as Logan received funding, the LHLP trial was nearing completion, and the Principal Investigator of LHLP was invited to sit on the Steering Committee that oversaw the allocation of the program funding. That committee was charged with identifying evidence-based chronic disease self-management initiatives that could be undertaken in the community. The Principal Investigator advocated for uptake in the local community of the LHLP based on it consistency with the funding goals. Consequently, the LHLP was adopted by the South East Primary HealthCare Network for delivery as part of the larger suite of programs offered under the Logan strategy. Central to its inclusion was the commitment of LHLP research staff to provide ongoing support for implementation, and to oversee its evaluation.

Documenting the Dissemination Context, the Target Group and Identifying the Relevant Program Content:

The first adaptation concerned the target group of the intervention. To avoid duplication of existing chronic disease services, and given the increasing focus on overweight and obesity in primary care, the South East Primary HealthCare Network resolved that the OHP should target physical activity, diet and modest weight loss in overweight primary care patients *without* chronic disease.

Due to these changes, new content around weight loss was incorporated into the intervention protocols and materials. The research team took the lead on these adaptations, which were based on a distillation of the evidence from previous reviews, were particularly concerned with program attributes that might enhance maintenance, and were developed in consultation with OHP program staff. Documenting precisely these changes and noting the relevant areas of difference compared with what was the case in the efficacy-study context is crucial to developing systematic accounts of behavior-change program dissemination.

Documenting Program Delivery

As the OHP was not being delivered in a research context, it was decided to allow more flexibility in program delivery, consistent with the norms of the clinical approach being used. Although maintaining the same call structure as the LHLP (a tapered call schedule over 12 months; weekly, fortnightly, then monthly phases), OHP telephone counselors had the discretion to tailor the frequency of calls according to individual participants' needs. Research staff assisted with the development of a database for participant and outcomes tracking.

Assessment of Outcomes in the Dissemination Context of Dealing with Those at High Risk

Like the LHLP, participant assessment in the OHP occurred at four time points (baseline, 4, 12, and 18 months) and was used to provide feedback to OHP program participants and for program evaluation.[52] While LHLP participant assessments were completed by computer-assisted telephone interviewers blinded to study condition, OHP budgetary constraints meant that the telephone counselors also completed assessment calls. To address limitations concerning the potential biases engendered by the collection of self-report data by program staff delivering the intervention, the OHP also collected clinical objective measures, including physician-measured weight, waist circumference, and blood pressure, which were not collected in the LHLP trial. The evaluation of this disseminated program required particular attention to the inevitable changes that take place in adapting the program from the efficacy-study context. Several adaptations to the original LHLP, rebadged by the South East Primary HealthCare Network as the OHP, were necessary to ensure feasibility and program "fit" within the adopting organizational context, based

largely on needs and availability of resources. Documenting the nature of such changes systematically is crucial to inform future efforts at designing for dissemination.

SUMMARY

The examples and perspectives on designing for dissemination in this chapter have dealt with two complementary and interrelated elements of Rose's[9,10] strategy of preventive medicine:

- Population health prevention strategy through designing for dissemination to promote evidence-based initiatives to influence health-risk behaviors in *settings that impact on large numbers of people.*
- Dissemination of evidence-based health behavior-change approaches for those with *major chronic diseases*

Box 7.1 identifies principles to guide designing for the dissemination of evidence-based environmental and policy initiatives, and the implementation and evaluation of dissemination initiatives for evidence-based health behavior-change programs.

This chapter has emphasized the need for research that is designed and implemented explicitly with dissemination in mind.[11,12] This has been illustrated in relation to environmental and policy initiatives to influence physical activity through active transport, and through the example of initiatives to reduce workplace sitting. The other element of this chapter, the broad-reach intervention-dissemination case study of a health behavior-change program, highlighted the need to maintain key elements of research quality in designing for dissemination: to the extent that is practically possible, a rigorous study design; the systematic tracking of implementation and related costs; and, the conduct of dose-response, maintenance and cost-effectiveness analyses.

These examples of designing for dissemination illustrate not only the exciting opportunities for real-world dissemination research, but also the resourcefulness and commitment required for success. Significant gaps remain to be bridged. Researchers' priorities are in the conduct of high-quality scientific investigation, and much less attention is paid to dissemination and communication of the findings and implications of their research.[11,12] Many challenges remain and many opportunities exist for strengthening the

---

BOX 7.1

SUMMARY OF KEY PRINCIPLES TO GUIDE DESIGNING FOR DISSEMINATION OF ENVIRONMENTAL INITIATIVES AND BROAD-REACH HEALTH BEHAVIOR PROGRAMS

ENVIRONMENTAL INITIATIVES

- Identify relevant and accessible evidence and communicate clear recommendations on the environmental attributes most likely to have beneficial impact.
- Promote a better understanding that multiple domains and levels of determinants need to be changed to have significant broad-reach impact on health behaviors.
- Build strong partnerships with influential instrumentalities outside of public health. Develop advocacy networks to guide and support evidence-based dissemination.

BROAD-REACH HEALTH BEHAVIOR PROGRAMS

- Partnerships with key stakeholders (funders and implementers)

  - Fit of program/intervention with organizational goals
  - Availability of ongoing resources to support sustained implementation (monetary and personnel)
  - On-the-ground constraints on program delivery
  - In-depth knowledge of target populations

- Rigorous study designs

  - Randomized designs where possible
  - Integration of outcomes important to informing funders and advancing science
  - Systematic tracking of resources needed for implementation and intervention
  - Maintaining program fidelity while being flexible and responsive

---

knowledge bases, concepts, and systems needed in designing for dissemination.

SUGGESTED READINGS AND WEBSITES

Readings

Glasgow RE, Emmons KM. How can we increase translation of research into practice? Types of evidence needed. *Annu Rev Public Health.* 2007;28(1):413–433.
Describes the forms of evidence that can be gathered in the context of dissemination research, emphasizing types of evidence that can best inform translation into practice.

Owen N, Glanz K, Sallis JF, Kelder S. Evidence-based approaches to dissemination and diffusion of physical activity interventions. *Am J Prev Med.* 2006;31(4)(suppl 1):35–44.
Describes examples of how broad-reach approaches to physical activity may be disseminated, drawing on dissemination models and approaches from other areas of public health.

Sallis JF, Owen N. Ecological models of health behavior. In: Glanz K, Rimer BK, Viswanath K, (Eds). *Health behavior theory research and practice.* 5th ed. San Francisco: Jossey-Bass; p. 43–64, 2015.
Describes an ecological model of health behavior, with a particular focus on the role of "behavior settings"— the social and physical attributes of environments that can facilitate and encourage some behaviors and prevent or constrain others. Understanding multiple levels of determination of health behaviors and the role of environmental attributes can inform designing for dissemination.

Goode AD, Owen N, Reeves M, Eakin E. Translation from research to practice: community dissemination of a telephone-delivered physical activity and dietary behavior change intervention. *Am J Health Promot.* 2012;26:253–259.
Presents a case study of the process by which a telephone-delivered dietary-change and physical activity intervention previously tested in a controlled trial was implemented in a socially disadvantaged community.

Selected Websites and Tools

Cancer Control P.L.A.N.E.T. http://cancercontrol-planet.cancer.gov/index.html.

Cancer Control P.L.A.N.E.T. acts as a portal to provide access to data and resources for designing, implementing and evaluating evidence-based cancer control programs. The site provides five steps (with links) for developing a comprehensive cancer control plan or program.

RE-AIM (Reach, Effectiveness, Adoption, Implementation, Maintenance). http://www.re-aim.org/

RE-AIM is a framework designed to enhance the quality, efficiency, and public health impact of efforts to translate research into practice. Practical measurement tools, guidelines on application, and background readings are provided.

Active Living Research (ALR). http://www.activelivingresearch.org/.

ALR is an initiative supported by the Robert Wood Johnson Foundation, focussed on the prevention of childhood obesity in low-income and high-risk groups. It describes how environment and policy research can be used to influence active living opportunities for children and families. The ALR website provides many useful links to accounts of research-translation activities.

REFERENCES

1. Sallis JF, Owen N, Fotheringham MJ. Behavioral epidemiology: A systematic framework to classify phases of research on health promotion and disease prevention. *Ann Behav Med.* 2000;22(4):294–298.

2. Owen N, Healy GN, Matthews CE, Dunstan DW. Too much sitting: the population health science of sedentary behavior. *Exerc Sport Sci Rev.* 2010;38(3):105–113.

3. Glasgow RE, Emmons KM. How can we increase translation of research into practice? Types of evidence needed. *Ann Rev Public Health.* 2007;28(1):413–433.

4. Green LW, Ottoson JM, Garcia C, Hiatt RA. Diffusion theory, and knowledge dissemination, utilization, and integration in public health. *Ann Rev Public Health.* 2009;30(1):151–174.

5. Orleans CT. Increasing the demand for and use of effective smoking-cessation treatments reaping the full health benefits of tobacco-control science and policy gains--in our lifetime. *Am J Prev Med.* 2007;33(6)(suppl 1):S340–S348.

6. Glasgow RE, Goldstein MG, Ockene JK, Pronk NP. Translating what we have learned into practice: principles and hypotheses for interventions addressing multiple behaviors in primary care. *Am J Prev Med.* 2004;27(2)(suppl 1):88–101.

7. Wandersman A, Duffy J, Flaspohler P, et al. Bridging the gap between prevention research and practice: the interactive systems framework for dissemination and implementation. *Am J Commun Psychol.* 2008;41(3-4):171–181.

8. Cameron R, Brown KS, Best JA. The dissemination of chronic disease prevention programs: linking science and practice. *Can J Public Health.* 1996;87(suppl 2):S50–S53.

9. Rose G. *The strategy of preventive medicine.* Oxford: Oxford University Press; 1992.

10. Rose G. Sick individuals and sick populations. *Int J Epidemiol.* 2001;30(3):427–432, 433–434.

11. Brownson RC, Jacobs JA, Tabak RG, Hoehner CM, Stamatakis KA. Designing for dissemination among public health researchers: findings from a national survey in the United States. *Am J Public Health.* 2013;103(9):1693–1699.

12. Tabak RG, Reis RS, Wilson P, Brownson RC. Dissemination of health-related research among scientists in three countries: access to resources and current practices. *BioMed Res Int.* 2015;2015:179156.

13. Cohen EL, Head KJ, McGladrey MJ, Hoover AG, Vanderpool RC, Bridger C, Carman A, Crosby RA, Darling E, Tucker-McLaughlin M, Winterbauer N. Designing for dissemination: lessons in message design from "1-2-3 Pap," *Health Commun.* 2015;30(2):196–207.

14. McDavitt B, Bogart LM, Mutchler MG, Wagner GJ, Green Jr HD, Lawrence SJ, Mutepfa KD, Nogg KA. Dissemination as dialogue: building trust and sharing research findings through community engagement. *Prev Chronic Dis.* 2016;13:E38.

15. Johnson K, Tuzzio L, Renz A, Baldwin LM, Parchman M. Decision-to-implement worksheet for evidence based interventions: from the WWAMI Region Practice and Research Network. *J Am Board Fam Med.* 2016;29:553–562.

16. Sallis JF, Owen N. *Physical activity and behavioral medicine.* Thousand Oaks, CA: Sage; 1999.

17. Sallis JF, Cerin E, Conway TL, Adams MA, Frank LD, Pratt M, Salvo D, Schipperijn J, Smith G, Cain KL, Davey R, Kerr J, Lai P-C, Mitas J, Reis R, Sarmiento OL, Schofield G, Troelsen J, Van Dyck D, De Bourdeaudhuij I, Owen N. Urban environments in 14 cities worldwide are related to physical activity. *Lancet.* 2016;387(10034):2207–2217.

18. Sallis JF, Floyd MF, Rodríguez DA, Saelens BE. Role of built environments in physical activity, obesity, and cardiovascular disease. *Circulation.* 2012;125:729–737.

19. Glanz K, Owen N, Wold JA. Perspectives on behavioral sciences research for disease prevention and

control in populations. *J Nat Inst Public Health (Japan)*. 2009;58(1):40–50.

20. Sallis JF, Owen N. Ecological models of health behavior. In: Glanz K, Rimer BK, Viswanath K, (Eds). *Health behavior theory research and practice*. 5th ed. San Francisco: Jossey-Bass; 2015:43–64.

21. Giles-Corti B, Timperio A, Bull F, Pikora T. Understanding physical activity environmental correlates: increased specificity for ecological models. *Exerc Sport Sci Rev*. 2005;33(4):175–181.

22. Owen N, Humpel N, Leslie E, Bauman A, Sallis JF. Understanding environmental influences on walking: review and research agenda. *Am J Prevent Med*. 2004;27(1):67–76.

23. Owen N, Healy GN, Mathews CE, Dunstan DW. Too much sitting: the population-health science of sedentary behavior. Exerc Sport Sci Rev. 2010;38(3):105–113.

24. Frank LD, Greenwald MJ, Winkelman S, Chapman J, Kavage S. Carbonless footprints: promoting health and climate stabilization through active transportation. *Prevent Med*. 2010;50(suppl 1):S99–S105.

25. Handy SL, Boarnet MG, Ewing R, Killingsworth RE. How the built environment affects physical activity: views from urban planning. *Am J Prev Med*. 2002;23(2)(suppl 1):64–73.

26. Frank LD, Schmid TL, Sallis JF, Chapman J, Saelens BE. Linking objectively measured physical activity with objectively measured urban form: findings from SMARTRAQ. *Am J Prev Med*. 2005;28(2)(suppl 2):117–125.

27. Owen N, Cerin E, Leslie E, et al. Neighborhood walkability and the walking behavior of Australian adults. *Ame J Prev Med*. 2007;33(5):387–395.

28. Koohsari MJ, Sugiyama T, Sahlqvist S, Mavoa S, Hadgraft N, Owen N. Neighborhood environmental attributes and adults' sedentary behaviors: review and research agenda. *Prev Med*. 2015;77:141–149.

29. Sugiyama T, Neuhaus M, Owen N. Active transport, the built environment and human health. In: Rassia S, Pardalos P, (Eds). *Sustainable environmental design in architecture: Impacts on health*. London: Springer; 2011:43–67.

30. Koohsari MJ, **Owen N**, Cerin E, Giles-Corti B, Sugiyama T. Walkability and walking for transport: characterizing the built environment using Space Syntax. *Int J Behav Nutr Phys Act*. 2016;13(121):1–9.

31. Koohsari M., Sugiyama T, Mavoa S, Villanueva K, Badland H, Giles-Corti B, **Owen, N**. Street network measures and adults walking for transport: application of space syntax. *Health Place*. 2016;38:89–95.

32. Cole R., Dunn P, Hunter I, Owen N. Sugiyama T. Walk Score and Australian adults' home-based walking for transport. *HealthPlace*. 2015;35:60–65.

33. Duncan DT. What's Your Walk Score®? *Am J Prev Med*. 2013;45:244–245.

34. Kerr J, Emond JA, Badland H, Reis R, Sarmiento O, Carlson J, Sallis JF, Cerin E, Cain K, Conway T, Schofield G, Macfarlane D, Christiansen L, Van Dyck D, Davey R, Aguinaga-Ontoso I, Salvo D, Sugiyama T, Owen N, Mitáš J, Natarajan L. Perceived neighborhood environmental attributes associated with walking and cycling for transport among adult residents of 17 Cities in 12 countries: the IPEN Study. *Environ Health Perspect*. 2016;1241(31):290–298.

35. Owen N. Sedentary behavior: understanding and influencing adults' prolonged sitting time. *Prevent Med*. 2012;55:535–539.

36. Dunstan DW, Kingwell BA, Larsen R, et al. Breaking up prolonged sitting reduces postprandial glucose and insulin responses. *Diabetes Care* 2012;35(5):976–983.

37. Hadgraft N, Dunstan D, Owen N. Models for understanding sedentary behavior. In Leitzmann M, Joche, C, Schmid, D, (Eds). *Sedentary behavior epidemiology*.

38. Hadgraft NT, Healy GN, Owen N, et al. Office workers' objectively assessed total and prolonged sitting time: individual-level correlates and worksite variations. *Prevent Med Rep*. 2016;4:184–191.

39. Gupta N, Christiansen CS, Hallman DM, et al. Is objectively measured sitting time associated with low back pain? A cross-sectional investigation in the NOMAD study. *PloS one*. 2015;10(3):e0121159.

40. Healy GN, Eakin EG, Lamontagne AD, et al. Reducing sitting time in office workers: short-term efficacy of a multicomponent intervention. *Prevent Me*. 2013;57(1):43–48.

41. Healy GN, Eakin EG, Owen N, et al. A Cluster RCT to reduce office workers' sitting time: impact on activity outcomes. *Med Sci Sports Exerc*. 2016;48(9):1787–1797.

42. Healy GN, Goode AD, Schultz D, et al. The BeUpstanding Program TM: scaling up the Stand Up Australia Workplace Intervention for translation into practice. *AIMS Public Health*. 2016;3(2):341–347.

43. Robinson M, Tilford S, Branney P, et al. Championing mental health at work: emerging practice from innovative projects in the UK. *Health Promot Int*. 2014;29(3):583–595.

44. Eakin EG, Reeves MM, Lawler SP, et al. The Logan Healthy Living Program: a cluster randomized trial of a telephone-delivered physical activity

and dietary behavior intervention for primary care patients with type 2 diabetes or hypertension from a socially disadvantaged community—rationale, design and recruitment. *Contemp Clin Trials.* 2008;29(3):439–454.

45. Kroeze W, Werkman A, Brug J. A systematic review of randomized trials on the effectiveness of computer-tailored education on physical activity and dietary behaviors. *Ann Behav Med.* 2006;31(3):205–223.

46. Fjeldsoe B, Neuhaus M, Winkler E, Eakin E. Systematic review of maintenance of behavior change following physical activity and dietary interventions. *Health Psychol.* 2011;30(1):99–109.

47. Eakin E, Reeves M, Lawler S, et al. Telephone counselling for physical activity and diet in primary care. *Am J Prev Med.* 2009;36(2):142–149.

48. Graves N, Barnett A, Halton KA, et al. Cost-effectiveness of a telephone-delivered intervention for physical activity and diet. *PLoS ONE.* 2009;4(9):e7135.

49. Goode AD, Winkler EAH, Lawler SP, Reeves MM, Owen N, Eakin EG. Telephone-delivered physical activity and dietary intervention for type 2 diabetes and hypertension: does intervention dose influence outcomes? *Am J Health Promot.* 2011;25(4):257–263.

50. Eakin E, Reeves M, Winkler E, Lawler S, Owen N. Maintenance of physical activity and dietary change following a telephone-delivered intervention. *Health Psychol.* 2010;29(6):566–573.

51. Goode AD, Eakin E. Dissemination of an evidence-based telephone-delivered lifestyle intervention: factors associated with successful implementation and evaluation. *Transl Behav Med.* 2013;3(4):351–356.

52. Goode A, Owen N, Reeves M, Eakin E. Translation from research to practice: Community dissemination of a telephone-delivered physical activity and dietary behavior change intervention. *Am J Health Promot,* 2012;26(4):253–259.

8

The Role of Organizational Processes in Dissemination and Implementation Research

GREGORY A. AARONS, JOANNA C. MOULLIN, AND MARK G. EHRHART

INTRODUCTION

The science of dissemination and implementation (D&I) is a swiftly growing and broad field that commonly involves change at multiple levels at both outer (i.e., system) and inner (i.e., organization) contexts of service systems and organizations.[1-5] The bulk of health, mental health, public health, and social services are delivered within or through organizations. One of the primary goals of this chapter is to support implementers and leaders within organizations in attending to and shaping the context in which implementation takes place in order to increase the likelihood of implementation success and long-term sustainment.[1] Such attention must be strategic, consistent, goal directed, and consider the interplay of outer context and inner context, and the motivations and needs of individuals and workgroups within the participating organizations.[1,2,4] Although the types of organizations are varied (e.g., for profit, nonprofit, public, private) and range from large (e.g., National Health Systems, health insurance companies, US Veterans Affairs healthcare system, County Health Departments) to small (e.g., single program community-based nonprofits), there are a number of common organizational constructs or processes likely to be associated with successful D&I of health care innovations and evidence-based practices (EBPs).[2,4]

It is becoming increasingly clear that organizational level issues are critical considerations in effective implementation, and there are likely complex interactions of multiple factors in successful D&I of EBPs.[6-8] As shown in Figure 8.1, each of the constructs addressed in this chapter may operate in ways that are unidirectional, bi-directional, or more likely, have multiple determinants and influences that operate reciprocally or as a function of complex interactions.

For example, within a given public or private organization, the organization's culture can be determined through leadership, structures, and procedures within the organization.[9] From a "bottom-up" perspective, the nature of the employees and their relationships, motives, and the influence of leaders at multiple levels can help to shape the culture of an organization.[9,10] For instance, transformational leadership and leaders' relationships with subordinates and others in an organization are differentially important during active implementation compared with stable operations.[11,12] Thus, it is important to consider not only how organizational factors can impact the implementation process, but also how implementation can impact organizational processes and functioning. For example, it may be that staff receptivity to EBP can impact the fidelity and integrity with which EBPs are delivered,[13,14] but the process of implementation in combination with the practice itself may impact the system or organization, its management, and its workforce.[15-17]

What is not captured in the figure that is also deserving of consideration is that change in organizational processes or routines (such as implementing new interventions) takes time. Further, some changes take more time than others, as learning is frequently incremental and iterative.[18] For example, changing a relatively circumscribed aspect of organizational support for EBP could involve strategies such as making summaries of peer-reviewed literature available to staff and could be relatively low threshold, low cost, and quickly implemented. However, more complicated goals, such as improving the effectiveness or efficiency of safety in emergency medicine departments, may involve numerous iterative changes or improvement cycles. In addition, such changes may be slowed or facilitated

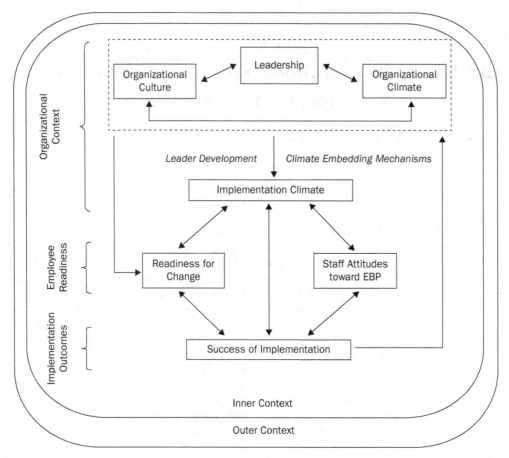

FIGURE 8.1 Multiple levels of organizational processes and implementation.

by the organizational culture of the hospital or department in which change is to take place.[19] Thus, the type and size of the system or organization and the type and scope of the change target can impact the need for more or less protracted change strategies, with the ultimate goal of incorporating evidence and EBP into usual care. Such changes may be fluid and require different time frames to become part of the ongoing organizational culture.[20]

Drawing from the implementation science, business, management, and organizational literatures, this chapter focuses on several of the more common and well-researched organizational constructs and processes that may impact uptake and sustainment of EBPs in organizations.

Our discussion of organizational issues in implementation begins by focusing on two related but distinct concepts: organizational culture and organizational climate. Subsequently, organizational climate will be divided into two types, general or "molar" organizational climate

and more focused or "strategic" climates, both of which can be tailored to D&I activities. Finally, organizational readiness for change, attitudes toward EBP, and a brief introduction to the field of improvement science will be explored. Each factor is considered in relation to the questions and challenges in health care, behavioral health, and social service settings, particularly in regard to how they can be applied to improvement and EBP implementation.

ORGANIZATIONAL CULTURE

An organization's culture is essentially what makes that organization unique from all others, including the core values instilled in the organization by its founder(s) and the organization's history of how it has survived through successes and failures. It includes the values for the services or products provided as well as how individuals and groups within the organization treat and interact with one another. Our working

TABLE 8.1 MULTPLE LEVELS AND CHARACTERISTICS OF ORGANIZATIONAL CULTURE

Source	Number of Layers	Layers
Schein[21]	3	Underlying Assumptions Espoused Values Artifacts
Rousseau[22]	5	Fundamental Assumptions Values Behavioral Norms Patterns of Behavior Artifacts

definition of organizational culture for this chapter comes from Schein,[9] who described organizational culture as the ". . . pattern of shared basic assumptions that was learned by a group as it solved its problems of external adaptation and internal integration, and that has worked well enough to be considered valid and, therefore, to be taught to new members as the correct way to perceive, think, and feel in relation to those problems."[9(p. 17)]

One way that scholars have discussed organizational culture is in terms of its layers or levels. Two examples are shown in Table 8.1. Frameworks along these lines specify outer layers that are more tangible and easily accessible (e.g., artifacts such as style of dress or the physical arrangement of space) but may have different meanings in different organizations. To truly understand these outer layers, Schein[21] and others have argued that one must gain a deeper understanding of the more deeply held, subjective, and less easily accessed values and assumptions that comprise inner layers.[9,22] Such basic shared assumptions are so deeply ingrained in the organization that its members may not be able to readily articulate them; thus, scholars have argued that both qualitative and quantitative methods must be used to truly understand an organization's culture.[9,22]

Adding to the complexity of defining culture and its levels, scholars vary in their models of the specific components or dimensions of organizational culture. Table 8.2 lists six different ways in which scholars have conceptualized organizational culture and notes the reference(s) cited for each approach. This is by no means an exhaustive list but is provided to give the reader a sense of some of the variability in conceptual models of organizational culture.

Part of the allure of the concept of organizational culture has been its connection to organizational performance. Its rise in popularity in the 1980s was linked to books such as those authored by Deal and Kennedy[32] and Peters and Waterman[33] that influenced executives to attempt to change their culture in order to increase organizational effectiveness. Unfortunately, most of those efforts did not result in much success, as organizational culture is rather resistant to change, and, as such, some have even questioned the link between organizational culture and organizational performance.[34] Nevertheless, there is evidence to suggest that organizations with cultures that are more supportive of employees and that are adaptable to changes in the environment are more effective in general.[35,36]

In the context of health care, although a recent systematic review of organizational culture change attempts[37] was unable to identify general and effective strategies for changing organizational culture (only two studies met criteria for inclusion, suggesting a need for more research in this regard), organizational culture has been identified as a key element in EBP adoption, implementation, and sustainment,[1,38-40] and has been linked to decreased infection rates in a hospital,[41] increased work satisfaction and organizational commitment in long-term care,[42] more positive attitudes toward EBPs,[43] and improved outcomes for youth in child welfare systems.[44] In addition, in the area of social and mental health services for children, Charles Glisson and colleagues have developed the ARC (Availability, Responsiveness, and Continuity) intervention, which uses trained change agents to change organizational culture and climate, and to support the implementation of innovative

TABLE 8.2 MEASURES OF ORGANIZATIONAL CULTURE

Source	# of Dimensions	Dimensions
Organizational Culture Inventory (Cooke & Rousseau)[23]	3	Constructive Culture Passive/Defensive Culture Aggressive/Defensive Culture
Denison[24,25]	4	Involvement Consistency Adaptability Mission
'Organizational Culture Profile (O'Reilly)[26,27]	8	Attention to Detail Outcome Orientation Aggressiveness Emphasis on Rewards Innovation Supportiveness Team Orientation Decisiveness
Organizational Culture Profile (Ashkanasy)[28]	10	Leadership Structure Innovation Job Performance Planning Communication Environment Humanistic Workplace Development of the Individual Socialization on Entry
Competing Values Framework (Cameron & Quinn)[29]	4	Clan Adhocracy Hierarchy Market
Organizational Social Context (Glisson)[30,31]	4	Proficiency Resistance Apathy Suppression

'Note: There are two different conceptual models of culture, both identified as the Organizational Culture Profile.

practices.[3] One major component of the ARC model is improving service provider behaviors and attitudes, including openness to EBP.[45] Change agents develop staff attitudes toward EBP by designating the targeted EBP as the solution to a previously perceived problem in the organization.[30] They also develop and maintain interest in new practices by providing information about EBP, resolving problems in the implementation process, and facilitating communication regarding implementation.[30] The ARC model has been associated with significantly improved client outcomes when implemented in conjunction with EBP, compared with implementation of EBP without the ARC model.[45] Specifically with regard to culture, the intervention's effects on provider intentions to adopt EBPs, perceived barriers to using EBPs, and EBP-related behaviors have been shown to be mediated by its effects on the overall organizational culture.[46,47]

ORGANIZATIONAL CLIMATE

The popularity of the study of organizational culture among organizational researchers throughout the 1980s and 90s was preceded by a time of high levels of interest in the construct of organizational climate from the late 1960s through the 1970s. The goal of the earliest research and writing on the topic of organizational climate was to describe the environment that emerged through the treatment of workers by their leaders. This, in turn, affected employee attitudes, motivations, and performance.[48,49] Over time, a number of differences emerged in how the organizational climate was conceptualized and studied, including in terms of level of analysis (individual vs. organizational unit), content (description vs. evaluation), focus (general vs. specific), and type of composition model (climate level vs. climate strength). Although a discussion of individual perceptions of climate (also known as psychological climate) and climate strength (variability in climate perceptions) are outside the scope of this chapter, the content and focus of organizational climate perceptions are particularly relevant. In response to early criticisms regarding overlap between the constructs of climate and job attitudes (e.g., job satisfaction),[50,51] some climate scholars have emphasized that climate involves employees' descriptions (but not evaluations) of the "events, practices, and procedures and the kinds of behaviors that get rewarded, supported, and expected in a setting."[52(p. 384)] Other climate researchers, particularly those who have studied climate in the context of mental health services, have emphasized climate as both perception of and affective response to employees' work environment.[30,53] In either case, it is important to note that climate is not merely defined by the presence of practices and procedures in the work environment. Rather, it is the perceived meaning inferred by employees through management practices and procedures that ultimately defines the climate of the organization.[53,54]

The other important distinction for this chapter that emerged early in the history of the climate literature was between molar (or generic) climate and focused or "strategic" climate. The molar approach typically involves an attempt to measure climate at a broad level across multiple dimensions, such as role stress, autonomy, leadership support, and warmth.[55] These dimensions generally refer to the extent to which management provides a positive experience for employees at work, and thus has also been described as a climate for employee well-being.[54] In contrast, the focused climate approach involves employee perceptions of the practices and procedures with regard to a specific criterion, whether it be a strategic outcome (e.g., climate for customer service, climate for safety) or an organizational process (e.g., ethics, fairness).[52] In other words, in contrast to molar climate that attempts to capture the general "feel" of the organization, the focused or strategic climate approach attempts to understand the extent to which employees perceive that management emphasizes a specific criterion of interest, whatever it may be. A relevant example is the notion of a climate for implementation of innovations in an organization,[56] discussed below as one type of strategic climate.

IMPLEMENTATION CLIMATE

The strategic climate approach to organizational climate is highly relevant for research on D&I.[57-59] Organizational culture and molar climate are important for successful implementation and for achieving successful clinical outcomes;[45,60,61] in fact, there is clear evidence that they are.[44,45,62] However, their role is important in laying the foundation for the development of an effective implementation climate. An implementation climate is defined as ". . . employees' shared perceptions of the importance of innovation implementation within the organization. . . [that] results from employees' shared experiences and observations of, and their information about and discussions about, their organization's implementation policies and practices."[63(p. 813)] It is important to note that implementation climate is distinct from a climate for innovation, which involves the extent to which the organization encourages and supports the development of new ideas and technologies[64,65] but does not capture how those ideas and technologies are actually implemented in the organization. Implementation climate focuses specifically on creating a fertile organizational context for putting a new innovation into practice. When management communicates the importance of the implementation of a new practice through its policies, procedures, and reward systems, employees are able to clearly understand that the leaders in the organization care about the implementation and use of the innovation, therefore enabling employees to better focus their energy and motivation for that goal. As a result, the overall implementation is more likely to succeed.[63,66,67]

There are many mechanisms through which leaders, managers, and supervisors can communicate the value of successful implementation. Recent research developing measures of implementation climate provides some insight into those mechanisms. For instance, Jacobs, Weiner, and Bunger (2014) drew from Klein et al.'s definition of implementation climate to measure the three dimensions of implementation climate: expectations, support, and rewards. Alternatively, Ehrhart, Aarons, and Farahnak's (2014) measure captures six dimensions of a climate for EBP implementation: (1) focus on EBP, (2) educational support for EBP, (3) recognition for EBP, (4) rewards for EBP, (5) selection for EBP, and (6) selection for openness. In either case, the idea is that when the organization aligns its policies, practices, and systems in support of implementation, employees have a clear understanding of what the organization's priorities are and will be more likely to behave accordingly. In the authors' own work on the implementation of EBPs in mental health agencies, they have witnessed a variety of means through which management communicates the value of EBP for the organization. For instance, in one agency, EBP guest speakers were brought in for staff and educational materials such as manuals were made readily available. Another agency's chief executive officer attended a regular team meeting to recognize their efforts in EBP implementation. In all of the participating agencies, leaders made a concerted effort to recognize staff for successfully implementing EBP, including thanking staff via e-mail and recognizing positive client outcomes in staff meetings. All of these strategies communicated to staff members that management valued the successful implementation of EBP, creating a more positive climate for EBP implementation.

It is important to note that if management enacted only one of these strategies, implementation would not be as likely to be successful in contrast to an organization that strategically employed a number of these aspects of implementation climate. More importantly, if management contradicts itself, for instance by talking about the importance of EBP but not providing appropriate supports or incentives for their proper use, then a strong implementation climate will not result. Thus, it is the concerted convergence of targeted strategies to promote EBP uptake that creates a positive EBP implementation climate.[62] The role of leaders is crucial in creating and implementing such strategies during the EBP implementation process, and thus we now turn to the research literature on leadership and its application to the field of implementation science.

LEADERSHIP

Leadership is one organizational contextual factor that has come under extensive investigation[68] across a range of private,[69] military,[70] medical,[71] mental health,[72,73] public health,[74] and nonprofit[75] settings. Leadership is a critical and important factor in implementation of community initiatives.[76] Of the many theories of leadership (see Avolio[77] for a review), one particularly useful and well-researched framework is the Full Range Leadership (FRL) Model.[78-81] According to this model, leadership behaviors fall into three broad categories, with more specific dimensions within each. The first, *transformational* leadership, includes those behaviors in which a leader attends to and develops followers to higher levels of performance and potential (individualized consideration), engages followers in thinking about issues in new ways (intellectual stimulation), communicates an appealing vision for the future (inspirational motivation), and becomes a trusted role model for staff (idealized influence).[82] *Transactional* leadership, the second category in the FRL model, involves exchanges between leaders and followers in which leaders reinforce or reward followers for engaging in certain behaviors and meeting practical and/or aspirational goals (contingent reward) as well as monitoring and correcting performance (passive or active management-by-exception). The final general category in the FRL model, *passive* or laissez faire leadership (i.e., nonleadership), refers to withdrawal behaviors on the part of the purported leader in which little exchange between the leader and follower is enacted. It is, however, not merely a nonimpactful or neutral set of behaviors, but is thought to represent an actively destructive abdication of responsibility.[83] Obviously, this is considered to be an ineffective style of leadership.

The FRL model has been subject to a high degree of scrutiny in many countries and cultures, and in many different types of organizations, and has been the subject of at least five meta-analyses[81,84-87] that support its predictive validity. Specifically, transformational leadership is positively associated with follower job satisfaction,[88] job well-being, individual follower performance,[89] group performance,[69,70,90] cohesive organizational culture,[91] decreased turnover,[92] absenteeism,[93] risk of injury,[90] and employee burnout.[91,94] The contingent reward dimension of transactional leadership is also associated with group performance[95] and individual follower performance.[89] Passive leadership is associated with poor job satisfaction and poor efficiency,[96] higher workplace stress, psychological distress, increased risk of bullying at work,[83] and lower safety climate and conscientiousness.[97] These findings have been supported across a broad range of organizational settings[86,98] and cultures,[88,99] including health care organizations and behavioral health organizations.[91,93,94,100,101] Furthermore, there is evidence for the importance of many dimensions of leadership in common with the FRL such as the role of participative and charismatic or value-based leadership across countries and cultures.[101,102]

Several studies have shown that leaders can be trained to display more transformational leadership behaviors. One approach stemming from the FRL model that has come under extensive investigation is the Full Range Leadership Program (FRLP),[103] a training that consists of leadership feedback and a personal development plan that is used during an initial 3-day workshop and a 2-day workshop 3 months later.[104] Several studies have shown the FRLP to be effective in increasing staff ratings of transformational leadership[105,106] and other positive organizational outcomes such as staff productivity, attendance, and prosocial behavior.[105] Several adaptations of the FRLP have also been found effective in improving transformational leadership,[107–109] including a more targeted 1-day leadership training.[110]

Leadership has also been shown to be a critical factor for organizational effectiveness in health care organizations.[39,73] Positive and effective leadership in health care systems can help to create climates that support quality of care and improve other economic, clinical, and humanistic outcomes. For example, Corrigan and colleagues[73] found a positive association between strong mental health program leadership and consumer satisfaction and quality of life. Moreover, leadership training that includes transformational leadership has been provided in order to improve safety climate, operationalized as the way in which managers balance the dynamic between safety and productivity.[111] Stronger transformational leadership has been associated with positive work attitudes in both for-profit and nonprofit organizations,[41] and more positive leadership in human service organizations has been associated with staff members' higher organizational

commitment.[42] In mental health settings, Aarons and colleagues[43] found that leadership had a positive relationship on therapeutic alliance through the mediator of a positive organizational climate. Glisson and Durick[112] identified leadership as a positive predictor of organizational commitment within human service organizations. In addition, transformational leadership has been positively associated with positive organizational culture and reduced burnout in mental health service teams,[91] and mental health providers report that they want their leaders to display a range of behaviors similar to those prescribed by the FRL model.[113]

In addition to research on general effective leadership in health settings, other work has focused on investigating the specific application of such leadership theory on the implementation of EBPs. For example, both transformational and transactional leadership have been shown to be positively associated with clinicians' receptivity toward the use of EBP.[114] In another example comparing leadership across settings, social care managers were found to have more positive attitudes toward EBP and to be more active implementation process managers in care for older adults.[115]

IMPLEMENTATION LEADERSHIP

Research on leadership and implementation has recently taken an integrated approach to the leadership and strategic climate literature by focusing on strategic leadership for implementation, or "implementation leadership." This research has delineated the specific behaviors leaders perform to support organizational implementation efforts. In developing their measure of implementation leadership, the Implementation Leadership Scale (ILS), Aarons and colleagues (2014)[115a] drew from the work of Ed Schein on embedding mechanisms[9] to identify the specific ways that leaders develop a strategic climate for implementation in their organizations. Using mixed qualitative and quantitative methods, they found that implementation leadership was comprised of four dimensions that include the leader being *knowledgeable* about the practice or innovation to be implemented, being *proactive* in anticipating implementation issues, being *supportive* of direct service providers in their efforts to use a new practice or innovation, and *persevering* through the ups-and-downs of the implementation process. Although the ILS was originally developed in allied health/mental health service settings, it has now been validated in substance abuse treatment, and child welfare settings, and validation is underway in other health care settings such as nursing.[116,117] Other work has independently formulated a model of implementation leadership for clinical guideline implementation,[118] as well as to integrate this work—the "Ottawa Model of Implementation Leadership (O-MILe)"—with the dimensions of the ILS in order to advance theory and ultimately to test these models for effectiveness in supporting implementation.[119] In addition, promising approaches are being used to integrate FRL—and specifically transformational leadership—in approaches to improving health manager implementation leadership and implementation effectiveness.[120] However, the challenge remains in getting leaders to use appropriate strategies and tactics for implementation that have the highest likelihood of success. In a 1986 study summarizing the results of 91 case studies of the "Tactics of Implementation," it was found that while "intervention tactics" were most successful, less than 20% of executives utilized this approach.[121] In contrast, approaches such as persuasion (75% of cases successful) and participation (17% of cases successful) were used much more frequently.[122]

One particularly critical issue for understanding how leaders influence implementation efforts is how the role of leadership varies across multiple levels within health and social service organizations.[123] Indeed, there are many commonalities across service sectors in how leadership manifests at different levels that must be considered for effective implementation to occur.[1,124] A recent study across 11 public sector allied health service systems found that outer context or system level leadership—closely matching dimensions of implementation leadership—was critical in implementation and sustainment, while FRL predicted sustainment at the team level within organizations.[122] At the same time, there may be important differences across levels that should be considered. For instance, strategies and policies often emerge from top management, and thus executive leaders are involved in decision-making processes for the adoption of EBPs, while lower level supervisors are involved in the day-to-day implementation of EBPs in their teams.[125] Thus, leadership at all levels in an organization should be considered so that there is congruence of message, reinforcement, and direction that is accessible and palpable for staff at the front line of services.[10]

Despite the importance of strong leadership across levels during EBP implementation, first-level leaders are often neglected when it comes to support in how to lead effectively and support organizational change.[10] Thus, first-level leaders may lack the management and leadership skills and requisite organizational standing and power necessary to develop positive organizational and implementation climates and effectively implement EBPs. This represents a critical gap between workforce readiness for EBP and the need to implement the most effective services for health and mental health care. In response to this gap in the literature, the authors have developed the Leadership and Organizational Change for Implementation (LOCI) intervention to simultaneously improve FRL and a positive EBP implementation climate. Acceptability and feasibility data for this intervention are promising,[126] and further tailoring and large-scale testing is underway to validate this approach to leadership development and improving organizational readiness and effectiveness in implementing EBPs.[127]

PERCEPTUAL DISTANCE AND ALIGNMENT

In line with the discussion highlighting the importance of considering multiple levels in the organization, research on leadership in health care has specifically begun to address the implications of alignment across levels. Most research in this domain has addressed the perceptual distance between the perceptions of the leader and the perceptions of his/her subordinates.[128] Alignment of perceptions within organizations occurs when employees, regardless of role, report similar views, values, or beliefs. Recent research suggests that the degree to which employees' perceptions align can have an impact on organizational dynamics and contribute to shaping an organization's culture and climate.[129,130] For example, Hasson and colleagues found that organizational learning improved where a leader and his or her team agreed on the level of organizational learning.[128,131,132] Aarons and colleagues found that "humble" leadership, where leaders rated themselves lower than their subordinates, was associated with more positive climate for performance feedback and organizational involvement compared with groups who agreed or where the leaders rated themselves higher on ILS than their followers.[132] In another study, organizational culture was found to suffer more when supervisors rated themselves more positively than providers, in contrast to when supervisors rated themselves lower than the provider ratings of the supervisor.[133] This is important because it is apparently not just average level of leadership that is important, but rather the dynamic relationship between leaders and followers that may impact organizational context. In addition to the perceptual distance between leaders and subordinates, other research has considered the alignment of perceptions across stakeholders in the implementation process. Hasson and colleagues found that staff describe their roles and the roles of others in implementation processes differently across various stakeholder groups in the organization.[134] In such cases, implementation strategies should be employed in an attempt to reduce the discrepancy and increase the communication and understanding of the staffs' roles and responsibilities.

At a system level, alignment occurs when there is perceptual agreement between stakeholders across organizations. In large system transformations, change may be required across several systems and within several organizations within those systems. A study investigating such a transformation looked at programs to improve the quality of care for elderly.[135] In such cases, organizational collaboration,[136,137] community based participatory research[138] or community-academic partnerships,[139] and learning collaboratives[140] are examples of methodologies that may be fruitful to increase perceptual alignment, ensure the perceptions of all stakeholders are accounted for, and select appropriate tailored implementation strategies across all contextual levels.[141]

ORGANIZATIONAL READINESS FOR CHANGE

An often discussed concern, that requires further research and attention, is the degree to which organizational readiness for change impacts implementation. The concept of organizational readiness for change arose from Lewin's 3-stage model of change, which advocates "unfreezing" the workings of an organization and creating the motivation and capacity to change.[142] Several scholars have supported the notion that when employees exhibit readiness to change, they expend greater effort during the process of implementation, are more invested in the change, and are more persistent in the face of obstacles to successfully implementing change.[143-147] As with culture and climate, organizational readiness for change is the subject of different definitions that focus on various aspects of organizations

including structure, process, equipment and technology, and staff attitudes. For the purposes of this chapter, organizational readiness for change includes (1) organizational members' psychological and behavioral motivation to implement a new innovation, technology, or EBP; (2) general organizational capacity; and (3) innovation-specific capacity.[148] Organizational readiness is widely regarded as an essential antecedent to successful implementation of change in health care and social service organizations.[142,149-153]

The first aspect of organizational readiness is organizational members' motivation to change. Motivation may be divided into two dimensions, collective commitment and collective efficacy.[154,155] Organizational commitment is the shared intention to implement, whereas collective efficacy is the shared belief that the organization has the capability to implement.

There are several interpersonal and social dynamics to consider when discussing staff motivation to change, as well as a number of theories that inform this issue. For example, social information processing asserts that members of a team look to one another for clues on issues such as change in an organization, and suggests that an individual's readiness to change may be shaped by the readiness of peers.[156] Social cognitive theory suggests that when organizational readiness for change is high, organizational members are more likely to initiate change and exert greater efforts and persistence for change.[157,158] Motivation theory adds that when organizational readiness for change is high, members will exhibit prosocial, change-related behaviors that exceed job requirements.[150,159] Based on these theories, researchers have explored mechanisms for creating readiness for change in organizations. Several key change beliefs that lead to improved staff commitment and efficacy for change have been identified.[150,160,161] Studies have focused on change beliefs and the extent to which they improve staff motivation to implement and subsequently implementation behaviors. Two hypothesized antecedents for organizational commitment to change are change valence and change discrepancy.[154] Change valence refers to whether employees think the change being implemented is beneficial or worthwhile for them personally.[150,161] Dimensions of change valence include perceived need, perceived benefit, perceived timeliness and perceived capability.[154] In an effort to create change valence among organizational members, agents should discuss with employees the positive results of the change (e.g., improved patient or client outcomes) as well as any negative consequences should the implementation fail (e.g., possible layoffs).[162] One potential benefit for many health care workers is the ability to include certification in a new intervention or technology on their resume, thus becoming more competitive in the job market.[163] Change discrepancy refers to employees' belief that implementation or change is needed due to a gap between the organization's current state and some desired end-state. Implementation facilitators or organizational change agents may use external contextual factors, such as changes in economic conditions or new competition in the field, in order to create discrepancy beliefs.[164] A counterintuitive strategy is that of creating and spreading dissatisfaction among employees so they will perceive the discrepancy indirectly, and come to perceive a need for change.[165] Once employees perceive a discrepancy in their workplace, they are likely to be motivated to lessen the discrepancy.

Along with collective commitment, collective change efficacy, or the degree to which employees think they are capable of implementing a change, shapes staff motivation to change. Change advocates should include employees in activities, such as planning meetings, in order to increase their collective confidence in their ability to implement and manage the change.[166] They should focus on communicating to employees that training and support will be available throughout the implementation process and through the sustainment phase.[155] Some agencies participating in a study funded by the Centers for Disease Control and Prevention, the "dynamic adaptation implementation project" (DAP) decreased their service providers' caseloads by about 50%, which allowed staff more time to prepare for and use the new intervention with clients.[167] However, it was also clear that these issues need to be balanced by outer context exigencies including productivity and workflow requirements. When employees are considering whether they are capable of implementing a new practice, they may consider the task demands, availability of resources (including staffing), and current situational factors.[150,168]

In addition to the psychological and behavioral dimension of organizational motivation, organizational readiness for change consists of two structurally related dimensions: organizational capacity and innovation-specific capacity.[148] General organizational capacity for change is the "attributes of a functioning organization and connections with other organizations."[148] Examples include leadership, organizational culture and climate, infrastructure, quality improvement processes, and staff openness to new practices. Innovation-specific capacity refers to an organization's resources (financial, material, human and informational), context, and processes that will support the introduction and integration of a specific innovation.[148,168] Examples include an organization having the necessary knowledge and skills, implementation climate, innovation champions, and implementation drivers. In addition, ongoing support beyond the implementation phase of integrating the new innovation is implied.[168]

An important influence on organizational readiness is principal support, in which formal leaders and opinion leaders in the organization are committed to the successful implementation of a given change. Support is included within innovation-specific capacity, although it may influence all three aspects of organizational readiness. This is highly related to the previously discussed notion of creating a positive implementation climate through strategic leader behaviors. Opinion leaders can promote organizational change, such as the implementation of EBP,[169] through the mechanisms described earlier. However, it is also beneficial to include employees in change efforts, as this has been shown to also increase motivation for organizational change.[170] A leader's ability to recognize and address individual staff members' motivations and attitudes[114] may also facilitate buy-in to strategic objectives such as EBP adoption and implementation.

Organizational readiness for change can lead to better staff buy-in and willingness to adopt organizational change. Staff require motivation and the innovation-specific capacity to implement change together with the organizational capacity and a supportive culture, climate, and leadership. As such, organizational readiness for change is complex and sets the stage for the implementation of EBP, and may specifically impact the most proximal predictor of implementation behaviors: staff attitudes toward EBP.

ATTITUDES TOWARD EVIDENCE-BASED PRACTICE

Staff and leader attitudes toward EBP are important aspects to consider when implementing manualized treatments in health care settings.[171] Early work on developing the Evidence-Based

Practice Attitude Scale (EBPAS) identified four primary dimensions (scale names in italics): (1) the intuitive *Appeal* of the EBP, (2) likelihood to adopt if *Requirements* were to do so, (3) the practitioners' *Openness* to new practices, and (4) perceived *Divergence* between EBP and current practice.[172,173] More recent work has identified eight additional dimensions including *Limitations* of EBPs, EBPs *Fit* with values and needs of client and clinician, perceptions of *Monitoring, Balance* between perceptions of clinical skills and science as important in service provision, time and administrative *Burden* with learning EBPs, *Job security* related to expertise in EBP, perceived *Organizational support*, and positive perceptions of receiving *Feedback*.[174,175]

Attitudes toward EBP can be predicted by a number of organizational characteristics including the culture and climate of an organization,[176] leadership,[11,72] and the level of organizational support for EBP that is provided by the organization.[62] In addition, Dobbins[177] has suggested that attitudes toward the use of research or an organizational "research culture" is a key factor influencing employee attitudes toward change. It is important to consider the role of attitudes along with other factors such as behavioral intentions,[178] provider self-efficacy[162] and motivations, incentives, and infrastructure to support effective provider implementation behaviors. In addition to the effects of attitudes on implementation behaviors, more positive attitudes toward evidence-based practice may also be linked to going above and beyond requirements to support implementation. Such "implementation citizenship behaviors" may include offering additional help and assistance to others during the implementation process, and keeping up with the latest updates and news on the implementation process and the evidence-based practice itself.[179]

IMPROVEMENT SCIENCE

Barriers to health care provision arise not only from the aforementioned factors such as lack of organizational readiness and a negative or ineffective culture or climate in organizations, but also from issues along classic process and quality dimensions of service delivery. Moreover, an improvement drive has been promulgated by policy reforms on managing outcomes and value, and the introduction of pay for performance remuneration schemes.[180] Too often, health care services fail to be efficient, timely, well organized, evidence-based, safe, patient/client-centered, and

consistent.[181] Thus, attempts have been made to improve health care and social services via process and quality improvement approaches, many of which are drawn from fields outside of health care.[182,183] Process improvement approaches are business management strategies that aim to improve efficiency by improving specific organizational processes usually for explicit outcomes or targets.[184] These efforts originated in the manufacturing sector, and became prominent with the advent of such approaches as Six Sigma[185] and Lean thinking.[186] Typically intended to reduce manufacturing defects and increase the speed of manufacturing production, process improvement strategies have also been applied to health care and social service delivery.[187]

As with implementation, the generalizability and application of improvement strategies can be challenging due to the high degree of variability in service delivery processes across different types of organizations and because cultural change within service organizations is particularly difficult.[188] Improvement efforts typically include an emphasis on the following basic principles: quality leadership, focus on process, continuous improvement, evidence-based decision making, and a systems approach to management.[181] According to the World Health Organization, process improvement is both a philosophy and a set of technical methods, which include a systematic review of delivery processes, operations research, teamwork improvement, the use of data and measurement, and the use of benchmarking.[189] Process improvement frequently relies on Plan-Do-Study-Act (PDSA) cycles that allow organizations to experiment with, implement, measure, and evaluate incremental change (or lack thereof) in relatively short periods of time.[181,184,190] Health care-specific process improvement strategies include reduction of medical errors,[191,192] decreases in admission and other wait times,[193] dissemination of clinical practices and guidelines,[194,195] improvement of patient discharge processes,[196] and improvement in hiring practices.[189,197]

One example of a widespread process improvement effort is the Institute for Healthcare Improvement's (IHI) Breakthrough Series, which intends to help health care organizations make specific clinical and operational process improvements. At the core of IHI quality improvement work is the Model for Improvement, which is a heuristic for learning from experience. This model incorporates three questions, What are we trying to accomplish?; How will we know that a change is an improvement?; What change can we make that will result in improvement?; and the PDSA cycle. The model encourages rapid-cycle testing as the process for achieving the change and goals.[183] Small tests of changes thought to lead to the improvement goal, over a short time frame, are initiated, evaluated, refined, and then extended to different contexts with ongoing testing.

Another type of process improvement, utilized in the VA system, is the Quality Enhancement Research Initiative (QUERI).[198,199] There are nine different QUERIs and each focuses on specific health or clinical care targets. For example, there are QUERI divisions to address chronic heart failure, diabetes, HIV/hepatitis, ischemic heart disease, mental health, polytrauma and blast-related injuries, spinal cord injury, stroke, and substance use disorders. The QUERI approach utilizes a six-step model focused on improving care through the implementation of new practices.[200] The six steps include identifying disease or health care problem, identifying the best practices or EBPs to address the problem, defining existing practice patterns and outcomes across the hospital or service system, identifying and implementing an intervention or interventions to implement and or promote best practices, using data to document that new practices improve outcomes, and documenting that outcomes are associated with improving the patient's quality of life.

Improvement science as a field of research has grown to study the gap between evidence and practice, with the ultimate goal to improve both health care organizations and health care outcomes.[201–203] Such growth has paralleled the growth in implementation science. Even though both of these fields have developed organically as cross-disciplinary fields from heterogeneous lists of publications, they also have remained relatively independent from each other without much cross-fertilization between the two.[202,204,205] Debate reigns about the distinction between implementation science and improvement science, although without doubt they share many traits and may be used synergistically.[153] An example of synergy of implementation and improvement science would be innovation improvement through adaptation to fit the context.[206] It could be argued that in any implementation effort there should be a degree of quality improvement as an innate part of fidelity/adaptation. From the perspective of implementation science, "quality improvement" may be the innovation being implemented[207–209]

or the implementation strategy for EBP implementation.[210] To improve quality of care may be the outcome of an innovation's implementation, and Continuous Quality Improvement or Total Quality Management may be seen as components of implementation and ongoing sustainability.[211] Methodologies that facilitate combining implementation science and improvement science include learning evaluation;[212] sequential, multiple assignment, randomized trials;[213] interrupted time-series, and process evaluations. The evidence from improvement processes and evaluations may then be utilized within implementation projects.

Despite the promises involved in the application of organizational improvement techniques to health care settings, several challenges remain. As with any implementation effort, these initiatives may occur in systems that are facing other competing priorities and demands. In addition, it may be difficult to embed and sustain quality improvement initiatives as part of the culture of the organizations. Optimally, process improvement will be integrated into the health care or social service system and not be seen as an external time-limited "program."[189] Finally, process improvement strategies may be expensive and time consuming, and require substantial commitment from stakeholders.

SUMMARY

Taken as a whole, both organizational characteristics and specific organizational strategies are important for the effective D&I of EBPs in health and allied health care settings, as well as mental health, alcohol/drug treatment, and social service settings. This chapter summarizes some of the most critical organizational factors and strategies likely to impact successful EBP implementation. There are myriad approaches to supporting organizational development and change—this chapter focuses on issues supported by relevant scientific literatures, particularly those germane to EBP implementation in health care and related settings.

Although a broad view of organizational issues related to D&I at first glance implicates contextual factors as paramount, the inner workings of organizations, workforce trends, health care providers, and consumers also impact uptake and use of scientific discovery in practice.[214,215] This "topography" of D&I provides the backdrop for the proposed phases of the implementation process including Exploration (consideration of whether to adopt or even consider an innovation), Preparation (preparing for implementation once the adoption decision is made), Implementation (enacting plans and working through emergent issues), and Sustainment (creating and supporting the structures and processes that will allow an implemented innovation to be maintained in a system or organization).[1,124] Considering D&I as a process with multiple phases has implications for how the various topographic levels (i.e., country, system, organization, provider, patient) may impact or be impacted by the D&I of evidence-based practices into routine care. Such bidirectional effects are key to conceptual models that recognize recipients of new technologies as not passive but as highly likely to react in various ways depending on characteristics of the context, the innovation to be implemented, and individual differences in health care providers and patients.[148]

Certain organizational factors are likely to be more or less important across the phases of implementation. For example, effective and committed leadership may be particularly important during Exploration and Adoption decision/Preparation phases.[1] Various organizational factors may have the most impact for particular types of D&I efforts or those focused on the unique aspects of a particular context. For example, leadership may impact D&I progress and process in diverse implementation contexts.[76] Focusing on improving organizational climate for implementation may also be more or less important for a particular team or workgroup that is implementing an EBP within an organization. For example, a given team might be implementing an EBP while the rest of the organization is continuing stable operations. Conversely, if the entire organization is becoming more committed to and focused on the use of EBP, then more global organizational culture and climate change strategies may be appropriate.

With the realization that development of organizational cultures, climates, and contexts supportive of EBP implementation takes time and concerted effort, there is hope that EBP implementation can be effectively pursued in diverse service settings. Understanding organizational context and applying organizational development strategies can aid in the improvement of health and mental health care, as well as social services. In order for patients and clients to benefit from care, the best interventions that science has to offer must be implemented effectively. Organizational change can lead to improved implementation outcomes[216,217] and ultimately improved clinical outcomes.[45] These goals can be achieved if we can create the organizational contexts that support EBP implementation.

Although the concepts and constructs discussed in this chapter appear at times to be quite abstract, it is important to remember that they are created and maintained by the behaviors, decisions, policies, and procedures developed and supported by people in the organization. In the same vein, they can be changed by individuals, groups, and teams with the vision, determination, and persistence to shepherd the organizational changes needed to implement and sustain EBPs. Any given implementation has the potential to improve the care needed by individuals, groups, and populations. It starts with a vision of how health care can be improved, and this can be global in scope or relate to a specific disease, its treatment, and specific subpopulations. Although there is evidence that EBPs tend to be robust across populations, it is important for organizations to make the changes necessary to deliver those interventions to the right people at the right time. This is done by people in organizations creating organizational contexts open to change and able to implement and sustain that change.

It is imperative that those responsible for the implementation of EBPs take action to first identify the organizational issues to address. Then effective organizational change strategies must be identified, utilized, and consistently applied in order to improve the culture and climate of the organization, to more effectively implement effective health care innovations and practices. The promise of this course of action is improved care, improved health, and improved lives for those we serve.

ACKNOWLEDGEMENTS

Preparation of this chapter was supported by NIMH grants R01MH072961, R01MH092950 and NIDA grant R01DA038466 (PI: Aarons).

SUGGESTED READINGS AND WEBSITES

Readings

Aarons GA, Ehrhart MG, Farahnak LR, Sklar M. Aligning leadership across systems and organizations to develop a strategic climate for evidence-based practice implementation. *Ann Rev Public Health.* 2014;35:255–274.

This paper presents a description of how leadership may be considered and used at health and allied health service system and organization levels, and how principles of leadership can inform shifting systems and organizations can be aligned to be more evidence-informed.

Ehrhart MG, Schneider B, Macey WH. *Organizational climate and culture: An introduction to theory, research, and practice.* New York; Routledge; 2014.
This book provides a comprehensive review of issues of organizational climate and culture including definitions, conceptualizations, debates, and research findings.

Klein KJ, Sorra JS. The challenge of innovation implementation. *Acad Manag Rev.* 1996;21:1055–1080.
This seminal article discusses implementation outcomes and presents a model in which implementation effectiveness is a function of organizational climate for implementation and fit of innovations with users' values.

Lee SY, Weiner BJ, Harrison MI, Belden CM. Organizational transformation: a systematic review of empirical research in health care and other industries. *Med Care Res Rev.* 2013;70(2):115–142.
This paper reviews transformational change in health and non–health care settings. The review describes antecedents, processes, and outcomes of change efforts and notes a "multiplicity" of factors that may affect organizational change.

Schein E.H., Schein, P. *Organizational culture and leadership.* 5th ed. Hoboken, NJ. John Wiley & Sons, Inc.; 2017.
This book provides a comprehensive review of organizational culture and climate, and leadership. The book describes the "embedding mechanisms" that leaders and organizations can use to demonstrate to employees what is expected, supported, and rewarded in the organization.

Weiner BJ, Amick H, Lee SD. Conceptualization and measurement of organizational readiness for change: A review of the literature in health services research and other fields. *Med Care Res Rev.* 2008;65:379–436.
A comprehensive review of organizational readiness for change based on research in various organizational contexts.

Websites and Tools

Leadership and Organizational Change for Implementation. http://implementationleadership.com/
This site provides description of a leadership and organizational change for implementation intervention, and provides related tools, assessments, and other resources. This includes access to the Implementation Leadership Scale (ILS), Implementation Climate Scale (ICS), Implementation Citizenship Behavior Scale (ICBS), and the Evidence-Based Practice Attitude Scale (EBPAS).

Institute for Healthcare Improvement. http://www.ihi.org/ihi
This site provides resources for process improvement in health care including education, resources, various topics in health care improvement, and descriptions of IHI work in the Umited States and globally.

Veterans Affairs Healthcare System Quality Enhancement Research Initiative (QUERI). http://www.queri.research.va.gov/
This site describes the VA QUERI program that supports a strategic process for implementing quality improvement initiatives.

Mind Garden. http://www.mindgarden.com/translead.htm#
This site provides information on the Multifactor Leadership Questionnaire. The authorized measures of the Full Range Leadership model are available from Mindgarden for research and/or applied purposes.

REFERENCES

1. Aarons GA, Hurlburt M, Horwitz SM. Advancing a conceptual model of evidence-based practice implementation in public service sectors. *Adm Policy Ment Health.* 2011;38(1):4–23.
2. Damschroder L, Aron D, Keith R, Kirsh S, Alexander J, Lowery J. Fostering implementation of health services research findings into practice: a consolidated framework for advancing implementation science. *Implement Sci.* 2009;4(1):50–64.
3. Glisson C, Schoenwald S. The ARC organizational and community intervention strategy for implementing evidence-based children's mental health treatments. *Ment Health Serv Res.* 2005;7(4):243–259.
4. Greenhalgh T, Robert G, Macfarlane F, Bate P, Kyriakidou O. Diffusion of innovations in service organizations: systematic review and recommendations. *Milbank Q.* 2004;82(4):581–629.
5. Rubin RM, Hurford MO, Hadley T, Matlin S, Weaver S, Evans AC. Synchronizing watches: the challenge of aligning implementation science and public systems. *Adm Policy Ment Health.* 2016;43(6):1023–1028.
6. Jacobs JA, Dodson EA, Baker EA, Deshpande AD, Brownson RC. Barriers to evidence-based decision making in public health: a national survey of chronic disease practitioners. *Public Health Rep.* 2010;125(5):736–742.
7. Ahearne M, Jelinek R, Mathieu J, Rapp A, Schillewaert N. A longitudinal examination of individual, organizational and contextual factors on technology adoption and job performance. In: Spotts HE, ed. *Creating and delivering value in marketing:* New York: Springer International Publishing; 2015:171–171.

8. Glasgow RE, Chambers D. Developing robust, sustainable, implementation systems using rigorous, rapid and relevant science. *Clin Transl Sci.* 2012;5(1):55.

9. Schein E. *Organizational culture and leadership.* 3rd ed. San Francisco: Jossey-Bass; 2004.

10. Priestland A, Hanig R. Developing first-level leaders. *Harv Bus Rev.* 2005;83(6):112–120.

11. Aarons GA, Sommerfeld DH, Willging CE. The soft underbelly of system change: the role of leadership and organizational climate in turnover during statewide behavioral health reform. *Psychol Serv.* 2011;8(4):269–281.

12. Aarons GA, Sommerfeld DH. *Transformational leadership, team climate for innovation, and staff attitudes toward adopting evidence-based practice.* Anaheim, CA: Academy of Management; 2008.

13. McLeod BD, Southam-Gerow MA, Weisz JR. Conceptual and methodological issues in treatment integrity measurement. *School Psych Rev.* 2009;38(4):541–546.

14. Taxman FS, Friedman PD. Fidelity and adherence at the transition point: Theoretically driven experiments. *J Exp Criminol.* 2009;5(3):219–226.

15. Aarons GA, Sommerfeld DH, Hecht DB, Silovsky JF, Chaffin MJ. The impact of evidence-based practice implementation and fidelity monitoring on staff turnover: Evidence for a protective effect. *J Consul. Clin Psychol.* 2009;77(2):270–280.

16. Aarons GA, Fettes DL, Flores LE, Sommerfeld DH. Evidence-based practice implementation and staff emotional exhaustion in children's services. *Behav Res Ther.* 2009;47(11):954–960.

17. Palinkas LA, Aarons GA. A view from the top: executive and management challenges in a statewide implementation of an evidence-based practice to reduce child neglect. *Int J Child Health Hum Dev.* 2009;2(1):47–55.

18. Sproull L. Organizational learning. In: Bird Schoonhoven C, Dobbin F, eds. *Standford's organization theory renaissance, 1970-2000.* Vol 28. Bingley, UK: Emerald Group Publishing Limited; 2010:59–69.

19. Van Noord I, Bruijne MC, Twisk WR. The relationship between patient safety culture and the implementation of organizational patient safety defences at emergency departments. *Int J Qua. Health Care.* 2010;22(3):162–169.

20. Nutley SM, Davies HTO. Making a reality of evidence-based practice: some lessons from the diffusion of innovations. *Public Money Manage.* 2001;20(4):35–42.

21. Schein EH. Organizational culture. *Am Psychol.* 1990;45(2):109–119.

22. Rousseau DM. Normative beliefs in fund-raising organizations: linking culture to organizational performance and individual responses. *Group Organ Stud.* 1990;15(4):448–460.

23. Cooke RA, Rousseau DM. Behavioral norms and expectations: A quantitative approach to the assessment of organizational culture. *Group Organ Manage.* 1988;13(3):245–273.

24. Denison DR. *Corporate culture and organizational effectiveness.* New York: Wiley; 1990.

25. Denison DR, Neale W. *Denison organizational culture survey.* Ann Arbor, MI: Denison Consulting; 2000.

26. Chatman J. Matching people and organizations: selection and socialization in public accounting firms. *Admin Sci Quart.* 1991;36:459–484.

27. O'Reilly CA, Chatman J, Caldwell DF. People and organizational culture: a profile comparison approach to assessing person-organization fit. *Acad Manage J* 1991;34(3):487–516.

28. Ashkanasy NM, Broadfoot LE, Falkus S. Questionnaire measures or organizational culture. In: Ashkanasy NM, Wilderom CPM, Peterson MF, eds. *Handbook of organizational culture and climate.* Thousand Oaks, CA: Sage; 2000.

29. Cameron KS, Quinn RE. *Diagnosing and changing organizational culture: Based on the competing values framework.* San Francisco: Jossey-Bass; 2006.

30. Glisson C. The organizational context of children's mental health services. *Clin Child Fam Psych.* 2002;5(4):233–253.

31. Glisson C, Landsverk J, Schoenwald S, et al. Assessing the organizational social context (OSC) of mental health services: implications for research and practice. *Adm Policy Ment Health.* 2008;35(1-2):98–113.

32. Deal TW, Kennedy AA. *Corporate cultures.* Reading, MA: Addison-Wesley; 1982.

33. Peters TJ, Waterman RH. *In search of excellence.* New York: Harper & Row; 1982.

34. Siehl C, Martin J. Organizational culture: The key to financial performance? In: Schneider B, ed. *Organizational climate and culture.* San Francisco: Jossey-Bass; 1990:241–281.

35. Kotter JP, Heskett JL. *Corporate culture and performance.* New York: The Free Press; 1992.

36. Wilderom CPM, Glunk U, Maslowski R. Organizational culture as a predictor of organizational performance. In: Ashkanasy NM, Wilderom CPM, Peterson MF, eds. *Handbook of organizational culture and climate.* Thousand Oaks, CA: Sage; 2000:193–209.

37. Parmelli E, Flodgren G, Beyer F, Baillie N, Schaafsma ME, Eccles MP. The effectiveness of strategies to change organisational culture to improve healthcare performance: a systematic review. *Implement Sci.* 2011;6(33).

38. Innis J, Dryden-Palmer K, Perreira T, Berta W. How do health care organizations take on best practices? A scoping literature review. *Int J Evid Based Healthc*. 2015;13(4):254–272.

39. Damschroder L, Hall CS, Gillon L, et al. The Consolidated Framework for Implementation Research (CFIR): progress to date, tools and resources, and plans for the future. *Implement Sci*. 2015;10 (Suppl 1):A12.

40. Gale NK, Shapiro J, McLeod H, Redwood S, Hewison A. Patients-people-place: developing a framework for researching organizational culture during health service redesign and change. *Implement Sci*. 2014;9:106.

41. Larson EL, Early E, Cloonan P, Sugrue S, Parides M. An organizational climate intervention associated with increased handwashing and decreased nosocomial infections. *Behav Med*. 2000;26(1):14–22.

42. Kinjerski V, Skrypnek BJ. The promise of spirit at work: Increasing job satisfaction and organizational commitment and reducing turnover and absenteeism in long-term care. *J Gerontol Nurs*. 2008;34(10):17–25.

43. Aarons GA, Glisson C, Green PD, et al. The organizational social context of mental health services and clinician attitudes toward evidence-based practice: a United States national study. *Implement Sci*. 2012;7(1):56–70.

44. Williams NJ, Glisson C. Testing a theory of organizational culture, climate and youth outcomes in child welfare systems: a United States national study. *Child Abuse Neglect*. 2014;38(4):757–767.

45. Glisson C, Schoenwald SK, Hemmelgarn A, et al. Randomized trial of MST and ARC in a two-level evidence-based treatment implementation strategy. *J Consult Clin Psychol*. 2010;78(4):537–550.

46. Glisson C, Williams NJ, Hemmelgarn A, Proctor E, Green P. Increasing clinicians' EBT exploration and preparation behavior in youth mental health services by changing organizational culture with ARC. *Behav Res Ther*. 2015;76:40–46.

47. Williams NJ, Glisson C, Hemmelgarn A, Green P. Mechanisms of change in the ARC organizational strategy: Increasing mental health clinicians' EBP adoption through improved organizational culture and capacity. *Adm Policy Ment Health*. 2016;44(2):269–283.

48. Lewin K, Lippitt R, White RK. Patterns of aggressive behavior in experimentally created "social climates." *J Soc Psychol*. 1939;10:271–299.

49. McGregor DM. *The human side of enterprise*. New York: McGraw-Hill; 1960.

50. Guion RM. A note on organizational climate. *Organ Behav Hum Perform*. 1973;9:120–125.

51. Johannesson RE. Some problems in the measurement of organizational climate. *Organ Behav Hum Perform*. 1973;10(1):118–144.

52. Schneider B. *Organizational climate and culture*. San Francisco, CA: Jossey-Bass; 1990.

53. James LR, Choi CC, Ko CHE, et al. Organizational and psychological climate: A review of theory and research. *Eur J Work Organ Psy*. 2008;17(1):5–32.

54. Schneider B, Ehrhart MG, Macey WA. Organizational climate research: Achievements and the road ahead. In: Ashkanasy NM, Wilderom CPM, Peterson MF, eds. *Handbook of organizational culture and climate*. 2nd ed. Newbury Park, CA: Sage Publications; 2011:29–49.

55. James LA, James LR. Integrating work environment perceptions: explorations into the measurement of meaning. *J Appl Psychol*. 1989;74(5):739–751.

56. Klein KJ, Sorra JS. The challenge of innovation implementation. *Acad Manage Rev*. 1996;21(4):1055–1080.

57. Weiner BJ, Belden CM, Bergmire DM, Johnston M. The meaning and measurement of implementation climate. *Implement Sci*. 2011;6:78–89.

58. Jacobs SR, Weiner BJ, Bunger AC. Context matters: measuring implementation climate among individuals and groups. *Implement Sci*. 2014;9(1):46.

59. Ehrhart MG, Aarons GA, Farahnak LR. Assessing the organizational context for EBP implementation: the development and validity testing of the Implementation Climate Scale (ICS). *Implement Sci*. 2014;9:157.

60. Glisson C, Hemmelgarn A. The effects of organizational climate and interorganizational coordination on the quality and outcomes of children's service systems. *Child Abuse Negl*. 1998;22(5):401–421.

61. Beidas RS, Wolk CL, Walsh LM, Evans AC, Hurford MO, Barg FK. A complementary marriage of perspectives: understanding organizational social context using mixed methods. *Implement Sci*. 2014;9(175).

62. Aarons GA, Sommerfeld DH, Walrath-Greene CM. Evidence-based practice implementation: the impact of public versus private sector organization type on organizational support, provider attitudes, and adoption of evidence-based practice. *Implement Sci*. 2009;4(1):83–96.

63. Klein KJ, Conn AB, Sorra JS. Implementing computerized technology: an organizational analysis. *J Appl Psychol*. 2001;86(5):811–824.

64. West MA, Wallace M. Innovation in health care teams. *Eur J Soc Psychol*. 1991;21:303–315.

65. Siegel SM, Kaemmerer WF. Measuring the perceived support for innovation in organizations. *J Appl Psychol*. 1978;63(5):553–562.

66. Drach-Zahavy A, Somech A, Granot M, Spitzer A. Can we win them all? Benefits and costs of structured and flexible innovation–implementations. *J Organ Behav*. 2004;25(2):217–234.

67. Holahan PJ, Aronson ZH, Jurkat MP, Schoorman FD. Implementing computer technology: a multiorganizational test of Klein and Sorra's model. *J Eng Technol Manage*. 2004;21(1):31–50.

68. Avolio BJ. Examining the Full Range Model of Leadership: Looking back to transform forward. In: Day DV, Zaccaro SJ, Halpin SM, eds. *Leader development for transforming organizations*. Mahwah, NJ: Lawrence Erlbaum Associates, Inc.; 2004.

69. Howell JM, Avolio BJ. Transformational leadership, transactional leadership, locus of control, and support for innovation: Key predictors of consolidated-business-unit performance. *J Appl Psychol*. 1993;78(6):891–902.

70. Bass BM, Avolio BJ, Jung DI, Berson Y. Predicting unit performance by assessing transformational and transactional leadership. *J Appl Psychol*. 2003;88(2):207–218.

71. McDaniel C, Wolf GA. Transformational leadership in nursing service: a test of theory. *J Nurs Adm*. 1992;22(2):60–65.

72. Aarons GA, Palinkas LA. Implementation of evidence-based practice in child welfare: service provider perspectives. *Adm Policy Ment Health*. 2007;34(4):411–419.

73. Corrigan PW, Garman AN. Transformational and transactional leadership skills for mental health teams. *Community Ment Health J*. 1999;35(4):301–312.

74. Brownson RC, Allen P, Duggan K, Stamatakis KA, Erwin PC. Fostering more-effective public health by identifying administrative evidence-based practices: a review of the literature. *Am J Prev Med*. 2012;43:309–319.

75. Drucker PF. *Managing the nonprofit organization*. New York: HarperCollins Publishers, Inc; 1990.

76. Goodman RM. A construct for building the capacity of community-based initiatives in racial and ethnic communities: a qualitative cross-case analysis. *J Public Health Manag. Pract*. 2009;15(2):E1–8.

77. Avolio BJ, Walumbwa FO, Weber TJ. Leadership: Current theories, research, and future directions. *Annu Rev Psychol*. 2009;60:421–449.

78. Bass BM, Avolio BJ. *The multifactor leadership questionnaire*. Palo Alto, CA: Consulting Psychologists Press; 1989.

79. Avolio BJ, Bass BM, Jung DI. Re-examining the components of transformational and transactional leadership using the Multifactor Leadership Questionnaire. *J Occup Organ Psychol*. 1999;72:441–462.

80. Jung D, Sosik JJ. Who are the spellbinders? Identifying personal attributes of charismatic leaders. *J Leadersh Stud*. 2010;12(4):1071–7919.

81. Judge TA, Piccolo RF. Transformational and transactional leadership: a meta-analytic test of their relative validity. *J Appl Psychol*. 2004;89(5):755–768.

82. Bass BM, Avolio BJ. *Training full range leadership*. Redwood City, CA: Mind Garden, Inc.; 1999.

83. Skogstad A, Einarsen S, Torsheim T, Aasland MS, Hetland H. The destructiveness of laissez-faire leadership behavior. *J Occup Health Psychol*. 2007;12(1):80–92.

84. DeGroot T, Kiker DS, Cross TC. A meta-analysis to review organizational outcomes related to charismatic leadership. *Can J Adm Sciences*. 2000;17(4):356–371.

85. Dumdum UR, Lowe KB, Avolio BJ. A meta-analysis of transformational and transactional leadership correlates of effectiveness and satisfaction: An update and extension. In: Avolio BJ, Yammarino FJ, eds. *Transformational and charismatic leadership: The road ahead*. Oxford, UK: Elsevier Science; 2002.

86. Lowe KB, Kroeck KG, Sivasubramaniam N. Effectiveness correlates of transformational and transactional leadership: a meta-analytic review of the MLQ literature. *Leadership Quart*. 1996;7(3):385–425.

87. Gasper JM. *Transformational leadership: An integrative review of the literature*, Kalamazoo, MI: Western Michigan University; 1992.

88. Walumbwa FO, Orwa B, Wang P, Lawler JJ. Transformational leadership, organizational commitment, and job satisfaction: a comparative study of Kenyan and U.S. financial firms. *Hum Resour Devel Q*. 2005;16(2):235–256.

89. MacKenzie SB, Podsakoff PM, Rich GA. Transformational and transactional leadership and salesperson performance. *J Acad Mark Science*. 2001;29(2):115–134.

90. Zohar D. Modifying supervisory practices to improve subunit safety: a leadership-based intervention model. *J Appl Psychol*. 2002;87(1):156–163.

91. Corrigan PW, Diwan S, Campion J, Rashid F. Transformational leadership and the mental health team. *Adm Policy Ment Health*. 2002;30(2):97–108.

92. Griffith J. Relation of principal transformational leadership to school staff job satisfaction, staff turnover, and school performance. *J Educ Adm*. 2004;42(3):333–356.

93. Kuoppala J, Lamminpaa A, Liira J, Vainio H. Leadership, job well-being, and health effects—A systematic review and meta-analysis. *J Occup Environ Med*. 2008;50(8):904–915.

94. Constable JF, Russell DW. The effect of social support and the work environment upon burnout among nurses. *J Human Stress*. 1986;12(1):20–26.

95. Geyer ALJ, Steyrer JM. Transformational leadership and objective performance in banks. *Appl Psychol: Int Rev*. 1998;47(3):397–420.

96. Frischer J, Larsson K. Laissez-faire in research education—An inquiry into a Swedish doctoral program. *High Educ Policy*. 2000;13:131–155.

97. Kelloway EK, Mullen J, Francis L. Divergent effects of transformational and passive leadership on employee safety. *J Occup Health Psychol*. 2006;11(1):76–86.

98. Antonakis J, Avolio BJ, Sivasubramaniam N. Context and leadership: an examination of the nine-factor full-range leadership theory using the Multifactor Leadership Questionnaire. *Leadership Quart*. 2003;14(3):261–295.

99. Koh WL, Steers RM, Terborg JR. The effects of transformational leadership on teacher attitudes and student performance in Singapore. *J Organ Behav*. 1995;16(4):319–333.

100. Garman AN, Davis-Lenane D, Corrigan PW. Factor structure of the transformational leadership model in human service teams. *J Organ Behav*. 2003;24(6):803–812.

101. House RJ, Dorfman PW, Javidan M, Hanges PJ, de Luque MFS. *Strategic leadership across cultures: GLOBE study of CEO leadership behavior and effectiveness in 24 countries*. Thousand Oaks, CA: Sage Publications; 2014.

102. Chhokar JS, Brodbeck FC, House RJ. *Culture and leadership across the world: The GLOBE book of in-depth studies of 25 societies*. Lawrence Erlbaum Associates, Taylor & Francis Group, 270 Madison Avenue, New York, NY 10016: Routledge; 2008.

103. Avolio BJ, Bass BM. *The full range of leadership development: Basic and advanced manuals*. Binghamton, NY: Bass, Avolio, & Associates; 1991.

104. Bass BM, Riggio RE. The development of transformational leadership. In: Bass BM, Riggio RE, eds. *Transformational leadership*. 2nd ed. Mahwah, NJ: Lawrence Erlbaum Associates, Inc.; 2006:142–166.

105. Crookall P. Management of inmate workshops: A field test of transformational and situational leadership. London, ON: University of Western Ontario; 1989.

106. Avolio BJ, Bass BM. *Evaluate the impact of transformational leadership training at individual, group, organizational and community levels. (Final report to the W. K. Kellog Foundation)*. Binghamton, NY: Binghamton University;1994.

107. Dvir T, Eden D, Avolio BJ, Shamir B. Impact of transformational leadership on follower development and performance: a field experiment. *Acad Manage J*. 2002;45(4):735–744.

108. Kelloway EK, Barling J, Helleur J. Enhancing transformational leadership: the role of training and feedback. *Leadership Org Dev J*. 2000;21:145–149.

109. Dettmann JR, Beehr T. Training transformational leadership: A field experiment in the non-profit sector. Meeting of the Society for Industrial and Organizational Psychology; 2004; Chicago, IL.

110. Barling J, Weber TJ, Kelloway EK. Effects of transformational leadership training on attitudinal and financial outcomes: a field experiment. *J Appl Psychol*. 1996;81(6):827–832.

111. von Thiele Schwarz U, Hasson H, Tafvelin S. Leadership training as an occupational health intervention: improved safety and sustained productivity. *Safety Sci*. 2016;81:35–45.

112. Glisson C, Durick M. Predictors of job satisfaction and organizational commitment in human service organizations. *Admin Sci Quart*. 1988;33(1):61–81.

113. Corrigan PW, Garman AN, Lam C, Leary M. What mental health teams want in their leaders. *Adm Policy Ment Health*. 1998;26(2):111–123.

114. Aarons GA. Transformational and transactional leadership: association with attitudes toward evidence-based practice. *Psychiatr Serv*. 2006;57(8):1162–1169.

115. Mosson R, Hasson H, Wallin L, Von Thiele Schwarz U. Exploring the role of line managers in implementing evidence-based practice in social services and older people care. *Br J Soc Work*. March 17, 2016.

115a. Aarons GA, Ehrhart MG, Farahnak LR. The implementation leadership scale (ILS): development of a brief measure of unit level implementation leadership. *Implementation Science*. 2014;9(1):45.

116. Aarons GA, Ehrhart MG, Torres EM, Finn NK, Roesch SC. Validation of the Implementation Leadership Scale (ILS) in substance use disorder treatment organizations. *J Subst Abuse Treat*. 2016;68:31–35.

117. Finn NK, Torres EM, Ehrhart MG, Roesch SC, Aarons GA. Cross-validation of the Implementation Leadership Scale (ILS) in child welfare service organizations. *Child Maltreat*. 2016;21(3):250–255.

118. Tistad M, Palmcrantz S, Wallin L, et al. Developing leadership in managers to facilitate the implementation of national guideline recommendations: a process evaluation of feasibility and usefulness. *Int J Health Policy Manag*. 2016;5(8):477–486.

119. Gifford WA, Graham ID, Ehrhart MG, Davies BL, Aarons GA. Ottawa Model of Implementation Leadership (O-MILe) and Implementation Leadership Scale (ILS): mapping concepts for developing and evaluating theory-based leadership interventions. *J Healthcare Leadership*. 2017:15–23.

120. Richter A, von Thiele Schwarz U, Lornudd C, Lundmark R, Mosson R, Hasson H. iLead—a transformational leadership intervention to train healthcare managers' implementation leadership. *Implement Sci*. 2016;11(1):108.

121. Nutt PC. Tactics of implementation. *Acad Manage J*. 1986;29(2):230–261.

122. Aarons GA, Green AE, Trott E, et al. The roles of system and organizational leadership in system-wide evidence-based intervention sustainment: a mixed-method study. *Adm Policy Ment Health*. 2016;43(6):991–1008.

123. Aarons GA, Wells RS, Zagursky K, Fettes DL, Palinkas LA. Implementing evidence-based practice in community mental health agencies: a multiple stakeholder analysis. *Am J Public Health*. 2009;99(11):2087–2095.

124. Mendel P, Meredith L, Schoenbaum M, Sherbourne C, Wells K. Interventions in organizational and community context: a framework for building evidence on dissemination and implementation in health services research. *Adm Policy Ment Health*. 2008;35(1-2):21–37.

125. Aarons GA, Ehrhart MG, Farahnak LR, Sklar M. Aligning leadership across systems and organizations to develop a strategic climate for evidence-based practice implementation. *Annu Rev Public Health*. 2014;35:255–274.

126. Aarons GA, Ehrhart MG, Farahnak LR, Hurlburt MS. Leadership and organizational change for implementation (LOCI): a randomized mixed method pilot study of a leadership and organization development intervention for evidence-based practice implementation. *Implement Sci*. 2015;10(1):11.

127. Aarons GA, Ehrhart MG, Moullin JC, Torres EM, Green AE. Testing the leadership and organizational change for implementation (LOCI) intervention in substance abuse treatment: a cluster randomized trial study protocol. *Implement Sci*. 2017;12(1):29.

128. Hasson H, Von Thiele Schwarz U, Nielsen K, Tafvelin S. Are we all in the same boat? The role of perceptual distance in organizational health interventions. *Stress Health*. 2016;32(4):294–303.

129. Silver Wolf DAP, Dulmus C, Maguin E, Keesler J, Powell BJ. Organizational leaders' and staff members' appraisals of their work

130. Beidas RS, Williams Jr. JW, Green AE, et al. Concordance between administrator and clinician ratings of organizational culture and climate. *Adm Policy Ment Health*. 2016:1–10.

131. Hasson H, Tafvelin S, Von Thiele Schwarz U. Comparing employees and managers' perceptions of organizational learning, health, and work performance. *Adv Develop Hum Res*. 2013;15(2):163–176.

132. Aarons GA, Ehrhart MG, Torres EM, Finn NK, Beidas RS. The humble leader: association of discrepancies in leader and follower ratings of implementation leadership with organizational climate in mental health organizations. *Psychiatr Serv*. 2016;appi–ps.

133. Aarons GA, Ehrhart MG, Farahnak LR, Sklar M, Horowitz J. Discrepancies in leader and follower ratings of transformational leadership: relationship with organizational culture in mental health. *Adm Policy Ment Health*. 2017;44(4):480–491.

134. Hasson H, Villaume K, Von Thiele Schwarz U, Palm K. Managing implementation: roles of line managers, senior managers, and human resource professionals in an occupational health intervention. *J Occup Environ Med*. 2014;56(1):58–65.

135. Nystrom ME, Strehlenert H, Hansson J, Hasson H. Strategies to facilitate implementation and sustainability of large system transformations: a case study of a national program for improving the quality of care for the elderly people. *BMC Health Services Research*. 2014;14(1):401.

136. Rycroft-Malone J, Burton CR, Bucknall T, Graham ID, Hutchinson AM, Stacey D. Collaboration and co-production of knowledge in healthcare: opportunities and challenges. *Int J Health Policy Manag*. 2016;5(4):221–223.

137. Kislov R, Harvey G, Walshe K. Collaborations for leadership in applied health research and care: lessons from the theory of communities of practice. *Implement Sci*. 2011;6(64).

138. Teal R, Bergmire DM, Johnston M, Weiner BJ. Implementing community-based provider participation in research: an empirical study *Implement Sci*. 2012;7(41).

139. Kislov R, Waterman H, Harvey G, Boaden R. Rethinking capacity building for knowledge mobilisation: developing multilevel capabilities in healthcare organisations. *Implement Sci*. 2014;9(166).

140. Bunger A, Hanson RF, Doogan NJ, Powell BJ, Cao Y, Dunn JC. Can learning collaboratives support implementation by rewiring

professional networks? *Adm. Policy Ment. Health.* 2016;43(1):79–92.

141. Powell BJ, Beidas RS, Rubin RM, et al. Applying the Policy Ecology Framework to Philadelphia's behavioral health transformation efforts. *Adm Policy Ment Health.* 2016;43(6):909–926.

142. Lewin K. Frontiers in group dynamics: Concept, method and reality in social science; social eqilibria and social change. *Hum Relat.* 1947;1(1):5–41.

143. Armenakis AA, Harris SG. Crafting a change message to create transformational readiness. *J Organ Change Manage.* 2002;15(2):169–183.

144. Beckhard R, Harris RT. *Organizational transitions: Managing complex change.* Reading, MA: Addison-Wesley; 1987.

145. Kimberly JR, Quinn RE. *Managing organizational transitions.* Homewood, IL: Irwin; 1984.

146. Kotter JP. *Leading change.* Cambridge. MA: Harvard Business School Press; 1996.

147. Michie S, van Stralen MM, West R. The behaviour change wheel: a new method for characterising and designing behaviour change interventions. *Implement Sci.* 2011;6(1):42.

148. Scaccia JP, Cook BS, Lamont A, et al. A practical implementation science heuristic for organizational readiness: R = MC². *J Commun Psychol.* 2015;43(4):484–501.

149. Lehman WEK, Greener JM, Simpson DD. Assessing organizational readiness for change. *J Subst Abuse Treat.* 2002;22(4):197–209.

150. Weiner BJ. A theory of organizational readiness for change. *Implement Sci.* 2009;4:67.

151. Weiner BJ, Amick H, Lee SD. Conceptualization and measurement of organizational readiness for change: a review of the literature in health services research and other fields. *Med Care Res Rev.* 2008;65:379–436.

152. Lundgren L, Amodeo M, Chassler D, Krull I, Sullivan L. Organizational readiness for change in community-based addiction treatment programs and adherence in implementing evidence-based practices: a national study. *J Subst Abuse Treat.* 2013;45(5):457–465.

153. Lehman WE, Simpson DD, Knight DK, Flynn PM. Integration of treatment innovation planning and implementation: strategic process models and organizational challenges. *Psychol Addict Behav.* 2011;25(2):252.

154. Shea CM, Jacobs SR, Esserman DA, Bruce K, Weiner BJ. Organizational readiness for implementing change: a psychometric assessment of a new measure. *Implement Sci.* 2014;9:7.

155. Nickel NC, Taylor EC, Labbok MH, Weiner BJ, Williamson NE. Applying organisation theory to understand barriers and facilitators to the implementation of Baby-Friendly: a multisite qualitative study *Midwifery.* 2013;29(8):956–964.

156. Griffin RW, Bateman TS, Wayne SJ, Head TC. Objective and social factors as determinants of task perceptions and responses: an integrated perspective and empirical investigation. *Acad Manage J.* 1987;30(3):501–523.

157. Bandura A. Social cognitive theory: an agentic perspective. *Annu Rev Psychol.* 2001;52:1–26.

158. Gist ME, Mitchell TR. Self-Efficacy: A theoretical analysis of its determinants and malleability. *Acad Manage Rev.* 1992;17(2):183–211.

159. Herscovitch L, Meyer JP. Commitment to organizational change: extension of a three-component model. *J Appl Psychol.* 2002;87(3):474–487.

160. Holt DT, Armenakis AA, Feild HS, Harris SG. Readiness for organizational change: the systematic development of a scale. *J Appl Behav Sci.* 2007;43(2):232–255.

161. Armenakis AA, Harris SG. Reflections: our journey in organizational change research and practice. *J Change Manage.* 2009;9(2):127–142.

162. Bandura A. Self-efficacy mechanism in human agency. *Am Psychol.* 1982;37(2):122–147.

163. Shaw RJ, Kaufman MA, Bosworth HB, et al. Organizational factors associated with readiness to implement and translate a primary care based telemedicine behavioral program to improve blood pressure control: the HTN-IMPROVE study. *Implement Sci.* 2013;8(106).

164. Pettigrew AM. Context and action in the transformation of the firm. *J Manage Stud.* 1987;24(6):649–670.

165. Jex SM, Spector PE. The generalizability of social information processing to organizational settings: a summary of two field experiments. *Percept Mot Skills.* 1989;69(3, Part 1):883–893.

166. Armenakis AA, Harris SG, Mossholder KW. Creating readiness for organizational change. *Hum Relat.* 1993;46(6):681–704.

167. Aarons GA, Green AE, Palinkas LA, et al. Dynamic adaptation process to implement an evidence-based child maltreatment intervention. *Implement Sci.* 2012;7(32):1–9.

168. Shea CM, Malone R, Weinberger M, et al. Assessing organizational capacity for achieving meaningful use of electronic health records. *Health Care Manage Rev.* 2014;39(2):124–133.

169. Doumit G, Gattellari M, Grimshaw J, O'Brien M. Local opinion leaders: effects on professional practice and health care outcomes. *Cochrane Database Syst Rev.* 2009(1).

170. Coch L, French JRP. Overcoming resistance to change. In: Burke WW, Lake DG, Paine

JW, eds. *Organization change: A comprehensive reader* (pp. 341–363). San Francisco, CA: Jossey-Bass; 2008.

171. Aarons GA. Mental health provider attitudes toward adoption of evidence-based practice: The Evidence-Based Practice Attitude Scale (EBPAS). *Ment Health Serv Res.* 2004;6(2):61–74.

172. Aarons GA, Glisson C, Hoagwood K, Kelleher K, Landsverk J, Cafri G. Psychometric properties and United States national norms of the Evidence-Based Practice Attitude Scale (EBPAS). *Psychol Assess.* 2010;22(2):356–365.

173. Silver Wolf DAP, Dulmus CN, Maguin E, Fava N. Refining the Evidence-Based Practice Attitude Scale: an alternative confirmatory factor analysis. *Soc Work Res.* 2014;38(1):47–58.

174. Aarons GA, Cafri G, Lugo L, Sawitzky A. Expanding the domains of attitudes towards evidence-based practice: the Evidence-based Practice Attitude Scale-50. *Adm Policy Ment Health.* 2012;39(5):331–340.

175. Rye M, Torres EM, Friborg O, Skre I, Aarons GA. The Evidence-based Practice Attitude Scale-36 (EPBAS-36): a brief and pragmatic measure of attitudes to evidence-based practice validated in Norwegian and U.S. samples. *Implement Sci.* 2017;12(1):44.

176. Aarons GA, Sawitzky AC. Organizational climate partially mediates the effect of culture on work attitudes and staff turnover in mental health services. *Adm Policy Ment Health.* 2006;33(3):289–301.

177. Dobbins M. Dissemination and use of research evidence for policy and practice: A framework for developing, implementing, and evaluating strategies. In: Rycroft-Malone J, Bucknall T, eds. *Models and frameworks for implementing evidence-based practice: Linking evidence to action.* Oxford: Wiley-Blackwell; 2010.

178. Ajzen I, Fishbein M. The influence of attitudes on behavior. In: Albarracín D, Johnson BT, Zanna MP, eds. *The handbook of attitudes.* Mahwah, NJ: Lawrence Erlbaum Associates, Inc.; 2005:173–222.

179. Ehrhart MG, Aarons GA, Farahnak LR. Going above and beyond for implementation: the development and validity testing of the Implementation Citizenship Behavior Scale (ICBS). *Implement Sci.* 2015;10(65).

180. Austin JM, Pronovost PJ. Improving performance on core processes of care. *Curr Opin Allergy Clin Immunol.* 2016;16(3):224–230.

181. Schneider A. How quality improvement in health care can help to achieve the Millennium Development Goals. *Bull World Health Organ.* 2006;84(4):259–260.

182. Berwick D. The science of improvement. *JAMA.* 2008;299(10):1182–1184.

183. Scoville R, Little K. *Comparing lean and quality improvement.* Cambridge, MA: Institute for Healthcare Improvement; 2014.

184. Evans AC, Rieckmann T, Fitzgerald MM, Gustafson DH. Teaching the NIATx model of process improvement as an evidence-based process. *J Teach Addict.* 2008;6(2):21–37.

185. Eckes G. *The six sigma revolution: How General Electric and others turned process into profits.* New York: John Wiley & Sons; 2000.

186. George ML. *Lean six sigma for service: How to use lean speed & six sigma quality to improve services and transactions.* New York: McGraw-Hill; 2003.

187. McCarty D, Gustafson DH, Wisdom JP, et al. The network for the improvement of addiction treatment (NIATx): enhancing access and retention. *Drug Alcohol Depend.* 2007;88(2-3):138–145.

188. Sehwail L, DeYong C. Six sigma in health care. *Leadersh Health Serv.* 2003;16(4):1–5.

189. Leatherman S, Ferris TG, Berwick D, Omaswa F, Crisp N. The role of quality improvement in strengthening health systems in developing countries. *Int J Qual Health Care.* 2010;22(4):237–243.

190. Ragsdale MA, Mueller J. Plan, do, study, act model to improve an orientation program. *J Nurs. Care Qual.* 2005;20(3):268–272.

191. Leape LL, Berwick DM. Five years after *To Err is Human*: What have we learned? *JAMA.* 2005;293(19):2384–2390.

192. Becher EC, Chassin MR. Improving quality, minimizing error: making it happen. A five-point plan and why we need it. *Health Aff.* 2001;20(3).

193. Boe DT, Riley W, Parsons H. Improving service delivery in a county health department WIC clinic: an applicaiton of statistical process control techniques. *Am J Public Health.* 2009;99(9):1619–1625.

194. Rosenheck RA. Organizational process: a missing link between research and practice. *Psychiatr Serv.* 2001;52:1607–1612.

195. Pearson ML, Wu S, Schaefer J, et al. Assessing the implementation of the chronic care model in quality improvement collaboratives. *Health Serv Res.* 2005;40(4):978–996.

196. Kim CS, Spahlinger DA, Kin JM, Billi JE. Lean health care: What can hospitals learn from a world-class automaker? *J Hosp Med.* 2006;1(3):191–199.

197. De Koning H, Verver JPS, van den Heuvel J, Bisgaard S, Does RJMM. Lean six sigma in healthcare. *J Heathcare Qual.* 2006;28(2):4–11.

198. Demakis JG, McQueen L, Kizer KW, Feussner JR. Quality Enhancement Research Initiative

(QUERI): a collaboration between research and clinical practice. *Med. Care.* 2000;38:17–25.

199. Rubenstein LV, Mittman BS, Yano EM, Mulrow CD. From understanding health care provider behavior to improving health care: the QUERI framework for quality improvement. *Med. Care.* 2000;38(6):129–141.

200. Goetz MB, Bowman C, Hoang T, Anaya H, Osborn T, Gifford AL. Implementing and evaluating a regional strategy to improve testing rates in VA patients at risk for HIV, utilizing the QUERI process as a guiding framework: QUERI series. *Implement Sci.* 2008;3(1).

201. Improvement Science Research Network. What is Improvement Science? 2017; https://isrn.net/about/improvement_science.asp.

202. Marshall M, Pronovost PJ, Dixon-Woods M. Promotion of improvement as a science. *Lancet.* 2013;381(9864):419–421.

203. Speroff T, Miles PV, Dougherty D, Mittman BS, Splaine ME. Introduction to the Academy for Healthcare Improvement conference on advancing the methods for healthcare quality improvement research. *Implement Sci.* 2013;8(Suppl 1):I1.

204. Rubenstein LV, Hempel S, Farmer MM, et al. Finding order in heterogeneity: types of quality-improvement intervention publications. *BMJ Qual. Saf.* 2008;17(6):403–408.

205. Grol R, Bosch MC, Hulscher MEJL, Eccles MP, Wensing M. Planning and studying improvement in patient care: the use of theoretical perspectives. *Milbank Q.* 2007;85(1):93–138.

206. Kislov R, Walshe K, Harvey G. Managing boundaries in primary care service improvement: a developmental approach to communities of practice. *Implement Sci.* 2012;7(1):97.

207. Patel B, Patel A, Jan S, et al. A multifaceted quality improvement intervention for CVD risk management in Australian primary healthcare: a protocol for a process evaluation. *Implement Sci.* 2014;9:187.

208. Quanbeck AR, Gustafson DH, Ford JH, et al. Disseminating quality improvement: study protocol for a large cluster-randomized trial. *Implement Sci.* 2011;6:44.

209. Alexander JA, Hearld LR. The science of quality improvement implementation: developing capacity to make a difference. *Med Care Res Rev.* 2011;49:S6-S20.

210. Vos L, Duckers MLA, Wagner C, van Merode GG. Applying the quality improvement collaborative method to process redesign: a multiple case study. *Implement Sci.* 2010;5(1):19.

211. Doyle C, Howe C, Woodcock RW, et al. Making change last: applying the NHS institute for innovation and improvement sustainability model to healthcare improvement. *Implement Sci.* 2013;8(1):127.

212. Balasubramanian BA, Cohen DJ, Davis MM, et al. Learning evaluation: blending quality improvement and implementation research methods to study healthcare innovations. *Implement Sci.* 2015;10(1):31.

213. Kilbourne AM, Almirall D, Eisenberg D, et al. Protocol: Adaptive Implementation of Effective Programs Trial (ADEPT): cluster randomized SMART trial comparing a standard versus enhanced implementation strategy to improve outcomes of a mood disorders program. *Implement Sci.* 2014;9(1):132.

214. Bond G, Drake R, McHugo G, Rapp C, Whitley R. Strategies for improving fidelity in the national evidence-based practices project. *Res Soc Work Pract.* 2009;19(5):569.

215. Torrey WC, Drake RE, Dixon L, et al. Implementing evidence-based practices for persons with severe mental illnesses. *Psychiatr Serv.* 2001;52(1):45–50.

216. Dadich A. From bench to bedside: methods that help clinicians use evidence-based practice. *Aust Psychol.* 2010;45(3):197–211.

217. Saldana L, Chamberlain P, Wang W, Brown CH. Predicting program start-up using the stages of implementation measure. *Adm. Policy Ment. Health.* 2011;39(6):419–425.

9

Systems Thinking and Dissemination and Implementation Research

BARBARA L. RILEY, CAMERON D. WILLIS, BEV HOLMES, DIANE T. FINEGOOD, ALLAN BEST, AND JESSIE-LEE D. MCISAAC

INTRODUCTION

Health issues are increasingly recognized as complex problems, deeply embedded within the fabric of society,[1] occurring in complex systems with multiple interacting components and unknowable behaviors.[2] This is no longer a new message among those working in academic, policy and practice settings, in which dialogue about complexity has increased over the last 20 years across a broad spectrum of health issues.[2-4]

In the health field, there is generally a shared understanding of complex problems. They are complex for many reasons. For example, they involve multiple interacting agents, the context in which they unfold keeps changing, and the manner in which things change does not conform to linear or simple patterns.[5]

There is also general agreement on what is needed to address complex health problems. Solutions to complex problems often require intervening at many different levels, using multiple strategies, and engaging multiple actors and organizations. In health, the most common and long-standing translation of this multilevel, multistrategy, multiactor view is the social ecological approach.[6,7] Multilevel refers to multiple levels within a social ecological system, including: individual, interpersonal, family, organizational, interorganizational/network, community, and societal levels. Multistrategy generally refers to a mix of educational, skill-building, policy, and media approaches. Multiactor refers to individuals and organizations from health and non-health sectors; public, private and charitable sectors; and research, policy and practice sectors. Other perspectives on how to address complex problems, primarily from nonhealth sectors, are gaining some attention in health and may have significant implications for dissemination and implementation (D&I) research. One perspective described later in this chapter is Meadows' "places to intervene" in complex systems.

Despite this general agreement on what constitutes complex problems and how to address them, there is wide variability in related language and actions. There are many institutes and centers whose efforts are guided by principles of complexity, implicitly or explicitly.[8] Yet a common language related to the complexity of health problems and the complex systems in which they play out does not exist,[9] and there is no agreed upon taxonomy of theories, methods, and tools that define and support the application of "systems thinking" in health.[5] Least well-developed is a focus on *solutions* to complex problems, and especially the nature and role of dissemination and implementation (D&I) research in contributing to these solutions. The most common response to complex problems—by practitioners in the health system and many academics—is to rely on reductionist thinking in an attempt to reduce complexity rather than consider characteristics of complex problems and the systems within which they are generated and reproduced.[10] A systems-oriented approach to D&I research is neither defined nor applied in any systematic way. Our reliance on scientific approaches that do not necessarily respect complexity is not serving us well in solving today's complex health problems, including chronic diseases and their underlying determinants.

This chapter aims to describe a potentially more effective scientific response to complexity, by proposing systems-oriented D&I research as part of the solution. By D&I research, we mean all research that is concerned with putting evidence into practice. Overarching aims for such research may include: describing and/or guiding the process of translating research into practice, understanding and/or explaining what influences implementation outcomes, and evaluating implementation.[11]

As a health community, how can we better align our D&I research with how we create solutions to complex health problems in both public and clinical health domains? This chapter explores ways to create this alignment, expanding the conversation initiated by others (e.g., Glasgow & Chambers, 2012).[12] To do so, the chapter describes what we refer to as systems thinking, and discusses implications of systems thinking for D&I research. It concludes with two applications of systems thinking in D&I research—one public health and one clinical health services example.

SYSTEMS THINKING

Systems thinking can be described as a way of seeing the world that respects attributes of systems and proposes how we can best work with them. As noted by Peters,[5] "systems thinking is an enterprise aimed at seeing how things are connected to each other within some notion of a whole entity." Systems thinking has diverse disciplinary origins including in (but not limited to) biology, physics, psychology, and computer science.[5] As a result of this diversity, there are many expressions of the theory of systems thinking, as well as its application through various lenses, perspectives, methods and tools. Examples of perspectives on taking effective action in complex systems include Meadow's[13] places to intervene or "leverage points," Wheatley's description of "influencing emergence,"[14] Greenhalgh and colleagues' ideas of "helping it happen,"[15] and Bar-Yam's notion of "making things work."[10]

Often, systems thinking is translated into sets of simple rules, principles, or critical features. From the authors' own experiences, some examples in health include: Best et al.'s simple rules for large system transformation (e.g., blend designated leadership with distributed leadership; establish feedback loops; attend to history);[16] Riley et al.'s principles of systems approaches in knowledge to action (e.g., establish and nurture relationships, coproduce and curate knowledge, create feedback loops);[8] Finegood et al.'s solutions to complex problems (e.g., individuals matter, match capacity to complexity, distribute decision, action and authority);[17] Willis et al.'s cross-cutting features of a systems approach to transformation

(e.g., a focus on relationships, a long-term vision, recognition of context),[18] and Holmes et al.'s actions to mobilize knowledge in complex systems, at the intervention level and beyond.[19] The authors' and others' efforts yield a mix of perspectives, attributes, principles, or approaches that represent variations on similar themes. Continuing to build on these efforts will ideally move us toward a more unified, complex systems-based theory of change, and thereby potentially enhance the application of systems thinking in D&I research.

Since this chapter is to provide an overview of systems thinking applied to D&I research in health, systems thinking is defined with this purpose in mind. Systems and their attributes are briefly described, followed by selective perspectives on ways to define the object of D&I (evidence-based interventions) and how to apply, sustain, and spread these interventions effectively (D&I strategies). The chapter concludes by describing three systems concepts that may help guide a systems-oriented D&I research agenda.

Systems and their Attributes

Systems are defined in different ways, including what they are, what they do, and how they behave. We adopt Meadow's[20] definition that most simply captures these various attributes: "a set of things (people, cells, molecules or whatever) interconnected in such a way that they produce their own pattern of behavior over time."

Systems can be thought of as simple, complicated, or complex,[21,22] all of which are relevant in the health field. For example, clinical reminder systems for physicians[23] could be considered simple, consisting as they do of basic issues of technique and terminology that, once mastered, contain a very high assurance of success.[24] Complicated systems demand more coordination and more specialized expertise than simple ones; in this sense, a medical surgery can be viewed as complicated. In complex systems there is no single point of control. Health systems are composed of individuals with varying degrees of influence whose goals and behaviors are likely to conflict.[25,26] Change occurs naturally and continuously as people within the system acquire new information that alters their understanding. Planned change in such a system is difficult because of these dynamic characteristics: nothing stands still while we intervene.[19] Such is the case with most public and clinical health problems in the 21st century, including tobacco use, other addictions, obesity, chronic disease management, and other noncommunicable diseases.[21,27,28] This understanding of systems fundamentally shapes how effective solutions are created, implemented, and evaluated. This chapter focuses on *complex systems*, since D&I research to solve complex problems in complex systems is increasingly recognized as important and is least developed.

D&I Objects and Strategies

As noted earlier, it is generally accepted that complex problems in society require a mix of effective interventions (i.e., the objects of D&I) by a diverse set of actors and organizations whose influence is in various settings ranging from the home, school, and work environments to communities, regions, and entire countries.[6,7,21] In health, the widespread adoption of social ecological models has usefully reinforced the need for multiple levels of influence (individual through societal), multiple strategies, and multiple actors. The most common application of social ecological models is to define evidence-based interventions as media, program, and policy approaches in a variety of settings, with sufficient evidence of effectiveness. D&I strategies are any actions at multiple levels (in a social ecological sense, at the individual, interpersonal, community, regional, national, global levels) that may support the adoption, implementation, sustainability and spread of evidence-based programs and policies by diverse sets of actors and organizations.

Systems thinking expands our view of how to think about the objects of D&I and strategies to apply them in practice. A perspective that may be particularly relevant to these D&I constructs is from systems thinker Donella Meadows. Meadows[13] described places to intervene in complex systems in the form of 12 levels. The top level is the paradigms under which a system operates (e.g., childhood obesity is a societal issue versus childhood obesity is an individual issue) and at the bottom are what she calls "structural elements," which consist of the set of actors and interventions as they are normally considered in the health field (e.g., media, program, and policy initiatives in various settings). At the top, changing paradigms is the hardest place to intervene, but the most effective. At the bottom, structural elements are the easiest to change, but by themselves the least effective. These "places to intervene" in complex systems invite us to consider a broader scope of the objects of D&I—evidence-based interventions—than the structural, sub-system

elements (according to Meadows) that are generally considered the primary objects of D&I. The same would be true for D&I strategies: how might the places to intervene (e.g., collaborative approaches, the "mindset" of the system, feedback loops) help inform strategies to improve the uptake, implementation, sustainability, and/or spread of evidence-based interventions?

Table 9.1 may help inform what are considered to be D&I objects and strategies from a systems perspective. In an effort to use Meadow's places to intervene as a novel framework to plan, analyze, and support systems thinking-based interventions, Finegood and colleagues[29] collapsed the 12 levels into 5 (Table 9.1). They have used this framework to assess initiatives to address obesity;[28] initiatives to make food systems healthy, green, fair, and affordable;[29] and as a tool underpinning efforts to engage in dialogues that support cross-sector partnership (unpublished observations). Much more work is needed to further develop the framework and determine its utility as either a planning or analytic tool. In this chapter, the primary purpose of the framework is to propose how systems thinking can be used to define D&I objects and strategies.

Empirical evidence is beginning to emerge that interventions informed by systems thinking can have positive effects. Leykum et al.[30] looked at the effectiveness of organizational interventions to improve care of Type II diabetes and found the number of complex system characteristics present was associated with effectiveness. Riley et al.[8] also found attention to complex systems principles in successful social innovations. Lanham et al.[31] showed that self-organization, while not completely controllable, can be influenced, and that improving interdependencies and sense-making among stakeholders is a strategy for facilitating self-organization processes that increase the probability of spreading effective practices across diverse settings. More of this kind of evidence is needed to inform evidence-based interventions and strategies to apply them from a systems perspective.

Systems Concepts to Guide a D&I Research Agenda

As noted, there is no single set of agreed upon systems concepts. This chapter privileges concepts that may usefully guide D&I research, and that build on the description of systems and their attributes, as well as how D&I objects and strategies may be defined. It focuses on a small set of systems

TABLE 9.1 SYSTEM LEVEL FRAMEWORK, ADAPTED FROM MEADOWS[13]

Level	Explanation
Paradigm	The system's "mindset," the deepest held, often unspoken beliefs about the way the system works. Goals, rules, and structures that govern the system arise out of the paradigm. Actions and ideas at this level propose to either shift or reinforce the existing paradigm. Intervention at this level is very difficult.
Goals	Targets that need to be achieved for the paradigm to shift. Actions at this level focus or change the aim of the system.
System structure	Elements that make up the system as a whole, including the subsystems, actors, and interconnections among these elements. The structure conforms to the system's goals and paradigms. Actions at this level can change the system structure by changing linkages within the system or incorporating new types of structural elements.
Feedback and delays	Feedback allows the system to regulate itself by providing information about the outcome of different actions back to the source of the actions. Feedback occurs when actions by one element of the system affect the flows into or out of that same element. Actions at this level attempt to create new, or increase the gain around existing, feedback loops. Adding new feedback loops or changing feedback delays can restructure the system.
Structural elements	The smaller subsystems, actors, and physical elements of the system, connected through feedback loops and communications. Actions at this level affect specific subsystems, actors, or elements of the system.

concepts and draws on existing definitions, to avoid adding even more diversity and confusion to the literature on definitions of systems thinking. Using these criteria, this chapter draws most explicitly on the work of Williams and Hummelbrunner[32] by highlighting relationships, multiple perspectives, and boundaries as three systems concepts that may inform D&I research efforts.

Relationships

Given the focus of systems thinking on "connectedness," relationships are considered one of the most well-established and familiar systems concepts.[4,32] For a given problem or situation, multiple relationships may exist, such as those between people—as individuals, organizations, or communities—as well as relationships between nonhuman entities such as financial and nonfinancial resources, equipment and infrastructure, policies and programs. Relationships may be between people or elements at the same level (e.g., health and education departments within a state-level government) or across multiple levels (e.g., local, state, and federal level governments).

Often, the relationships between levels in a social ecological sense are most critical to

effective D&I, yet are also the most difficult to initiate, sustain, or modify.[33] Relationships within and among interventions and contextual factors influencing them are also centrally important for seeking solutions to complex health problems. A systems lens helps to focus on the structure of relationships; the processes that exist between elements within that structure; the nature of the relationships (e.g., are they strong, weak, fast, slow, collaborative, combative); and the value the relationships provide for each entity in the relationship. These are the mid-level places to intervene according to Meadows, which include incentives and punishments, information flows, and feedback loops. Efforts to better understand relationships requires attention to how relationships influence observed patterns of action or behavior; the tendency for nonlinear effects often resulting from feedback; and the influence of contexts on relationships and how this limits our ability to transplant solutions across settings.

Multiple Perspectives

Working in complex systems recognizes that multiple perspectives exist on a given situation. These perspectives are expressed in the different languages, actions, behaviors and traditions of diverse (heterogeneous) stakeholders, which are themselves driven by different logics, histories, and motivations. For any given issue or situation, many and varied perspectives may exist, at individual through to familial, organizational, community, or societal levels. A systems lens promotes the importance of recognizing and understanding these diverse perspectives, not just on what a given situation is, but also on how stakeholders view potential alternative futures, what is open to change, what is not, and why.

Meadows puts "perspective" at the top of her hierarchy for places to intervene with the most potential impact. The paradigm or "mind-set out of which the system arises" is potentially the most influential place to intervene, because our deeply held beliefs drive our goals and how we organize our systems around them. Meadows suggests that there is only one leverage point higher than changing paradigms and that is the effort to transcend paradigms and recognize that no perspective is right.

Making explicit the factors that motivate stakeholder action and behavior can be a powerful tool enabling system change as well as greater explanatory and predictive capacities. Focusing on perspective forces us to make explicit our own assumptions, judgements, and mental models at the same time as we are attempting to make sense of each other's. Understanding multiple perspectives supports the establishment of cross-sector, cross-silo networks and teams (e.g., public-private partnerships in health),[34] and to distribute decision-making, action and authority in ways that capitalize on variation.[10] A focus on multiple perspectives also encourages valuing a broad scope of evidence that reflects diverse vantage points (e.g., practice knowledge in addition to knowledge gained through scientific observations).

Boundaries

While seeing "wholes" is a critical feature of systems thinking, in reality, boundaries need to be placed around a situation in order to make that situation manageable.[35] Where boundaries are drawn and by whom has important implications for how we view a situation, whose perspective matters, and who or what is most important. Boundaries reflect values, assumptions, and perspectives on what or who is within or outside a boundary; what or who is relevant to a situation; and what or who is important to a situation. In complex systems, Plsek and Greenhalgh[2] remind us that "fuzzy" boundaries are often a reality. Nonetheless, efforts to make explicit where and why we draw boundaries helps to reveal these different values, assumptions, and perspectives, which may have minor or major impacts (e.g., determining who receives a resource or not). Being explicit and transparent about boundaries also has implications for how a situation is approached, and the expectations we have for what kinds of changes may result. Choices about boundaries influence the composition of networks and teams that join forces to address complex health problems, and also choices about what is best done at local, regional, and global levels. Boundaries also influence whose interests are served with research, what information will be most relevant to meet their needs, and when those needs will be met throughout the research process (e.g., short-term learning cycles, findings shared once the research is completed).

IMPLICATIONS OF SYSTEMS THINKING FOR D&I RESEARCH

Informed by the previous sections in this chapter, there are many possible implications of systems thinking for D&I research. In this section, we highlight those that may be most instructive for defining an overall systems orientation to D&I research in health. We focus on four features that may be most useful to consider when designing, conducting, and using D&I research. These features are: the research purpose and questions, conceptual frameworks, study designs and methods, and the research process. Selective implications for each of these features are shown in Box 9.1.

As noted in Box 9.1, a systems thinking approach influences the overall purpose of research and types of research questions that are asked about D&I. By respecting the dynamic nature of complex systems and related system concepts, research goals and questions tend to focus on how best to *improve* the effectiveness of interventions and D&I strategies, either in the same or different contexts, and how to optimize the "fit" between interventions and their contexts.[36] For example, questions may seek to better understand the contexts for implementation, how these contexts interact with different features of an intervention, and what constitutes meaningful measures of implementation effectiveness and for whom. As such, these questions also prompt consideration of the

---

BOX 9.1

SOME IMPLICATIONS OF SYSTEMS THINKING FOR D&I RESEARCH

RESEARCH PURPOSE AND QUESTIONS

- Research focuses more on improving (rather than proving) the effectiveness of interventions under changing conditions.
- Questions are framed by first defining the evidence-based intervention(s) and D&I strategies, and emphasizing relationships, perspectives, and boundaries in relation to these constructs.
- Outcomes of interest to diverse stakeholders (science, policy, practice) are relevant and valued.
- Questions tend to explore the relationship and "fit" between interventions and contexts (i.e., questions of adaptation rather than attribution and fidelity of the intervention).

CONCEPTUAL FRAMEWORKS

- Frameworks emphasize relationships, including context, actors, actions and outcomes.
- They are holistic and integrative rather than reductionist.
- Frameworks acknowledge power imbalances among relationships, as well as system incentives and disincentives.

STUDY DESIGNS AND METHODS

- A variety of study designs may be used: experimental, quasi-experimental, nonexperimental.
- Approaches such as natural experiments, simulations and comparative case studies may be most suitable.
- Emphasis is placed on shared measurement systems that enable understanding intervention success in different contexts and from different perspectives.
- Different types of evidence (scientific, practice, contextual) are valued.
- Measures for concepts like complexity, capacity, connectedness, and trust may need to be developed.

RESEARCH PROCESS

- Emphasis will be on participatory and coproduction approaches.
- Studies will consider relevant and timely feedback loops.

---

relationships that are of most interest to explore, the perspectives that need to be captured in relation to implementation questions, and the boundaries these perspectives place on what and who is considered relevant to implementation.

The conceptual frameworks guiding systems approaches to D&I therefore encourage engagement and examination of context, as well as features of the intervention and D&I strategies. They promote a more holistic understanding of D&I, inclusive of diverse perspectives. Examples of such frameworks include the Dynamic Sustainability Framework,[36] systems models for knowledge to action,[37] the ABLe Change Framework,[38] and the Linking Systems Framework.[39]

Informed by these frameworks, D&I researchers may choose from any number of study designs, including experimental, quasi-experimental or nonexperimental designs. Consistent with all types of research, the most appropriate design and methods will be those that best answer the research questions. While this may seem obvious, a possible misperception is that systems approaches to D&I research are limited to methods and tools of systems science. They are not. Even so, assuming the D&I in health community will continue to increase its engagement with systems thinking and its applications to D&I research, greater use of system tools[40] may be seen. Some of these tools focus explicitly and directly on relationships (e.g., network analyses and causal loop diagrams), capturing diverse perspectives (e.g., concept mapping) and making explicit choices about the boundaries of an issue (e.g., network analysis and system dynamics modeling). Chapter 10 discusses the application of a subset of systems science methods. Whether branded as methods of systems science or not, all designs and methods used to address systems-oriented D&I research questions must respect the diversity of actors and structures, and also the need for them to work together. As a result, methods tend to emphasize shared measurement across diverse settings. Common measures are used to compare and contrast the combination of contexts, implementation, and results of interventions and how these change over time. Methods also value and promote a plurality of evidence, including that derived from practical experience, in addition to evidence derived from empirical studies.[41]

Influencing all aspects of research is the process used to initiate, design, execute, interpret, and use research findings. Systems approaches to D&I research emphasize a coproduction process, which engages relevant stakeholders at all stages of research. This coproduced, highly participatory approach is central to valuing multiple perspectives, while also needing to consider boundaries for whose perspectives will be included for particular D&I research studies. Decisions about these boundaries will also influence plans for how research is used, including who participates in the interpretation of findings, and who receives results from the research, at what time, in what form and for what purpose.

Despite recent increases in the application of systems thinking in D&I health research, such applications are still limited. This is not surprising given the initial focus on gaining conceptual clarity on systems thinking; and these efforts continue. Applications of systems thinking may be accelerated by sharing examples of D&I research that reflect systems thinking. To contribute to this goal, the next section provides two examples of D&I research in which the authors were directly involved.

APPLICATIONS OF SYSTEMS THINKING TO D&I RESEARCH IN HEALTH

Here are two illustrations to demonstrate the applicability of systems thinking to D&I research across a range of health issues. The first illustration is from the area of public health, and the second from clinical health services.

Case Study #1: A Learning and Improvement Strategy for the Public Health Agency of Canada's Multisectoral Partnerships Approach

The Public Health Agency of Canada (the Agency) provides national oversight for public health initiatives in Canada. In 2013, the Agency launched the *Multi-sectoral Partnerships to Promote Healthy Living and Prevent Chronic Disease* approach (MSPA), which reconceptualised the Agency's funding portfolio to more effectively support multisectoral approaches.[42] The MSPA aims to improve the capacity of government and non-government partners in designing and delivering preventive health activities; to improve the use of public funds through a pay for performance strategy; and to leverage partner funding in all programs.[43] Through the MSPA, each funded project is required to secure matched funding from nongovernment partners, as well as engage the skills, competencies, and capacities of all partner organizations. Since its launch, the MSPA approach has funded 23 projects, each involving strategic mixes of multi-sector organizations including for-profit private sector organizations, not-for-profit organizations, and research based partners. To date, individual projects have focused on evidence-based interventions that address physical inactivity, unhealthy eating, tobacco use, and injuries. Many projects focus on established interventions suitable for scaling up to new populations, settings, or jurisdictions. In contrast, other projects are at earlier stages of development, with a focus on exploring innovative approaches and methods. The MSPA requires the Agency to take an active role in identifying and engaging potential partners, brokering relationships, and bringing together often disparate organizations to collaborate toward chronic disease prevention.

With the introduction of the MSPA, the Agency recognized the opportunity to invest in D&I research; a real-time learning and improvement strategy that would benefit both continuous program improvement, as well as contribute to the evidence base on multisectoral approaches in prevention.[43] In partnership with the Propel Centre for Population Health Impact (Propel), the Agency has developed a Learning and Improvement

Strategy to assist in program implementation. This strategy has a primary focus on the overall initiative level, rather than specific multisectoral projects, and helps to highlight some of the features of a systems approach to dissemination and implementation science. As a result, the MSPA is considered here as the object of D&I, with the Learning and Improvement Strategy as part of an overall implementation strategy.

Research Purpose and Questions

The MSPA's Learning and Improvement Strategy was developed in partnership with Agency staff, to ensure that research questions were addressing the perspectives of staff on priority learning needs. Through consultations with Agency staff, key learning needs were identified that related to better understanding which outcomes multisectoral partnerships are thought to influence and the pathways by which they influence those outcomes, highlighting key relationships between contexts, actions, and outcomes. In addition, Agency staff expressed interest in examining the perspectives of partners regarding their motivations to engage in partnerships for chronic disease prevention, as well as ways to shift the boundaries of evaluation to include both *expected* and *unexpected* effects associated with partnership implementation. Finally, Agency consultations identified a need to better understand how relationships with diverse organizational partners enable diverse resources to be leveraged for chronic disease prevention.[43] To address these learning needs, evidence from a range of sources is considered relevant, including published research, models of inter-sectoral action, and direct partner experiences.[44]

Conceptual Frameworks

The Agency's approach to learning and improvement was seen as a complement to ongoing evaluation strategies already in use by Agency teams. In contrast to these evaluation approaches, the Learning and Improvement Strategy drew on conceptual models related to learning cycles,[45] continuous improvement,[46] and developmental evaluation.[47] A review of conceptual frameworks was specifically undertaken as part of the Learning and Improvement Strategy, which examined key frameworks focused on multisectoral action and partnership approaches.[43] This literature highlighted the macro, meso, and micro level perspectives that exist on partnership approaches, and the different boundaries around internal (to partnerships) and external frames

of reference that need to be considered when exploring implementation questions. While the overall Learning and Improvement Strategy was informed by a variety of frameworks, specific substudies conducted as part of the strategy drew on a range of study-specific frameworks. For example, in examining the resources leveraged through the MSPA, the perspectives offered by frameworks focused on collaborative value[48,49] and network resources[50] were found to be highly instructive. These frameworks were used to refine and bound research questions and methods, interpret findings, and help shape how the relational characteristics of the MSPA could be examined. This diversity in conceptual frameworks recognizes that no one framework is likely to contain the full range of perspectives necessary to guide or understand the implementation of complex, multicomponent initiatives such as the MSPA.

Study Design and Methods

As noted, the Learning and Improvement Strategy was informed by concepts from adult learning including learning cycles, which enabled specific questions to be designed, data to be gathered, and feedback to Agency staff in ways that promote continuous program improvement. In addressing specific learning needs, a range of study designs and methods were selected. For examining the pathways by which partnerships create value, a literature-based study was conducted with results summarized using causal loop diagrams that described the relationships between contributing factors.[43] For exploring the unanticipated effects of multisectoral partnerships, a focused set of perspectives were gathered using a comparative case study approach and in-depth qualitative interviews with organizational representatives from three diverse partnerships.[51] To describe how the MSPA leverages and shares diverse resources among partners, the boundaries were broadened to capture the perspectives of all organizational members of the MSPA (in this case, through an on-line partnership survey).[52] Finally, to capture the tacit wisdom of Agency staff in brokering what are complex relationships, a qualitative study involving focus groups and individual interviews is being conducted. These diverse approaches to gathering and understanding the structures, processes, outcomes, and contexts of partnership work highlight the flexibility required to apply and learn from systems approaches in implementation.

Research Process

As noted, the Learning and Improvement Strategy was developed in partnership between Agency staff and a research intensive organization (Propel). In designing the strategy, this partnership was critical for ensuring the strategy was both locally and policy relevant to the needs of the Agency, as well as grounded in relevant and recent evidence on multisectoral action and continuous learning. Both perspectives are needed to ensure the strategy is able to generate data that can drive improvement and contribute to the evidence base on multisectoral approaches in prevention.

Each study conducted as part of the Learning and Improvement Strategy intentionally seeks to gain both a depth and breadth of perspectives from a range of participants, including those internal to the Agency as well as external to the Agency (i.e., partners involved in MSP projects). For some projects, this engagement has proved relatively straightforward (e.g., examining the unanticipated effects of partnerships),[43] while for other areas of focus, engaging project partners has proved more challenging (e.g., completing a brief on-line survey).[52] In part, these challenges may reflect issues to do with the research tool itself (i.e., the survey), relative importance in relation to the busy workloads of partners, the strength of relationships between the research team and study participants, or signify potential "boundary" issues that reflect if and how different organizations recognize their role in a broader partnership initiative. Ultimately, the process of engaging in research is recognized as an intervention itself, helping to reveal where energy and interest may exist, as well as where potential barriers and challenges may need to be overcome.

Summary for Case Study #1

The MSPA provides one example of a large scale, complex initiative, and which specifically adopts a public–private partnership approach to chronic disease prevention. To advance the implementation of the MSPA, a real-time Learning and Improvement Strategy was developed, helping Agency staff learn about priority learning needs during its implementation. Informed by a systems lens, the Learning and Improvement Strategy has evolved into a highly participatory approach, which adopts various study designs, applies a range of conceptual frameworks, and addresses research questions of value to practitioners and researchers alike. As governments continue to

invest in innovation and experimentation agendas, opportunities to learn from practice through initiatives such as the Learning and Improvement Strategy may prove highly beneficial.

Case Study #2: The British Columbia Ministry of Health's Clinical Care Management Initiative

The British Columbia Ministry of Health's Clinical Care Management (CCM) initiative provides the context for describing a systems approach to D&I research in a health care setting. CCM aims to implement an evidence-informed, guideline-driven approach to clinical care management (i.e., the D&I object), resulting in improved quality of care and patient outcomes. Given the widely documented challenges in guideline implementation,[53] the InSource Research Group conducted a study focused on the province-wide implementation of clinical guidelines in varying contexts (i.e., D&I strategies). Insights from this study fed into a broader effort to understand the requirements for achieving large system change in clinical care settings.

Research Purpose and Questions

The questions and objectives framing this research exhibit many of the characteristics of those described in Box 9.1. High-level questions focused on identifying and describing those factors and mechanisms that enable and constrain the implementation of clinical guidelines in British Columbia, examining how these mechanisms operate across varied clinical care settings. These questions are relational in nature, requiring an understanding of varied perspectives in explaining differences in guideline implementation. Objectives for the work highlighted the need to gather diverse perspectives on the enablers, constraints, and barriers to implementation, including the critical role of context in influencing implementation. Standardized data collection protocols helped to set the boundaries around what data were considered relevant, and the analysis approach explicitly focused on the interactions or relationships among variables and local context using a thematic analysis.

Conceptual Frameworks

In contrast to case study #1, this study was guided by a general model of complex adaptive systems, with use of two more specific approaches: realist evaluation and system dynamics mapping.

Included in both were explicit efforts to gather context sensitive data. Realist evaluation, as described by Pawson,[41] focuses on understanding what works, for whom, why, and under what conditions. Realist approaches recognize the role of "mechanisms" that link aspects of context to desired outcomes. Mechanisms are largely reactions to particular stimuli, are often in the minds of people (e.g., belief in the effectiveness of a particular course of action; commitment to a cause), and are activated or fired as a result of actions shifting or changing contexts. In examining the implementation of clinical guidelines, this research generated multiple configurations of contexts-mechanisms-outcome combinations, from which higher level principles and dynamics can be inferred. Dynamics mapping offers an additional lens for understanding interactions among elements of a system by providing realistic scenarios in which causes and effects influence each other with dynamic, evolving feedback. Maps use arrows to show how different factors either enable or dampen the influence of study participant-generated variables like "patient concerns" or "competing priorities." The maps foster group knowledge and understanding, and provide a concise view of the system complexity to guide improvement work.

Study Design and Methods

Consistent with a general model of complex systems, and guided by a realist approach, the study design and methods employed in this case example emphasized a highly iterative and engaged process, as well as the use of specific system tools. Primary data collection was accompanied by iterative analysis with ongoing validation of results using literature and practitioner experience. Data collection involved a range of methods, including email surveys, individual interviews, and focus groups. Email surveys were used to gain initial insights into the enablers and inhibitors of guideline implementation across British Columbia's health authorities, as well as to inform the questions for initial interviews, and to identify a subset of guideline domains to examine. Key informant interviews further explored enablers and constraints on implementation, but broadened the boundaries of inquiry to include how culture and context influence implementation efforts. Focus groups allowed informants to engage with, test, and refine the themes emerging from individual key informant interviews. A focused literature review was conducted in order to support data

analysis. Findings from this targeted review identified limited literature focused on guidelines implementation, but also novel methods and insights that were woven into the project.

Data analyses favored an ongoing and iterative approach, using both thematic analyses as well as visual displays of relationships between variable. These approaches recognize the diverse perspectives that affect guideline implementation, the need to gather both individual and relation-based insights, and the utility of both visual and narrative analytical techniques to bring meaning to data. In particular, the diagrams helped to reveal the critical relationships that influence guideline implementation, including the roles of culture, leadership, and capacity, as well as the boundaries between guideline implementation in specific topic domains (e.g., sepsis) and the broader system in which such implementation efforts interact.

Research Process

Consistent with the first case example, this study highlights a partnered approach involving government agencies, health care organizations and providers, and a systems research group. This process was grounded in a continuous improvement orientation that explicitly attempted to link learning with action. Stakeholder engagement was critical, including those from the Ministry of Health, health authorities, specialist and primary care physicians, as well as the British Columbia Patient Safety & Quality Council. A participatory approach to project governance allowed these various partners to engage in and contribute to the research, doing so through theme-specific clinical expert groups, as well as the overall CCM steering committee. Working with these groups, a subset of three clinical guideline domains was identified as the foundations of this work that would provide transferable lessons and insights across guideline areas.

The research process intentionally generated two sets of recommendations in order to meet distinct but related audiences and needs. The first specifically related to CCM and the implementation of guidelines across contexts. These recommendations highlight the importance of identifying and engaging local champions; allowing for guideline adaptation and interpretation; promoting internal networks; and avoiding change fatigue. The second provided higher level guidance for large system change efforts, that reinforced a range of activities such as the importance of preparation for substantial change efforts; creating a clear path through complexity; and strengthening knowledge management. Both sets of recommendations, while useful independently, speak to the different perspectives that influence guideline implementation in complex systems. Ultimately, both need to be considered for successful implementation.

Summary for Case Study #2
Participation of diverse stakeholder groups using multiple methods ensured a shared understanding and recommendations to guide system improvement. The mapping process highlighted ways in which key factors operate differently for varying clinical procedures and local contexts. Key factors affecting leadership, culture, and management shed light on critical elements for implementation and change strategy. One of the most important findings was the importance of aligning policymaker, executive, and practitioner perspectives to improve implementation.

SUMMARY
Increasingly, the literature highlights the benefits of systems thinking in approaching D&I efforts and associated research in health. This chapter aims to contribute to this literature by bringing an action orientation; defining and applying systems thinking in ways that will advance and accelerate D&I research and the improvements it seeks to support. The chapter draws attention to features of systems thinking that are most pertinent to D&I research, including how we think about D&I objects and strategies. It covers main features of D&I research—its purpose and questions, conceptual frameworks, study designs and methods, and the research process. In doing so, it provides an overview of a systems-oriented approach to D&I research. This overview is context for chapter 10, which provides an in-depth look at specific systems science methods that are part of a toolkit to answer systems-oriented research questions. The two D&I research examples offered demonstrate the applicability of the approaches described in this chapter across a range of health issues, especially the complex health problems—of today and the foreseeable future—that cause the greatest health, social, and economic burden to individuals and societies worldwide.

ACKNOWLEDGMENTS
The authors wish to thank Eric d'Avernas (Propel) for providing research support. Author contributions were supported by grants from the Canadian Cancer Society to BLR (grant 2011-701019), and JDM (grant 703878), and from an NHMRC Sidney Sax Fellowship to CDW (grant 1013165).

SUGGESTED READINGS AND WEBSITES

Readings
Finegood D. The complex systems science of obesity. In: Cawley J, ed. *The social science of obesity.* New York: Oxford University Press; 2011:208–236.
This chapter considers obesity as a complex problem and illustrates the various characteristics that make obesity complex. It considers the usual responses to complexity and solutions appropriate for complex problems. Two frameworks for intervention are also presented.

Holmes, B. J., Best, A., Davies, H., Hunter, D., Kelly, M. P., Marshall, M., & Rycroft-Malone, J. Mobilising knowledge in complex health systems: a call to action. *Evidence Policy* 2016; https://doi.org/10.1332/174426416X14712553750311
This call to action blends theoretical, empirical and experiential knowledge to identify a set of six recommended actions to strengthen knowledge mobilization in complex systems. The recommendations provide a broader context within which a systems-oriented approach to D&I research can be situated. http://www.ingentaconnect.com/content/tpp/ep/pre-prints/content-evp_094

Meadows, DH. *Thinking in systems: A primer.* White River Junction: VT: Chelsea Green Publishing; 2008.
Published posthumously, this succinct primer describes a shift in systems thinking that can be applied to local and international contexts alike. Meadows asserts that understanding the relationship between structure and behavior can produce a new, improved way of thinking about systems.

Rittel H, Webber M. Dilemmas in a general theory of planning. *Policy Sciences.* 1973;4: 155–169.
The search for the scientific bases of many societal problems is bound to fail, say Rittel and Webber, because these are "wicked" problems in the sense that they are difficult to define and locate. The authors describe ten properties of such problems to which attention must be paid in the identification of actions towards their resolution.

Sterman J. Learning from evidence in a complex world. *Am J Public Health.* 2006;96:505–514.
Using evidence-based practices should result in more effective policies and practices, but too often policies intended to promote health do just the opposite. Sterman uses principles of systems thinking and simulation

modeling to help researchers and policymakers better understand existing evidence and how to create real, positive changes in public health.

Websites and Tools

http://www.msfhr.org/our-work/activities/knowledge-translation

Knowledge mobilization resources from British Columbia's (and affiliation for author BH) Michael Smith Foundation for Health Research.

https://i2insights.org/

A blog on integration and implementation insights.

http://www.oxfordbibliographies.com.proxy.lib.sfu.ca/view/document/obo-9780199756797/obo-9780199756797-0049.xml?rskey=yXwIEh&result=1&q=finegood#firstMatch

Materials on complexity and systems thinking from the New England Complex Systems Institute.

http://www.managementassistance.org/systems-grantmaking-guide

A resource for funders who want to change the way they grant to be aligned with a systems approach.

REFERENCES

1. Kreuter MW, De Rosa C, Howze EH, Baldwin GT. Understanding wicked problems: a key to advancing environmental health promotion. *Health Educ Behav.* 2004;31(4):441–454.

2. Plsek PE, Greenhalgh T. Complexity science: the challenge of complexity in health care. *BMJ.* 2001;323(7313):625–628.

3. Bar-Yam Y, Bar-Yam S, Bertrand KZ, et al. A complex systems science approach to healthcare costs and quality. *Handb Syst Complex Health.* 2012:1–47.

4. Kannampallil TG, Schauer GF, Cohen T, Patel VL. Considering complexity in healthcare systems. *J Biomed Inform.* 2011;44(6):943–947.

5. Peters DH. The application of systems thinking in health: why use systems thinking? *Health Res Policy Syst.* 2014;12:51.

6. McLeroy KR, Bibeau D, Steckler A, Glanz K. An ecological perspective on health promotion programs. *Health Educ Q.* 1988;15(4):351–377.

7. Stokols D, Allen J, Bellingham RL. The social ecology of health promotion: implications for research and practice. *Am J Health Promot.* 1996;10(4):247–251.

8. Riley BL, Robinson KL, Gamble J, et al. Knowledge to action for solving complex problems: insights from a review of nine international cases. *Health Promot Chronic Dis Prev Can.* 2015;35(3):47–53.

9. Wutzke S, Morrice E, Benton M, Wilson A. Systems approaches for chronic disease prevention: sound logic and empirical evidence, but is this view shared outside of academia? *Public Health Res Pract.* 2016;26(3).

10. Bar-Yam Y. *Making things work: Solving complex problems in a complex world.* Cambridge, MA: Knowledge Press; 2004.

11. Nilsen P. Making sense of implementation theories, models and frameworks. *Implement Sci.* 2015;10:53.

12. Glasgow RE, Chambers D. Developing robust, sustainable, implementation systems using rigorous, rapid and relevant science. *Clin Transl Sci.* 2012;5(1):48–55.

13. Meadows DH. Leverage points: Places to intervene in a system. http://www.sustainer.org/pubs/Leverage_Points.pdf. 1999.

14. Wheatley M, Frieze D. Using emergence to take social innovation to scale. *The Berkana Institute.* 2006:1–7.

15. Greenhalgh T, Robert G, Macfarlane F, Bate P, Kyriakidou O. Diffusion of innovations in service organizations: systematic review and recommendations. *Milbank Q.* 2004;82(4):581–629.

16. Best A, Greenhalgh T, Lewis S, Saul JE, Carroll S, Bitz J. Large-system transformation in health care: a realist review. *Milbank Q.* 2012;90(3):421–456.

17. Finegood DT, Karanfil O, Matteson CL. Getting from analysis to action: framing obesity research, policy and practice with a solution-oriented complex systems lens. *Healthc Pap.* 2008;9(1):36–41; discussion 62–67.

18. Willis CD, Best A, Riley B, Herbert CP, Millar J, Howland D. Systems thinking for transformational change in health. *Evid Policy.* 2014;10(1):113–126.

19. Holmes BJ, Best A, Davies H, et al. Mobilising knowledge in complex health systems: a call to action. *Evid Policy.* 2016. https://doi.org/10.1332/174426416X14712553750311

20. Meadows DH. *Thinking in systems: A primer.* White River Junction, VT: Chelsea Green Publishing; 2008.

21. Finegood D. The complex systems science of obesity. In: Cawley J, ed. *The social science of obesity.* New York: Oxford University Press; 2011.

22. Westley F, Zimmerman B, Patton MQ. *Getting to maybe: How the world is changed.* Toronto: Random House of Canada; 2007.

23. Nease DE, Jr., Green LA. ClinfoTracker: a generalizable prompting tool for primary care. *J Am Board Fam Pract.* 2003;16(2):115–123.

24. Glouberman S, Zimmerman B. Complicated and Complex Systems: What Would Successful Reform of Medicare Look Like? *Discussion Paper No 8.* 2002.

25. Hunter DJ. Role of politics in understanding complex, messy health systems: an essay by David J Hunter. *BMJ.* 2015;350:h1214.

26. Rouse W. Managing complexity: disease control as a complex adaptive system. *Inf Knowl Syst Manag.* 2000;2(2):143–165.

27. Borland R, Young D, Coghill K, Zhang JY. The tobacco use management system: analyzing tobacco control from a systems perspective. *Am J Public Health.* 2010;100(7):1229–1236.

28. Johnston LM, Matteson CL, Finegood DT. Systems science and obesity policy: a novel framework for analyzing and rethinking population-level planning. *Am J Public Health.* 2014;104(7):1270–1278.

29. Malhi L, Karanfil O, Merth T, Acheson M, Palmer A, Finegood DT. Places to intervene to make complex food systems more healthy, green, fair, and affordable. *J Hunger Environ Nutr.* 2009;4(3-4):466–476.

30. Leykum LK, Pugh J, Lawrence V, et al. Organizational interventions employing principles of complexity science have improved outcomes for patients with Type II diabetes. *Implement Sci.* 2007;2:28.

31. Lanham HJ, Leykum LK, Taylor BS, McCannon CJ, Lindberg C, Lester RT. How complexity science can inform scale-up and spread in health care: understanding the role of self-organization in variation across local contexts. *Soc Sci Med.* 2013;93:194–202.

32. Williams B, Hummelbrunner R. *Systems concepts in action: A practitioner's toolkit.* Stanford, CA: Stanford University Press; 2011.

33. Best A, Berland A, Herbert C, et al. Using systems thinking to support clinical system transformation. *J Health Organ Manag.* 2016;30(3):302–323.

34. Johnston LM, Finegood DT. Cross-sector partnerships and public health: challenges and opportunities for addressing obesity and noncommunicable diseases through engagement with the private sector. *Annu Rev Public Health.* 2015;36:255–271.

35. Checkland P, Scholes J. *Soft systems methodology in action.* Chichester, UK: Wiley; 1990.

36. Chambers DA, Glasgow RE, Stange KC. The dynamic sustainability framework: addressing the paradox of sustainment amid ongoing change. *Implement Sci.* 2013;8:117.

37. Best A, Holmes B. Systems thinking, knowledge and action: towards better models and methods. *Evid Policy.* 2010;6(2):145–159.

38. Foster-Fishman PG, Nowell B, Yang H. Putting the system back into systems change: a framework for understanding and changing organizational and community systems. *Am J Community Psychol.* 2007;39(3-4):197–215.

39. Robinson K, Elliott SJ, Driedger SM, et al. Using linking systems to build capacity and enhance dissemination in heart health promotion: a Canadian multiple-case study. *Health Educ Res.* 2005;20(5):499–513.

40. Willis CD, Mitton C, Gordon J, Best A. System tools for system change. *BMJ Qual Saf.* 2012;21(3):250–262.

41. Pawson R. *The Science of evaluation: A realist manifesto.* London: Sage; 2013.

42. Public Health Agency of Canada. Multi-sectoral Partnerships to Promote Healthy Living and Prevent Chronic Disease. 2014; http://www.phac-aspc.gc.ca/fo-fc/mspphl-pppmvs-eng.php. Accessed May 5, 2014.

43. Willis CD, Greene JK, Abramowicz A, Riley BL. Strengthening the evidence and action on multi-sectoral partnerships in public health: an action research initiative. *Health Promot Chron.* 2016;36(6):101–111.

44. Willis CD, Greene JK, Riley BL. Understanding and improving multi-sectoral partnerships for chronic disease prevention: blending conceptual and practical insights. *Evid Policy.* 2017;(In Press).

45. Kolb DA. *Experiential learning: Experience as the source of learning and development.* Eaglewood Cliffs, NJ: Prentice Hall; 1984.

46. Deming WE. *Out of the crisis.* Cambridge, MA: MIT Press; 2000.

47. Patton MQ. Developmental evaluation. *Eval Pract.* 1994;15(3):311–319.

48. Austin JE, Seitanidi MM. Collaborative value creation: a review of partnering between nonprofits and businesses: Part I. Value creation spectrum and collaboration stages. *Nonprof Volunt Sec Q.* 2012;41(5):726–758.

49. Austin JE, Seitanidi MM. Collaborative value creation: a review of partnering between nonprofits and businesses. Part 2: Partnership processes and outcomes. *Nonprof Volunt Sec Q.* 2012;41(6):929–968.

50. Gulati R, Lavie D, Madhavan R. How do networks matter? The performance effects of interorganiztional networks. *Res Organ Behav.* 2011;31:207–224.

51. Willis CD, Corrigan C, Stockton L, Greene JK, Riley BL. Exploring the unanticipated effects of multi-sectoral partnerships in chronic disease prevention. *Health Policy.* 2017;121(2):158–168.

52. Patton R, Stockton L, Willis C, Riley B. *Multi-sectoral partnerships for chronic disease prevention: motivations, contributions and resource value.* Waterloo, ON: Propel Centre for Population Health Impact, University of Waterloo; 2016.

53. Watkins K, Wood H, Schneider CR, Clifford R. Effectiveness of implementation strategies for clinical guidelines to community pharmacy: a systematic review. *Implement Sci.* 2015;10:151.

10

Systems Science Methods in Dissemination and Implementation Research

DOUGLAS A. LUKE, ALEXANDRA B. MORSHED,
VIRGINIA R. MCKAY, AND TODD B. COMBS

INTRODUCTION

The still relatively new field of dissemination and implementation (D&I) science is addressing new types of research questions focusing on how society can better reap the benefits of its investments in public health and healthcare research, by delivering scientific discoveries into the clinic and community. With these research challenges come requirements for alternative types of analytic methods and study designs. More specifically, there are philosophical, theoretical, and substantive reasons why dissemination & implementation researchers should make greater use of systems science methods such as those described in this chapter.

The Argument from Philosophy of Science

Early methodological work in the social sciences derived from positivist epistemology. The desire to establish firm foundations for causal explanations led to experimental methods and our Popperian approach to hypothesis testing that are common in basic scientific research.[1] Despite philosophical movement away from positivism, the social sciences have held onto scientific methods that emphasize control and randomization, and that value internal validity over external validity. Newer epistemological frameworks that include holism, functionalism, and structuralism and which emphasize the influence of multiple social-level forces on individual behavior suggest new methodological approaches that balance internal and external validity and can help identify contextual effects, behavioral dynamics, and causal mechanisms.[2,3] All of these concepts are relevant and useful for studying the complex, dynamic systems that embody D&I processes and outcomes.

The Argument from Theory

Despite the relative youth of D&I as a distinctive discipline, many important theoretical and conceptual advances have been made and used to guide research[4] (see also chapters 3 and 5). However, the most widely used theories are in the form of conceptual frameworks, rather than more fully fleshed out theories or models.[5] These are still quite useful; for example, RE-AIM,[6] the Consolidated Framework for Implementation Research (CFIR),[7] and the Implementation Outcomes framework[8] identify important concepts and conceptual domains (e.g., reach, acceptability, inner and outer settings). These frameworks are mostly silent, however, on how these concepts relate to each other. For example, how exactly do outer settings act to constrain innersetting behavior, and how do the interactions between inner and outer settings enhance or inhibit successful implementation? Future theoretical development in the D&I sphere would be supported by studies utilizing the sorts of methods that can identify and elaborate on these domain interrelationships.

Figure 10.1 presents a socioecological framework for understanding D&I processes, which is adapted from Glass and McAtee (2006).[9] This framework is also a schematic, much like CFIR.[7] However, it highlights two important characteristics of D&I phenomena that need to be articulated by rich D&I theories and studied using the sorts of methods that are the subject of this chapter. First, D&I processes are embedded in a hierarchical socioecological system (left-hand arrow from lower to higher). Second, these processes play out over time. Traditional analytic methods are fairly limited in their ability to handle these types of multilevel systems, with heterogeneous

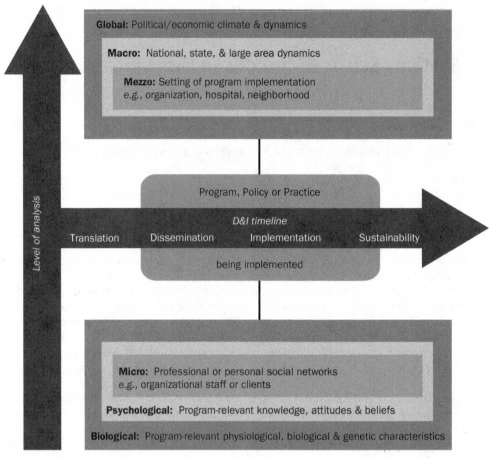

FIGURE 10.1 Socioecological framework for understanding dissemination and implementation processes. (Adapted from Glass & McAtee.[9])

actors (e.g., persons and organizations), who are interacting and changing dynamically over time.

The Argument from Phenomenology

As suggested earlier and argued at greater length in chapter 9, dissemination & implementation itself comprises a complex system made up of interacting parts, and those parts are diverse collections of people, settings, and organizations. More so than in many other areas of the social and health sciences, studying these complex systems as phenomena in and of themselves using traditional experimental and quasi-experimental designs is challenging. Even when traditional tools of the experimentalist's art such as randomization can be used, the results are often limited to "we discovered it worked for this program, at this site, and at this point in time." Learning about how or why a particular dissemination

or implementation approach did in fact work requires a different set of tools; tools that can illuminate dynamic processes, map social and organizational relationships; identify feedback mechanisms; forecast future system behavior; and delineate the interactions between system actors and their social/organizational environments.

Chapter Roadmap

Systems science models and methods have been developed in a wide variety of disciplines including sociology, business, political science, organizational behavior, computer science, and engineering. They have been used increasingly in public health to study and develop new practices and policies in such areas as global pandemics, vaccination system preparation, tobacco control, cancer, and obesity.[10] In public health, three broad types of methods have been used most often: social network analysis, system dynamics, and agent-based modeling. The rest of this chapter introduces each of these methods, explains how they are appropriate tools for D&I, provides entry points to a broader literature, and illustrates each method with a brief case study.

SOCIAL NETWORK ANALYSIS

Social network analysis focuses on the relationship between objects rather than on the objects themselves—a view of social phenomena fundamentally different from many types of social science investigation.[11] Because of this focus, network analysis is one of the most useful strategies for studying context, social processes, and social structure.[12] Social network analysis has been used widely in public health and health sciences to study infectious disease transmission, information flows, social influences on health behavior, organizational systems, and diffusion of innovations.[13] Suggested by the research translation "pipeline model,"[14] D&I processes can be viewed as a type of information transmission. A new scientific discovery, medical procedure, policy formulation, or other innovation is a piece of information that needs to be transferred to a different part of society and put to use. A network analytic model of D&I focused on the structural and relational aspects of dissemination or implementation can be used both to *study* and *shape* processes and outcomes.

Social Network Analysis Fundamentals

Social network analysis typically includes three interconnected methodological strategies: description, visualization, and modeling. Network *description* focuses on the nodes (objects) and the ties (relationships) that connect them. Nodes (also called actors, members, or vertexes) can be almost any type of social entity—a person, organization, country, etc. Ties (also called links, arcs, or edges) can be many things—friendship, money exchange, an email, or disease transmission. Networks and their ties can signal directed or nondirected relationships. For example, money is given by one individual (a node) and received by another, typically indicating a directed tie. Many other types of ties are nondirected. For example, two (or more) organizations work together on a common project, and it may not make sense to assign direction to the collaboration. Network structures and characteristics can evolve over time; for example, local

departments of health might initially be connected mainly through a centralized department at the state or national level, but over time develop and strengthen ties with other local departments through common programs, goals, or challenges.

Network *visualization* is useful for exploring descriptive properties of nodes and ties and for demonstrating overall analytic network characteristics. Key characteristics of networks include density (proportion of observed ties to total possible ties) and diameter (longest path between any two nodes). Figure 10.2 shows the pattern of dissemination ties that connect the public health agencies making up the tobacco control program in Indiana.[15] Nodes in network graphs can be differentiated by color, and the agencies here are distinguished by agency type. The network has a diameter of two, indicating that information must pass through at most two nodes to travel from any given agency to another. Its density is 0.32, meaning that around one third of all possible connections are present. This is not to say, however, that perfect density (density = 1) indicates a *better* or more effective network of people or organizations for dissemination or implementation. Network analyses have found the opposite: relatively less dense networks may be more efficient at disseminating information and implementing prevention programs, as denser networks tend to focus inward and are less open to information and community resources provided by weak ties outside the core network.[16] Both network descriptive statistics and visualizations are important for understanding the structural characteristics of this public health system.

Individual nodes also have analytic characteristics, most of which describe their relative prominence in the network. Key among node properties are degree (the number of ties) and betweenness centrality (the extent to which a node bridges otherwise unconnected nodes). In Figure 10.2 the nodes are sized by betweenness centrality, and the lead organization is the largest node, indicating that it bridges more pairs of unconnected nodes than any other, making it a critical element in network sustainability.

Network *modeling* has been made possible through statistical and computational advances over the last decade that use exponential random graph modeling (ERGM).[17,18] ERGM predicts the likelihood of ties between nodes using characteristics of individual or pairs of nodes (e.g., people, organizations). Newer modeling strategies incorporate the ability to model changing node and tie

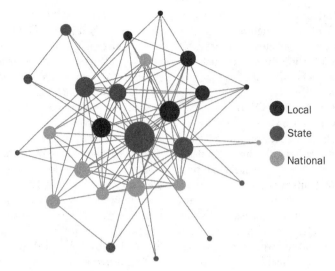

FIGURE 10.2 Indiana Tobacco Control Dissemination Network.
(Adapted from Luke et al.[15])

characteristics in the longitudinal evolution of networks.[19] For those interested in more in-depth treatment of network analysis, see Wasserman & Faust, Valente, or de Nooy.[20–22]

Applications for Dissemination & Implementation Research

Social network analysis has been particularly useful when applied to the theory of Diffusion of Innovations[23] (see also chapter 2), perhaps the most important and influential theoretical framework in D&I research. Pioneering work in Diffusion of Innovations emphasized different types of members and distinguished them by the time at which they adopted new innovations into clinical or community practice (i.e., early, middle, and late adopters). After some time, observers began to look beyond simple temporal ordering to focus on the structural characteristics that distinguish opinion leaders (individuals who may expedite the diffusion process) from early adopters (those who may adopt an innovation quickly but may not influence others to do so). Network analysis focusing on the structural and relational aspects of diffusion has helped shed light on this issue.[24] As an example, *threshold models* have been developed that suggest the likelihood of a particular individual (or agency, institution, etc.) adopting an innovation is dependent upon the proportion of others in her network who have already done so.[25] One study of healthy cities found that health care professionals were more

likely to ride bicycles to work if opinion leaders did so, *or* if a certain proportion of others in their social networks switched to bicycles for commuting.[26]

More recently, D&I research has turned from examining the adoption of innovations toward long-term implementation and sustainability of innovations. Feldstein & Glasgow's Practical, Robust Implementation and Sustainability Model (PRISM) incorporates the role of social networks (both organization- and patient-based) when studying the implementation of interventions as important tools for understanding predictors of adoption, implementation, and maintenance outcomes.[27] In a successful application of the PRISM model, Beck and colleagues further demonstrated the usefulness of network analysis.[28] First, organizational advice-seeking patterns among clinicians and staff at two health maintenance organization sites were identified and next, network maps were used to help drive the subsequent implementation of a new well-child care intervention. More generally, Valente and colleagues have illustrated how network analysis might be applied at each of the four stages of program implementation.[29]

Network modeling has also been applied to dissemination in the context of public health. The study from which Figure 10.2 originated found through ERGM that state tobacco control programs and partners were more likely to disseminate CDC Best Practices if state organizations, advocacy groups, and advisory agencies had existing contact- or collaboration-based ties.[15] In another study, Harris et al. examined influence within the U.S. Department of Health and Human Services via ERGM and found that certain individual or shared characteristics (e.g., job rank, agency affiliations) were associated with greater organizational influence.[30]

Network Analysis in Dissemination & Implementation Research: a Brief Case Study

During the planning stages for implementing a cancer screening prevention program in the Peel region of Ontario, Canada, Lobb and colleagues[31] observed that reaching South Asian immigrant populations, almost one third of the region's population, was a challenge for cancer screening programs in the region. Based on this observation, they developed an implementation strategy designed to improve reach. The researchers worked with stakeholders to identify 22 organizations that comprised the cancer screening network for South Asians in the region, including hospitals, governmental and nongovernmental agencies, clinical service providers, and community service providers who specifically provided social (nonclinical) services to South Asians.

Through surveys of the organizations, three different types of networks were identified and observed: communication, collaboration, and

referral networks. Ties in the communication network represented any contact, and ties in the collaboration network were based on organizations that worked together on a common goal. The referral network included directional ties that denoted which organizations referred clients to the others.

Relevance to Dissemination & Implementation Research

Figure 10.3 shows the referral network from the study. The network map shows that the two hospitals in the region were centrally positioned in the referral network, more so than the provincial screening lead. The community service providers as well as the community health centers were on the periphery and not well connected. These were valuable findings to inform intervention planning since the provincial lead was intended to lead dissemination of program information, because community health centers are vital in providing services to vulnerable populations who might otherwise not receive any, and since community service organizations were explicitly linked to the region's South Asian population. Another specific and important finding was that neither of the two community health centers was linked directly to the provincial cancer screening lead, suggesting that communication of screening program changes from either core agency might take unnecessary time to reach the community health centers.

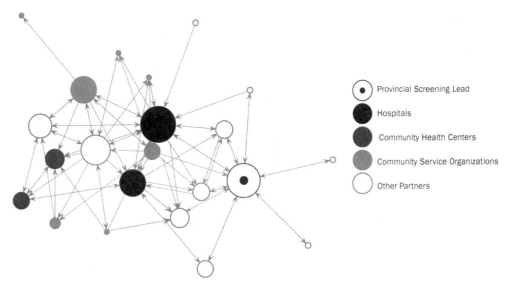

FIGURE 10.3 Referral network in cancer screening intervention planning study.

(Adapted from Lobb et al.[31])

These system insights would have gone unnoticed in the absence of a focus on the networks and connections among organizations serving South Asians and those providing cancer screening services. Especially important was the knowledge of relationships between community health centers and community service organizations and their place in the greater cancer screening network. Equipped with this information, stakeholders were able to include all relevant types of organizations in intervention planning and focus on strengthening weak ties and utilizing existing ones.

SYSTEM DYNAMICS MODELING

System dynamics (SD) models and accompanying analyses represent complex systems as having underlying generalizable structures that produce specific patterns of system behavior over time. System dynamicists look for solutions to complex problems from the feedback mechanisms within these systems rather than from influences external to the system.[32-36] A D&I research study using traditional analytic approaches may examine whether an implementation strategy results in a greater number of patients receiving EB treatment. An SD simulation study, on the other hand, may explore the system structure that leads to a sharp increase in patients served followed by a gradual collapse in service reach (an example of a dynamic system behavior) or to identify areas of leverage (i.e., places to intervene in a system) that would most efficiently change the behavior pattern of the system in the desired direction.[35,37] System dynamics is complementary to network analysis and agent-based modeling (see later), but SD models are typically presented at the aggregate level, tend to have broader boundaries, and can incorporate more variables even in the absence of concrete estimates for parameters.[10,38,39] Developed in the 1950s by Jay W. Forrester,[40] SD has been widely applied to population health, urban, social, ecological, and organizational management problems.[41-43]

System Dynamics Fundamentals

The core elements of system dynamics are the concepts of *endogenous feedback* and *accumulation* of quantities (e.g., information, energy, people, trust) in a system over time.[32,33] Endogenous feedback is present when a change at one point of the system *feeds back* onto itself, creating an endogenous (i.e., within system) feedback loop.[32,34]

An example of a feedback loop is the number of infected people in a community increasing the rate of infection, which in turn increases the number of infected people. These feedback loops can be reinforcing (when the original change is amplified by the succeeding changes as in the example, leading to a vicious or virtuous cycle) or balancing (when the succeeding changes balance the initial change). SD models represent accumulation using stocks (levels of accumulation) and flows (rates of change in the stocks). For example, in a mental health treatment system, the number of patients waiting for an intake interview represents a stock, while the rate of intake interviews conducted by the clinic represents a flow of people out of this stock. An important influence on flows within a system are delays, for example the average time it takes to conduct an intake interview, which contribute to the dynamic complexity and instability of the system.[32,33] Together feedback, accumulation, and delays are responsible for specific patterns of behaviors of systems, such as exponential growth, overshoot and collapse, oscillation, or S-shaped growth.[32]

Dynamic hypotheses, which posit that given feedback structures result in specific system behaviors over time, can be expressed conceptually using diagrams and mathematically using simulation software. SD simulation models utilize a system of ordinary differential equations to model systems over specific time horizons at an aggregate level. The initial values, relationships between variables, and constants are specified using existing theoretical and empirical literature, surveillance and administrative data, stakeholder estimates, and other sources.[33,44]

The process of problem articulation, dynamic hypothesis formulation, model quantification, confidence building, and policy analysis is iterative and strengthened by the participation of stakeholders.[32,45,46] Group model building methods have emerged within the broader SD field to provide steps and tools to meaningfully engage stakeholders in creation of system structures and, in some group model building practices, in development of simulation models.[46,47] Community based system dynamics, a community participatory practice of group model building, specifically focuses this engagement on community members with the goal of building a public constituency for addressing root causes of dynamic social problems.[47]

Due to their aggregate and compartmentalized nature, SD models are less able to capture heterogeneity in the system, and adding additional sources of heterogeneity to the model is time-intensive, as it often changes the system structure. SD models also utilize a top-down perspective that is not well suited to examining how individual-level behaviors generate system-wide behaviors.[48] For those interested in more in-depth treatment of SD methods, see Sterman, Rahmandad et al., or Vennix.[32,46,49]

Applications in Dissemination & Implementation Research

SD methods are applicable to several areas of D&I research. First, they are useful in developing and testing dynamic D&I theories. Some D&I models and frameworks include recursive influences between processes and concepts (e.g., Conceptual Model for the Diffusion of Innovations in Service Organizations, Conceptual Model for Evidence-Based Implementation in Public Service Sectors, 4E's Process Theory [50-52]) but do not explicitly model them. SD allows for the specification and quantification of the feedback mechanisms, accumulations, and delays that drive the behavior of D&I systems but are normally difficult to conceptualize.[32,53] As stated by Jay Forrester, "a simulation model is a theory describing the structure and interrelationships of a system,"[54] and through iterative model assessments, modelers can challenge theoretical assumptions, uncover and address flaws, and identify the limitations of the theory.[53] At each step of model specification (e.g., from conceptual models to stock-and-flow diagrams to simulation models), theories are necessarily refined and made more precise. Lich and colleagues illustrated the utility of SD diagramming in understanding complex factors influencing translation efforts of tobacco prevention research at five stages of knowledge translation.[55] The work of Hovmand and Gillespie[56] serves as an example of combining previously quantified theories of organizational change and management to create a new simulated theoretical model of how organizations respond to implementation of evidence-based interventions and what accounts for these responses.

Well-developed SD simulation models can serve as virtual laboratories for examining D&I dynamics in a multitude of contexts. Hovmand and Gillespie[56] simulated 2,312 scenarios of organizations with differing initial characteristics to determine what types of organizations were able to improve their performance after implementing evidence-based interventions. In another study, Miller and colleagues[57] examined nine strategies for increasing the reach of an EB HIV prevention program. They found that although some strategies improved reach, they did not stabilize the service delivery system that was experiencing patterns of overshoot and collapse, placing the service organizations into long-term states of uncertainty. Virtual laboratories capture the feedback and accumulation present in systems and allow for examining how strategies or interventions work under differing conditions that would otherwise be difficult, costly, time consuming, or unethical to manipulate in the real world.[32,53] In addition, contextualizing D&I problems within specific practice contexts using SD produces knowledge that is practice-based and thus particularly relevant to D&I science.[58-60]

When modeling is carried out with participation of key stakeholders, SD methods can themselves serve as implementation strategies useful for building buy-in, developing relationships, and prioritizing implementation actions.[61,62] The strong emphasis in SD on engagement of stakeholders[33,47] lends itself particularly well to engagement of multidisciplinary actors necessary for producing D&I knowledge.[58,63] As a process, group model building is effective in creating individual (e.g., improved insight, commitment to conclusions) and group outcomes (e.g., improved communication, consensus, cohesion).[62] Models can serve as boundary objects, which are tangible representations of structures or processes, partially interpretable across disciplinary, organizational, social, or cultural distinctions, and which all participants can modify.[64] These objects facilitate the negotiation of knowledge, development of shared vocabulary around a problem, and alignment of goals.[60,65] In addition, SD simulation models are useful tools for communication with policymakers, frontline providers, and other decision-makers regarding the scope and root causes of health problems, projected magnitude and timing of impact of policy alternatives, and setting of reasonable goals for action.[42,66,67]

System Dynamics in Dissemination & Implementation Research: a Brief Case Study

Implementation scientists from the Veterans Health Administration (VA) National Center for Post Traumatic Stress Disorder (PTSD) carried out a study in partnership with the VA Palo Alto Healthcare System.[68] The project used SD

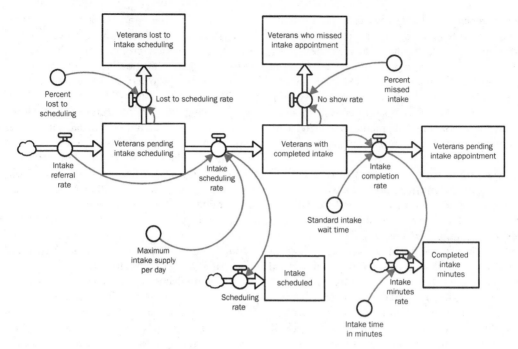

FIGURE 10.4 Stock and flow diagram.

(Adapted from Zimmerman et al.[68] system dynamics model of mental health service provision in a system of VA clinics.)

modeling to test two evidence-based practice (EBP) implementation strategies to increase the number of patients initiating and completing treatment for depression and PTSD compared with services as usual. Through repeated engagement with the service delivery teams, the researchers iteratively developed a model comprised of the accumulation and flow of patients through distinct service provision categories in the clinic over time and included several feedback loops between model elements (Figure 10.4). Two strategies selected by stakeholders were tested: (1) shortening intake evaluation from 90 to 60 minutes, and (2) streamlining intake procedures by eliminating participation in an EBP information group prior to treatment. The first implementation strategy resulted in an additional 796 scheduled and 424 completed EBP sessions per year. The second implementation strategy resulted in an additional 758 completed EBP sessions. For both strategies, generalist teams experienced higher reach than specialty mental health programs. Improvement in services was observed around week 21 of implementation, which is important information for making decisions on when to discontinue a strategy.

Relevance to Dissemination & Implementation Research

This case study illustrates the value of SD modeling for identifying and testing evidence-based implementation strategies in complex service provision settings. Simulation of several implementation options in a virtual model is faster and less costly than implementing and evaluating these strategies in real-world settings and allows for better informed decision-making. Explicit modeling also allows researchers and practitioners to unpack assumptions about the dynamic structure of the implementation context.[53] The study's qualitative results indicated that clinic staff had differing hypotheses about which strategies would improve EBP reach, indicating that building consensus was necessary. The study authors also noted that "clinicians and managers can be disabused of ineffectual notions more efficiently if they have developed confidence in the usefulness of the model, than simply discussing policies and procedures without modeling."[68] This suggests that the participatory nature of the model development process was key in creating buy-in for the model. This allowed for what Sterman calls double-loop learning,[53] where model building and simulation results challenge stakeholders' mental models, leading to improved decision-making, and ultimately, better implementation.

AGENT-BASED MODELING

Agent-based models (ABMs) are computational simulations modeling individual actors that behave according to a set of rules within an environment over time.[10] The models are used to examine how the accumulation of these small individual-level behaviors gives rise to system-level outcomes, often called emergence, that may be qualitatively different from the behavior of any one individual within the system.[69] Early models within the social sciences have illuminated social phenomena, such as emergence of collective social benefit out of cooperation among individuals[70] or neighborhood segregation arising out of slight preferences for others similar to oneself.[71] This generative ability (using simple individual behaviors to generate complex system phenomena) of ABM is a distinguishing feature compared with other simulation approaches. ABM is a relatively new approach compared with other simulation techniques, but models developed for public health purposes are on the rise, especially to examine infectious[72-74] and chronic disease.[75,76]

Agent-Based Modeling Fundamentals

The basic steps for agent-based modeling are (1) model construction, (2) calibration and validation, and (3) analyses.[69,77] ABMs are constructed from three basic components: individuals or agents, their environment, and rules that define how agents interact with one another and with their environment. Agents can represent homogeneous or heterogeneous types of system members, and they exhibit a variety of behaviors defined by a set of decision rules. The environment is the physical or social space where agents engage in the behavior of interest. A key feature of ABMs is explicitly representing the interaction among individuals or between individuals and the environment. Many have modeled interaction between individuals and a physical environment, such as how neighborhood location and household income can influence diet choices and quality.[78] More recently, ABMs representing the interaction between individuals and the social environment, such as how population norms influence obesity among individuals,[75] have been useful for demonstrating the influence of social factors on population health. Aside from these fundamental components, the potential agent

characteristics and behaviors, environments, and relationships that can be represented are virtually unlimited. However, researchers must carefully choose the parameters incorporated in a model. The disaggregated nature of ABMs can quickly produce a myriad of parameters and growth in complexity that subsequently makes interpreting the outcomes of an ABM difficult. Last, time can be represented in ABMs according to any scale (e.g., days, weeks, or years). Although ABMs do model changes in systems over time, the predictive ability of ABMs wanes the further out in modeled time due to the dynamic nature of the system represented.[69,79]

After a baseline ABM is developed, a model is calibrated and validated. These are techniques used to help ensure a model is generating relevant outcomes via plausible mechanisms and that the model is a valid representation of the real system of interest. For a detailed discussion of model construction, calibration, and validation, see Hammond (2015) as well as the references in Table 10.2. Empirical data, including qualitative and quantitative data, can be used to inform all aspects of ABM development.[80,81] The amount and specificity of data needed to inform model development reflects the extent to which an ABM is intended to realistically represent a specific system. The realism of ABMs falls along a spectrum that ranges from highly abstract to highly specific (see Figure 10.5).[79] Within public health, ABMs tend toward the specific, since public health researchers, including D&I researchers, generally address specific health issues in real contexts. As a rule of thumb, more data are needed to inform ABMs intended to accurately reflect real contexts, but where data are not available, a researcher may incorporate randomness and error into ABMs to account for uncertainty.

As a final step, the ABM outcomes of interest are analyzed using both descriptive and statistical approaches, to identify important aspects of the behavioral dynamics and outcomes of the model. Another analytic approach of ABMs is using the simulation as an experimental laboratory where the researcher can systematically manipulate variables of interest at regular intervals and analyze primary outcomes of repeated iterations.[84] Using this experiment-like approach helps researchers analyze conditions that may be difficult to conduct in real-life settings. For those interested in more in-depth treatment of ABM, see Bonabeau, Fioretti, or Burke et al.[85-87]

TABLE 10.1 SUMMARY OF APPROACHES

	Network Analysis	System Dynamics	Agent-Based Modeling
Characteristics			
Basic building blocks	• Nodes • Ties	• Feedback loops • Stocks and flows	• Agents • Agent behavior
Interactions & dynamics	• Node↔node • Tie creation/dissolution • Changing node/tie characteristics	• Feedback structure • Accumulation of stocks • System delays	• Agent↔agent • Agent↔environment • Behavioral changes
Insights & outcomes	• Identification and characterization of most efficient information pathways • Social influences on decision-making	• System behavioral patterns • Structural sources of system behavior • Areas of leverage for changing system behavior patterns	• Individual-level adaptations • Emergence of system-level patterns • Unexpected outcomes
Potential challenges & limitations	• Mapping complete networks is dependent on stakeholder participation • Limited ability to model dynamics over time	• Top-down perspective less able to address individual behavior • Difficult to capture large amounts of heterogeneity	• Exponentially growing complexity • Predictive ability lessens further out in modeled time

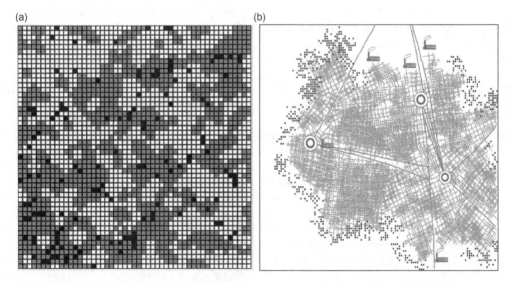

(a)   (b)

FIGURE 10.5 Illustrations of two ABMs from the Netlogo modeling library demonstrating different levels of abstraction. Model a (left) is a highly abstracted model designed to examine the development of neighborhood segregation where agents are represented by different shades of dots within a grid. Model b (right) is a more realistic model designed to study migrant settlement in a realistic urban landscape based on human geography with centers of commerce (*circles*), an urban street design (*lines*), residential settlements (*small dark squares*) and factory locations (*buildings with smoke plumes*).

(Model a from Wilensky;[82] Model b from De Leon et al.[83])

Applications for Dissemination & Implementation Research

ABMs relevant to D&I science are increasingly available and the approach shows promise in its applicability to D&I research questions. Dissemination and implementation of EBPs represent key challenges within D&I where ABM may be particularly relevant, and offer several benefits over other experimental or computational designs.

There is a long tradition of using ABMs to examine the diffusion process.[88,89] ABMs are helpful for investigating how particular actors within a system, such as opinion leaders or innovation champions, improve or hinder the movement of EBPs across a system. ABMs have also been used to understand how different interventions addressing the same issue diffuse differently, based on the system structure and intervention characteristics. For example, Dunn and Gallego constructed an ABM to examine the dissemination of competing EBPs within a health care system based on geographic and network data of the Australian healthcare system.[89] Organizations closer to others, socially or geographically, were more likely to adopt higher quality practices, which led to unintentional disparities in service quality by region. These ABM results illuminate how disparities in the quality of care can arise unintentionally and unexpectedly from system structure and diffusion process.

ABMs are particularly useful because characteristics of physical and social environments influence health outcomes. D&I researchers often work in real contexts where manipulating real settings is difficult and randomization is impossible or unethical. ABMs can aid in understanding differences that might emerge from different implementation choices, and the importance of EBP implementation relative to the influence of environmental contexts on individual and community outcomes. ABMs in D&I research in health have focused on the implementation of one policy in multiple contexts,[90–93] the implementation of multiple interventions to address a single problem,[92,94] or the influence of a single intervention on multiple, yet conceptually distinct, outcomes.[95,96]

Agent-Based Modeling in Dissemination & Implementation Research: a Brief Case Study

Yang and colleagues developed an ABM to assess multiple interventions designed to improve active travel to school.[95,96] While they examined multiple approaches and community characteristics relevant to active school travel, the focus here is on their examination of implementation approaches for a walking school bus intervention within hypothetical cities of various population densities. The ABM was a simulated city with multiple schools and a grid road system. The primary agents were children who lived within a distance of a designated school. Children decided if they wanted to walk to school based on a personal preference for active travel (i.e., biking or walking), willingness to walk a distance to school, and their parents' perceived safety of the route to school. Children may join the walking school bus, walk on their own, or take some other means to school (e.g., a parent drives the child to school in a car).

The authors used the ABM to assess the influence of a walking school bus route, an education intervention designed to improve attitudes toward active travel to school, or both interventions in combination. The authors tested each approach in a variety of communities with different population densities (and thus, varying numbers of students per school). Results suggested that the success of either intervention—alone or in combination—was dependent on community context, and that the magnitude of difference seen across communities varied for interventions (Figure 10.6). While each intervention alone was beneficial for all communities, the walking school bus showed the greatest increase in the least densely populated communities: student participation in active travel doubled. For the educational intervention alone, results were more equitable, with student participation increasing by about two thirds across community types. Modeling the potentially synergistic effects of simultaneous interventions in an ABM revealed that all communities enjoyed the most benefits from dual implementation, and this scenario was the only case where at least 20% of students in every type of community engaged in active travel.

Relevance to Dissemination & Implementation Research

This model demonstrates many of the characteristics and strengths of ABM for D&I. The model is made up of multiple heterogeneous actors, in this case children, who make decisions based on personal characteristics, the social environment, and the physical environment. The researchers modeled multiple interventions across multiple

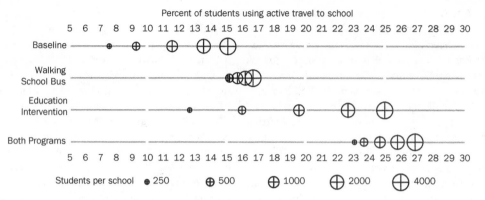

FIGURE 10.6 Results of walking school bus ABM.

(Adapted from Table 1 in Yang et al.[96])

community contexts to assess how environment may influence intervention success. The ABM served as an experimental laboratory where researchers could manipulate both the interventions and the community in a systematic way that would otherwise be difficult, costly, or impossible. Although the ABM cannot predict the success of the same or a similar intervention in a specific real community, the results could be used to implement interventions that are more likely to be successful, given community characteristics, and eliminate possibilities that show relatively little value. Furthermore, the positive interaction between the intervention, social environment, and individuals to produce a qualitatively different outcome at the community level is a hallmark of ABMs. They demonstrated the potential synergistic benefit of implementing multiple interventions designed to address the same overarching issue but through different approaches.

SUMMARY

As we have seen, numerous analysis and modeling tools that take into account the natural complexity of systems and D&I processes are available, and the use of them is increasing over time.[60] The characteristics, potential insights, and limitations of each modeling approach are summarized in Table 10.1. It is important to note that modeling from a systems perspective, like all modeling approaches, requires assumptions about variables to include (or exclude), and hypothesized relationships dictate the quality of the model and the utility of the results. As such, using theory and empirical data to inform model design is paramount.

Systems thinking and methods remain underutilized in D&I despite demonstrations of the utility of incorporating systems thinking and methods into D&I studies (e.g., Leykum, et al., 2007).[97] How can interested D&I researchers make greater use of these approaches? The following are a number of suggestions, based on the authors' own experiences working at the intersection of dissemination & implementation science and systems science.

- As with any research method, its appropriateness is determined by its fit with the theories and research questions driving the study. Systems methods are more likely to be appropriate when the D&I research is being guided by systems thinking.[37]
- Systems approaches can be integrated into more traditional study designs; however full-scale integration of systems modeling requires careful attention from the start of the research design process.
- The results of systems modeling are more likely to be valid and useful when they involve a wide variety of stakeholders in all phases of the modeling and incorporate theories, data, and perspectives from multiple disciplines.[47,98]
- Although the systems methods discussed here are presented separately, they are often combined. For example, the Cancer Intervention and Surveillance Monitoring Network combined an ABM that generated individual smoking histories for the entire United States, with a higher-level SD model used to forecast effects of cancer

TABLE 10.2 USEFUL RESOURCES FOR SYSTEMS SCIENCE METHODS FOR D&I RESEARCH

	Network Analysis	System Dynamics	Agent-based Modeling
Professional Associations	• International Network for Social Network Analysis *insna.org*	•Systems Dynamics Society *systemdynamics.org*	• Network for Computational Modeling in Social & Ecological Sciences *comses.net*
Major Conferences	• International Conference on Advances in Social Networks Analysis and Mining *asonam.cpsc.ucalgary.ca* • Sunbelt Conference *insna.org*	• International System Dynamics Society *conference.systemdynamics.org* • Innovations in Collaborative Modeling *modeling.outreach.msu.edu*	• International Conference on Social Computing, Behavioral-Cultural Modeling & Prediction *sbp-brims.org* • Social Simulation Conference *openabm.org* Swarmfest *swarm.org*
Major Journals	• *Applied Network Science appliednetsci.springeropen.com* • *Journal of Complex Networks comnet.oxfordjournals.org* • *Network Science cambridge.org/core/journals/network-science*	• *Journal of the Operational Research Society theorsociety.com/Pages/Publications/JORS.aspx* • *System Dynamics Review systemdynamics.org/publications/system-dynamics-review* • *Systems Research & Behavioral Science wiley.com/WileyCDA/WileyTitle/productCd-SRBS.html*	• *Advances in Complex Systems worldscientific.com/page/acs/aims-scope* • *Complex Adaptive Systems Modeling casmodeling.springeropen.com* • *Journal of Artificial Societies and Social Simulation jasss.soc.surrey.ac.uk*
Software	• Pajek *mrvar.fdv.uni-lj.si/pajek* • R, packages: igraph, RSiena, statnet, visNetwork *r-project.org* • UCINET *sites.google.com/site/ucinetsoftware/home*	• AnyLogic *http://www.anylogic.com/* • Stella/iThink*iseesystems.com/store/products/stella-architect.aspx* • Vensim *vensim.com*	• Mason *cs.gmu.edu/~eclab/projects/mason/#Features* • Netlogo *ccl.northwestern.edu/netlogo* • Repast *repast.github.io/repast_simphony.html*
Online Training	• Social Network Analysis, archived course tutorials, Borgatti *sites.google.com/site/mgt780sna* • Video Tutorial on Social Network Analysis using R, Goodreau & Hunter *rs.resalliance.org/2009/12/16/video-tutorial-on-social-network-analysis-using-r*	• System Dynamics Modeling for Health Policy: Collected Videos, Audio, Slides and Examples Models, Osgood *cs.usask.ca/faculty/ndo885/Classes/ConsensusSD/Lectures.html* • System Dynamics Self Study 15.988, Forrester http://www.ocw.mit.edu/courses/sloan-school-of-management/15-988-system-dynamics-self-study-fall-1998-spring-1999	• Agent-Based Models, various tutorials *agent-based-models.com/blog/resources/tutorials* • Modeling Tutorials, OpenABM *openabm.org/page/modeling-tutorials* • Online Guide for Newcomers to Agent-Based Modeling in the Social Sciences, Axelrod & Tesfatsion *econ.iastate.edu/tesfatsi/abmread.ht* • Complexity Explorer *complexityexplorer.org*

(continued)

TABLE 10.2 CONTINUED

	Network Analysis	System Dynamics	Agent-based Modeling
Overview Books	• Wasserman S & Faust K. 1994. *Social Network Analysis: Methods & Applications* • Valente TW. 2010 *Social Networks and Health: Models, Methods & Applications* • Newman MEJ. 2010. *Networks: An Introduction*	• Morecroft JD. 2015. *Strategic Modelling and Business Dynamics: A Feedback Systems Approach* • Rahmandad H & Oliva R. 2015. *Analytical Methods for Dynamic Modelers* • Sterman JD. 2000. *Business Dynamics: Systems Thinking and Modeling in Complex World*	• Epstein JM. 2006. *Generative Social Science: Studies in Agent-Based Computational Modeling* • Gilbert N. 2008. *Agent-Based Models* • Railsback SF & Grimm V. 2011. *Agent-Based and Individual-Based Modeling: A Practical Introduction*

control interventions on population health (Holford, et al., 2014). Modern ABMs often incorporate social network data and knowledge to model the influence of "social spaces" on actor behavior and dynamics (Alam & Geller, 2012; Lanham, et al., 2014).[99, 100] In fact, because the three methods reviewed here are complementary modeling approaches, generating solutions to D&I problems using multiple methods is likely to improve the quality of the solutions.[36]

• Finally, there is a wide variety of resources available that can facilitate and accelerate understanding of systems science methods. See Table 10.2 for a concise list of professional associations, major conferences, professional journals, software packages, and important books devoted to the methods covered in this chapter.

SUGGESTED READINGS AND WEBSITES

Readings
See Table 10.2

Selected Websites and Tools
See Table 10.2

REFERENCES

1. Rosenberg A. *Philosophy of social science.* 5th ed. Boulder, CO: Westview Press; 2016.
2. Hedström P, Ylikoski P. Causal mechanisms in the social sciences. *Ann Rev Sociol.* 2010;36(1):49-67.
3. Porpora DV. Four concepts of social structure. *J Theory Soc Behav.* 1989;19(2):195-211.
4. Tabak RG, Khoong EC, Chambers DA, Brownson RC. Bridging research and practice. *Am J Prev Med.* 2012;43(3):337-350.
5. Ostrom E. Beyond markets and states: polycentric governance of complex economic systems. *Transnat Corp Rev.* 2010;2(2):12.
6. Glasgow RE, Vogt TM, Boles SM. Evaluating the public health impact of health promotion interventions: the RE-AIM framework. *Am J Public Health.* 1999;89(9):1322-1327.
7. Damschroder LJ, Hagedorn HJ. A guiding framework and approach for implementation research in substance use disorders treatment. *Psychol Addict Behav.* 2011;25(2):194-205.
8. Proctor E, Silmere H, Raghavan R, et al. Outcomes for implementation research: conceptual distinctions, measurement challenges, and research agenda. *Adm Policy Ment Health.* 2011;38(2):65-76.
9. Glass TA, McAtee MJ. Behavioral science at the crossroads in public health: extending horizons, envisioning the future. *Soc Sci Med.* 2006;62(7):1650-1671.
10. Luke DA, Stamatakis KA. Systems science methods in public health: dynamics, networks, and agents. *Ann Rev Public Health.* 2012;33:357-376.
11. Monge PR, Contractor NS. Theories of communication networks. Oxford: Oxford University Press; 2003.
12. Luke DA. Getting the big picture in community science: methods that capture context. *Am J Community Psychol.* 2005;35(3-4):185-200.

13. Luke DA, Harris JK. Network analysis in public health: history, methods, and applications. *Annu Rev Public Health.* 2007;28:69–93.

14. Kleinman MS, Mold JW. Defining the components of the research pipeline. *Clin Transl Sci.* 2009;2(4):312–314.

15. Luke DA, Wald LM, Carothers BJ, Bach LE, Harris JK. Network influences on dissemination of evidence-based guidelines in state tobacco control programs. *Health Educ Behav.* 2013;40(1 Suppl):33S-42S.

16. Brown CH, Kellam SG, Kaupert S, et al. Partnerships for the design, conduct, and analysis of effectiveness, and implementation research: experiences of the prevention science and methodology group. *Adm Policy Ment Health.* 2012;39(4):301–316.

17. O'Malley AJ, Marsden PV. The analysis of social networks. *Health Serv Outcomes Res Methodol.* 2008;8(4):222–269.

18. Harris JK. *An introduction to exponential random graph modeling.* Los Angeles: SAGE; 2014.

19. Snijders TAB, van de Bunt GG, Steglich CEG. Introduction to stochastic actor-based models for network dynamics. *Soc Networks.* 2010;32(1):44–60.

20. de Nooy W, Mrvar A, Batagelj V. *Exploratory social network analysis with Pajek.* Rev. and expanded 2nd ed. New York: Cambridge University Press; 2011.

21. Valente TW. *Social networks and health: Models, methods, and applications.* New York: Oxford University Press; 2010.

22. Wasserman S, Faust K. *Social network analysis: Methods and applications.* Cambridge: Cambridge University Press; 1994.

23. Rogers EM. *Diffusion of innovations.* 5th ed. New York: Free Press; 2003.

24. Valente TW. *Network models of the diffusion of innovations.* Cresskill, N.J.: Hampton Press; 1995.

25. Granovetter M. Threshold models of collective behavior. *Am J Sociol.* 1978;83(6):1420–1443.

26. Benito del Pozo P, Serrano N, Marqués-Sánchez P. Social networks and healthy cities: spreading good practices based on a spanish case study. Geographical Review. 2016:n/a-n/a.

27. Feldstein AC, Glasgow RE. A practical, robust implementation and sustainability model (PRISM) for integrating research findings into practice. *Jt Comm J Qual Patient Saf.* 2008;34(4):228–243.

28. Beck A, Bergman DA, Rahm AK, Dearing JW, Glasgow RE. Using implementation and dissemination concepts to spread 21st-century well-child care at a health maintenance organization. *Permanente J.* 2009;13(3):8.

29. Valente TW, Palinkas LA, Czaja S, Chu KH, Brown CH. Social network analysis for program implementation. *PLoS One.* 2015;10(6):e0131712.

30. Harris JK, Carothers BJ, Wald LM, Shelton SC, Leischow SJ. Interpersonal influence among public health leaders in the United States department of health and human services. *J Public Health Res.* 17 2012;1(1):67–74.

31. Lobb R, Carothers BJ, Lofters AK. Using organizational network analysis to plan cancer screening programs for vulnerable populations. *Am J Public Health.* 2014;104(2):358–364.

32. Sterman J. *Business dynamics: systems thinking and modeling for a complex world.* Boston: Irwin/McGraw-Hill; 2000.

33. Forrester JW. *Industrial dynamics.* Cambridge, MA: M.I.T. Press; 1961.

34. Richardson GP. Reflections on the foundations of system dynamics. *Syst Dyn Rev.* 2011;27:219–243.

35. Meadows DH, Robinson JM. *The electronic oracle: Computer models and social decisions.* Chichester, UK: Wiley; 1985.

36. Hovmand PS, Sato J, Kuhlberg J, Chung S. Introduction to system dynamics for applied social sciences. Manuscript in preparation.

37. Meadows DH, Wright D. *Thinking in systems: A primer.* White River Junction, VT: Chelsea Green Publishing; 2008.

38. Hammond RA. Complex systems modeling for obesity research. *Prev Chronic Dis.* 2009;6(3):A97.

39. Homer JB, Hirsch GB. System dynamics modeling for public health: background and opportunities. *Am J Public Health.* Mar 2006;96(3):452–458.

40. Forrester JW. System dynamics—a personal view of the first fifty years. *Syst Dyn Rev.* 2007;23:345–358.

41. Haase D, Schwarz N. Simulation models on human–nature interactions in urban landscapes: a review including spatial economics, system dynamics, cellular automata and agent-based approaches. *Liv Rev Landsc Res.* 2009;3(2):1-45.

42. Homer J, Milstein B, Wile K, et al. Simulating and evaluating local interventions to improve cardiovascular health. *Prev Chronic Dis.* 2010;7(1) LA18.

43. Mingers J, White L. A review of the recent contribution of systems thinking to operational research and management science. *Eur J Oper Res.* 2010;207(3):1147–1161.

44. Forrester JW. Information sources for modeling the national economy. *J Am Stat Assoc.* 1980;75(371):555–566.

45. Homer JB. Why we iterate: scientific modeling in theory and practice. *Syst Dynam Rev.* 1996;12(1):1–19.

46. Vennix JAM. *Group model building: Facilitating team learning using system dynamics.* Chichester, UK: Wiley; 1996.

47. Hovmand PS. *Community based system dynamics.* New York: Springer; 2014.

48. Marshall DA, Burgos-Liz L, Ijzerman MJ, et al. Selecting a dynamic simulation modeling method for health care delivery research—Part 2: Report of the ISPOR Dynamic Simulation Modeling Emerging Good Practices Task Force. *Value Health.* 2015;18(2):147–160.

49. Rahmandad H, Oliva R, Osgood ND, eds. *Analytical methods for dynamic modelers.* Cambridge, MA: The MIT Press; 2015.

50. Greenhalgh T, Robert G, Macfarlane F, Bate P, Kyriakidou O. Diffusion of innovations in service organizations: systematic review and recommendations. *Milbank Q.* 2004;82(4):581–629.

51. Aarons GA, Hurlburt M, Horwitz SM. Advancing a conceptual model of evidence-based practice implementation in public service sectors. *Adm Policy Men Health Ment Health Serv Res.* 2011;38(1):4–23.

52. Pronovost P, Berenholtz S, Needham D. Translating evidence into practice: a model for large scale knowledge translation. *BMJ.* 2008;337(7676).

53. Sterman JD. Learning from evidence in a complex world. *Am J Public Health.* 2006;96(3):505–514.

54. Forrester JW. *Urban dynamics.* Cambridge, MA: MIT. Press; 1969.

55. Lich KH, Frerichs L, Fishbein D, Bobashev G, Pentz MA. Translating research into prevention of high-risk behaviors in the presence of complex systems: definitions and systems frameworks. *TBM.* 2016;6(1):17–31.

56. Hovmand PS, Gillespie DF. Implementation of evidence-based practice and organizational performance. *J Behav Health Serv Res.* 2010;37(1):79–94.

57. Miller RL, Levine RL, McNall MA, Khamarko K, Valenti MT. A dynamic model of client recruitment and retention in community-based HIV prevention programs. *Health Promot Pract.* 2011;12(1):135–146.

58. Glasgow RE, Emmons KM. How can we increase translation of research into practice? Types of evidence needed. *Ann Rev Public Health.* 2007;28:413–433.

59. Green LW. Public health asks of systems science: To advance our evidence-based practice, can you help us get more practice-based evidence? *Am J Public Health.* 2006;96(3):406–409.

60. Northridge ME, Metcalf SS. Enhancing implementation science by applying best principles of systems science. *Health Res Policy Syst.* 2016;14(1):74.

61. Powell BJ, McMillen JC, Proctor EK, et al. A compilation of strategies for implementing clinical innovations in health and mental health. *Med Care Res Rev.* 2012;69(2):123–157.

62. Scott RJ, Cavana RY, Cameron D. Recent evidence on the effectiveness of group model building. *Eur J Oper Res.* 2016;249(3):908–918.

63. Holmes BJ, Finegood DT, Riley BL, Best A. Systems thinking in dissemination and implementation research. In: Brownson RC, Colditz GA, Proctor EK, eds. *Dissemination and implementation research in health: Translating science to practice.* New York: Oxford University Press; 2012;175–191.

64. Black LJ, Andersen DF. Using visual representations as boundary objects to resolve conflict in collaborative model-building applications. *Syst Res Behav Sci.* 2012;29:194–208.

65. Black LJ. When visuals are boundary objects in system dynamics work. *Syst Dynam Rev.* 2013;29(2):70–86.

66. Thompson KM, Tebbens RJD. Using system dynamics to develop policies that matter: global management of poliomyelitis and beyond. *Syst Dynam Rev.* 2008;24(4):433–449.

67. Lich KH, Tian Y, Beadles CA, et al. Strategic planning to reduce the burden of stroke among veterans using simulation modeling to inform decision making. *Stroke.* 2014;45(7):2078–2084.

68. Zimmerman L, Lounsbury DW, Rosen CS, Kimerling R, Trafton JA, Lindley SE. Participatory system dynamics modeling: increasing stakeholder engagement and precision to improve implementation planning in systems. *Adm Policy Ment Health.* 2016;43(6):834–849.

69. Gilbert N. *Agent-based models.* Thousand Oaks, CA: Sage; 2008.

70. Axelrod R. Launching "the evolution of cooperation." *J Theor Biol.* 2012;299:21–24.

71. Spielman S, Harrison P. The co-evolution of residential segregation and the built environment at the turn of the 20th century: a schelling model. *T GIS.* 2014;18(1):25–45.

72. Doroshenko A, Qian W, Osgood ND. Evaluation of outbreak response immunization in the control of pertussis using agent-based modeling. *Peer J.* 2016;4:e2337.

73. Wares JR, Lawson B, Shemin D, D'Agata EMC. Evaluating infection prevention strategies in outpatient dialysis units using agent-based modeling. *PLoS ONE.* 2016;11(5):e0153820.

74. Parker J, Epstein JM. A distributed platform for global-scale agent-based models of disease transmission. *ACM Trans Model Comput Simul.* 2011;22(1):2.

75. Hammond RA, Ornstein JT. A model of social influence on body mass index. *Ann N Y Acad Sci.* 2014;1331:3.4–42

76. Nianogo RA, Arah OA. Agent-based modeling of noncommunicable diseases: a systematic review. *Am J Public Health*. 2015;105(3):e20–e31.

77. Hammond RA. Considerations and best practices in agent-based modeling to inform policy. 2015.

78. Auchincloss AH, Garcia LMT. Brief introductory guide to agent-based modeling and an illustration from urban health research. *Cadernos de Saúde Pública*. 2015;31:65–78.

79. Hoffer L. Unreal models of real behavior: the agent-based modeling experience. *Pract Anthropol*. 2013;35(1):19–23.

80. Ip EH, Rahmandad H, Shoham DA, et al. Reconciling statistical and systems science approaches to public health. *Health Educ Behav*. 2013;40(1 suppl):123S-131S.

81. Chattoe-Brown E. Using agent based modelling to integrate data on attitude change. *Sociol Res Online*. 2014;19(1):16.

82. Wilensky U. *NetLogo segregation Model*. Evanston, IL: Center for Connected Learning and Computer-Based Modeling at Northwestern University; 1997.

83. De Leon FD, Felsen M, Wilensky U. *NetLogo Urban Suite—Tijuana Bordertowns model*. Evanston, IL: Center for Connected Learning and Computer-Based Modeling at Northwestern University; 2007.

84. Loomis J, Bond C, Harpman D. The potential of agent-based modelling for performing economic analysis of adaptive natural resource management. *J Nat Resourc Pol Res*. 2008;1(1):35–48.

85. Bonabeau E. Agent-based modeling: methods and techniques for simulating human systems. *Proc Natl Acad Sci U S A*. 2002;99 Suppl 3:7280–7287.

86. Burke JG, Lich KH, Neal JW, Meissner HI, Yonas M, Mabry PL. Enhancing dissemination and implementation research using systems science methods. *Int J Behav Med*. 2015;22(3):283–291.

87. Fioretti G. Agent-based simulation models in organization science. *Organ Res Methods*. 2013;16(2):227–242.

88. Kiesling E, Günther M, Stummer C, Wakolbinger LM. Agent-based simulation of innovation diffusion: a review. *Cent Eur J Oper Res*. 2012;20(2):183–230.

89. Dunn AG, Gallego B. Diffusion of competing innovations: the effects of network structure on the provision of healthcare. *J Artif Soceties Soc Simul*. 2010;13(4).

90. Orr MG, Galea S, Riddle M, Kaplan GA. Reducing racial disparities in obesity: simulating the effects of improved education and social network influence on diet behavior. *Ann Epidemiol*. 2014;24(8):563–569.

91. Auchincloss AH, Riolo RL, Brown DG, Cook J, Diez Roux AV. An agent-based model of income inequalities in diet in the context of residential segregation. *Am J Prev Med*. 2011;40(3):303–311.

92. Brookmeyer R, Boren D, Baral SD, et al. Combination HIV prevention among MSM in South Africa: results from agent-based modeling. *PLoS ONE*. 2014;9(11):e112668.

93. Hoffer L, Alam SJ. "Copping" in heroin markets: the hidden information costs of indirect sales and why they matter. In Greenberg AM, Kennedy WG, Bos ND, eds. *Social computing, behavioral-cultural modeling and prediction*. Heidelberg: Springer; 2013:83–92.

94. Luke DA, Hammond RA, Combs T, et al. Tobacco town: using computational modeling to study effects of policies designed to reduce tobacco retailer density. *Am J Public Health*. 2017 May;107(5):740–746.

95. Yang Y, Diez-Roux A. Using an agent-based model to simulate children's active travel to school. *Int J Behav Nutr Phys Act*. 2013;10(10.1186):1479–5868.

96. Yang Y, Diez-Roux A, Evenson KR, Colabianchi N. Examining the impact of the walking school bus with an agent-based model. *Am J Public Health*. 2014/07/01 2014;104(7):1196–1203.

97. Leykum LK, Pugh J, Lawrence V, et al. Organizational interventions employing principles of complexity science have improved outcomes for patients with Type II diabetes. *Implement Sci*. 28 2007;2:28.

98. IOM (Institute of Medicine). *Assessing the use of agent-based models for tobacco regulation*. Washington, DC: The National Academies Press; 2015.

99. Alam SJ, Geller A. Networks in agent-based social simulation. In Heppenstall AJ, Crooks AT, See LM, Batty M, eds. *Agent-based models of geographical systems*. Netherlands: Springer; 2012:199–216.

100. Lanham MJ, Morgan GP, Carley KM. Social Network Modeling and Agent-Based Simulation in Support of Crisis De-Escalation. *IEEE Transactions on Systems, Man, and Cybernetics: Systems*. 2014;44(1):103–110.

Participatory Approaches for Study Design and Analysis in Dissemination and Implementation Research

MEREDITH MINKLER, ALICIA L. SALVATORE, AND CHARLOTTE CHANG

INTRODUCTION

The past half century has witnessed greatly increased recognition of the importance of community and other stakeholder participation for improving health research.[1-4] Growing interest in closing the gap between research and practice has brought further attention to the benefits of participatory approaches for the dissemination and implementation of research findings.[1,5,6] With its commitment to action as an integral part of the research process, community-based participatory research (CBPR) has demonstrated particular promise for helping translate study findings into programs, practices, and policies to promote health. In this chapter, CBPR is used as an umbrella term for an orientation to research that goes by many names (among them participatory action research, community-partnered research, and participatory research) and that have in common a commitment to combining research, participation, education, and action.[1,7,8]

As classically defined by Green and his colleagues[1] CBPR is "systematic investigation, with the participation of those affected by the issue being studied, for the purposes of education and taking action or effecting change." Building on this definition, as well as earlier work by Israel et al.,[3] the Kellogg Community Health Scholars Program[9] crafted a definition that further situates CBPR within the context of efforts to study and address health inequities. In this expanded definition, CBPR is "A collaborative process that equitably involves all partners in the research process and recognizes the unique strengths that each brings. CBPR begins with a research topic of importance to the community with the aim of combining knowledge and action for social change to improve community health and eliminate health disparities."[9] This partnership orientation to research has become recognized as an important means through which the distance between research and action might be more effectively bridged.[10] Indeed, as Horowitz and her colleagues point out, "CBPR may be the ultimate form of translational research . . . moving discoveries bi-directionally from bench to bedside to *el barrio* (the community) to organizations and policy makers."[11] Although CBPR is not possible or applicable in all research contexts, when it is appropriate, much value can be added to the research process, and subsequent dissemination and implementation of findings through high-level community and other stakeholder participation. As discussed later, the level of community engagement in research takes place along a continuum, from limited consultation on specific aspects of the study to co-collaboration at every step in the process.

For readers unfamiliar with CBPR, this chapter seeks to demonstrate the value added from community participation to the research process itself. It also shows how CBPR methods are useful in the dissemination and implementation (D&I) of research findings and some of the lessons from CBPR for D&I research. Since the large and growing literature on CBPR cannot be covered in a single chapter, entry points into this scholarship are provided. After briefly describing a continuum of such participation, the discussion is focused, in particular, on CBPR. Challenges that can play out in participatory research are discussed, followed by a more detailed examination of the specific ways in which a CBPR approach can enhance the D&I of research findings through collaborative design, analysis, dissemination and research translation. A case study is presented of a community-university-health department CBPR project, in which all three of the authors were involved, that endeavored to study and improve the health and working conditions of restaurant workers in San

Francisco's Chinatown District. Methods used to involve all partners in study design, data analysis, and translation of findings into action, as well as some of the benefits of doing so, are discussed. Finally, key lessons learned through this and other CBPR efforts are shared, and their implications for improving the breadth and effectiveness of the critical dissemination and implementation phases of research are summarized.

CONTINUUM OF PARTICIPATION IN RESEARCH

Community and other stakeholder participation in research can be seen as occurring along a continuum, with benefits accruing at each stage, and the most substantial value added often occurring at the farthest end of the continuum. Balazs and Morello-Frosch's[12] "continuum of community participation in research" is illustrative (Figure 11.1).

At one end is what American Indian author and activist V. Deloria[13] called "helicopter research," in which outsiders design and execute a study and community members simply take part as subjects, if at all. In helicopter research, there is no intentional dissemination of findings to the community, nor any use of the findings to benefit participants. Higher level, though still fairly minimal engagement, occurs when pre-and postdata collection is used to "actively solicit" the opinions of participants, who may be involved, as well, in the dissemination of study findings.[12] Finally, at the other end of the continuum, community partners are engaged at each stage of the research process. These include helping identify a problem or issue of deep local relevance; designing the

study, including the use of culturally and socially appropriate research methods; engaging in data collection and interpretation; determining the appropriateness and effectiveness of interventions dissemination; and using findings to help affect change. As Balazs and Morello-Frosch[12] note, such high-level community engagement can increase the "relevance, rigor and reach" of the research. Simultaneously, authentic partnership with community members can increase mutual learning and local control over the research process.

As suggested, in the ideal case—what Trickett[14] calls CBPR as "world view"—the research is initiated and driven by the community partner, or by an authentic partnership of community, academic, and other stakeholders. Yet investigator-initiated and managed studies that emphasize sincere collaboration and partnership with community and other partners can also substantially increase the relevance and efficacy of the research, resulting in greater community buy-in and trust; better tailored interventions; enhanced efficacy in data collection and interpretation; and more effective dissemination and translation of findings into programs and policies to address identified problems.[2,5-7]

When feasible and appropriate, CBPR may be particularly well suited to translational research aimed at studying and addressing health disparities.[2,5,15-17] Although it also presents substantial challenges, including the time- and labor- intensive nature of the work and ethical challenges, among them more complicated IRBs[12,] and a tangle of "everyday ethics,"[18] this orientation to research has achieved growing attention both in North America and globally.

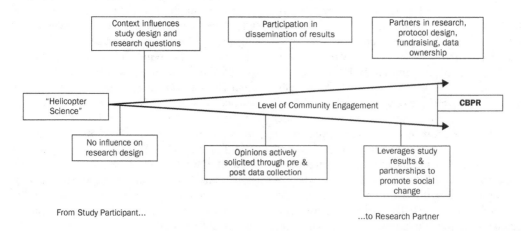

FIGURE 11.1 Continuum of community participation in research.

(Reprinted with permission from Balazs and Morello-Frosch.[12])

CBPR APPROACHES AND PRINCIPLES

The research dimension of CBPR can involve a wide range of qualitative and quantitative methods. Developing and administering community surveys or focus groups; conducting walkability assessments or air monitoring; using geographic information systems mapping; conducting secondary data analysis, and using randomized controlled trials (RCTs) to assess intervention effectiveness, all have been used by as part of CBPR efforts.[5,19,20] Regardless of the particular research methods used, however, what is unique about this orientation to research is *how* the research is conceptualized and conducted;[4] the heavy accent placed on genuine community and stakeholder engagement throughout the process; and the use of findings to help bring about change.

CBPR Principles

Eleven principles of CBPR, described in Box 11.1, help to further articulate how CBPR differs from more traditional "top-down" approaches to research and is consistent with translational research that is indeed "community-based," rather than merely "community-placed." Israel and her community and academic colleagues[3,20] developed nine guiding principles of CBPR that are widely used to inform and guide the process of CBPR. Two other principles, added subsequently by Minkler and Wallerstein[7,8] are also critical to this work. Although translational research partnerships wishing to utilize CBPR should adapt these principles (or develop new ones), as appropriate, given their own unique contexts, these eleven principles may be helpful in providing initial guidance.

Following these principles may help strengthen the quality of data and the statistical power of analysis. Yet as Green and Glasgow[23] point out, although CBPR improves one facet of external validity—its relevance to "end users" of findings in a particular community—CBPR may make it less relevant to other communities. The more we make a study locally relevant,

---

BOX 11.1

PRINCIPLES OF COMMUNITY-BASED PARTICIPATORY RESEARCH

1. Recognizes community as a unit of identity, whether community is defined in geographic, racial/ethnic, or other terms
2. Builds on strengths and resources within the community
3. Facilitates a collaborative, equitable partnership in all phases of research, involving an empowering and power-sharing process that attends to social inequalities
4. Fosters colearning and capacity building among all partners
5. Integrates and achieves a balance between knowledge generation and intervention for the mutual benefit of all partners
6. Focuses on the local relevance of public health problems and on ecological perspectives that attend to the multiple determinants of health
7. Involves systems development using a cyclical and iterative process
8. Disseminates results to all partners and involves them in the wider dissemination of results
9. Involves a long-term process and commitment to sustainability
10. Openly addresses issues of race, ethnicity, racism, and other social divides, and embodies "cultural humility,"[21] recognizing that while no one can be truly "competent" in another's culture, we can demonstrate a commitment to self-reflection and critique, working to redress power imbalances and to develop authentic partnerships
11. Works to assure research vigor and validity by also "broaden[ing] the bandwidth and validity"[22] to insure that the *research question* is valid (coming from, or being of importance to the community) and that different "ways of knowing," including community lay knowledge, are valued alongside more traditional scientific sources of knowledge.[22]

tailoring it to a particular population or community group, the more we make it ungeneralizable beyond that setting and population. Such research remains important and relevant to others, however, in that it was made more applicable to typical circumstances, rather than settings that are "artificially constructed and controlled" for academic purposes [23] (see also Schillinger et al.,[24] and chapter 18). We turn now to the more specific ways in which CBPR may add value to community-based translational research.

BENEFITS OF CBPR FOR IMPROVING D&I RESEARCH QUALITY AND RELEVANCE

A CBPR orientation to inquiry has the potential to strengthen research quality at each step of the process, many of which have direct relevance for study design and analysis as well as the dissemination and implementation of findings. Although there are fewer examples of CBPR in D&I research specifically, the strengths of CBPR, highlighted in the following, are increasingly being stressed as a way to remedy the "lack of 'fit'" between an intervention design on the one hand and, on the other hand, the realities inherent to community and practice settings, and the information needed by policymakers. Such mismatch often leads to poor or only modest uptake and implementation.[23]

CBPR Can Help Ensure the Relevance of the Research Topic

When "bench to bedside" or "bench to curbside" translational research is not seen by patients or communities as holding relevance for their lives and contexts, even the most elegant of research designs may fail to achieve their intended effects. Although the far end of the CBPR continuum involves communities or other stakeholders in identifying the topic to be studied, engaging such partners early in the process can help to ensure that even investigator-driven research is locally relevant and likely to yield useful results. Stanford University's Chronic Disease Self-Management Program was initially tested through numerous peer -reviewed RCTs,[25] yet whether this program would have relevance to American Indian/Alaska Natives, (AI/AN) who are believed to have among the highest rates of diabetes globally, was open to question. A community advisory board (CAB) of American Indians with diabetes in Santa Clara County, CA worked closely with Jernigan and her academic colleagues,[26] and suggested that the program did have relevance but would need to be culturally adapted. The proposed changes included beginning each weekly session with a blessing and smudging ceremony, increasing session length to allow time for storytelling, and incorporating the image of a dream catcher into the program's visual of the symptom cycle.[26] With these changes, the pilot program, had a 100% retention rate, with impressive changes in a variety of disease symptoms and self-management behaviors.[26] Based on these successes, the program was adapted for dissemination over the Internet[27]—a medium widely used by American Indians across the United States since a major, cross tribal newspaper is most easily accessed on line. An active member of the original CAB, moreover, went on to play a leadership role with the CAB for a PCORI-funded RCT of an enhanced diabetes prevention program for urban AI/AN. With new CBPR academic partners at Stanford University School of Medicine,[28] this elder helped build on his earlier experience and that of other CAB members, working with the academic partners in developing such new elements as a focus on historical trauma and the use of digital storytelling and other methods that complemented American Indian traditions and beliefs.[28]

CBPR Can Enhance the Quality, Validity, Sensitivity, and Practicality of Research Instruments by Involving the Local Knowledge of Community Members

Surveys and other research instruments that lack cultural sensitivity or that appear naive or ill-suited to the community being studied can reinforce feelings of disconnection, and sometimes be hurtful or insulting. Community insights into how to rephrase questions, or what type of research instrument may be best suited to a given community (e.g., focus groups versus in-depth interviews) can improve recruitment and retention[7,17,20,29] and, as Cargo and Mercer[5] point out, help in "reducing measurement error from survey and interview questions that are not culturally aligned." In the oft-cited Healthy Homes Project in Seattle-Kings County, Washington,[30] Community Health Workers administering a standard baseline survey to assess exposure to indoor asthma triggers noted that, despite earlier pretesting, questions about whether residents smoked at home were not sensitive enough to pick up whether or not *others* were smoking inside the house, and survey modifications resulted. As the study's epidemiologists pointed out, "Any loss in the ability to make 'pure' baseline and exit comparisons may have been outweighed by the higher quality of the exit data" as a result of community partner input.[30] The integration of different types of information and knowledge through CBPR's inclusion of local knowledge and multiple stakeholder perspectives is particularly relevant to D&I research, which, as Glasgow and Emmons[10] and Green[31] point out, has largely employed a narrow and researcher-determined perspective as to what constitutes "evidence."[10,31]

CBPR Can Enhance the Likelihood of Overcoming the Distrust of Research by Communities That Traditionally Have Been the "Subjects" of Such Research by Bringing Together Partners with Different Skills, Knowledge, And Expertise to Address Complex Problems

The earlier mentioned "helicopter research"[13]— imposed most often on American Indian, African American, Latino and other marginalized communities of color and frequently embedded in a context of decades or centuries of oppression, including unethical research, at the hands of the dominant population—has engendered deep distrust.[7,13,32,33] Openly acknowledging and discussing this history, and its current forms and consequences, while actively working to build trust and "terms of engagement" that stress community determination and high-level partnership, can help build a foundation necessary for authentic CBPR.

By Increasing the Relevance of Research Interventions, CBPR can Increase the Likelihood of Success

When community input is earnestly sought and valued, interventions may deviate from what the outside researchers originally had in mind.[23,31,34] Yet such changes may have positive effects for relevance and adaptation, improving external validity in the process.[23,31] Further, the participation of community members, practitioners, and policymakers can enhance the probability of an intervention's adoption, "closing the gap between discovery and delivery."[23] Community Partners in Care, an RCT to improve the relevance of quality improvement approaches to depression care among African Americans, was planned using

a community-partnered participatory research approach,[35] and was implemented in Los Angeles, CA, following these same participatory research principles and practices. The inclusion of multiple stakeholders, including a wide network of agencies, policymakers, and the arts community (since community partners identified the arts as providing culturally appropriate avenues for opening discussion about the stigma of depression), led to robust community engagement model and some encouraging results when compared with a more traditional service model.[36]

CBPR Can Improve Data Analysis and Interpretation by Enhancing our Understanding of the Meaning of Study Findings Through the Contribution of Lay Knowledge

Although community members often have neither the time for nor the interest in being engaged in hands-on data analysis,[7,20,36] their help in reviewing and interpreting preliminary findings may add important nuance and deeper understandings of study results. In an effort to study and address food insecurity in San Francisco's low-income Tenderloin neighborhood, academic members of a CBPR partnership interviewed the owners of local corner stores about their attitudes toward "healthy retail." Through this approach, merchants are incentivized for decreasing selling space devoted to alcohol and tobacco, while increasing space for fresh produce and other nutritious foods. Although the academic researchers found many useful themes in their qualitative data analysis, community partners, trained in coding redacted interview transcripts, both provided additional support for the initial themes identified and added context and new understandings (e.g., regarding degree of merchants' expressed identification with the community and their willingness to change their business model) that added important nuance to our understanding of merchants' attitudes and behaviors.

CBPR Can Improve the Potential for Disseminating Findings to Diverse Audiences and Translating Evidence-Based Research into Sustainable Changes in Programs, Practices and Policies

Publication of CBPR translational research studies in peer-reviewed journals is critical, particularly in building the evidence base for the efficacy of this approach in achieving health outcomes.[5,16,17] Community and other stakeholder partners, however, can identify additional dissemination channels (e.g., ethnic media, patient-focused magazines in doctors' offices, relevant community events), for more effectively reaching key community members and decision-makers with the findings. A number of CBPR projects also have created workbooks or replication manuals to assist other partnerships interested in adapting and utilizing their approaches, and many of these, along with myriad other resources, are now available online through the Community Tool Box (http://ctb.ku.edu) and Community-Campus Partnerships for Health (www.ccph.info). The combination of community engagement and relevant scientific research further can pack substantial political punch, helping to effect policy and systems level changes conducive to more health-promoting environments.[37] Successful CBPR efforts in two low-resource San Francisco neighborhoods with little access to fresh fruits and vegetables not only led to community-based efforts to pilot corner store conversions to healthy retail, but also helped secure the passage of a 2013 municipal ordinance creating the "Healthy Retail SF" program.[38,39] To date, 9 corner stores have been incentivized and redesigned through the program, reducing to less than 20% selling space for alcohol and tobacco combined and increasing to at least 35% the space allotted to fresh produce. Regular store assessment data collected by community partner researchers and of monthly point-of-sale data from merchants, have documented a 25% increase in fresh produce sales in participating stores, with slower but still impressive declines in tobacco and alcohol advertising, availability, and sales.[40]

ETHICAL AND METHODOLOGICAL CHALLENGES

Although CBPR can indeed help enhance the quality and relevance of translational research, including making substantial contributions to research design and analysis, this approach also raises difficult ethical and methodological challenges meriting attention.[7,18,33] Community and other stakeholders thus may make recommendations that would weaken the rigor of study instruments (e.g., altering validated scales) or propose changes in study design that may weaken the science, for example, when community members

object to an RCT or staggered design that may be needed to prove whether the intervention had an effect. To avoid such difficulties, many partnerships now begin by developing memorandums of understanding (MOUs) and/or holding colearning workshops where the meaning of terms like validity and research rigor are explored from both academic and community perspectives, and decisions made ahead of time about how difficult issues will be handled. Partnerships further have benefited by the development of tools, such as Mercer and Green et al.'s[41] reliability-tested guidelines for assessing partnership process and progress along multiple dimensions, and tools developed by Israel and her colleagues[42] and Butterfoss and Kegler,[43] which also have been widely adapted and used.

When trained community members are engaged in conducting interviews or administering surveys, perceptions of bias may be raised. In communities characterized by high levels of distrust borne of years of discriminatory treatment, however, as in some rural parts of the southern United States, involving outside researchers in face-to-face data gathering may be unrealistic, especially initially. Creative ways of dealing with such problems, such as having residents of neighboring communities accompany and introduce university researchers in door-to-door surveys may help in building trust and increasing participation rates.[44]

In the data interpretation and dissemination phases of translational research, ethical and methodological challenges also may arise if community partners are seen as having an "axe to grind" that could lead them to present findings selectively to further their community's best interests. Additionally, if data emerge that could cast the community in an unfavorable light,[45, 46] thorny questions of community ownership and decision-making processes may ensue. As in other stages of the research process, colearning sessions and trainings on the importance of accurately collecting, analyzing, and reporting findings, as well as frank discussions of community and outside researcher roles and responsibilities in this regard, are critical. At the same time, instruments such as Flicker et al.'s[46] recommendations for institutional review boards reviewing participatory research, may be useful to CBPR partnerships in asking hard questions up front, including, for example, "what will be done if findings emerge that are unflattering to the community?" As noted earlier, process appraisal instruments that CBPR partnerships can use throughout the research process,[41-43] and careful MOUs between partners can aid in preventing or openly confronting such challenges when they arise. Several ethical and methodological challenges and how they were addressed are highlighted in the case study that follows.

CBPR CASE EXAMPLE: THE SAN FRANCISCO CHINATOWN RESTAURANT WORKER STUDY

The Chinatown Restaurant Worker Study was a CBPR effort to examine and address the health and working conditions of restaurant workers in San Francisco's Chinatown. Nationwide, workers in the restaurant industry face high rates of injury and other challenges such as low wages and few benefits, limited opportunities for upward mobility or wage increases, and other types of occupational injustice.[47] Studying the relationships between restaurant work and worker health is particularly important for immigrant workers, who comprise a large portion of this workforce and who may experience disproportionately greater rates of illness and injury due to immigration concerns, language barriers, and lack of awareness of US workplace regulations.[47,48] Given that restaurants are the largest employer of Chinese immigrants, one of the largest and most rapidly growing immigrant populations in the United States,[49] research and intervention efforts with Chinese restaurant workers are critical. San Francisco's Chinatown, home to almost 5,000 people and more than 100 restaurants, offered an important setting in which to study and address the working conditions and health of this important community.

Building on strong mutual interest in promoting the health and welfare of Chinatown restaurant workers, a partnership was developed in 2007 comprised of a community-based organization (the Chinese Progressive Association [CPA]); two universities (the University of California, Berkeley School of Public Health, including UC Berkeley's Labor Occupational Health Program [LOHP], and the University of California San Francisco School of Medicine), and a local health department (the San Francisco Department of Public Health's Occupational and Environmental Health Section). Many of the partners had worked previously together on other CBPR projects and the project coordinator (a university partner) was a founding member of CPA and a former resident of Chinatown. These existing relationships greatly facilitated the establishment of the partnership as well as initial trust between partners.[50]

The community-university-health department collaborative aimed to follow CBPR principles[3,8] and included an ongoing participatory evaluation of partnership process and effectiveness.[51,52] A 12-member Steering Committee was formed, comprised of representatives from each partner organization and tasked with serving as the project's primary coordinating and decision-making body. Over the course of the project, nine current and former immigrant Chinese restaurant workers participated in a Restaurant Worker Leadership Group (RWLG), which was established with the goal of facilitating in-depth participation from restaurant workers throughout all phases of the project.

A CBPR grant from the National Institute for Occupational Safety and Health supported partnership development, an ecologic study of Chinatown restaurant worker health and safety, described in more detail later; a participatory evaluation of the partnership; and some dissemination activities. In keeping with its CBPR orientation, the Chinatown project kept the "final" phases of CBPR—dissemination and translation of findings into action—at the forefront of planning from the study's onset. For example, the team sought additional funding early in the project from a large philanthropic organization, The California Endowment, which supports and encourages CBPR and policy-level intervention. This additional funding went directed to the CPA and enabled the partnership to more broadly disseminate study findings and translate research findings into programs and policies to promote worker health. The long history and success of the community partner, CPA, in organizing and advocacy made it well suited to lead these expanded dissemination and translational activities and to serve as lead agency on the new grant.

Participation in Study Design

Partners' collaboration in study design began during grant writing and intensified once study funds, the Steering Committee, and the RWLG were all in place. Consistent with partners' values and CBPR principles, and recognizing the multilevel nature of factors influencing restaurant worker health, the Chinatown study employed an ecologic design. The study was comprised of a community-based cross-sectional survey of Chinatown restaurant workers conducted by trained worker partners. It also included standardized observations of hazards to workers in Chinatown restaurants conducted by health department staff.[53] All partners, including RWLG members, actively participated in working groups to develop data collection protocols and study instruments. Involving all partners in study development required significant time and commitment from all partners. In addition, considerable resources were needed for critical services such as translation of documents into Chinese and English and simultaneous interpretation into Cantonese or English at project team meetings.

To more effectively involve RWLG members, Chinatown restaurant workers with no prior research experience, an 8-week training was held at the beginning of the study on topics such as workplace health and safety, workers' rights, research goals, and research-related topics such as confidentiality, informed consent, and survey administration. After the initial training, the RWLG met biweekly to provide feedback on study instruments, develop a recruitment plan for the worker survey, and prepare to pilot test the survey instrument. Interactive activities such as risk mapping,[54-55] neighborhood mapping, and mock food inspections in a simulated kitchen were used to enhance workers' participation.

The instruments developed by the collaborative are described in the following with some examples of how the involvement of diverse partners improved their quality, and thereby enhanced their application and outcomes.

Worker Survey

A standardized questionnaire was developed to measure Chinatown restaurant workers' health and work experiences. A draft instrument, created with inputs from all partners, was reviewed and revised by the RWLG and then finalized after piloting with 15 restaurant workers. The participation of CPA in the development of the questionnaire resulted in many additions to the original draft created by university partners. These included questions designed to learn more about the broader context of workers' lives (e.g., wages, housing, health and social service utilization, and workers' civic engagement). The RWLG's participation in survey development resulted in some important wording additions to standardized scales (e.g., explaining such idioms as "butterflies in my stomach"), as well as new questions to document previously ignored hardships in their work

environments such as harassment, violence, and wage and tip theft.[50, 51]

Procedures for survey recruitment and administration similarly were collaboratively developed by all partners. The participation of CPA and the RWLG, in particular, was critical for anticipating possible risks to participants (e.g., worker retaliation) and developing a protocol that assuaged participants' fears and safeguarded their identities. Members of the RWLG and 17 additional community members who were hired as surveyors went through intensive training in informed consent and study procedures prior to their involvement in recruiting participants and administering the survey.[51]

Restaurant Observations

A 13-item observational survey, the Restaurant Worker Safety Checklist, was developed to collect restaurant-level information about the presence of required labor law postings, occupational hazards, and safety measures, equipment, and behaviors. The health department partner, the San Francisco Department of Public Health (SFDPH), took the lead on the development of the checklist,[53] with additional inputs from community and academic partners and health department food inspection staff. RWLG members' recommendations resulted in important improvements to the final tool. As they pointed out, for example, the checklist should not only assess whether posters detailing Occupational Safety and Health Administration's regulations and San Francisco's wage ordinance were present but also whether Chinese language versions were posted. Further, the checklist should not just assess whether first aid kits were visible but document whether they were fully stocked (82% of restaurants did not have fully stocked kits).[51,53]

The SFDPH was solely responsible for the administration of the checklist. However, community and university partners shadowed health department staff during checklist piloting. This enhanced partners' understanding of the types of challenges present in restaurants that affect both data collection and worker health.

Participation in Data Analysis and Interpretation

The collaborative was successful in exceeding research targets. Surveys were completed with 433 restaurant workers and observational data using the Restaurant Worker Safety Checklist were collected by health department staff in 98%

of Chinatown restaurants that were open for business at the time of data collection (n = 106 of 108 possible restaurants). Once data were collected, the partnership followed an agreed upon process for preparing and analyzing the findings. This process included all partners and was designed to build upon partners' existing skills and expertise (e.g., data analysis and knowledge of local context) as well as codeveloping and enhancing additional skills necessary for improved interpretation of study results (e.g., "outsiders" understanding of local culture and context and RWLG members' knowledge of how to read data tables).

University partners took the lead in preparing and analyzing the survey data, and health department partners did so for the observational restaurant-level data. During the analysis period, preliminary results were routinely shared with all partners through email communications and presentations at Steering Committee, RWLG, and other project meetings. A critical component of the analysis phases of the study was the ongoing involvement of restaurant workers in data interpretation. Six monthly data interpretation workshops were held with the RWLG members at CPA's office in Chinatown. These workshops, conducted in Chinese by CPA staff and the project coordinator with additional support from other university and health department partners, employed hands-on learning to teach RWLG members to speak "data language" and to facilitate their participation in the interpretation of checklist and survey findings.

RWLG members provided many insights into the data not originally apparent to other partners. For example, when considering findings indicating that cooks wore long-sleeved shirts or cook jackets in only 10% of restaurant observations conducted, RWLG members suggested that, in addition to the high kitchen temperatures, this was likely due to Chinese male cooks' viewing of burns and cuts as "badges of honor."[51] Similarly, RWLG members helped identify and provide context for some survey findings that they believed to be over-reported due to workers' fears of employer retaliation or misinterpretation. For example, the RWLG doubted that 58% of restaurant worker respondents actually received paid sick days, as reported, explaining, "When people ask for a day off, they work another day later . . . workers often understand this [having to make up a day for taking a sick day] as sick leave." Similarly, the RWLG explained that some of the statistics related to health, such as

general health status and work-related injuries, were likely underestimated due to the fact that many workers would only report major problems "like cancer." One member summed up this phenomenon, saying that Chinese workers think that "unless you're *really* sick, you're healthy." RWLG members felt that the same phenomenon resulted in an underreporting of abusive treatment at work such as being yelled at (reported by 42%). RWLG felt that those responding in the affirmative were probably only those for whom the "yelling had made them cry," explaining that they are constantly being yelled at by their supervisors.[51]

The in-depth participation of all partners in data analysis and interpretation resulted in all partners, including restaurant workers themselves, having a detailed knowledge of study findings. This greatly enhanced equitable and high-level involvement in dissemination of study results as well as the use of data in the creation of translational strategies, discussed below.

Community and Stakeholder Participation in Disseminating and Translating Results into Programs and Policies

In contrast to the research phase of the study, in which the researchers, in many ways, took the lead on guiding activities, the community and health department partners led in the "final phase" of the Chinatown CBPR effort. The partnership's dissemination plan included sharing study findings through both scientific and lay/ethic media as well as targeted meetings with restaurant workers, restaurant owners, and key policy and decision-makers. Recognizing that diverse purposes and audiences would require different types of communications, the partnership created several different reports to share findings: (1) a report of worker survey findings authored by university partners;[56] (2) a report of restaurant observation findings written by health department partners;[57] and (3) a comprehensive, visually appealing and action-oriented, report authored by CPA[58] that draws from the two previous reports to lay out a vision for improving working conditions for a healthy Chinatown. The collaborative's dissemination activities, like other CBPR efforts,[59,60] were guided by agreements regarding publication and presentation established early in the study. These guidelines emphasize co-ownership of data and co-authorship. To date, all partners have participated in presenting study findings and have served as co-authors on the peer-reviewed papers published to date.[51, 52, 61]

Multiple efforts were undertaken to translate study findings into sustainable improvements for Chinatown restaurant workers. As a result of the significant lack of labor law posting documented in this study (e.g., only 15% of observed restaurants had posted workers' compensation in English and 8% in Chinese; just 24% had the city's sick leave regulation posted in English and 23% in Chinese), and the results of a subsequent study to examine compliance with labor law posting in restaurants within and beyond Chinatown, SFDPH began requiring proof of workers' compensation insurance coverage for all new and change-of-business health permits. The health department also took additional steps to assess citywide compliance with these policies. For example, as a result of study findings that 50% of Chinatown restaurant workers did not receive minimum wage, 52% reported not receiving paid sick leave, 40% didn't received mandated work breaks, and 97% did not receive the City's required health care coverage,[61] SFDPH sent formal letters to regulatory bodies such as the local Office of Labor Standards Enforcement (OSLE) to share study findings and request collaboration in improving enforcement of these laws. OLSE and SFDPH ultimately began coordinating efforts to identify and revoke the health permits of labor law violators.

CPA led a number of efforts to implement or support action interventions based on study findings that demonstrated the existence of widespread wage theft and other regulatory violations, which culminated in the groundbreaking passage of a citywide anti-wage theft enforcement ordinance. Half of all workers surveyed reported earning below the legal minimum wage, three quarters did not receive legally required overtime pay, and 64% did not receive any mandated health and safety training at work. CPA held a press event to launch its action-oriented report[58] of study findings in September 2010, with many project partners and close to 170 community members, neighborhood organization representatives, media personnel, and policymakers in attendance. The event received widespread media coverage in local newspapers, television and radio programs, as well as online. Subsequently, CPA cofounded the Progressive Workers Alliance (PWA), which initiated a Low Wage Worker Bill of Rights organizing campaign to create support for policy change. At a kickoff event on the steps of the City Hall in Spring 2011, CPA and the PWA introduced a multipronged policy approach to preventing or redressing wage theft and related violations, as well as improving worker education and protection for employer retaliation. When speaking on the bill he cosponsored, a prominent local Supervisor remarked, "I am proud to be introducing local legislation that is drawn from action-based research and bottom-up grassroots organizing that will help strengthen labor law enforcement in San Francisco and give workers a meaningful voice in stopping wage theft in our city." The Board of Supervisors unanimously passed the bill in 2011, and then again unanimously passed legislation creating a dedicated Wage Theft Ordinance Task Force to promote enforcement in 2012. These policy actions, along with increased capacity of the community organization resulting from the project, would prove pivotal to CPA's success in several important organizing efforts that followed, including one involving a $4 million settlement between a restaurant and its workers in 2014.[62]

CPA additionally engaged in extensive community education efforts that included monthly worker teas and exchanges with other workers and worker rights groups around San Francisco and nationally (e.g., at the U.S. Social Forum). Further, since no study of this magnitude had previously been conducted with Chinese restaurant workers in the Umited States, and since restaurants remain the largest employer of immigrant Chinese workers throughout the nation,[49] study findings have been cited by worker centers and other organizations in New York, Los Angeles, and other major cities. Finally, the community capacity that CPA was able to build during the study through the acquisition of a major grant, increased visibility, and particularly through new worker partners engaged through the project who would serve as part of CPA's community leadership core for years to come, has contributed to the organization's expanded ability to organize and lead on economic and racial justice movements both locally and nationally.

Other dissemination activities undertaken by members of the partnership included efforts by the Labor Occupational Health Program and the SFDPH to investigate the potential for disseminating the Restaurant Worker Checklist to other health departments within California. The sharing of the final report of restaurant observation findings and the project's observational check list tool through the SFDPH's website, and articles and book chapters published about various dimensions of the study from the check list[50, 52] to the worker leadership development processes[63] to analysis of policy change success,[61] also are expected to help facilitate the dissemination process.

Lessons Learned and Implications for D&I Research

The Chinatown Restaurant Worker Project in many ways exemplifies the potential value of CBPR for improving the relevance of research and enhancing the dissemination and implementation of findings through collaborative design, analysis, dissemination, and research translation. Drawing on this and other participatory research case studies, as well as the now substantial body of literature in the field of CBPR, we present key lessons learned and their implications for research dissemination and implementation.

Through the codevelopment of research priorities and design with community and other stakeholders, CBPR can help ensure that the research is relevant to the community, potentially helping improve its external validity.[64] Further, such cogeneration of research topics and study design can enhance buy-in and shared commitment on the part of all partners in moving from research to action. In the Chinatown CBPR study and numerous others,[6,7,20,31,66] the participation of community partners in the design of research instruments resulted in the generation of new survey items and improved data gathering tools that in turn proved critical to a fuller understanding of the topic under investigation—and the design of subsequent research-based action.

Inclusion of multiple stakeholders, including but not limited to a strong community partner, also is advised. As illustrated in the Chinatown case study, having as a partner a local health department can be important for gaining entrée into the community and to environments (i.e., worksites) that otherwise would likely be "off limits." Further, including as partners one or more policymakers, and/or having a strong policy mentor, may be critical for those partnerships wishing to help affect broader, systems-level change. In West Oakland, California, a CBPR partnership to study and address the large number of diesel trucks driving through and idling in a low-income portside community, profited early on by including a local city council member as a policy mentor and active partner. By holding monthly meetings in the councilor's office, where study findings were discussed and a proposed new truck route ordinance designed, the partnership was able to get many disparate stakeholders to the table, and several subsequent policy wins followed in part as a result.[67]

The special benefits of a participatory approach for dissemination of study findings through diverse channels and to multiple audiences also should be underscored. Publication of study methods and findings in respected peer-reviewed journals is, of course, critical, both for extending the study's reach and underscoring its scientific merit. Yet as Canadian scholar Dennis Raphel is fond of asking, "If an article is published in *Social Science and Medicine* but nobody reads it, does it exist?" A prolific scholar himself, Raphel's message is not to *avoid* publishing, but rather to ensure that we don't stop there. Many CBPR partnerships, including the Chinatown study, have a special subcommittee that helps to ensure the wide dissemination of findings through a diversified strategy. Proposed journal articles and abstracts for presentations at professional meetings, typically with community partner co-authors, are reviewed by these committees. But attention also is focused on effective use of the mass media (including local language newspapers), presentations at community forums, development of policy briefs based on study findings, and other nonacademic means of disseminating findings to promote education and action. The involvement of multiple stakeholders, especially those "in" the community, increases the capacity to disseminate findings in a meaningful and culturally appropriate way.

Furthermore, as in the Chinatown project, the inclusion of a health department may enhance the partnerships' ability to speak the "language" of, and have greater success in engaging, regulators and policymakers in organizational- and policy-level interventions to address research findings. As an inherently collaborative and colearning process, CBPR enhances the expertise and capacity of all partners for culturally appropriate research and prevention that addresses contextual factors. While university partners bring research expertise to the table, the inclusion of community and health department partners, who often are more skilled in organizing and policy advocacy than their academic counterparts, can be critical for ensuring that findings are translated more broadly into innovative actions to address social, economic, and political determinants of health. Such actions may be more likely to result in sustainable and long-term impacts than more traditional health and public health interventions.[40,68]

Ethical and methodological challenges will almost invariably emerge in the course of a CBPR effort—a fact that underscores the importance of preparing, in advance via MOUs or less formal mechanisms, as well as encouraging ongoing dialogue around tough issues such as funding and workload equity. Although as noted, useful instruments have been developed to help guide such discussions,[41-43] the unique composition and needs of each partnership suggest the utility of tailoring such tools, or devising new ones, to best serve a particular partnership.

Among the most challenging aspects of CBPR, with special relevance to D&I research, is that this orientation to research requires a long-term commitment from all partners. In addition to the added time involved in front-end partnership building and maintenance (e.g., involving numerous steering committee and advisory board meetings, community meetings, retreats, etc.), the translation and action phases of such work may often not take place until after the funded research period. In a Harlem, New York based CBPR effort to promote the successful community reintegration of former substance abusing inmates, several key policy victories were achieved only well after the project's federal support had ended. Had the Harlem Community and Academic Partnership members not continued to work together, the impressive policy changes to which they contributed, including legislation mandating discharge planning services, help finding housing and drug treatment services, and reinstatement of Medicaid coverage immediately upon release from prison or jail, might never have been achieved.[68] Complicated issues take time to understand and address, and rarely align neatly with academic or community partner timetables.

Successful translation and use of CBPR findings also may require obtaining additional funding, including some from nongovernmental and other sources that can constrict or preclude advocacy on behalf of relevant legislation. In the Chinatown case study, substantial supplemental funding from a large and progressive foundation committed to policy-level change, with the community partner as the lead agency, proved particularly suited for translating study finding into policy-level interventions. Yet philanthropic organizations differ in their support for policy

related activities, and CBPR partnerships whose goals include action on the legislative level should determine in advance whether and to what extent their funding source(s) will support and/or even allow such activity.

SUMMARY

An inherently action-focused research orientation, CBPR is particularly wellsuited to D&I research. As suggested in this chapter, although CBPR is not relevant in all or even most research contexts, when there is goodness-of-fit between this orientation to research and a proposed study, significant value can be added to both the processes and outcomes of the research. Prominent among the latter are enhanced dissemination and implementation of findings through the authentic engagement of community partners and other stakeholders throughout. In the discussion of CBPR, and the use of the Chinatown Restaurant Worker Study to illustrate its principles in action, this chapter has highlighted many of the benefits CBPR can offer to research and its dissemination and implementation. Drawing on this and other CBPR case studies and literature, the authors also have suggested a number of implications that CBPR holds for dissemination and implementation research and bridging the gap between research and practice.

In concluding, the authors would like to emphasize an additional and important strength that CBPR offers for reducing health disparities. When conducted in accordance with its key tenets and principles, CBPR can be an important paradigm for promoting not only health equity in the sense of distributive justice, but also the "procedural justice"[69] necessary for real change to take place, and be sustained over time. Procedural justice has been described as involving "equitable processes through which low-income communities of color, rural residents, and other marginalized groups can have a seat at the table—and stay at the table—having a real voice in decision-making affecting their lives."[37] In the words of one RWLG member from the Chinatown study, involvement in a CBPR study and its subsequent translational efforts can yield, "courage to confront problems in [our] community." Through reciprocal capacity building of diverse partners; the establishment of "structures for participation"; and the provision, especially for underrepresented communities, of a "place" for their voices to be heard and a way to make change,[37] CBPR can be a potent mechanism for addressing some of the social and other inequalities at the heart of many health disparities.

SUGGESTED READINGS AND WEBSITES

Readings

Cargo M, Mercer SL. The value and challenges of participatory research: strengthening its practice. *Annu Rev Public Health.* 2008;29:325–350.

This thorough and sophisticated article on CBPR in the health field provides a critical review of the literature, followed by an "integrative practice framework" highlighting key domains including values and drivers (such as knowledge transfer and self-determination), partnership processes, and the interpretation and application of research outcomes.

Wallerstein N, Duran B, Oetzel, J and Minkler M, *Community-based participatory research for health: Advancing social and health equity.* 3rd ed. NY: Wiley and Sons; 2017.

The first major volume on CBPR in the health field in the United States this co-edited text, now in its 3rd edition, includes 23 chapters and 12 appendixes covering a wide range of theoretical, methodological, ethical, and practical issues and tools, with a special emphasis on policy and other health-related outcomes. Key topics include the theoretical and practice roots of CBPR; a conceptual pathways model of CBPR contexts, dynamics, and outcome; issues of power, race and racism, and trust in working cross-culturally; ethical and methodological challenges; participatory evaluation; and CBPR as a strategy for policy change. Numerous case studies and practical tools are included.

Selected Websites and Tools

The Community Tool Box. (http://ctb.ku.edu)
Created by the Work Group for Community Health and Development at the University of Kansas, and over 9,000 pages in length, this well-organized website offers numerous tools for participatory community assessment and evaluation, as well as other aspects of CBPR and related approaches.

Campus Community Partnerships for Health. ccph. info@gmail.com
CCPH is a nonprofit membership organization that promotes health equity and social justice through partnerships between communities and universities. The CCPH website and large list serve provide numerous updates about funding and job opportunities, useful tools, forthcoming meetings and other events.

REFERENCES

1. Green L, George M, Daniel M, et al. *Study of participatory research in health promotion.* Ottawa: The Royal Society of Canada; 1994.

2. De Las Nueces D, Hacker K, DiGirolamo A, Hicks LS. A systematic review of community-based participatory research to enhance clinical trials in racial and ethnic minority groups. *Health Serv Res.* 2012;47(3pt2):1363–1386.

3. Israel BA, Schulz AJ, Parker EA, Becker AB. Review of community-based research: assessing partnership approaches to improve public health. *Annu Rev Public Health.* 1998;19:173–202.

4. Cornwall A, Jewkes R. What is participatory research? *Soc Sci Med.* 1995;41(12):1667–1676.

5. Cargo M, Mercer SL. The value and challenges of participatory research: strengthening its practice. *Annu Rev Public Health.* 2008;29:325–350.

6. Cacari-Stone L, Wallerstein N Cacari-Stone L., Wallerstein, N., Garcia A. P, & Minkler M. The promise of community-based participatory research for health equity: a conceptual model for bridging evidence with policy. *Am J Public Health,* 2014;104(9):1615–1623.

7. Minkler M. Enhancing data quality, relevance and use through Community-Based Participatory Research. In Cytron N, Petit K and Kinglsey GT, senior eds. *What counts? Harvesting data for America's communities* (245–259). Washington DC: Federal Reserve Bank of San Francicso and the Urban Institute; 2014:245–259.

8. Wallerstein N, Duran B, Oetzel J, Minkler M. Introduction to CBPR. In: Wallerstein N, Duran B, Oetzel J, Minkler M, eds. *Community-based participatory research for health: Advancing social and health equity.* 3rd ed. San Francisco: Wiley and Sons; 2017: In Press.

9. W.K. Kellogg Foundation Community Health Scholars Program. *Stories of Impact* [brochure]. Ann Arbor, MI: University of Michigan, School of Public Health, Community Health Scholars Program, National Program Office; 2001.

10. Glasgow RE, Emmons KM. How can we increase translation of research into practice? Types of evidence needed. *Annu Rev Public Health.* 2007;28:413–433.

11. Horowitz CR, Robinson M, Seifer S. Community-based participatory research from the margin to the mainstream: are Researchers Prepared? *Circulation.* 2009;119:2633–2642.

12. Balazs CL, Morello-Frosch R. The three R's: how community based participatory research strengthens the rigor, relevance and reach of science. *Environ Justice.* 2013;6(1):9–16. doi: 10.1089/env.2012.0017

13. Deloria V, Jr Commentary: research, redskins, and reality. *Am Indian Q.* 1991;15(4):457–468.

14. Trickett EJ. Community-based participatory research as worldview or instrumental strategy: is it lost in translation(al) research? *Am J Public Health.* 2011;101(8):1353–1355.

15. Cyril S, Smith BJ, Possamai-Inesedy A, Renzaho AMN. Exploring the role of community engagement in improving the health of disadvantaged populations: a systematic review. *Global Health Action*. 2015;8:29842. doi: 10.3402/gha.v3408.29842.

16. O'Mara-Eves A, Brunton G, Oliver S, Kavanagh J, Jamal F, Thomas J. The effectiveness of community engagement in public health interventions for disadvantaged groups: a meta-analysis. *BMC Public Health*. 2015;15(1):129.

17. Salimi Y, Shahandeh K, Malekafzali H, et al. Is community-based participatory research (cbpr) useful? A systematic review on papers in a decade. *Int J Prev Med*. 2012;3(6):386–393.

18. Banks, S, Armstrong, A, Carter, K, Graham, H, Hayward, P, Henry, P et al. Everyday ethics in community-based participatory research, *Contemp Soc Sci*. 2013;8(3):263–277. doi: 10.1080/21582041.2013.769618

19. Corburn, J and Karanja, I. Informal settlements and a relational view of health. *Health Promot Int*. 2014;31(2) 258–269. doi: 10.1093/heapro/dau100

20. Israel BA, Eng E, Schultz A, Parker E. *Methods in community-based participatory research for health*. 2nd ed. San Francisco, CA: Jossey-Bass; 2012.

21. Tervalon M, Murray-Garcia J. Cultural humility versus cultural competence: a critical distinction in defining physician training outcomes in multicultural education. *J Health Care Poor Underserved*. 1998;9(2):117–125.

22. Reason P, Bradbury H. *Handbook of action research: Participative inquiry and practice (Concise ed.)*. Thousand Oaks, CA: Sage; 2008.

23. Green, LW and Glasgow, RE. Evaluating the relevance, generalization and applicability of research: issues in external validation and and translation methodology. *Eval Health Prof*. 2006; 29(1):126–153.

24. Schillinger D. An introduction to effectiveness, dissemination and implementation research. In: P. Fleisher and E. Goldstein e, eds. *UCSF Clinical and Translational Science Institute (CTSI) Resource Manuals and Guides to Community-Engaged Research*. San Francisco: Clinical Translational Science Institute Community Engagement Program, University of California San Francisco; 2010: 1–12.

25. Lorig KR, Sobel DS, Ritter PL, Laurent D, Hobbs M. Effect of a self-management program on patients with chronic disease. *Eff Clin Pract*. 2001;4(6):256–262.

26. Jernigan VB. Community-based participatory research with Native American communities: the Chronic Disease Self-Management Program. *Health Promot Pract*.2010;11(6):888–899.

27. Jernigan VB, Lorig K. The Internet diabetes self-management workshop for American Indians and Alaska Natives. *Health Promot Pract*. 2011;12(2):261–270.

28. Rosas LG, Vasquez JJ, Naderi R, Jeffery N, Hedlin H, Qin F et al., Development and evaluation of an enhanced diabetes prevention program with psychosocial support for urban American Indians and Alaska Natives: a randomized controlled trial" *Contemp Clin Trials J*. 2016;50:28–36. doi: 10.1016/j.cct.2016.06.015.

29. Kaplan SA, Dillman KN, Calman N, Billings J. Opening doors and building capacity: employing a community-based approach to surveying. *J Urban Heatlh*. 2004;81:291–300.

30. Kreiger J, Allen C, Robersts J, Ross L, Takaro T. What's with the wheezing? Methods used by the Seattle-King County Healthy Homes Project to assess exposure to indoor asthma triggers. In: Israel BA, Eng E, Schultz A, Parker E, eds. *Methods in community-based participatory research for health*. San Francisco, CA: Jossey-Bass; 2005:230–250.

31. Green LW, Glasgow RE, Atkins D, Stange K. Making evidence from research more relevant, useful, and actionable in policy, program planning, and practice: Slips "twixt cup and lip." *Am J Prev Med*. 2009;37(6S1):S187–S191.

32. Williams DR, Mohammed SA. Racism and health II: A needed research agenda for effective interventions. *Am Behav Sci*. 2013;57(8). doi: 10.1177/0002764213487341.

33. Buchanan D, Miller F, Wallerstein N. Ethical issues in community-based participatory research: balancing rigorous research with community participation in community intervention studies. *Prog Comm Hlth Partn*. 2007;1.2:153–160.

34. Jones D, Franklin C, Butler BT, Williams P, Wells KB, Rodriguez MA. The Building Wellness project: a case history of partnership, power sharing, and compromise. *Ethn Dis*. 2006;16(1 Suppl 1):S54–S66.

35. Bowen C, Jones L, Dixon EL, Miranda J, Wells K. Using a community partnered participatory research approach to implement a randomized controlled trial: planning community partners in care. *J Health Care Poor Underserved*. 2009;21(780–795).

36. Cashman SB, Adeky S, Allen A,III, Corburn, J, Israel, BA et al. The power and the promise: working with communities to analyze data, interpret findings and get to outcomes. *Am J Public Health*. 2008;98(8):1407–1417. doi: 10.2105/AJPH.2007.113571

37. Minkler M. Linking Science and Policy Through community-based participatory research to

eliminate health disparities. *Am J Public Health.* 2010;100(Suppl 1):S81–S87.

38. Vasquez VB, Lanza D, Hennessey-Lavery S, Facente S, Halpin HA, Minkler M. Addressing food security through public policy action in a community-based participatory research partnership. *Health Promot Pract.* 2007;8(4):342–349.

39. Flood J, Minkler M, Estrada J, Hennessey-Lavery S and Falbe J. Healthy Retail as a strategy for tobacco control and food justice: a case study of collective impact. *Health Educ Behav.* 2015;42(5):654–668.

40. Hennessey-Lavery S. Building Healthy Corner Stores and Healthy Communities. Healthy Retail SF Report 2016. Office of Economic and Workforce Development (OEWD) and Department of Public Health. http://oewd.org/sites/default/files/Documents/HRSF_Package_8.5x11-v10.pdf Accessed 1-31-17.

41. Mercer SL, Green LW, Cargo M, et al. Reliability-tested guidelines for assessing participatory research projects. In: Minkler M, Wallerstein N, eds. *Community-based participatory research for health: from process to outcomes.* San Franciso, CA: Jossey-Bass; 2nd ed. 2008:408–418.

42. Israel BA, Lantz PM, McGranaghan RJ, Guzman JR, Lichtenstein, R and Z Rowe. Closed-Ended Survey Questionnaire: Detroit Community-Academic Urban Research Center, Detroit URC Board Evluation 1997-2007. In: Israel BA, Eng E, Schultz A, Parker E, eds. *Methods in Community-Based Participatory Research for Health.* 2nd ed. San Francisco, CA: Jossey-Bass; 2013:627–638.

43. Butterfoss, FD and Kegler, MC. A Community Model for Coalition Action. In: Minkler M, ed. Community Organizing for Health and Welfare, 3rd ed. New Brucswick, NJ; Rutgers University Press: 309–328.

44. Farquhar S, Wing S. *Methodological and ethical considerations in community-driven environmental justice research: Two case studies from rural North Carolina.* In: Minkler M, Wallerstein N, eds. *Community-based participatory research: from process to outcome.* 2nd ed. San Francisco, CA: Jossey-Bass; 2008:263–280.

45. Flicker S, Travers R and Guta A. Broadening the bandwidth of ethics. In: Wallerstein N, Duran B, Oetzel J, Minkler M, eds. *Community-based participatory research for health: Advancing social and health equity.* 3rd ed. San Francisco: Wiley and Sons; 2017; In Press.

46. Flicker S, Travers R, Guta A, McDonald S and Meagher A. Ethical Dilemmas in Community-Based Participatory Research: Recommendations for Institutional Review Boards. *Journal of Urban Health: Bulletin of the New York Academy of Medicine.* 2007;84(4). doi:10.1007/s11524-007-9165-7.

47. Jayaraman S. *Behind the kitchen door.* Ithaca:,NY: ILR Press, 2013.

48. Restaurant Opportunities Center of New York (ROC-NY). *Behind the kitchen door: Pervasive inequality in New York's thriving restaurant industry.* New York: Restaurant Opportunities Center of New York and the New York City Restaurant Industry Coalition; 2005.

49. U.S. Census Bureau. *American Community Survey San Francisco, CA General Demographic Characteristics: 2004.* Suitland, MD: Author; 2004.

50. Minkler M, Tau Lee P, Tom A, et al. Using community-based participatory research to design and initiate a study on immigrant worker health and safety in San Francisco's Chinatown restaurants. *Am J Ind Med.* 2010;53(4):361–371.

51. Chang C, Minkler M, Salvatore A, Lee P, Gaydos M, Liu S. Studying and addressing urban immigrant restaurant worker health and safety in San Francisco's Chinatown District: A CBPR case study. *J Urban Health.* 2013;80(6):1026–1040.

52. Chang C, Salvatore A, Lee P, et al. Adapting to context in community-based participatory research: "participatory starting points" in a Chinese immigrant worker community. *Am J Community Psychol.* 2013;51(3-4):480–491.

53. Gaydos M, Bhatia R, Morales A, et al. Promoting health and safety in San Francisco's Chinatown Restaurants: findings and lessons learned from a pilot observational checklist. *Public Health Rep.* 2011;126(Suppl 3):62–69.

54. Mujica J. Coloring the hazards: risk maps research and education to fight health hazards. *Am J Ind Med.* 1992;22(5):767–770.

55. Brown MP. Risk mapping as a tool for community-based participatory research and organizing. In: Minkler M, Wallerstein N, eds. *Community-based participatory research for health.* 2nd ed. San Francisco, CA: Jossey-Bass; 2008:453–458.

56. San Francisco Department of Public Health. *Health and safety in San Francisco's Chinatown Restaurants: Findings from an observational survey.* San Francisco: Author; 2009.

57. Salvatore AL, Krause N. *Health and working conditions of restaurant workers in San Francisco's Chinatown: Report of survey findings.*: UC Berkeley and UC San Francisco; 2010.

58. Chinese Progressive Association. *Check please!: Health and working conditions in San Francisco Chinatown Restaurants.* San Francisco: Author; 2010.

59. Wing S, Horton RA, Muhammad N, Grant GR, Mansoureh T, et al. Integrating epidemiology, education, and organizing for

environmental justice: community health effects of industrial hog operations. *Am J Public Health.* 2008;98(8):1390–1397.

60. Parker E, Israel B, Robins T, et al. Evaluation of Community Action Against Asthma: a community health worker intervention to improve children's asthma-related health by reducing household environmental triggers for asthma. *Health Educ Behav.* 2008;35(3):376–395.

61. Minkler M, Salvatore AL, Chang C, et al. Wage Theft as a neglected public health problem: an overview and case study from San Francisco's Chinatown District. *Am J Public Health.* 2014;104(6):1010–1020.

62. Hua V. The dim sum revolution. *San Francisco Magazine.* 2015;62(4).

63. Chang C, AL S, Lee P, Liu S, Minkler M. Popular education, participatory research, and community organizing with immigrant workers in Chinatown Restaurants: A case study. In: Minkler M, ed. *Community organizing and community building for health and welfare.* 3rd ed. Rutgers, NJ: Rutgers University Press; 2012.

64. Green LW, Glasgow RE, Atkins D, Stange K. Making evidence from research more relevant, useful, and actionable in policy, program planning, and practice: Slips "twixt cup and lip." *Am J Prev Med.* 2009;37(6S1)S187–S191.

65. Minkler M, Garcia, A, Rubin, V, Wallerstein, N. *Community-based participatory research: A strategy for building healthy communities and promoting health through policy change.* Oakland, CA: PolicyLink; 2012.

66. Morello-Frosch R, Pastor MJ, Sadd J, Porras C, Prichard M. *Citizens, science and data judo: Leveraging secondary data analysis to build a community-academic collaborative for environmental justice in Southern California.* In: Israel BA, Eng E, Schultz A, Parker E, eds. *Methods in community -based participatory research for health.* San Francisco, CA: Jossey-Bass; 2005: 371–393.

67. Gonzalez P, Minkler M, Gordon M, Garica A, et al. Community-based—participatory research and policy advocacy to reduce diesel exposure in West Oakland, California. *Am J Public Health.* 2011;101 Suppl 1:S166–S175.

68. Minkler M, Freudenberg N. From community-based participatory research to policy change. In: Fitzgerald H, Burack C, Seifer S, eds. *Handbook for engaged scholarship: contemporary landscapes, future directions Vol. 2: Institutional Change.* East Lansing, MI.: Michigan State University; 2013:275–294.

69. Kuehn R. A taxonomy of environmental justice. *Environ Law Reporter.* 2000;30(10681–10703).

12

Enhancing Dissemination Though Marketing and Distribution Systems

A Vision for Public Health

JOSEPH T. STEENSMA, MATTHEW W. KREUTER,
CHRISTOPHER M. CASEY, AND JAY M. BERNHARDT

INTRODUCTION

The long lag time between discovery of new knowledge and its application in public health and clinical settings is well documented[1] and described in numerous other chapters in this book. Along this evidence-to-practice cycle, there is no shortage of evidence-based approaches and empirically supported programs to enhance the public's health,[2,3] but there are few *systems* in place to bring these discoveries to the attention of practitioners and into use in practice settings. In business, the process of taking a product or service from the point of development to the point of use by consumers is carried out by a *marketing and distribution system*.[4] In previous work, the authors have argued that marketing and distribution responsibilities within the broad public health system are largely unassigned, underemphasized and/or underfunded for disseminating effective public health programs, and without them widespread adoption of evidence-based approaches is unlikely.[5] By understanding and applying fundamentals of marketing, efforts to disseminate public health solutions could be more effective. This chapter builds on our earlier work by (1) providing a framework from which to understand marketing, (2) proposing three specific components of a marketing and distribution system for evidence-based public health practices, and (3) describing how the potential benefits of such a system could be evaluated through dissemination research.

A CASE STUDY

In the late 1990s, a team of public health researchers in St. Louis, MO created the ABC Immunization Calendar. It was a simple computer software program designed to help community health centers boost low rates of immunization among babies and toddlers. The program used information from new parents and a digital photograph of their baby to create personalized monthly calendars that were given to the family during their baby's first 2 years of life. The calendars provided health and developmental information matched to the baby's age and reminders of the baby's next appointment in the vaccination series. Each time the parent and baby returned for a required vaccination, the program would take a new picture of the baby and print more months of the calendar (to cover the period leading to the next vaccination).

The program was well received in a pilot study[6] and increased child vaccination rates from 65% to 82% in an efficacy trial.[7] Based on these results, the research team obtained dissemination grant funding and adapted the program for widespread use.[8] A survey was conducted among potential user organizations to determine what computer platform and operating systems they were using. The ABC software was then reprogrammed to maximize compatibility with existing infrastructure. A user's guide was developed to help organizations install and use the program. An implementation guide was developed to help organizations decide how to integrate the program into their standard procedures and implement it. A promotional brochure with sample calendars and published articles was created and distributed at national meetings and to any person or organization that expressed interest. Training was provided, and some computer equipment was made available on loan. These efforts led to four Federally Qualified Health Centers (FQHCs) in the St. Louis area adopting the ABC Immunization Calendar. The program was delivered to thousands of families, and some centers used the program for many years.

Was the ABC Immunization Calendar a dissemination success? The research team adhered closely to conventional wisdom about translating public health science into practice. The intervention was tested for feasibility, acceptability, and efficacy in real-world settings. When positive results were found, the research team identified potential adopters, learned about their practice settings, and adapted the program accordingly. They created instruction manuals to help adopters use the software and to customize an implementation plan for their organization. They provided training and technical assistance. Local organizations adopted and used the program. But there are 7,500 FQHCs in the United States, reaching 17 million Americans. The ABC Immunization Calendar was adopted by four of them. In the grand scheme of things, the program's impact on the public's health was negligible.

Why didn't a program that's fast, easy, cheap and effective find a home in more FQHCs? What should the research team have done differently to maximize its adoption and use? This story illustrates the limitations of current approaches to disseminating evidence-based programs and the need for marketing and distribution systems to support those efforts. For example, it's not the case that 7,496 FQHCs rejected the ABC Immunization Calendar. Rather, they *never even heard of it*. And if they had heard of it and wanted to adopt it, how would they obtain a copy? Could a small, university-based research team duplicate and distribute software and instruction manuals to hundreds or thousands of potential adopters? Could such a team also provide timely training and technical assistance to a mass of users? Are they trained to do this? Would they know how to set up such an operation? Would they *want* to do it? Would their university reward them for spending time on this? Thus, even well-intentioned, dissemination-minded researchers trying to do the right thing and following recommendations that are nearly universally accepted today will run up against demands that they are not trained to understand or address, lack the capacity to carry out, and are not viewed as central to the mission of the organizations where they work.

FROM SOCIETAL NEEDS TO CUSTOMERS AND EVERYTHING IN BETWEEN

In the example, the Immunization Calendar program was developed to meet a specific societal need. There was a need to increase childhood vaccination rates, and a solution was developed that appeared to meet this need in an efficient and effective manner. In spite of its advantages, there was not widespread uptake of the solution. To understand why this was the case, it is useful to understand how solutions are developed, marketed, and ultimately adopted by end-users.

The old axiom that "necessity is the mother of invention" is accurate: most great advancements (in public health and otherwise) were made because society had an unmet need and enough people were impacted by the need to create a viable market for a solution. Unmet needs have costs associated with them, both personal and societal, and innovations bring value when the sum of their costs and benefits exceed the costs of the unmet need.[9]

If a need is big enough there may be several people or entities trying to innovate around that need. In the academic realm we often refer to these people as "colleagues," in business we call them "the competition." In theory, as more competitors move in to solve a problem, the market becomes more efficient as competitors jostle to have consumers adopt their products or services.[10] This is how markets are born and how they should behave. In a perfect world, the most valuable solutions persist, while less valuable solutions join laserdiscs and Betamax video tapes in the dustbin of failed innovations.

Note that value and effectiveness are not synonymous. Value is a product of effectiveness and cost. For example, "Solution A" might have a very low cost and good (but not great) effectiveness, whereas "Solution B" is slightly more effective, but ten times the cost. In this example, for most people "Solution A" is likely to be perceived as providing more value than "Solution B." As illustrated in the case of Immunization Calendars, however, even valuable innovations can fail to achieve widespread uptake. Is this evidence that market approaches don't apply in the context of research dissemination, or is there something beyond the value a solution brings to the market that needs to be taken into account?

A Framework

We have already established that all nearly innovations start with a need, but how does an innovation go from addressing a "theoretical need" to "widespread adoption" with actual customers? This is the real challenge for a dissemination oriented scientist; finding customers. It is incorrect to think of potential customers (users, clients) as any person or entity that might benefit from a particular solution. Rather, potential customers are a subset of that population, who have characteristics that make them amenable to trying a particular solution and have the means to adopt the solution.

Failure to properly identify customers is the undoing of many valuable innovations. These principles are partially grounded in diffusion theory[11](see chapter 3) and should be applied early in the research process so that innovations (often in the form of evidence-based interventions) can be better designed for dissemination (see chapter 7).[12]

To identify a customer one can ask these five questions (Figure 12.1):

- What is the need/problem?
- Who deals with the need/problem?
- How are they dealing with the need or problem?

- In what ways is your solution better?
- Who would value the ways in which your solution is better?

Although the questions are simple and straightforward, the answers are often complicated. But the answers will reveal critically important information:

- By identifying the problem one has identified the societal need.
- By identifying who deals with the problem, one has identified the market for the solution.
- By identifying the ways in which the market deals with the problem, one has identified the competition for their product or service.
- By identifying in what ways one's product or service is better, one has identified where the value lies. This is called *the value proposition*.
- If one can identify who would perceive the most benefit from the value proposition, one has identified the potential customers for the solution.

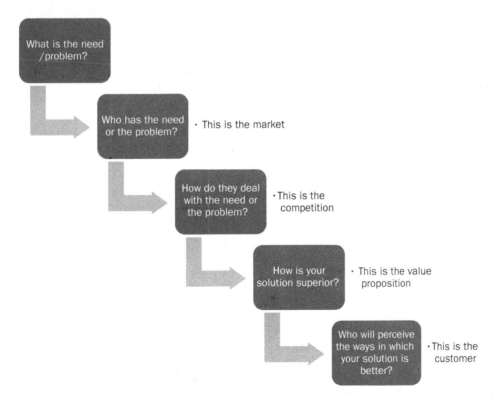

FIGURE 12.1 Five questions to identify customers, competitors, and a value proposition.

Returning to the Immunization Calendars example, researchers had identified the need and the market was clearly defined. Further, they understood how the market was dealing with the issue and had a service that was valuable. Researchers often have a deep understanding of the problems they are trying to solve and, at least sometimes, who in society is dealing with the problem. That said, in the Immunization Calendar case the researchers had not articulated a value proposition in the context of other alternatives, nor did they know who would value the Immunization Calendars over alternatives, one of which is maintaining the status quo. In other words, who are their target customers? Is it FQHCs? Public health departments? Social service agencies? New parents? The market for the service had been defined, but the customer had not. A better definition of the customer helps identify the proper channel(s) for reaching the customer.

The immunization calendar case elucidates common challenges for dissemination-oriented researchers. As challenging as it is to produce, deliver, and support innovations such as the immunization calendar, it is equally difficult to understand the competitive landscape and identify which segments of the market represent the best prospects for potential customers. Creating valuable solutions to society's challenges is not enough to garner widespread uptake if those solutions are unknown to those who would value them most and/or the solutions cannot be delivered effectively.

In short, the immunization calendar was not lacking in potential value to society, it was lacking in the areas of marketing and distribution. One way to address such deficiencies would be to better prepare individual researchers to think and act as marketers. Alternatively, public health might establish marketing and distribution systems designed to accelerate movement of proven solutions into practice.

A Marketing and Distribution Perspective

Marketing and distribution systems are designed to bring products and services from their point of development to their point of use. This typically occurs through a system of interconnected organizations or intermediaries.[4] Collectively, these intermediaries identify potential users, promote the product to them, provide them with easy access to the product through convenient (and usually local) channels, allow them to see and use the product before acquiring it, help them acquire it, and support the product after purchase if the buyer has questions or problems.[13] Without such systems, every "producer" would have to interact directly with every potential customer or user to promote, distribute, and support a product or program. As illustrated by the previous case example, such interaction would be impractical and inefficient, and in business practice it is rare.

In understanding how a marketing and distribution system might improve dissemination of evidence-based interventions into public health practice, three key characteristics of the business model stand out. First, there is specialization of labor. It is not expected that the person (or organization) that developed a product will be the same one that manufactures it, distributes it, promotes it, sells it, services it, and supports the users that buy it.

Second, each of these responsibilities is assigned. It is the primary responsibility of someone (or some organization) to assure that its part of the distribution chain is fulfilled. It is someone's job. If it's not carried out, they don't get paid.

Finally, all parts of the process are integrated. Even when carried out by different individuals (or organizations), these efforts are highly coordinated. In public health, most steps in the marketing and distribution process are unassigned, underemphasized, and underfunded. If they are undertaken at all, it is usually only as one of many responsibilities of someone who may lack the training or resources to do it well. And rarely are there financial or other tangible incentives for distributing or adopting evidence-based public health programs and services.

A SYSTEM FOR PUBLIC HEALTH

In the remainder of this chapter, three parts of a marketing and distribution system that could help bring more evidence-based interventions into public health practice are proposed and discussed. These are: (1) user review panels; (2) design and marketing teams; and (3) dissemination field agents. After each is described, a model system is presented that would incorporate all three in an integrated fashion.

User Review Panels

For several years *American Idol* was one of the most popular TV shows in the United States. On the show, aspiring singers competed to earn a recording contract. To identify contestants for the program, auditions were held in cities across the country. Tens of thousands of hopeful contestants waited hours to sing before a panel of judges comprised of professionals from the music industry. Only a dozen or so were chosen to be finalists and invited to appear on the TV program. Once on the program, these contestants performed and were critiqued by celebrity judges. Each week the TV audience voted for their favorite performer. The contestant who received the fewest votes was eliminated from the competition. This continued until there was only one contestant remaining, the winner. *American Idol* then invested heavily in developing, marketing, and promoting the music and career of this singer.

American Idol's process and format illustrates key differences between expert reviews and user reviews. Selecting the most talented 12 to 18 singers from 10,000+ aspirants was done by *expert review*. The judges evaluated auditioning singers based on a range of criteria they believe predicted success. This is not unlike the process of systematic evidence reviews in public health, wherein teams of scholars (i.e., experts) evaluate the strength of scientific findings for different types of interventions. Those with strong and consistent supporting evidence are "selected," and recommended for use in practice.

On *American Idol*, expert reviews were also provided after each song performed by a contestant. These critiques provided voters in the TV audience with some additional information on which they might base their decisions. But the viewing audience ultimately determined who won and lost. This is *user review*. Members of the voting audience were "users" because they would be the ones who purchased (or didn't) the music recorded by the winner. In essence, their votes reflect market demand for one singer versus another.

On *American Idol*, it's striking how often this market demand diverged from expert critiques. Why is that? One explanation is that not all viewers value the same things as music experts. Assuming that all of the finalists have a very high level of talent (and therefore a high likelihood of career success), it makes sense to leave this decision to market demand. We can apply the same logic to the process of disseminating evidence-based public health programs and strategies. When expert review has provided a menu of proven solutions, adopters and users (i.e., the market) will determine which, if any, meet their

own unique needs and preferences. Knowing this, and in the absence of high cost in-depth marketing research on intermediaries and end users, we should consider how to integrate formal user review processes into dissemination efforts in order to better identify potential customers/users.

We start with two assumptions: (1) not all evidence-based interventions will work equally well in real-world practice settings; and (2) there are insufficient resources to develop every successful (i.e., empirically supported) prototype into a program or policy for active dissemination to adopters. Thus, a primary goal of user review panels in public health dissemination would be to identify those evidence-based programs and approaches that adopters really want and believe can be implemented. In other words, identify programs and approaches likely to be in high demand by different market segments. Just like the winner of *American Idol*, this subset of evidence-based interventions would then receive priority treatment and resources to be developed, adapted and promoted for wider use. Programs and approaches not selected for focused development and marketing could still be adopted and used, but would not benefit from the same attention and resources.

Depending on the nature and type of evidence-based interventions being considered (and therefore, the types of organizations—*customers*—likely to adopt a particular program or approach), user review panels might include representatives from community-based organizations, schools, city planners, policy makers, state and local health departments, Federally Qualified Health Centers, health care systems, primary care providers, health foundations, and other organizations. These panels would review types of evidence-based based interventions (e.g., client reminder systems) as well as specific programs within each type. They could rate each on criteria like ease of use, organizational fit, implementation burden, acceptability to clients or patients, feasibility, as well as classic predictors of adoption such as relative advantage and trialability as described by Rogers (2003).[14] Interventions rated as most promising by a user review panel would be turned over to a design and marketing team to prepare them for widespread use and active promotion.

Design and Marketing Teams

At a 2002 *Designing for Dissemination* conference of invited researchers, practitioners, and intermediaries from across the United States, researchers were consistently the least likely to believe that translation and dissemination of research findings was their responsibility, felt unprepared in the science of dissemination and communication, and expressed that their interests and strengths were in areas other than translational work.[15] Researchers' interests and skills in translational science have grown in the 15 years since this meeting, although nearly one third of public health scientists surveyed rated their dissemination efforts as poor.[16] Formal training in disciplines related to the design, marketing, and distribution of public health programs and services is still uncommon, and there are few if any incentives—financial or otherwise—for researchers to actively disseminate their evidence-based public health programs.[17]

As noted in chapter 16 in this book and elsewhere,[18] greater attention to external validity during research design, analysis, and dissemination can help researchers and practitioners design programs that have higher translational potential. While agreeing that greater understanding of these steps would enhance the translational efforts of scientists, the authors argue that design and marketing functions are sufficiently important and complex and they require specialized expertise and dedicated personnel.

Although the details may vary case by case, there is a general sequence of actions that design and marketing teams carry out to make a promising product—like an evidence-based intervention—ready for the market. *Market research* is used to learn as much as possible about organizations or individuals that might adopt an intervention. What are their goals? How would this intervention help them achieve those goals? How would they use the intervention? How would it be integrated within their current client flow, operations, systems, and processes? Who within the organization would make the decision whether or not to adopt the intervention? Who would be responsible for implementing it? What are their concerns about the intervention? What would they change about the intervention?

Responses to questions like these would inform a wide range of design and distribution functions. For example, products routinely undergo *adaptation* or *reformulation* to maximize their appeal to potential users. If market research shows that potential adopters of a particular public health intervention are excited about feature X or concerned about feature Y, a smart design team

would adapt the intervention accordingly. Also, it is often the case that the version of a program used in research under controlled conditions is not yet ready for use in practice settings. Knowing how, by whom, and for what purposes it will be used will help a design team reshape and package the program for use in specific nonresearch settings. In the world of dissemination, success and failure is not measured in p-values and effect sizes, it is measured in uptake and satisfaction. To be successful in this context, an intervention must be malleable and the developers must be willing to continually refine (or even redefine) the intervention to maximize their customers' value.

Using *audience segmentation*, a design team can distinguish between different subgroups of users and create targeted marketing and distribution strategies for each. Audience segments might be defined by organization type (e.g., schools, public health departments, Federally Qualified Health Centers), populations served, intended use of the intervention, or any combination of these and other characteristics. What's important is that the characteristics shared within each subgroup, or segment, lead to distinct, actionable strategies for promoting and distributing the evidence-based intervention to specific types of potential customers. For example, different message strategies (e.g., "cost-effective" vs. "clients love it"), messengers (e.g., trusted peers vs. trade associations), and channels (e.g., conferences vs. online communities) might be indicated for different segments.

A design and marketing team would not only create the dissemination strategy, but would execute it as well. This would include many critical operational functions, including building partnerships; establishing a distribution system; providing training, technical assistance, and user support services; coordinating and evaluating the overall process; and creating tangible incentives and rewards for adoption. These and other operational functions of a marketing and distribution system have been described in the authors' previous work.[5] The question is not *whether* these functions are needed to more effectively disseminate evidence-based public health interventions, but rather *who* will perform them.[13] For the most part, they are currently unassigned. It is unrealistic to expect public health researchers to possess the skills and have the time and/or the organizational support that would be needed to do these tasks well. A dedicated public health design and marketing team would have both.

Dissemination Field Agents

What do real estate agents, travel agents, and talent agents have in common? Each has specialized expertise and provides assistance with complex tasks that are often unfamiliar to those who use their services. They do this through direct contact—in person, by phone, and/or electronically—with their clients. These interactions are usually goal directed: buying or selling a house, planning a trip, negotiating a contract.

In public health, a corps of dissemination field agents could operate in a similar fashion, as a kind of evidence-based public health sales force. These specialists would have extensive knowledge of evidence-based interventions and expertise in how to adapt and implement the interventions in different settings and for different populations. They would work closely and proactively with customers to help them understand and choose from available strategies. They could provide detailed information about specific evidence-based programs, approaches, or policies across health topics and practice settings. If an organization decided to try an intervention, dissemination field agents would help them prepare and succeed by providing training and ongoing technical assistance to adapt, implement, and evaluate the evidence-based program, practice, or policy they chose.

Additionally, they could provide valuable feedback to the design team about customers and their changing needs and preferences. Such agents would be the "boots on the ground" listening to the voice of the customer and providing needed feedback to the team. These field agents would have similar training and functions as the knowledge brokers described in chapter 2.

Elements of this approach have shown promise. New York City's Public Health Detailing Program aims to help primary care providers improve patient care related to key public health challenges like vaccination, cancer screening, obesity, and HIV testing.[19,20] Program representatives—*agents*, in our terminology—work in three communities with a high burden of poor health. They meet with doctors, physician assistants, nurse practitioners, and administrators to promote clinical preventive services and chronic disease management, and to distribute "detailing action kits" that include evidence summaries, patient education materials, other small media, referral forms, chart stickers, community resource guides, and lists of service providers. Other public health efforts like this, modeled after physician detailing by pharmaceutical representatives, have been around for at least 40 years,[21] though mostly on a local level.

Nationally, the National Cancer Institute's Cancer Information Service (CIS) created the Partnership Program to help put cancer control science into practice to eliminate health disparities.[22] The CIS hired and trained 45 partnership coordinators in 35 states. These staff developed relationships with local, regional, and national organizations for the purposes of sharing information and networking, jointly developing cancer control projects using evidence-based approaches in minority and medically underserved populations, and increasing the capacity of partners to move science into practice. With its national scope, emphasis on translating science into practice, and coordination under a single administrative unit (CIS), elements of the Partnership Program could be followed in establishing a corps of dissemination field agents. However, despite a promising start and numerous successes, the Program was short-lived and replaced by NCI's National Outreach Network.[23]

AN INTEGRATED APPROACH

How would these three recommendations—*User Review Panels, Design and Marketing Teams, and Dissemination Field Agents*—come together in a coordinated marketing and distribution system to bring more evidence-based interventions into public health practice? Here's one vision. Imagine a new administrative unit within one of the nation's public health agencies being charged with accelerating the translation of science to practice. A first step would be to identify the universe of evidence-based approaches and practices. This is easier today than it ever has been, with a growing number of inventories of effective programs as well as systematic evidence reviews like The Community Guide.[24]

User review panels would be charged with narrowing this pool of eligible interventions to a smaller set that addresses genuine user demand in ways that are highly appealing to potential adopters. Because the scope of this task would be great, it may be necessary to impose some initial restrictions, like focusing on evidence-based approaches that address leading causes of death and disease or setting up separate panels for specific practice settings and/or health problems. These user reviews would necessarily be ongoing, but would provide periodic priority rankings

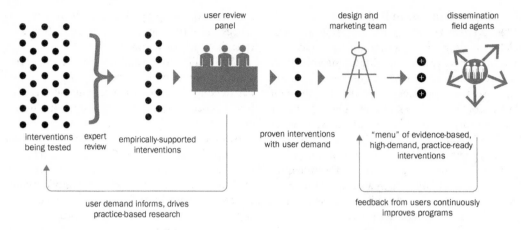

FIGURE 12.2 Marketing Teams and Dissemination Field Agents in a new system for moving evidence-based programs into public health practice.

of which evidence-based interventions were in greatest demand. A major collateral benefit of this process would be that its results, when shared, could redirect the efforts of public health scientists to better meet the needs of practice organizations, and even suggest specific partnerships for practice-based research.

These priority rankings would set the agenda for a *design and marketing team*. Starting with the highest priority interventions, the team would work closely with developers and potential adopters to: (1) define specific target audiences most likely to adopt each program; (2) make the programs ready for use in practice by these targeted adopters; and (3) develop strategies to effectively promote the program to these groups. Over time, the number of programs would grow. The result of these efforts would be an ever-expanding menu of evidence-based, high-demand, practice-ready programs. As user demand shifted (e.g., for emerging public health challenges), the items on the menu would expand accordingly.

This "menu" would establish the parameters of activity for a corps of *dissemination field agents*. Initially, agents would execute the plans of the design and marketing team. They would seek out organizations identified as potential adopters and share with them the menu of programs designed for their unique practice setting. They would aim to establish positive relationships with organizations, ideally viewed as trusted and competent sources of information about evidence-based public health and prevention programs. When organizations express interest in one or more menu item, agents would shift their focus

to providing technical assistance and support for implementation. One of the great advantages of having a field corps is that its members will quickly gain first-hand knowledge of the strengths and limitations of programs in different settings, and the challenges and solutions related to implementation. This invaluable information would inform ongoing and iterative activities of the design and marketing team via a formal feedback loop. It would also create a network of agents that could help each other (and each other's clients) by sharing their experiences.

Figure 12.2 illustrates how user review panels, design and marketing teams, and dissemination field agents might be linked in an integrated approach to disseminating evidence-based public health programs.

SUMMARY
It is undersstood that the vision of taking a more market-oriented approach to dissemination likely raises more questions than it answers. Who would build and operate such a system? Who would pay for it? Would researchers who have developed and evaluated public health interventions cooperate in sharing their programs and products? What tangible incentives can be created at each step of the process to encourage dissemination and adoption? What would constitute success for such an effort and how would we measure it? All are important questions and worthy of thoughtful answers that match their complexity. Doing so is beyond the scope of this chapter, but ongoing in our work. The authors hope the ideas presented here will stimulate others' thinking about systems

and infrastructure to enhance dissemination, and welcome critiques, refinement and additions to our proposed model.

SUGGESTED READINGS AND WEBSITES

Readings

Kreuter MW, Bernhardt J. Reframing the dissemination challenge: a marketing and distribution perspective. *Am J Public Health,* 2009;99(12):2123–2127.
Critiques current approaches to disseminating evidence-based public health programs and explains how and why a marketing and distribution system would enhance these efforts.

Kotler P, Keller KL. *Marketing management.* Harlow, England: Pearson Education Limited; 2016.
A useful introduction from an author with extensive experience in health and social marketing.

Larson K, Levy J, Rome MG, Matte TD, Silver LD, Frieden TR. Public health detailing: a strategy to improve the delivery of clinical preventive services in New York City. *Public Health Reps.* 2006;121(3):228–234.
Describes application of an "agent" model intervention to facilitate implementation of public health practices in primary care settings.

Ribisl KM, Leeman J, Glasser AM. Pricing behavior interventions to promote adoption: lessons from the marketing and business literature. *Am J Prevent Med.* 2014;46(6):653–659.
Outlines a new approach to public health interventions in which developers design effective and affordable interventions to fit an organization's budget.

Woolf SH, Purnell JQ, Simon SM, Zimmerman EB, Camberos GJ, Haley A, et al. Translating evidence into population health improvement: strategies and barriers. *Annu Rev Public Health.* 2015;36:463–482.
Reviews the four principles for successfully influencing population health, citing national and local examples.

Selected Websites and Tools

Cancer Control P.L.A.N.E.T. http://cancercontrol-planet.cancer.gov/index.html.
Cancer Control P.L.A.N.E.T. acts as a portal to provide access to data and resources for designing, implementing, and evaluating evidence-based cancer control programs. The site provides five steps (with links) for developing a comprehensive cancer control plan or program.

Diffusion of effective behavioral interventions. http://effectiveinterventions.org/en/home.aspx
Provides an inventory of effective HIV and STD prevention and control programs, as well as information on how to use them.

REFERENCES

1. Green L, Ottoson J, Garcia C, Hiatt R. Diffusion theory and knowledge dissemination, utilization and integration. *Annu Rev Public Health.* 2009;30:151–174.
2. Zaza S, Briss P, Harris K, eds. *The guide to community preventive services: What works to promote health?* New York: Oxford University Press; 2005.
3. The Cochrane Collaboration. http://www.cochrane.org/. Accessed August 28, 2010.
4. Coughlan A, Anderson E, Stern L, El-Ansary A. *Marketing channels.* Upper Saddle River, NJ: Pearson Prentice Hall; 2006.
5. Kreuter M, Bernhardt J. Reframing the dissemination challenge: a marketing and distribution perspective. *Am J Public Health.* 2009;99(12):2123–2127.
6. Kreuter M, Vehige E, McGuire A. Using computer-tailored calendars to promote childhood immunization. *Public Health Rep.* 1996;111(2):176–178.
7. Kreuter M, Caburnay C, Chen J, Donlin M. Effectiveness of individually tailored calendars in promoting childhood immunization in urban public health centers. *Am J Public Health.* 2004;94(1):122–127.
8. Caburnay C, Kreuter M, Donlin M. Disseminating effective health promotion programs from prevention research to community organizations. *J Public Health Manag Pract.* 2001;7(2):81–89.
9. Porter ME, Kramer MR. Creating shared value: How to reinvent capitalism- and unleash a wave of innovation and growth. *Harvard Business Review,* Jan-Feb 2011:17.
10. Bishop M. *Essential economics: An A to Z guide.* New York: Bloomberg Press; 2009: 63.
11. Rogers EM. *Diffusion of innovations.* New York: Free Press; 2003.
12. Brownson RC, Jacobs JA, Tabak RG, Hoehner CM, Stamatakis KA. Designing for dissemination among public health researchers: findings from a national survey in the United States. *Am J Public Health.* 2013;103:1693–1699.
13. Kotler P. *Marketing management.* Upper Saddle River, NJ: Prentice Hall; 2000.
14. Rogers E. *Diffusion of innovations.* 5th ed. New York: Free Press; 2003.
15. National Cancer Institute. *Conference summary report, Designing for dissemination,* September 19-20. Washington, DC: Author; 2002.
16. Tabak, R. G., Stamatakis, K. A., Jacobs, J. A., & Brownson, R. C. What predicts dissemination efforts among public health researchers in the United States?. *Public Health Rep.* 2014;129(4):361–368.
17. McKay AB, Stamatakis KA, Jacobs JA, Tabak RG, Brownson RC. The role of researchers in

dissemination evidence to public health practice settings: a cross-sectional study. *Health Res Policy Syst,* 2016;14:42.

18. Klesges L, Estabrooks P, Dzewaltowski D, Bull S, Glasgow R. Beginning with the application in mind: designing and planning health behavior change interventions to enhance dissemination. *Ann Behav Med.* 2005;29:S66-S75.

19. Larson K, Levy J, Rome M, Matte T, Silver L, Frieden T. Public health detailing: a strategy to improve the delivery of clinical preventive services in New York city. *Public Health Rep.* 2006;121(3):228–234.

20. Frieden TR, Bassett MT, Thorpe LE, Farley TA. Public health in New York City, 2002-2007: confronting epidemics of the modern era. *Int J Epidemiol.* 2008;37(5):966–977.

21. Butler B, Godfrey Erskine E (1970). Public health detailing: selling ideas to the private practitioner in his office. *Am J Public Health.* 1970;60(10):1996–2002.

22. LaPorta M, Hagood H, Kornfeld J, Treimann J. Partnerships as a means of reaching special populations: evaluating the NCI's CIS Partnership Program. *J Cancer Educ.* 2007;22:S35–S40.

23. Robinson B. NCI plans to expand outreach through community-based research programs. *NCI Cancer Bulletin.* 2009;6(16): 9.

24. Task Force on Community Preventive Services. *The guide to community preventive services: What works to promote health?* New York: Oxford University Press; 2005.

13

Design and Analysis in Dissemination and Implementation Research

JOHN LANDSVERK, C. HENDRICKS BROWN, JUSTIN D. SMITH,
PATRICIA CHAMBERLAIN, GEOFFREY M. CURRAN, LAWRENCE PALINKAS,
MITSUNORI OGIHARA, SARA CZAJA, JEREMY D. GOLDHABER-FIEBERT,
WOUTER VERMEER, LISA SALDANA, JENNIFER A. ROLLS REUTZ,
AND SARAH MCCUE HORWITZ

INTRODUCTION

Dissemination and implementation research has evolved into an emerging field, implementation science, as exemplified by the launching of the journal *Implementation Science* in 2006, and the annual Dissemination and Implementation conferences, initiated in 2007. Not surprisingly, progress in this emerging science is uneven, with a greater volume of empirical studies mounted in the physical health care field than in the fields of mental health, substance use, or social services, due largely to medicine's early focus on quality of care and, more recently, on comparative effectiveness. However, despite these important scientific efforts, there remains a lack of consensus on methodological approaches to the study of dissemination and implementation processes and especially tests of implementation strategies.[1] To begin to address these deficiencies, this chapter reviews design issues for dissemination and implementation research, and also presents an overview of some of the analytic approaches to dissemination and implementation research, recognizing that this analytic work is still at an early stage of development. Finally, the chapter presents a case study of research that crosses three of four recognized dissemination and implementation phases and illustrates a number of design and analysis issues.

Note the following major changes in the 2nd edition as compared with the 1st edition. In the 2nd edition, the discussion of mixed methods designs has been removed and integrated in a new 2nd edition chapter 20 on mixed methods

evaluation in dissemination and implementation science. Similarly, the discussion of system science approaches, specifically, system dynamics method and agent-based modeling, has been removed from this chapter and integrated with social network analysis into chapter 10. However, the role of general simulation in designing D&I studies has been retained and expanded. Third, a section on hybrid designs has been added in this 2nd edition chapter. Fourth, the concept of preimplementation designs has been linked with simulation modeling related to the exploration and adoption/preparation stages of D&I research. Finally, this chapter incorporates the classification of D&I designs recently put forth by Brown and colleagues,[2] which encompasses three overarching categories of designs based on the type of comparison.

FOCUS OF DISSEMINATION AND IMPLEMENTATION RESEARCH

A useful organizing heuristic is to conceptualize dissemination and implementation studies (D&I) in relation to two other stages of research, efficacy and effectiveness. Nicely captured in the 2009 National Research Council and Institute of Medicine report on *Preventing Mental, Emotional, and Behavioral Disorders Among Young People* [3] (shown in Figure 13.1) and adapted from that report and a recent typology;[2] D&I studies are the last stage of research in the science to practice continuum, preceded by efficacy and effectiveness studies that are distinct from and address different questions from D&I studies. The figure also demonstrates that distinct phases (albeit somewhat overlapping) exist within the D&I stage, characterized as exploration, adoption/preparation, implementation, and sustainment similar to the EPIS model proposed by Aarons and colleagues.[4] In the exploratory phase, we focus on preimplementation factors including deciding on what evidence-based intervention would be most appropriate. In the adoption/preparation phase, we are interested in factors related to the formal decision to implement, or strategies to increase adoption of an intervention or program. The next phase is implementation (or implementation fidelity), which involves strategies for improving program fidelity in the field, and finally sustainment (and moving to scale), involving strategies to maintain delivery of the intervention or extend its use in communities or organizations. D&I trials are also distinct from efficacy and effectiveness trials as it concerns the independent variable that is manipulated, which are referred to as implementation strategies.

Note that this research model typology represented in Figure 13.1 is also reflected in the NIH Roadmap initiative for re-engineering the clinical research enterprise currently driving the translational research initiative at the NIH.[5-7] The Roadmap initiative has identified three types of research leading to improvements in the public health of our nation, namely, basic research that informs the development of clinical interventions (e.g., biochemistry, neurosciences), treatment development that crafts the interventions and tests them in carefully controlled efficacy trials, and what has come to be known as service system and implementation research, where treatments and interventions are brought into and tested in usual care settings.[8] Based on this tripartite division, the Roadmap further identified two translation steps that would be critical for moving from the findings of basic science to improvements in the quality of health care delivered in community, clinical, and other delivery settings. The first translation step brings together interdisciplinary teams that integrate the science work being done in the basic sciences and treatment development

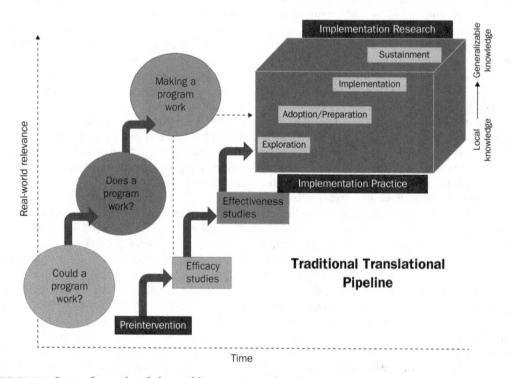

FIGURE 13.1 Stages of research and phases of dissemination and implementation.

(Adapted from "Figure 11-1 Stages of research in prevention research cycle" in Chapter 11: Implementation and Dissemination of Prevention Programs (2009) in National Research Council and Institute of Medicine. Preventing Mental, Emotional, and Behavioral Disorders among Young People. Washington DC: The National Academies Press, p. 326 and Brown CH, et al. (2017). An Overview of Research and Evaluation Designs for Dissemination and Implementation. Annual Rev Public Health. 2017; 38:1–22.)

science, such as translating neuroscience and basic behavior research findings into new treatments. The focus of the second translation phase is to translate evidence-based treatments into service delivery settings and sectors in local communities, and it is this second step that we identify as the D&I research enterprise.[9]

Next, briefly defined and described are three facets of D&I research in order to better frame the discussion of evaluation designs and related analytic issues covered in the remainder of this chapter.

Implementation Strategies

Central to understanding the distinctiveness of D&I research is the concept of implementation strategies. Implementation strategies are multicomponent interventions on and within the service delivery system that are aimed at increasing the adoption of new practices into routine care. Powell and colleagues[10] identified 73 discrete components of implementation strategies currently in use in the literature that have at least minimal support for their effectiveness. Concept mapping was then used to categorize these strategies into nine broad domains with varying numbers of discrete strategies in each.[11] These domains are: Engage consumers, Use evaluative and iterative strategies, Change infrastructure, Adapt and tailor to the context, Develop stakeholder interrelationships, Utilize financial strategies, Support clinicians, Provide interactive assistance, and Train and educate stakeholders. It is rare that a single discrete component of a strategy is used in implementation research. Rather, a package of component strategies is typically selected to address multiple barriers to adoption and implementation. However, when testing and evaluating the effects of implementation, key differences in strategies are the focus. For example, multiple strategies might be used to implement a behavioral intervention to increase testing for HIV among high-risk populations seen in community-based primary care clinics. These could include engaging key stakeholders, training clinicians, and incentivizing use of the intervention.

In the context of a trial to evaluate the penetration rate of HIV testing across clinics, the researcher might vary the amount or type of training the clinicians receive or change the way in which the intervention is embedded within the system (e.g., colocated testing vs. referral to an external STI testing center), with all other strategies held equal across systems. A comparison of these two alternatives would then isolate the effects of a strategy that is manipulated by the research team across units (i.e., the independent variable). It is the effects of these implementation strategies on proximal outcomes, processes, and outputs of the service delivery system and, in some cases that are explained in detail later, the distal patient-level outcomes, that are commonly under investigation in D&I research.

Evaluating Implementation Outcomes, Processes, and Outputs

Outcomes of implementation research are covered more fully in other chapters of this second edition, but an overview is useful here in the context of our discussion of research designs. Inherent in the definition of implementation strategies is the goal of increasing adoption, which can be conceptualized as a finite event (e.g., a new innovation is implemented) or an ongoing process (e.g., the intent of a service system to adopt a new innovation). However, outcomes in implementation research extend into many areas that affect the adoption and sustained delivery of a new innovation and the efficiency by which adoption occurs. To date, Proctor and colleagues[12] provide the most comprehensive taxonomy of implementation outcomes and place them in the greater context of service delivery system outcomes, using the Institute of Medicine's Standards of Care[13] and the distal clinical outcomes at the level of the individual. Among the implementation outcomes are acceptability, adoption, appropriateness, cost, feasibility, fidelity, reach or penetration, and sustainment. These are viewed as the direct outcomes resulting from the use of implementation strategies, which, in turn, affect service system outcomes and patient-level clinical outcomes, such as symptom severity.

Not explicit in such a taxonomy is that some outcomes are more germane to particular phases of implementation research.[14] For example, in the early phases of the EPIS model in Figure 13.1, primary outcomes might be acceptability, appropriateness, and feasibility, whereas during implementation, assessments of cost, fidelity, and penetration are possible and considered key outcomes. Likewise outcomes of acceptability, fidelity, and cost, which are relevant to adoption/ preparation and implementation phases, all can have lasting effect on sustainment, the 4th and final phase.

Beyond the Proctor taxonomy are measures that evaluate the efficiency and success of the implementation process itself. A prime example of this type of measurement system is the Stages of Implementation Completion (SIC).[15] The SIC is intended to be individualized to specific innovations and service contexts, as it concerns the stages to be completed and the specific activities within each stage. Some examples of stages include, readiness planning, hiring and training of staff, service delivery, and consultation. Each stage contains three or more activities defined by the implementation broker and implementing site, often in consultation with the innovation developer, as being important within a given stage. The SIC measure is focused on critical, observable indicators involving speed, quality, and quantity. These include the completion of key implementation stages, the time spent in each stage, the numbers of the population served, and the proportion of activities completed in each stage. These dimensions can then be used to compare the outcomes between sites. An example of this type of application is provided in the context of the CAL-OH study later in this chapter.[16,17]

Research Questions in D&I

The four phases of D&I research in Figure 13.1 correspond to fundamentally different research questions. In particular, the exploration phase focuses on identifying or enlarging the set of organizations or communities that express interest in using or making available a particular innovation (e.g., intervention or program). One may be interested in the sheer number of settings that express interest through a passive dissemination process, or we may want to identify whether some communities, say those serving high proportions of minority or poor populations, are differentially interested in using a certain program.[18] Early D&I research focused extensively on the characterization of barriers and facilitators to implementation, which remains a key consideration today but is often not viewed as a novel research question given the sheer amount of literature in this area to inform future research. Today, when new research begins, implementation readiness and capacity assessment that occurs during the adoption/preparation phase typically addresses this question in a particular study and informs the choice of which implementation strategies are needed.

We can summarize how D&I research is distinct from other research stages. In contrast to the traditional research questions of efficacy research, which routinely examines overall impact in a relatively homogeneous target population and of effectiveness research, which routinely asks who benefits and for how long in more realistic settings, D&I research questions focus primarily on whether different strategies for informing communities or delivery of an intervention increase the speed of implementation, the quality of program delivery, and/or the quantity or degree of access or penetration of the intervention. One can view these characteristics of speed, quality, and quantity as leading to measurable quantities that can be used to monitor the implementation process. Implementation success would generally be measured by attainment of certain milestones, such as a decision that a community or organization adopts a program, certification that an agency has been credentialed, or other appropriate milestones that can be measured using standardized measures of implementation. Through these milestone measures, we can assess the speed with which implementation takes place. The other two dimensions of quality, and quantity are also considered as critical to evaluating implementation strategies. For example, quality can refer to the fidelity or competence in program delivery, and quantity can refer to how many of the target population are served (similar to concepts of reach covered in chapter 19). Consequently, it is recommended that the study designs, assessment instruments, analytical strategies, and analytic tools for D&I research all should relate to speed, quality, or quantity of implementation. Given the different purposes for D&I research compared with efficacy or effectiveness, it is likely that they may require different research designs or different emphases as they navigate the tension all evaluations have between internal and external validity.

While specific research questions regarding D&I research may most efficiently be addressed by a unique research design, there may remain questions about effectiveness of newly implemented interventions that are worth answering anew. Indeed, hybrid designs,[19] which address research questions related to both implementation and effectiveness simultaneously in one study, are being used much more frequently than they have in the past.[20,21] Hybrid designs are discussed more fully later in this chapter. Finally, note that the primary focus of this 2nd edition chapter is on implementation without a separate discussion about designs in dissemination research, because dissemination research has not developed a body of research designs distinct from or as extensive as that for implementation research.

PREIMPLEMENTATION METHODS

The process of implementing new innovations in real-world systems is complex and involves numerous decisions on the part of the implementation evaluators and key decision makers in the system. Factors that are commonly considered during preimplementation, which coincides with the exploration and adoption/preparation phases of the EPIS framework in Figure 13.1, include the selection of the innovation to be implemented, the potential implementation strategies used, the population of both providers and patients to be targeted, the expected reach of an innovation within a particular setting given such factors as the characteristics of the population being served, the number of providers that will deliver the innovation, and other resources being allocated. Each of these factors has an influence on the overall impact of the effort and the speed that maximal impact is achieved. Given the plethora of potential options facing implementers, and the need to consider costs and efficiency, certain modeling approaches can be useful during preimplementation, and rarely will there be much reliance on new, rather than existing empirical studies. Policy makers face similar questions when crafting legislation, regulations, and other endorsements of specific and general practices. Attention to these factors occurs during exploration when needs and capacities are evaluated for different alternatives.

At times the number of choices in the exploratory phase is small, such as a situation where policymakers have dictated a certain evidence-based program is to be used. One such example is the recent requirement that states must use set-aside funding to implement the Coordinated Specialty Care model, based on the RAISE project[22] to address the mental health needs of adolescents and young adults who are experiencing psychotic symptoms.[23]

When there are a relatively limited number of possible intervention and implementation delivery choices, some straightforward tools can help guide effective decision-making. Often decision analysis is combined with an economic analysis, supporting not only overall decision analysis, but also cost-effectiveness analyses or cost-benefit analyses that explicitly acknowledge the reality of budget constraints and other limited resources, identifying those interventions

that can feasibly maximize the decision makers' objectives. Economic calculations for different HIV prevention programs, for example, can be compared to provide guidance on efficient use of limited funds[24] or other resources.[25-27] Linear programming tools have been developed to aid health departments in allocating limited resources for HIV prevention, for example.[28]

However, when there are no strict limits on programs or implementation strategies, the exploratory phase can consist of many different choices, as the number of factors to be considered during pre-implementation yields a parameter space whose size is determined by the product of the number of levels considered in each factor. On top of this factorial explosion in possibilities, models of real-world implementation behavior generally need to take into account interacting processes and agents, resulting in behaviors that are often nonlinear and highly context specific. A full description of such a system with complex behavior requires a scope that is generally infeasible to achieve using traditional experimental methods. There are several simulation approaches, under the heading of systems science,[29] that have been used to model such complex behavior in implementation,[30] including system dynamics,[31] network science, and agent-based modeling[32] (see chapter 10). These methods have informed us about strategies to prevent, for example, the spread of HIV through sexual networks.[33] A wide range of questions can be addressed using these simulation models, yet they mostly consider a variety of scenarios of how an implementation scales from the local to the system level. As these computer simulations can be easily scaled up, they enable capturing long-term, systemic impacts of a wide range of specified alternative scenarios, and comparison among them to provide recommendations about the best actions to take. It is important to note that such analyses provide their greatest value when they are employed in an iterative fashion, allowing policymakers to consider a variety of what-if scenarios and to evaluate multiple decisions holistically.

This section on preimplementation simulation designs focuses on two simulation approaches showing how decision analysis with microsimulations and agent-based modeling can be used to address this mismatch in scope and guide implementation research during the pre-implementation stages. Decision analysis represents a significant advance to project the needs of an agency and potential of a novel intervention to address a given service need. It employs computer-based models that simulate behaviors within a system. Using either microsimulations or agent-based modeling, this behavior is specified on the micro-level, in contrast to system-dynamics models, which consider dynamics on the system level alone. Specifying behavior on the micro level allows the heterogeneity in the system to be embraced, rather than to be controlled for or averaged out.

Microsimulation as a decision-support tool is well suited to supporting human service policy-makers (such as child welfare directors and managers) as they confront the challenges of complex, real-world operations,[34] as it can help identify policies and interventions that are most likely to achieve a set of desired objectives given current uncertainties. Indeed, decision analyses have been used successfully to consider complex decisions involving health conditions with long time courses and multiple outcomes. Such analyses have considered the prevention and management of HIV/AIDS, cardiovascular disease, diabetes, and HPV and cervical cancer.[35-40] For example, relying in part on model-based cost-effectiveness analyses, the Institute of Medicine recommended a shift from funding programs based on high AIDS prevalence to targeting prevention efforts to subgroups at high risk of infection.[41]

In the context of ongoing Child Welfare services, evidence-based interventions' superior effectiveness must be considered with respect to how well they enhance safety, permanence, and well-being and to any additional resources required to implement and maintain them at levels ensuring effectiveness. As decision-makers contemplate these interventions, they require actionable information to overcome uncertainty as to whether the long-term benefits and averted costs of evidence-based interventions justify the investment. With over 1 million children served by the US child welfare system at a cost of $20 billion annually, the use of evidence-based interventions has the potential to improve the health and well-being of a large, vulnerable population in a more cost-effective manner. However, substantial investments may be required to incorporate such interventions into child welfare agencies requiring evidence to support these decisions as they weigh the various trade-offs.[42]

An excellent illustration of the use of decision analysis is provided by Goldhaber-Fiebert and colleagues. The authors used a computer-based microsimulation model to evaluate the effect of implementing one such evidence-based foster parent training intervention: KEEP (Keeping Foster Parents Trained and Supported).[43] The microsimulation computed policy-relevant outcomes such as increased rates of adoption and reunification (positive exits) along with improved foster care placement stability (e.g., reduced lateral foster placement changes and reduced negative exits to group care) resulting from the application of KEEP. The microsimulation incorporated data on children in foster care from randomized controlled trials of KEEP[44,45] as well as large, population-representative longitudinal studies (e.g., National Survey of Child and Adolescent Well-Being), using multivariate Cox proportional hazard models and bootstrapping to provide estimates of the rates of foster care placement change, the main covariates that determine these rates, and their associated uncertainty.

The detailed microsimulation developed for this analysis simulated large cohorts of individual children whose characteristics matched those of the actual foster care populations within the US child welfare system. The model then followed these "simulated individuals" on their paths through the system, tracking their placement changes and allowing past experiences to influence their future risks of placement change and exit. This approach permitted the consideration of the rich, complex effects of each individual's experience in the system of over time, identifying cumulative benefits to KEEP, emphasizing higher-risk groups of children who may differentially benefit from the application of the intervention, and gauging the heterogeneous mediating effects that different state child welfare systems could have on KEEP. The paper demonstrated decision analytic methods to employ existing data to project policy-relevant child welfare outcomes related to permanence and stability. Decision-analytic microsimulation modeling is a feasible and useful methodology to inform challenging child welfare policy decisions and can be extended to consider multiple evidence-based interventions and outcomes.

Another recent example highlights how agent-based modeling can be used to study policy impacts.[46] In particular it focuses on the effects of various CDC guidelines for PrEP (preexposure prophylaxis) prescription on HIV prevalence. In this study the authors use existing field data to create a realistic system interacting agents, men who have sex with men, and simulate not only how HIV spreads among that population but also how different implementations of CDC guidelines for PrEP prescription affect this spreading process. The simulation incorporates a heterogeneous population of 10,000 agents with variations in sexual activity, risk behaviors, testing frequencies, and adherence levels. A second agent-based modeling approach highlights the importance of STI testing as a critical factor determining intervention success.[47]

These examples highlight the power of simulation for implementation during the preimplementation stage. It highlights this method as a scalable tool for doing virtual experiments, scanning the parameter space, and conducting consequent scenario analysis based on the outcomes, but the potential goes well beyond that. Decision analysis using simulation can also identify the factors critical for successful implementation, inform which populations to target and the differences to be expected for various target populations, and identify tipping points in the system, which can inform the amount of resources needed to achieve the desired impact.

RANDOMIZED AND NONRANDOMIZED IMPLEMENTATION DESIGNS FOR ADOPTION/ PREPARATION, IMPLEMENTATION, AND SUSTAINMENT PHASES

Historically, basic science and treatment research as partners in the first translation step have relied heavily on what has come to be known as the "gold standard" of designs; namely, the randomized controlled trial (RCT), involving randomization at the person level. In the efficacy phase the primary aim is to determine whether an intervention has impact on its intended target. A great deal of methods development has been devoted to the use of RCTs to evaluate program efficacy for medical[48] and behavioral research.[49] While effectiveness research also has played an important role in the science to practice continuum, group-based randomized trials are generally needed for these more complex longitudinal designs that often include multiple levels in the analysis.[50,51] In one of the few comprehensive discussions of the distinction between efficacy and effectiveness trials, Flay in 1986[52] noted that "whereas efficacy trials are concerned with testing whether a treatment or procedure does more good than harm when delivered under optimum

conditions, effectiveness trials are concerned with testing whether a treatment does more good than harm when delivered via a real-world program."[52]

It is not accidental that Flay's language on D&I includes a discussion of random assignment to different approaches for delivery. Flay's perspective then was that randomized trials could be used for such research, but such designs would need to differ from individually based RCTs.[2] There are circumstances where randomization may not be feasible or acceptable[53] and alternatives may be proposed to the randomized design such as "interrupted time series," "multiple baseline across settings" or "regression-discontinuity" designs. For example, Brown and colleagues have argued that incorporating randomization across time and place in roll-out trials can be acceptable for both communities and researchers.[20,50,54]

This section reviews the major issues in designs for D&I research, with a particular focus on randomization and alternatives to randomized designs, and also discusses the emerging development of hybrid, adaptive, and staging designs as well as mixed method designs. This is followed by a section that discusses power calculations in multilevel implementation designs and the use of analytic strategies such as mediation and moderation. Although little work in the use of mediation and moderation analyses in D&I research exists to date, the section lays out the need for this approach if we are to better understand the mechanisms and limitations of implementation strategies. Finally, this chapter addresses a rapidly emerging set of tools for dissemination and implementation research under the label of system science and then concludes with a case example of a rigorous and complex study in California of the impact of two implementation strategies for a 51-county roll-out of the robust, evidence-based intervention "Treatment Foster Care Oregon."

This emphasis on randomized designs in implementation research is supported by a paper that reviewed types of designs published on D&I research in nonmedical care service systems, namely child welfare and child mental health.[55] Using standardized search strategies, nine relevant studies were identified, all involving randomization, eight at a single level and one at 2 levels (treatment intervention vs. control, and intervention strategy vs. control). Note that randomized designs constitute the majority of implementation studies that met the criteria of some kind of control or comparison condition. Also note that approximately 1 in 10 studies reviewed by EPOC used an interrupted time series design as an alternative to randomization. This is one of the four alternatives to randomization reviewed by Glasgow and colleagues.[53]

The classification of D&I designs put forth by Brown and colleagues[2] encompasses three overarching categories of designs based on the type of comparison.

Within-Site Designs: that is, evaluation of an implementation project focused on change within a single site. This classification includes two types of within-site designs. The weaker design is the post design, where changes in the system's health care processes and utilization are evaluated after the introduction of an evidence-based practice. The more rigorous variant, the pre-post design, adds an evaluation of preimplementation data, which can then be compared to postimplementation data to infer effects. Interrupted time series designs in the EPOC framework[56] are a slight methodological improvement on the within-site design that simply requires additional measurement and analytic techniques that account for trend, serial dependence, and other characteristics of such data.[57] All these within-site design variants are considered quasi-experimental.

Between-Site Designs: that is, evaluation that compares outcomes, outputs, and processes between two or more sites where a novel intervention is being implemented. A basic type of study in this category is a head-to-head comparison of two implementation strategies for a specific intervention that occurs in two different sites or two groups of sites—randomly assigned when applicable. A variant of this design could be to assign different units or wards within an organization and compare the effectiveness of different implementation strategies. A useful rule of thumb is that randomization should be at the "level of implementation," meaning the level where the full impact of the strategy is designed to occur.[58] Brown and colleagues[2] also discuss special cases of this family of between-site designs: factorial designs; double randomized, two-level nested designs; and site selection of implementation strategies using a decision support strategy, as opposed to an a priori randomization that forces sites to use a certain implementation strategy.

Within- and Between-Site Comparison Designs: that is, sites begin as one implementation condition and move to another. The most common example of this design is a roll-out randomized implementation trial, which is similar to the stepped-wedge[59] and dynamic wait-listed design[54] that has been used in effectiveness research for decades. In such designs, sites are randomized to a time to crossover from implementation as usual to the use of the implementation strategy. In this way, each site serves as its own control (within-site) and can be compared with the performance of other sites (between-site). A number of variants to this design are possible, including clustering sites to start at different time points and pairwise-enrollment roll-out designs.[60] The roll-out trial is particularly palatable to community organizations, as they are assured of receiving the active implementation strategy at some point in the trial as opposed to serving solely as a control site. Last, in situations with a very small number of units to randomize, power can be increased and the experimental design can be strengthened by using randomized multiple-baseline designs,[61] which come from the single-subject experimental design tradition.

The observed dominance of D&I research designs with randomization supports the benefits of such designs for addressing common threats to interpretation of study findings. However, it is well to consider the nature of threats to the integrity of a randomized trial for dissemination and implementation research before further reviewing a range of design options for D&I research.

Often, one emphasizes characteristics of well-conducted research studies or trials in order to guide researchers into conducting studies that will lead to accurate scientific inferences. While this is helpful, the authors believe this is too optimistic a perspective, since research needs more than an overly optimistic "glass half-full" attitude to make appropriate conclusions. Indeed, a study can do many things right, but fail in just one way and thereby put all its inferences at risk. The critical scientific paradigm for assigning observed differences by condition to an implementation's effect is that the only systematic factor that differs by intervention condition is the assigned intervention. For example, an implementation trial can carry out an appropriate randomization of communities to one of two implementation conditions, use valid and reliable measures, and conduct statistical analyses that correctly take into account intraclass clustering within communities. But if community leaders in one arm of the trial are more likely to refuse to be interviewed or drop out more frequently, this effect on the quality of the inferences can never be compensated by other good parts of the study. To reduce the potential for such imbalance, and to hold an implementation design in place, requires a strong and active partnership between communities, institutions, and researchers.[62,63] Following, we list some of the factors that are known to affect the quality of inferences.[64] with special attention to implementation and dissemination research.

Random assignment is the obvious choice for insuring that implementation condition is fairly distributed (sometimes with blocking into similar communities followed by random assignment within these blocks). While some have suggested that random assignment is not appropriate for implementation research, our review indicates that there have been a sizeable number of such randomized implementation trials conducted, and they do have an important place in this research agenda. The usual alternative is a comparative study where one or more select communities apply a specified implementation procedure while other communities, often selected afterwards, are used as comparison. The problem with this design is that it hopelessly confounds two factors: the implementation itself as well as community readiness, since only those communities that are "ready" are prepared to implement. One can never distinguish whether the differences in communities is due to one of these factors or both. An alternative design is a roll-out design[20] where communities that express their willingness are randomized to the timing of implementation. Such a dynamic wait-listed design[54,65] has been used in the comparison of two implementation strategies for an evidence-based intervention for foster care to be described later in the case study.[18,66,67]

A second major threat to an implementation trial is a failure to use valid and reliable measures to assess implementation outcomes (also see chapter 14). Because the implementation process is inherently multilevel, it is critical to assess impact across the appropriate levels. One potential flaw can occur if one only measures the distal outcome on a target population that is served, since these may not be comparable across intervention conditions. For example, suppose an implementation strategy is designed to increase the number of youth who receive an evidence-based program. If we compare findings from those youth in communities randomized to the new implementation strategy to those using implementation as usual, it is quite possible for systematic differences to occur between those

target youth who are exposed to different interventions. There is no mechanism to guarantee that those who receive the intervention are equivalent, and it may be that the expansion of service delivery brings in more or less challenging populations that are served. Analytic strategies that use propensity scores to adjust for differences at the nonrandomized level could be considered.[68,69] There is ordinarily no need to adjust for covariates at the higher level where randomization occurs because randomization preserves balance.

While there are enormous benefits to randomization, the multilevel nature of D&I research creates issues for typical randomization at the individual level designs. Figure 13.2 shows a classic multilevel structure with four levels that Shortell has suggested for change in assessing performance improvement in organizations.[70] While randomization can and is being done at levels higher than the individual, there is an issue in having sufficient power as one moves to higher levels with diminishing units to be used in a randomized design (see later section on calculation of power in multilevel designs Selected Websites and Tools). Since power is so critical to the use of randomized designs, it is reasonable to consider quasi-experimental designs without randomization for D&I research. This clearly is the thrust of Glasgow and colleagues[53] in their 2005 article on practical designs. Another useful source for the alternative designs and the trade-offs between randomized and nonrandomized designs is the *Handbook of practical program evaluation*,[71] edited by Wholey, Hatry, and Newcomer, especially the contrasting chapters on "Quasi-experimentation"[72] by Reichardt and Mark, and the chapter on "Using randomized experiments"[73] by Pierre. Note that Reichardt and Mark describe four prototypical quasi-experimental study designs: (1) before-after; (2) interrupted time-series; (3) nonequivalent group; and (4) regression-discontinuity designs. Their rendering of alternative designs is quite comparable to the EPOC classification of designs in implementation research and to the discussion of alternative designs by Glasgow and colleagues.[53]

Also worth noting are important recent studies that have compared the results between randomized experiments and observational studies. These have included both examples of strong divergence between observational studies and experimental studies, such as found in studies of hormone replacement therapy,[74] as well as examples where the results were remarkably

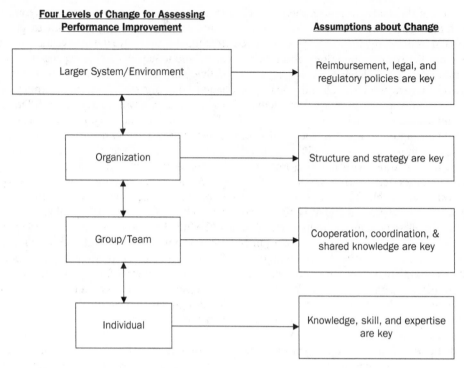

FIGURE 13.2 Four levels of change and assumptions about change.
(Adapted from: Shortell SM.[70])

consistent. Notable is the paper published in 2000 by Concato, Shah, and Horwitz [75] that examined meta-analyses of randomized controlled trials and meta-analyses of either cohort or case-control studies on the same intervention. Across interventions addressing five very different medical conditions, the authors found remarkable similarity between in the results between the two types of designs, which are perceived to be quite different in the hierarchy of evidence. The authors concluded that "The results of well-designed observational studies (with either a cohort or a case-control design) do not systematically overestimate the magnitude of the effects of treatment as compared to those in randomized, controlled trials on the same topic" (p. 1887). A later study published in 2008 by Cook, Shadish, and Wong[76] came to the same conclusion when comparing the results from randomized experiments and regression-discontinuity designs. In both papers, the authors argued that the quality of the observational studies had to be high to be comparable to the results in randomized designs. This line of research informs the emerging field of implementation science by suggesting that observational studies may also be seriously considered.[77]

RETHINKING RANDOMIZED DESIGNS

An alternative approach to problems with use of classic RCT designs, so important in efficacy and effectiveness research stages, is to rethink how randomized designs can be adapted to meet the special needs of research across the four phases of D&I research. The next section discusses some of this rethinking, by considering nontraditional ways of using random assignment in D&I research.

Random assignment provides a method for making fair comparisons between intervention conditions, but the standard procedure for assigning individuals as well as organizations or communities often is impractical to administer, unacceptable to stakeholders, or irrelevant to the major research question.[78] This section describes ways that nontraditional means of using random assignment can still be used to address important dissemination and implementation questions. One fundamental way of using random assignment involves the timing of delivery of an intervention. Often communities are uncomfortable withholding an intervention completely from a subpopulation, especially if the intervention is preventive in nature, holds little apparent risk of being iatrogenic, or addresses a major health problem in a community. In such a situation, researchers may suggest the use of a wait-listed design, which allows half the units to receive the intervention first, followed by the second set receiving it later. Communities are often more comfortable with this design compared with one involving a traditional control condition, and such a design can be used to address whether proximal impact on implementation targets (e.g., program adoption, fidelity, and reach into a target population) occurs. However, such standard wait-listed designs are inherently inefficient because the data from the second half of the study when the wait-listed group receives the intervention is weak or of negligible use in answering questions on implementation and dissemination.

An alternative class of designs for dissemination and implementation is a roll-out randomized design,[60] which are sometimes described as dynamic wait-listed[54] or stepped-wedge,[79,80] although historically these have been used much more in effectiveness than implementation research. When used to study implementation, these designs randomly assign units, which may be schools[54,65] or larger settings such as counties,[50,66,67] to different "start" times and/or types of implementation strategies. Starting with a small number of units assigned at the first time point, eventually all of the units receive an active implementation strategy. Because the timing is random and measurement occurs before and after implementation, one can track whether intended changes occur both across time and across condition for most outcomes and outputs on most if not all the units. This type of design has been used to test two implementation strategies for an evidence-based program in foster care.[16,66,67] There are three appealing features about this roll-out design compared with traditional wait-listed designs. First, the statistical power is substantially greater for the roll-out design in answering many relevant research questions.[54,60] Second, it is often not practical to train a large number of communities in an intervention all at once, and the roll-out feature nicely focuses on a small manageable number who can receive the training attention that they need. Third, the use of multiple times for assignment provides more robustness of the design to influence by exogenous factors, such as economic downturns, that could otherwise destroy any chance to make inferences if its

timing occurred at the most critical time in the assignment to training.

The authors recommend that a roll-out design be considered when an implementation program is being introduced into a set of communities as part of a federal, statewide, or local policy change.[20,54,65] Such roll-out trials could be of high utility in implementation research (see 1st edition chapter 12). As an example of an appropriate use of such a trial, consider examining the following typical strategy for improving the quality and effectiveness of services by improving the training of mental health counselors. There are four levels that we need to pay attention to: the level of the client who receives services, the therapist who delivers the services, the supervisor whose job it is to improve service delivery within a mental health agency, and the agency itself.

Let us consider an implementation strategy that changes the supervision practices of therapists within agencies. A first question is what level of randomization should be used to provide maximum utility to understanding whether a new supervision strategy is effective relative to that now being used. We can consider randomizing at any and all four levels from the client to the agency, but many of these levels will not be very useful. A key step is to identify what the most salient "level of intervention" is being examined; here we are fundamentally interested in how the use of a new supervision program will affect outcomes downstream, and therefore the key level of intervention is at the supervisor level; this is the first level where we would expect behavior to change. An empirically validated rule is the following: whenever possible one should randomize at the level of intervention, since randomization at lower levels (e.g., therapist) would contort supervisors from using new techniques to train therapists in the standard condition, and randomization at higher levels (e.g., agency) will generally result in major reductions in power.[58] If we do randomize at the level of the supervisor within an agency, then the agency is considered a "blocking factor." Blocking is a well-known way of reducing variability and thereby increasing power. In a roll-out design, we would randomly determine the order and timing of training of supervisors and consequently their transmission of new behaviors to their supervisee therapists and in turn their own clients.

To assess impact in this trial design, we would likely want to measure behaviors of the supervising process (supervisor–therapist interactions), as well as of the therapeutic session itself (therapist–client), and perhaps at the level of the client target behavior as well. All three of these measures would normally be assessed over time. Thus the design in this study would typically involve multiple observation/coding times for supervisors before and after they were trained to deliver a different type of supervision, multiple observation/coding times for their respective therapists, and multiple observation times for different clients across time. Three levels of analysis could be done, with the first examining changes in supervisor behavior across time before and after training; the second involving therapist-client behavior, also coded in terms of how therapist behavior with clients related to the timing of the supervisory training they received, and third the behavior of the clients themselves. To connect these three analyses, we would conduct mediation analyses, which are presented later in this paper.

The sample size for such a trial may be nested at several levels. For example, sample size determination may include the number of agencies, number of supervisors in each agency, the distribution of the number of therapists who receive supervision within these agencies, and finally the number of clients served by each therapist. Characteristics of timing include when supervisors in each agency receive training, the number of observation points in each supervision, the number of observation points for each therapist in interacting with a client, and the baseline and follow-up times for assessing client behavior. To make sure that there is sufficient power in this design to answer all three questions of impact on supervisor behavior, on therapist behavior, and on client behavior, as well as on mediational pathways, we would need to carry out a sophisticated study of how statistical power relates to these sample sizes and timing. While there are programs that allow one to compute power in multilevel designs,[81,82] to date the calculations for dynamic wait-listed designs are generally only available to do by simulation (see later section on power calculations Selected Websites and Tools).

RETHINKING STAGES OF RESEARCH WITH HYBRID DESIGNS

An innovative approach to implementation research design was published in 2012 by Geoffrey Curran and colleagues titled "Effectiveness-Implementation Hybrid Designs: Combining Elements of Clinical Effectiveness and Implementation Research to Enhance Public Health Impact."[19] The authors were all involved with the Veteran's Administration QUERI program in an early federal agency approach to the development and use of implementation science approaches to improving the quality of care in the VA health system. As the title of this section indicates, the 2012 paper is grounded in a rethinking of the stages of research in the "traditional research pipeline," where the steps from efficacy to effectiveness to implementation were seen as discrete stages, each of which was expected to be "completed" before the next stage was begun. Adhering to the pipeline meant that the implementation research stage was seldom entered in until the work and outcomes of the efficacy and effectiveness stages were finished. The traditional pipeline also suggested that the level of evidence issue had been concluded with proof of a strong evidence base "now ready for implementation" and provided no guidance for what to do with interventions with less than stellar evidence but which might have already shown robustness in fit for real-world service systems.

The concept of hybrid designs, which blends the two stages of effectiveness and implementation, was originally proposed as a way to increase the speed of moving research findings into routine adoption. The authors argued that one did not need to wait for the "perfect" effectiveness data before moving to implementation research and that it was possible to "backfill" effectiveness data while testing implementation strategies. Further, the hybrid concept shed light on the critical question of how clinical/prevention outcomes might relate to level of adoption and rate of fidelity—which can only be known when we have data from "both sides," or simultaneously from effectiveness and implementation types of data. The notion to blend effectiveness and implementation research also encourages consideration of building for "implementability" as early as you can in the development of interventions (e.g., considering service delivery issues such as geographic context, staffing, technology, and "dose"), seeking end-user input and partnership before initiating effectiveness trials, and using implementation frameworks in design of components (e.g., CFIR framework).[83] The sample size for such a trial may be nested at several levels. For example, sample size determination may include the number of agencies, number of supervisors in each agency, the distribution of the number of therapists who receive supervision within these

Types of Hybrids

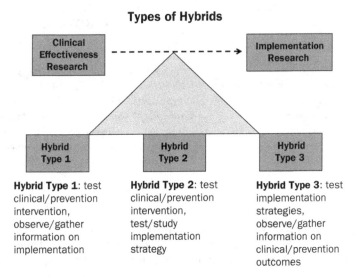

Hybrid Type 1: test clinical/prevention intervention, observe/gather information on implementation

Hybrid Type 2: test clinical/prevention intervention, test/study implementation strategy

Hybrid Type 3: test implementation strategies, observe/gather information on clinical/prevention outcomes

FIGURE 13.3 Types of hybrids.

(Adapted from: Curran GM. Research Questions and Design Considerations: Effectiveness to Implementation. Presented at the University of Wisconsin, Dissemination and Implementation Short Course Program, Madison, WI, October 2016.)

agencies, and finally the number of clients served by each therapist.

The language of hybrid designs requires some consistency in terminology. This section uses the term "intervention" to refer to the clinical/prevention practice and the term "strategy" to refer to the implementation-support activities/tools. Because both are interventions, usually the term "effectiveness" is used when referring to clinical/prevention outcomes and the term "impact" when describing implementation outcomes.

The 2012 paper by Curran and colleagues proposed three types of hybrid designs, which are shown in Figure 13.3. Hybrid Type 1 tests intervention effectiveness while gathering information on implementation issues, and Hybrid Type 3 tests implementation strategies while gathering information on clinical/prevention outcomes. Hybrid Type 2 tests the clinical/prevention intervention while also studying an implementation strategy or strategies. This typology suggests that the emphasis on effectiveness outcomes is greatest in the first type and the emphasis on implementation strategy outcomes is greatest in the third type.

Another way to clarify the distinction between the types is presented in Table 13.1, which indicates what is the primary aim and secondary aim for each type. Note here that Curran et al.'s 2012 paper is included in the suggested readings for this chapter, and the reader is recommended to

consider not only the text of the article but also the detailed tables that lay out the key terms and definitions, the characteristics of the three "ideal" types, and very detailed characteristics and key challenges for each type. In addition, the article provides published examples of empirical studies that used a specific type of hybrid design. However, it is important to consider that these are "ideal" types and specific proportions of emphasis on effectiveness and implementation issues may vary considerably among studies that indicate they used a specific type.

An important consideration for the three types of hybrid designs is the locus of randomization and power estimation, which in turn impacts overall study cost. Because the primary aim for Type 1 is clinical/prevention effectiveness, randomization would be at the individual patient/client level with appropriate power calculations. Consequently, the burden of study cost would be primarily driven by the effectiveness part of the study, while the implementation-focused activities would deploy less expensive processes such as surveys and qualitative interviews. The reverse would likely be done for a Hybrid Type 3 design, where randomization will take place at the level of organization or units within service organizations (e.g., providers or clinics). This typically means that adequate power is more difficult to achieve. The burden of cost and the adequacy of power for implementation impact may be

TABLE 13.1 HYBRID TYPES AND STUDY AIMS

Study Characteristic	Hybrid Type I	Hybrid Type II	Hybrid Type III
Research Aims	*Primary Aim:* Determine effectiveness of an intervention *Secondary Aim:* Better understand context for implementation	*Primary Aim:* Determine effectiveness of an intervention *Co-Primary* Aim:* Determine feasibility and/ or (potential) impact of an implementation strategy *or "secondary"...	*Primary Aim:* Determine impact of an implementation strategy *Secondary Aim:* Assess clinical outcomes associated with implementation

increased if secondary data sources are available for the effectiveness outcomes (e.g., administrative data routinely collected or electronic health records).

Recently, Curran and colleagues have been conducting a structured review of published studies and have come up with more than 80 papers that report using hybrid designs.[84] While a more detailed summary of the manuscripts and an accompanying set of revised recommendations for hybrid designs will be forthcoming, a brief set of findings and recommendations from the review are offered here. Concerning Type 1, currently published examples in the literature range from conventional effectiveness studies with limited exploratory measurement of barriers/facilitators to implementation (more common) to more intensive parallel process evaluations guided by implementation frameworks explaining effectiveness findings and elucidating implementation factors (less common). Concerning Type 2, the majority of published examples thus far embed a patient-level effectiveness trial nested with a pilot study of an implementation strategy (non-randomized). Very few "dual-randomized" designs are being used. Concerning Type 3, currently published examples indicate an array of targets for randomization (e.g., providers, clinics, systems) with clinical/prevention outcomes almost exclusively being collected/observed through medical record review or administrative data (nonprimary data collection at this level). A common design element is the comparison between an indicated "implementation-as-usual" strategy versus a more intensive strategy in terms of "dose" and/or number of components in a strategy. Three clear needs for the field moving forward with hybrid designs are for studies to (1) use implementation theories/frameworks explicitly to guide key aspects of the research, for example,

implementation process, strategy development, and measurements of outcomes;[85] (2) better differentiate between intervention components and implementation strategy components; and (3) fully describe the package of activities making up the implementation strategy (or strategies) under study using published terminology (e.g., see Waltz et al., 2015[11]).

SPECIAL ISSUES IN DESIGN AND ANALYSIS OF D&I RESEARCH

Power and Sample Size Calculations

The simpler tables that exist for calculating statistical power and sample size are typically not appropriate for implementation studies because of the multilevel or clustering and longitudinal nature of the data. Two online tools are often useful for these calculations, the Optimal Design system available through the W.T. Grant Foundation, and the RMASS program developed by the Center for Health Statistics at the University of Chicago. Websites for both are listed at the end of this chapter.

Randomization at Single versus Multiple Levels in D&I Research

Designs that involve multiple levels of random assignment or allocation are often useful in increasing the precision of inferences. For example, to examine sustainability of a classroom-based intervention, the authors randomized first grade teachers and classrooms within schools to the timing of training. This was the primary unit of intervention for this study. To compare early versus later training in this classroom-based intervention design, we would essentially rely on the average differences within schools for classrooms that had early versus late training. However, we knew that because schools ordinarily assign students with like ability in the same classrooms, called ability tracking, classrooms within schools would typically not be well matched. Therefore, a design that tried to compare outcomes for the one or two early-trained teachers in each school to those who were trained later would have to introduce a large heterogeneity in classrooms unless children were matched into similar classrooms within schools. This in fact was done by random assignment of all children to classroom as they were enrolled in the school,[86] and this design greatly increased the statistical power over a design that did not have balanced classrooms.[58,87] Such designs that use random assignment of groups at one level and random allocation of individuals into these groups can provide substantial improvement in power.

An alternative way to use randomization is to randomize units at two levels to different types of interventions. For example, a system-level intervention can be tested by random assignment of agencies to different intervention strategies, say to business as usual versus a new system for monitoring fidelity and providing correctives. A client-based intervention can be tested against standard practice by randomly assigning clients to these conditions within each agency. Such a two-level intervention design is known as a "split plot," and is commonly used in industrial experiments[88] but is suitable for implementation trials as well. It can be used to compare overall effect of the implementation strategy, overall effects of the client-based intervention, and their interaction. An example of such a design for implementation studies is given by Chambers.[89]

Pilot Studies and Estimating Effect Size

In developing a new implementation strategy, it is often very sensible to conduct a small-scale study to examine feasibility and assess sources of variation to determine the size one would need to have a fully powered study. While this is a useful approach, some caution is advised, especially with the estimation of effect sizes from a pilot study. As pointed out by Kraemer,[90] the precision of an effect size estimate from a pilot study is much lower than that in a fully powered study, and consequently, considerable uncertainty in power is introduced when this estimated effect size from the pilot study is entered into power calculation programs. It is possible to use these pilot studies to get some useful information about the magnitude of different sources of variance,[20] but the intended magnitude of the effect that one is aiming to achieve should best be determined by clinical relevance, rather than the estimated value obtained from the pilot study.

Analyzing for Mechanisms Through Mediation

A major task for D&I method development is to determine new mediation analysis methods for implementation modeling. There will be many challenging causality questions, particularly around how to best handle protocol deviations in implementation trials. One of these challenges will be to deal with the possibility of differential attrition in intervention agents in the intervention arms. For example, teachers who are successfully trained in an EBP such as the Good Behavior Game that promotes improved classroom behavior may be less frustrated with teaching and less likely to leave the profession.[91] Such attrition differences can become manifest in a longitudinal comparison of teachers who have been trained in this intervention versus those not trained,[21] and may be one explanation of persistent intervention effects.

This work also needs to incorporate innovative developments in causal inference for mediation models, that is, principal stratification (PS).[92-104] Traditional PS causal modeling characterizes subgroups that are responders to an intervention as well as nonresponders[92,95,97] and can assess the magnitude and extent of different impact that these subgroups experience. PS techniques are also closely connected to latent variable modeling and mediation analysis,[105-110] and these latent variable approaches can be used for evaluating intervention impact and examining rates of differential response across intervention conditions.[111] There is, however, a need to extend these methods to take into account repeated measures over time and multilevel modeling. As one example, Brown and colleagues have proposed developing two-level PS to account for different strata of intervention agents' (e.g., teachers') response to training. Like traditional PS, teachers could be classified into always successful managers of their classroom whether or not they received intervention training, always unsuccessful even if given training, and responders to the training. Also like PS, in implementation trials we cannot know any teacher's classification exactly, since we can only observe their response to the training or no training condition. However, causal inferences for outcomes of *youth*, who are exposed to these teachers, are indeed possible in randomized trials. The authors have identified a class of such two-level PS models using the Georgia Gatekeeper Trial[112] and are developing and testing several approaches in implementation research.

Finally, work needs to consider application of existing methods for multistage follow-up[50,113] to evaluate the effect of prevention programs on severe levels of drug abuse, an area that has not received sufficient attention in the literature in many evaluations. These applications for new trials will involve epidemiologic assessment of the strength of antecedent risk factors, that is, multiple drug use in adolescence, on later severe abuse. While the method is straightforward, it will require complex calculations to take into account unknown levels of differential attrition and any direct effects from program to drug abuse that do not involve drug use.

TWO SYSTEM SCIENCE APPROACHES IN D&I: SYSTEM ENGINEERING AND INTELLIGENT DATA ANALYSIS

The term "system science" refers to a transdisciplinary approach to understanding how interactions between elementary units produce complex patterns and, using the NIH/OBSSR definition, take into account the "complexity, dynamic nature, and emergent phenomena." System science methods typically include social network analysis, agent-based modeling, and systems dynamics (see chapter 10) as well as other tools such as decision analysis and systems engineering. These system science methods are critical to moving implementation research forward as a science for the following reasons. First, implementation is inherently interactional, across multilevels within systems as well as between systems, and only when different systems function together can we expect implementation to succeed. The system science methods discussed directly deal with interactions, in contrast to, say, traditional statistical modeling involving standard regression modeling, which assumes complete independence, or multilevel growth modeling, which allows correlation across persons and time but does not explicitly model these processes. Second, implementation process data, which are essential in research to monitor progress, are heavily dependent on interactions

between actors, as exemplified in the development of community-researcher partnerships.[62,63] Third, implementation process data also are essential for communities, organizations, and service systems themselves to provide monitoring and feedback for quality improvement. Most of today's research level implementation process data are very expensive for these systems to collect. Consequently, we need to develop cost-effective ways to assemble quality implementation process data, conduct analyses on these data, and integrate this into a monitoring and feedback system. The authors fully anticipate that such systems can be built by automating these steps as much as possible. Systems science methods will need to be used for all these purposes. Described in the following are system science methods not included in chapter 10, and brief illustrations of how they can be used in implementation.

Systems Engineering

Systems engineering refers[114] to the processes of identifying and manipulating the properties of a system as a whole rather than by its component parts. Systems engineering is both a discipline and process to guide the development, implementation, and evaluation of complex systems.[115] A system is an aggregation of components structurally organized to accomplish a set of goals or objectives. All systems have the following characteristics: a structure, interacting components, inputs and outputs, goals and objectives. Systems are dynamic in that each system component has an effect on the other components.[116]

System optimization requires design consideration of all components of a system, in contrast to a more traditional reductionist approach focusing on individual components. Attempts to design a system without considering the dynamic physical and social environments where the system operates will degrade system performance. For example, if a school-based prevention program competes for time against instruction, output would be low. *Task analysis* is one systems engineering tool used to characterize the implementation process and necessary resource and skill requirements. It was successfully applied to describe 15 complex intervention programs in the Resources for Alzheimer's Caregiver Health program conducted by Czaja and colleagues.[117] Another system engineering tool is the *Analytic Hierarchy Process.*[118] This can be used to capture decision-making within systems. By focusing on the decision process and establishing priorities, the Analytic Hierarchy Process can identify critical attributes of an intervention and areas where an intervention might be modified or adapted.[119]

It is not well known that strategies for implementation vary dramatically. We have been struck by the vast different approaches that have been used in different implementation strategies. To compare these alternatives, a full characterization of different strategies is required, and that requires the use of a standard procedure for eliciting intended implementation strategies as well as identifying where inefficiencies and other problems exist. The use of task analysis and the analytic hierarchical process and related techniques provides the ability to develop an ordering of priorities in decision-making to distinguish different implementation models in theory and practice.

Intelligent Data Analysis

Intelligent data analysis refers to advanced computational methods to automate the generation of meaning from text, video, or audio signals. These techniques can be used to reduce large amounts of process data on implementation that come in digitized form. Most implementation process data that are typically collected in agencies, such as number of people attending meetings or self-ratings of fidelity, are only crude indicators of the implementation process. However, there are other sources of information on the implementation process that are rarely codified but can be converted to analyzable data. Notably, these include audio and videotaped training as well as program delivery sessions. Such information is highly useful for supervision, but often just a small portion of this information is ever used. Automated signal processing and feature extraction of videotapes are possible using intelligent data analysis, and the outcomes of such methods would help to identify specific ways to improve facilitator fidelity.

As one illustration of the use of intelligent data analysis, consider the availability of contact logs, process notes, emails, and other communications to monitor implementation. Automated generation of meaning from text is one important tool to convert information that generally requires time-consuming human judgment. If we were able to automate the process of transferring such information into meaningful data on the implementation process, it would result in a major savings in costs for agencies and service providers. The transfer of text to meaningful terms involves intelligent data analysis. Similar to psychometrics,

computer science research has used latent variables via the Hidden Markov Model (HMM) to derive meaning from text information. In HMM, there is a time-dependent process governed by state changes and its associated state-dependent distribution that produces observations at each step (e.g., in speech a syllable is a state and the sound is the observation). In HMM the goal is to estimate the number of states, the state transition matrix, and the state-dependent distributions of observations.[120] A more advanced Latent Semantic Indexing method models implicit meanings behind texts[121,122] and has been used extensively in research, including our own,[123,124] to classify and categorize documents (i.e., automatic groupings). A general assumption is that the documents come from a set of unknown categories and the words and phrases appearing in the documents are produced by category-dependent distributions. Given a set of observed data, these methods construct matrices that explain document generation and word/phrase generation using iterative optimization and/or matrix decomposition. Note that completely automated systems for converting text to meaning are not likely to succeed by themselves. However, intelligent data analysis provides not only a best classification based on similarity to correctly classified text information, but also a probability assessment of this correct classification. Thus we can discriminate between text that is clearly classified and text that may be incorrectly classified. By screening these texts, we can concentrate the high-cost human interaction on those messages that have uncertain classification, greatly limiting the cost involved in producing valid implementation process data.

CASE STUDY: COMMUNITY DEVELOPMENT TEAMS TO SCALE-UP TREATMENT FOSTER CARE OREGON (TFCO) IN CALIFORNIA

Background

Each year, 87,000 children and adolescents are placed in group, residential, and institutional care settings in the United States (http://www.childwelfare.gov/pubs/factsheets/foster/), with over 15,000 in California. While there is some quasi-experimental evidence to support positive short-term effects for highly structured and individualized group care models such as Teaching Family Homes,[125] the majority of studies have linked placement in group and residential care with increased odds of an array of negative outcomes such as increased odds of association with delinquent peers,[126] delinquency,[127] isolation from family, and lowered odds of reunification.[128] Group home placements are also expensive, consuming 43% of the substitute care dollars in California in 2001. Treatment Foster Care Oregon (TFCO) was developed as an alternative to group and residential care for children and adolescents with severe emotional, behavioral, and mental health problems being placed through juvenile justice and child welfare systems. In TFCO, the child/teen is placed singly in a highly trained and supported community foster home where they and their family (biological, adoptive) receive intensive clinical services. A series of randomized trials have shown significantly better outcomes for participants in TFCO versus group care,[129,130] leading TFCO to be designated as a top tier evidence-based model by multiple scientific advisory boards and organizations.[131-134] TFCO has been implemented in over 90 agencies in the United States and Europe since 2001. However, these agencies likely do not reflect typical publically funded service systems; they are early innovators.[135] In fact, it is estimated that 90% of public systems do not implement evidence-based practice models. It is these non-early adopting agencies that are the focus of this case study.

Context

The California Institute of Mental Health (now California Institute for Behavioral Health Solutions; CIBHS) originated the Community Development Team (CDT) model[136] to increase the number of California counties that successfully adopt, implement, and sustain evidence-based practices. CDTs operate through several well-specified mechanisms including multicounty team meetings, expert local consultation, peer-to-peer exchanges, and regular multicounty conference calls. Forty California counties that were non-early adopters of TFCO were invited to participate in an NIMH-funded randomized trial to scale-up TFCO in California, and all agreed to be part of this trial. After matching counties on demographic characteristics (e.g., size, % minority, poverty, previous use of mental health funding) into three cohorts of 12 to 14 counties, a two-step randomization process was used. Counties were first randomized to condition (CDT or Individualized or standard "as usual" implementation). Then they were randomized again to one of three timeframes for implementation start date that spanned across 3 years. Randomization to start date allowed the management of issues related to implementation capacity, as training all counties at once was impossible. The random assignment of counties to cohort also increased protection against the influence of exogenous factors.[54]

Measurement and Analytic Framework

A primary research question relates to whether participation in the CDT condition improves the adoption, implementation, fidelity/adherence, and sustainability of TFCO. Secondarily, contextual and organizational factors are hypothesized to mediate the association between experimental condition and implementation outcomes. For example, as a result of participating in the CDTs, counties are expected to make better progress due to more positive attitudes toward the TFCO model and supportive organizational climates. However, regardless of experimental condition, those counties with higher scores on the hypothesized mediators are expected to achieve better implementation outcomes.

One of the main implementation outcomes to be examined is how long it takes for a county to place their first child in a TFCO home, an event that comes after the decision by multiple social service systems in the county to adopt TFCO, the selection and training of agency workers to support TFCO, and the selection and training of a foster parent in TFCO. Survival analysis techniques were used, including Cox regression modeling,[137] to compare the time it takes for placement for CDT and standard setting counties. Survival analysis is well suited for these data, as cohorts will vary in the amount of time that they have been involved in the study, thereby creating an outcome measure that is right-censored. Survival analyses will use the entire time period available for each cohort (4.5 years for Cohort 1; 2.5 years for Cohort 2; and 1.5 years for Cohort 3). By modeling how the hazard rate depends on intervention status and other covariates, a formal test can be conducted to assess the CDT intervention impact. An unusual feature in this study is that the outcomes for counties in the CDT groups could be correlated because they work together in a peer-to-peer setting. In contrast, those counties assigned to the standard implementation condition are expected to have outcomes that are independent To account for how this clustering effect in the CDT group affects the standard error and testing of the intervention, the Generalized Estimating Equation sandwich-type variance estimator will be used to adjust for non-independence in Cox regression modeling, using techniques similar to those employed previously in schizophrenia studies where family factors caused clustering.[138-140] These methods correct for nonindependence; test statistics can be based on exact tests where the distribution under the null is simulated and critical values are thereby obtained.

In addition to the time to first placement, implementation progress is measured using a Stages of Implementation Completion (SIC) scale developed for this trial that includes both time-based and quality indicators of completion of each of eight implementation stages: (1) Engagement, (2) Feasibility, (3) Readiness planning, (4) Staff hired/trained, (5) Fidelity monitoring system in place, (6) Services and consultation begins, (7) Adherence and competence tracked and feedback, and (8) Certification/licensure. Activities are specified at each stage and measured using dates of accomplishment and quality ratings. Progression through each stage involves unique (although sometimes overlapping) groups of constituents. For example, leaders of child welfare, mental health, and juvenile justice systems first explore the possibility of implementation (stage 1), and access the feasibility/fit of the model for their local circumstances (stage 2). If the determination to proceed is made, system leaders are likely to step back from the process and involve others who will be directly involved in the active implementation and in the planning (stage 3). During active implementation when staff are hired and trained (stage 4) and fidelity monitoring is set up (stage 5), intervention and agency staff are the primary agents involved, not the system leadership. Therefore the SIC is populated by data from a variety of agents at the various stages. Quality of participation ratings are made within several of the SIC stages.[15,66] Interestingly, this real-world implementation instrument reflects, quite closely, the theoretical model developed by Aarons et al.[3] and adds considerable support for the importance of different factors at various stages of the implementation process.

In addition to the SIC time to completion and quality of completion ratings, qualitative measures aimed at adding to the understanding of what factors influence decision makers to adopt evidence-based models are being examined. Palinkas found that the social networks of system

leaders played a key role in their decision to adopt during the exploration stage. Network size and density (the number of reported links divided by the maximum number of possible links) was not associated with the size of the county, but was significantly associated with stage of participation; individuals in counties that were considering participation in the Cal-40 study had larger and more dense networks than individuals in counties that had already made a decision to participate or not participate.[141] For those who had agreed to participate or were considering participation, information about TFCO and the Cal-40 study was obtained from presentations given by CIBHS representatives at state or regional meetings, direct contact by CIBHS with county agency directors, direct contact by other agency directors within the county, or staff within the agency. In addition, how leaders interpret and make use of evidence is being examined, including what sources of information they find credible, where they obtain information, and what types of evidence they see as relevant. The findings from the qualitative measures will enhance and extend the SIC outcomes by providing insights into specific mechanisms that drive decisions to adopt/not adopt.

Design

This implementation trial began by inviting all California county service agencies that had not previously adopted TFCO to participate. Of the 40 so-called non-early adopting California counties invited to participate, none declined and 39 consented to at least consider implementing TFCO. No counties objected to the randomization to condition, but several noted that the time frame to which they were assigned did not fit their circumstances.[142] Counties with more children placed in care and those that had more positive organizational climates consented to participate more quickly.[18] The study was extended to include 11 additional Ohio counties that are not early adopters of TFCO. Recruitment, enrollment, and randomization methods used in Ohio mirrored those used in California. The design used a roll-out head-to-head comparison of two implementation strategies, a standard approach that engaged individual counties, and a Community Development Team learning collaborative consisting of six to eight counties working together. Both arms delivered TFCO. Counties were assigned randomly to which implementation strategy and which year they began implementing TFCO. The SIC was used to assess the duration, speed, quality, and quantity of implementation. Because of these multiple dimensions, a composite score was chosen, derived from principal components analysis, as our primary outcome. Analyses used mixed models with random effects to take into account cohort effects as well as clustering of counties inherent in the Community Development Team approach, and readers are referred to the primary outcome publication for further details.[16]

SUMMARY

A wide variety of dissemination and implementation designs are now being used to evaluate and improve health systems and outcomes. This chapter discusses randomized and nonrandomized designs for the traditional translational research continuum or pipeline, which builds on existing efficacy and effectiveness trials to examine how one or more evidence-based clinical/prevention interventions are adopted, scaled up, and sustained in community or service delivery systems. The chapter also considers other designs, including hybrid designs that combine effectiveness and implementation research, and designs that use simulation modeling. A case example of a recent large scale implementation study is presented as an example of measurement and design considerations in dissemination and implementation research. The chapter provides suggested readings and websites useful for design decisions.

ACKNOWLEDGEMENTS

Support for this chapter was provided by the following grant funded by the National Institute of Mental Health and the National Institute on Drug Abuse: P30 MH074678, P30 DA027828, DA019984, MH040859, DA024370, P30 MH068579, and MH080916.

SUGGESTED READINGS AND WEBSITES

Readings

Berwick D. The science of improvement. *JAMA*. 2008;299(10):1182.
This article describes four recommended changes in the use of health care evidence that would speed along health care and practice improvements: (1) use a range of scientific methodologies, considering both mechanisms and contexts; (2) reconsider thresholds for action on evidence, making incremental changes; (3) reconsider concepts of trust and bias; and (4) engage both academics and patient caregivers with respect.

Brown CH, Curran G, Palinkas LA, et al. An overview of research and evaluation designs for dissemination and implementation. *Ann Rev Public Health*. 2017;38:1–22.
This article provides an overview of state-of-the-science experimental and quasi-experimental research designs for D&I. Three broad categories are discussed: (1) within-site designs; (2) between-site designs; and (3) within- and between-site comparison designs.

Brown CH, Wyman PA, Guo J, Peña J. Dynamic wait-listed designs for randomized trials: new designs for prevention of youth suicide. *Clin Trials*. 2006;3(3):259–271.
This article describes a modification to the traditional wait-listed design, in which random assignment occurs multiple times during a trial, thus enabling subjects to receive the intervention. Still, these designs can only be used to assess short-term impact, and there is no control group left as a comparison.

Brown CH, Ten Have TR, Jo B, et al. Adaptive designs for randomized trials in public health. *Annu Rev Public Health*. 2009;30:1–25.
Suggests adaptations to the traditional randomized trial. In this article, "adaptive design" refers to a trial in which characteristics of the study, such as assignment to an intervention or control group, change during the data collection process.

Curran G.M, Bauer M, Mittman B, Pyne J.M., Stetler C. (2012) Effectiveness-implementation hybrid designs: combining elements of clinical effectiveness and implementation research to enhance public health impact. *Med Care*. 2012;50(3)217–226.
This paper presents the concept of hybrid designs that are especially appropriate for implementation research and discuss the three basic types of such designs.

Flay B. Efficacy and effectiveness trials (and other phases of research) in the development of health promotion programs. *Prev Med*. 1986;15(5):451–474.
This early work from Flay provides a useful overview of the concepts of efficacy and effectiveness. While the science of translational research has evolved considerably over the past three decades, many of the principles from Flay's article remain highly relevant.

Glasgow R, Magid D, Beck A, Ritzwoller D, Estabrooks PA. Practical clinical trials for translating research to practice: design and measurement recommendations. *Med Care*. 2005;43(6):551.
Building on the influential work of Tunis et al. on practical clinical trials (PCTs), this article provides examples of conducting PCTs with enhanced external validity, without sacrificing internal validity. The authors suggest that in order to reduce the gap between academia and real-world practice, it is necessary to increase the relevance of PCTs for appropriate audiences.

Landsverk J, Brown C, Rolls Reutz J, Palinkas L, Horwitz S. Design elements in implementation research: a structured review of child welfare and child mental health studies. *Adm Policy Ment Health Ment Health Serv Res.* 2011,38(1):54–63.

This paper discusses the need for the development of methodological approaches to the study of implementation processes and tests of implementation strategies through a structured review of nine studies. The authors present limitations of randomized designs and potential design alternatives to consider.

Pierre RG St. Using randomized experiments. In: Wholey J, Hatry H, Newcomer K, eds. *Handbook of practical program evaluation.* San Francisco: Jossey-Bass Inc.; 2004: 150–175.

In this chapter, Pierre considers the recent push to use randomized experiments for obtaining evidence. He offers recommendations for using and designing randomized experiments, as well as how they should be executed and evaluated.

Reichardt C, Mark M. Quasi-experimentation. In: Wholey J, Hatry H, Newcomer K, eds. *Handbook of practical program evaluation.* San Francisco: Jossey-Bass Inc.; 2004: 126–149.

In this chapter, Reichardt & Mark consider four quasi-experimental designs: before-after, interrupted time series, nonequivalent group, and regression-discontinuity. They describe the strengths and weaknesses of each design, as well as threats to validity.

West SG, Duan N, Pequegnat W, et al. Alternatives to the randomized controlled trial. *Am J Public Health.* 2008;98(8):1359–1366.

The authors consider alternatives to the randomized controlled trial that also allow for drawing causal inferences. They describe the strengths and weaknesses of each design, including threats to validity and the strategies that can be used to diminish those threats.

Selected Websites and Tools

http://wtgrantfoundation.org/resource/optimal-design-with-empirical-information-od

Optimal Design is a software package, developed by Stephen Raudenbush and colleagues, which helps researchers determine sample size, statistical power, and optimal allocation of resources for multilevel and longitudinal studies. This includes group-randomized trials, also called setting-level experiments. Version 2.0 was released in summer 2009. The software, a description of the updates from the previous version, and a manual containing software documentation are available for download.

http://www.rmass.org

The **RMASS** program computes sample size for three-level mixed-effects linear regression models for the analysis of clustered longitudinal data. Three-level designs are used in many areas, but in particular, multicenter randomized longitudinal clinical trials in medical or health-related research. In this case, level 1 represents measurement occasion, level 2 represents subject, and level 3 represents center. The model allows for random effects of the time trends at both the subject level and the center level. The sample size determinations in this program are based on the requirements for a test of treatment by time interaction(s) for designs based on either subject-level or cluster-level randomization. The approach is general with respect to sampling proportions and number of groups, and it allows for differential attrition rates over time.

http://cepim.northwestern.edu

The **Center for Prevention Implementation Methodology for Drug Abuse and HIV (Ce-PIM)** website provides a range of publications and presentations on implementation principles, measures, designs, and analyses

http://epoc.cochrane.org/

The **Cochrane Effective Practice and Organisation of Care (EPOC) Group** is a Review Group of The Cochrane Collaboration—an international network of people helping health care providers, policymakers, patients, their advocates and carers make well-informed decisions about human health care by preparing and publishing systematic reviews. The research focus of the EPOC Group are interventions designed to improve the delivery, practice, and organization of health care services. The EPOC editorial base is located in Ottawa, Canada with satellite centers in Norway, Australia, and England.

https://cyberseminar.cancercontrolplanet.org/implementationscience/

The **Implementation Science Webinar Series** is sponsored by the National Cancer Institute (NCI) Division of Cancer Control & Population Sciences. In 2013 the Implementation Science Team started a webinar series focused on advanced dissemination and implementation research topics, including *design and analysis issues.* Each session includes approximately 40 minutes for presentation(s) by leaders in the field as well as 20 minutes for engaged discussion and Q&A. The website lists topics and session titles for upcoming sessions or archived sessions.

REFERENCES

1. Proctor E, Landsverk J, Aarons G, Chambers D, Glisson C, Mittman B. Implementation research in mental health services: an emerging science with conceptual, methodological, and training challenges. *Adm Policy Ment Health Ment Health Serv Res.* 2009;36(1):24–34.

2. Brown CH, Curran G, Palinkas LA, et al. An overview of research and evaluation designs for dissemination and implementation. *Annu Rev Public Health*. 2017;38:1–22.

3. National Research Council and Institute of Medicine; Committee on Prevention of Mental Disorders and Substance Abuse Among Children, Youth, and Young Adults: Research Advances and Promising Interventions; Board on Children, Youth, and Families; Division of Behavioral and Social Sciences and Education, Mary Ellen O'Connell, Thomas Boat; Warner KE, eds. *Preventing mental, emotional, and behavioral disorders among young people: Progress and possibilities*. Washington, DC: National Academy Press; 2009.

4. Aarons GA, Hurlburt M, Horwitz SM. Advancing a conceptual model of evidence-based practice implementation in public service sectors. *Adm Policy Ment Health Ment Health Serv Res*. 2011;38(1):4–23.

5. Zerhouni E. The NIH roadmap. *Science*. 2003;302(5642):63–72.

6. Zerhouni E. Translational and clinical science--time for a new vision. *N Engl J Med*. 2005;353(15):1621.

7. Culliton B. Extracting knowledge from science: a conversation with Elias Zerhouni. *Health Affairs*. 2006;25(3):w94.

8. Westfall J, Mold J, Fagnan L. Practice-based research--" Blue Highways" on the NIH roadmap. *JAMA*. 2007;297(4):403.

9. Spoth R, Rohrbach LA, Greenberg M, et al. Addressing core challenges for the next generation of type 2 translation research and systems: the translation science to population impact (TSci Impact) framework. *Prev Sci*. 2013;14(4):319–351.

10. Powell BJ, Waltz TJ, Chinman MJ, et al. A refined compilation of implementation strategies: results from the Expert Recommendations for Implementing Change (ERIC) project. *Implement Sci*. 2015;10(1):21.

11. Waltz TJ, Powell BJ, Matthieu MM, et al. Use of concept mapping to characterize relationships among implementation strategies and assess their feasibility and importance: results from the Expert Recommendations for Implementing Change (ERIC) study. *Implement Sci*. 2015;10(1):109.

12. Proctor E, Silmere H, Raghavan R, et al. Outcomes for implementation research: conceptual distinctions, measurement challenges, and research agenda. *Adm Policy Ment Health Ment Health Serv Res*. 2011;38(2):65–76.

13. Institute of Medicine Committee on Crossing the Quality Chasm: Adaptation to Mental Health and Addictive Disorders. *Improving the quality of health care for mental and substance-use conditions*. Wahington, DC: National Academy Press; 2006.

14. Smith J, Polaha J. Using implementation science to guide the integration of evidence-based family interventions into primary care. *Fam Syst Health*. 2017;35(2):125–135.

15. Chamberlain P, Brown CH, Saldana L. Observational measure of implementation progress in community based settings: the stages of implementation completion (*SIC*). *Implement Sci*. 2011;6(1):116.

16. Brown CH, Chamberlain P, Saldana L, Wang W, Padgett C, Cruden G. Evaluation of two implementation strategies in fifty-one counties in two states: results of a cluster randomized implementation trial. *Implement Sci*. 2015;9:134.

17. Wang D, Ogihara M, Gallo C, et al. Automatic classification of communication logs into implementation stages via text analysis. *Implement Sci*. 2016;11(1):119.

18. Wang W, Saldana L, Brown CH, Chamberlain P. Factors that influenced county system leaders to implement an evidence-based program: a baseline survey within a randomized controlled trial. *Implement Sci*. 2010;5(1):72.

19. Curran GM, Bauer M, Mittman B, Pyne JM, Stetler C. Effectiveness-implementation hybrid designs: combining elements of clinical effectiveness and implementation research to enhance public health impact. *Med Care*. 2012;50(3):217.

20. Brown CH, Ten Have TR, Jo B, et al. Adaptive designs for randomized trials in public health. *Annu Rev Public Health*. 2009;30:1–25.

21. Poduska J, Kellam S, Brown C, et al. Study protocol for a group randomized controlled trial of a classroom-based intervention aimed at preventing early risk factors for drug abuse: integrating effectiveness and implementation research. *Implement Sci*. 2009;4(1):56.

22. Dixon LB, Goldman HH, Bennett ME, et al. Implementing coordinated specialty care for early psychosis: the RAISE Connection Program. *Psychiatr Serv*. 2015;66(7):691–698.

23. Kane JM, Robinson DG, Schooler NR, et al. Comprehensive versus usual community care for first-episode psychosis: 2-year outcomes from the NIMH RAISE early treatment program. *Am J Psychiatry*. 2015;173(4):362–372.

24. Holtgrave DR. *Handbook of economic evaluation of HIV prevention programs*. New York: Springer Science & Business Media; 1998.

25. Baltussen R, Niessen L. Priority setting of health interventions: the need for multi-criteria decision analysis. *Cost Effect Resource Alloc*. 2006;4(1):14.

26. Alonso-Coello P, Schünemann HJ, Moberg J, et al. GRADE Evidence to Decision (EtD) frameworks: a systematic and transparent approach to making well informed healthcare choices. 1: Introduction. *BMJ.* 2016;353:i2016.

27. Haddix AC, Teutsch SM, Corso PS. *Prevention effectiveness: A guide to decision analysis and economic evaluation.* New York: Oxford University Press; 2003.

28. Yaylali E, Farnham PG, Schneider KL, et al. From theory to practice: implementation of a resource allocation model in health departments. *J Public Health Manag Practice.* 2016;22(6):567.

29. Lich KH, Ginexi EM, Osgood ND, Mabry PL. A call to address complexity in prevention science research. *Preven Sci.* 2013;14(3):279–289.

30. Northridge ME, Metcalf SS. Enhancing implementation science by applying best principles of systems science. *Health Res Policy Syst.* 2016;14(1):74.

31. Lich KH, Frerichs L, Fishbein D, Bobashev G, Pentz MA. Translating research into prevention of high-risk behaviors in the presence of complex systems: definitions and systems frameworks. *Transl Behav Med.* 2016;6(1):17–31.

32. Weiss CH, Poncela-Casasnovas J, Glaser JI, et al. Adoption of a high-impact innovation in a homogeneous population. *Phys Rev.* 2014;4(4):041008.

33. Liljeros F, Edling CR, Amaral LAN, Stanley HE, Åberg Y. The web of human sexual contacts. *Nature.* 2001;411(6840):907–908.

34. Gold MR, Siegel JE, Russell LB, Weinstein MC, eds. *Cost-effectiveness in health and medicine.* New York: Oxford University Press; 1996.

35. Frazier AL, Colditz GA, Fuchs CS, Kuntz KM. Cost-effectiveness of screening for colorectal cancer in the general population. *JAMA.* 2000;284(15):1954.

36. Gaspoz JM, Coxson PG, Goldman PA, et al. Cost effectiveness of aspirin, clopidogrel, or both for secondary prevention of coronary heart disease. *N Engl J Med.* 2002;346(23):1800.

37. Goldhaber-Fiebert JD, Stout NK, Salomon JA, Kuntz KM, Goldie SJ. Cost-effectiveness of cervical cancer screening with human papillomavirus DNA testing and HPV-16, 18 vaccination. *J Nat Cancer Inst.* 2008;100(5):308.

38. CDC Diabetes Cost-effectiveness Group. Cost-effectiveness of intensive glycemic control, intensified hypertension control, and serum cholesterol level reduction for type 2 diabetes. *JAMA.* 2002;287(19):2542–2551.

39. Sanders GD, Bayoumi AM, Sundaram V, et al. Cost-effectiveness of screening for HIV in the era of highly active antiretroviral therapy. *N Engl J Med.* 2005;352(6):570.

40. Tosteson ANA, Stout NK, Fryback DG, et al. Cost-effectiveness of digital mammography breast cancer screening. *Ann Intern Med.* 2008;148(1):1.

41. Ruiz MS. *No time to lose: Getting more from HIV prevention.* Washingtonm DC: National Academies Press; 2001.

42. Goldhaber-Fiebert JD, Snowden LR, Wulczyn F, Landsverk J, Horwitz SM. Economic evaluation research in the context of child welfare policy: a structured literature review and recommendations. *Child Abuse Neglect.* 2011;35(9):722–740.

43. Price JM, Chamberlain P, Landsverk J, Reid J. KEEP foster parent training intervention: model description and effectiveness. *Child Fam Soc Work.* 2009;14(2):233–242.

44. Price J, Chamberlain P, Landsverk J, Reid J, Leve L, Laurent H. Effects of a foster parent training intervention on placement changes of children in foster care. *Child Maltreatment.* 2008;13(1):64.

45. Chamberlain P, Price J, Reid J, Landsverk J. Cascading implementation of a foster and kinship parent intervention. *Child Welfare.* 2008;87(5):27–48.

46. Jenness SM, Goodreau SM, Rosenberg E, et al. Impact of the Centers for Disease Control's HIV preexposure prophylaxis guidelines for men who have sex with men in the United States. *J Infect Dis.* 2016;214(12):1800–1807.

47. Beck EC, Birkett M, Armbruster B, Mustanski B. A data-driven simulation of HIV spread among young men who have sex with men: the role of age and race mixing, and STIs. *J Aacquir Immune Defic Syndr.* 2015;70(2):186.

48. Friedman LM, Furberg C, DeMets DL. *Fundamentals of clinical trials.* 3rd ed. New York: Springer; 1998.

49. Torgerson D, Torgerson C. Designing and running randomised trials in health and the social sciences. Basingstoke, UK: Palgrave Macmillan; 2008.

50. Brown CH, Wang W, Kellam SG, et al. Methods for testing theory and evaluating impact in randomized field trials: intent-to-treat analyses for integrating the perspectives of person, place, and time. *Drug Alcohol Depend.* 2008;95(Suppl 1):S74-S104. Supplementary data associated with this article can be found, in the online version, at doi:110.1016/j.drugalcdep.2008.1001.1005.

51. Murray DM. *Design and analysis of group-randomized trials.* Vol 29. New York: Oxford University Press; 1998.

52. Flay B. Efficacy and effectiveness trials (and other phases of research) in the development of health promotion programs. *Prevent Med.* 1986;15(5):451–474.

53. Glasgow R, Magid D, Beck A, Ritzwoller D, Estabrooks P. Practical clinical trials for translating research to practice: design and measurement recommendations. *Med Care.* 2005;43(6):551.

54. Brown CH, Wyman PA, Guo J, Peña J. Dynamic wait-listed designs for randomized trials: new designs for prevention of youth suicide. *Clin Trials.* 2006;3(3):259–271.

55. Landsverk J, Brown C, Rolls Reutz J, Palinkas L, Horwitz S. Design elements in implementation research: a structured review of child welfare and child mental health studies. *Adm Policy Ment Health Ment Health Serv Res.* 2011:1–10.

56. Effective Practice and Organisation of Care (EPOC). EPOC Resources for review authors. Oslo: Norwegian Knowledge Centre for the Health Services; 2015: http://epoc.cochrane.org/epoc-specific-resources-review-authors.

57. Smith JD. Single-case experimental designs: a systematic review of published research and current standards. *Psychol Methods.* 2012;17(4):510.

58. Brown CH, Liao J. Principles for designing randomized preventive trials in mental health: an emerging developmental epidemiology paradigm. *Am J Commun Psychol.* 1999;27(5):673–710.

59. Brown CA, Lilford RJ. The stepped wedge trial design: a systematic review. *BMC Med Res Methodol.* 2006;6(1):54.

60. Wyman PA, Henry D, Knoblauch S, Brown CH. Designs for testing group-based interventions with limited numbers of social units: the dynamic wait-listed and regression point displacement designs. *Prev Sci.* 2015;16(7):956–966.

61. Kratochwill TR, Levin JR. Enhancing the scientific credibility of single-case intervention research: randomization to the rescue. *Psychol Methods.* 2010;15(2):124.

62. Brown CH, Kellam SG, Kaupert S, et al. Partnerships for the design, conduct, and analysis of effectiveness, and implementation research: experiences of the Prevention Science and Methodology Group. *Adm Policy Ment Health Ment Health Serv Res.* 2012;39(4):301–316.

63. Chamberlain P, Roberts R, Jones H, Marsenich L, Sosna T, Price JM. Three collaborative models for scaling up evidence-based practices. *Adm Policy Ment Health Ment Health Serv Res.* 2012;39(4):278–290.

64. Brown CH, Berndt D, Brinales JM, Zong X, Bhagwat D. Evaluating the evidence of effectiveness for preventive interventions: using a registry system to influence policy through science. *Addict Behav.* 2000;25(6):955–964.

65. Brown CH, Wyman PA, Brinales JM, Gibbons RD. The role of randomized trials in testing interventions for the prevention of youth suicide. *Int Rev Psychiatry.* 2007;19(6):617–631.

66. Chamberlain P, Saldana L, Brown CH, Leve LD. Implementation of multidimensional treatment foster care in California: A randomized trial of an evidence-based practice In: Roberts-DeGennaro M, Fogel S, eds. *Empirically supported interventions for community and organizational change*: Chicago: Lyceum Books, Inc.; 2010:218–234

67. Chamberlain P, Brown C, Saldana L, et al. Engaging and recruiting counties in an experiment on implementing evidence-based practice in California. *Admin Policy Ment Hlth Ment Hlth Res.* 2008;35:250–260.

68. Marcus SM, Gibbons RD. Estimating the efficacy of receiving treatment in randomized clinical trials with noncompliance. *Health Serv Outc Res Methodol.* 2001;2(3-4):247–257.

69. Stuart EA, Green KM. Using full matching to estimate causal effects in nonexperimental studies: examining the relationship between adolescent marijuana use and adult outcomes. *Dev Psychol.* 2008;44(2):395–406.

70. Shortell SM. Increasing value: a research agenda for addressing the managerial and organizational challenges facing health care delivery in the United States. *Med Care Res Rev.* 2004;61(3 suppl):12S–30S.

71. Wholey J, Hatry H, Newcomer K, eds. *Handbook of practical program evaluation.* San Francisco: Jossey-Bass Inc; 2004.

72. Reichardt C, Mark M. Quasi-experimentation. In: Wholey J, Hatry H, Newcomer K, eds. *Handbook of practical program evaluation.* San Francisco: Jossey-Bass Inc; 2004:126–149.

73. Pierre R. St, Using randomized experiments. In: Wholey J, Hatry H, Newcomer K, eds. *Handbook of practical program evaluation.* San Francisco: Jossey-Bass Inc; 2004:150–176.

74. Barrett-Connor E, Grady D, Stefanick M. The rise and fall of menopausal hormone therapy. *Annu Rev Public Health.* 2004;26:115–140.

75. Concato J, Shah N, Horwitz R. Randomized, controlled trials, observational studies, and the hierarchy of research designs. *NEngl J Med.* 2000;342(25):1887.

76. Cook T, Shadish W, Wong V. Three conditions under which experiments and observational studies produce comparable causal estimates: new findings from within-study comparisons. *J Policy Anal Manage.* 2008;27(4):724–750.

77. Concato J, Lawler EV, Lew RA, Gaziano JM, Aslan M, Huang GD. Observational methods in comparative effectiveness research. *Am J Med.* 2010;123(12):e16–e23.

78. West SG, Duan N, Pequegnat W, et al. Alternatives to the randomized controlled trial. *Am J Public Health*. 2008;98(8):1359–1366.

79. Brown CA, Lilford RJ. The stepped wedge trial design: a systematic review. *BMC Med Res Methodol*. 2006;6:54.

80. Bonell CP, Hargreaves J, Cousens S, et al. Alternatives to randomisation in the evaluation of public health interventions: design challenges and solutions. *J Epidemiol Commun Health*. 2011;65(7):582–587.

81. Raudenbush SW, Liu X. Statistical power and optimal design for multisite randomized trials. *Psychol Methods*. 2000;5(2):199–213.

82. Bhaumik DK, Roy A, Aryal S, et al. Sample size determination for studies with repeated continuous outcomes. *Psychiatr Ann*. 2008;38(12):765–771.

83. Damschroder LJ, Aron DC, Keith RE, Kirsh SR, Alexander JA, Lowery JC. Fostering implementation of health services research findings into practice: a consolidated framework for advancing implementation science. *Implement Sci*. 2009;4:50.

84. Curran GM, Mittman BS, Landes S, Pyne J. Effectiveness-Implementation Hybrid Designs: Clarification, Refinements, and Additional Guidance Based on a Systematic Review and Reports from the Field. 8th Annual Conference on the Science of Dissemination and Implementation in Health; December 2015, December 2015; Washington, DC.

85. Nilsen P. Making sense of implementation theories, models and frameworks. *Implement Sci*. 2015;10(1):53.

86. Brown CH, Kellam SG, Ialongo N, Poduska J, Ford C. Prevention of aggressive behavior through middle school using a first grade classroom-based Intervention In: Tsuang MT, Lyons MJ, Stone WS, eds. *Towards prevention and early intervention of major mental and substance abuse disorders* Arlington, VA: American Psychiatric Publishing, Inc.; 2007: 347–370.

87. Kellam SG, Brown CH, Poduska JM, et al. Effects of a universal classroom behavior management program in first and second grades on young adult behavioral, psychiatric, and social outcomes. *Drug Alcohol Depend*. 2008;95(Suppl 1):S5-S28. Supplementary data associated with this article can be found,in the online version, at doi: 10.1016/j.drugalcdep.2008.1001.1004.

88. Jones B, Nachtsheim CJ. Split-plot design: what, why, and how. *J Qual Technol*. 2009;41(4):340–361.

89. Chambers DA. Advancing the science of implementation: a workshop summary. *Adm Policy Ment Health Ment Health Serv Res*. 2008;35(1-2):3–10.

90. Kraemer HC, Mintz J, Noda A, Tinklenberg J, Yesavage JA. Caution regarding the use of pilot studies to guide power calculations for study proposals. *Arch Gen Psychiatry*. 2006;63(5):484–489.

91. Kellam SG, Ling X, Merisca R, Brown CH, Ialongo N. The effect of the level of aggression in the first grade classroom on the course and malleability of aggressive behavior into middle school. *Dev Psychopathol*. 1998;10(2):165–185.

92. Frangakis CE, Rubin DB. Principal stratification in causal inference. *Biometrics*. 2002;58:21–29.

93. Greenland S, Lanes S, Jara M. Estimating effects from randomized trials with discontinuations: the need for intent to treat design and G-estimation. *Clin Trials*. 2007;5:5–13.

94. Robins JM, Greenland S. Identifiability and exchangeability for direct and indirect effects. *Epidemiology*. 1992;3:143–155.

95. Barnard J, Frangakis CE, Hill JL, Rubin DB. Principal stratification approach to broken randomized experiments: a case study of school choice vouchers in New York City/Comment/ Rejoinder. *J Am Stat Assoc*. 2003;98(462):299–323.

96. Frangakis CE, Brookmeyer RS, Varadhan R, Safaeian M, Vlahov D, Strathdee SA. Methodology for Evaluating a Partially Controlled Longitudinal Treatment Using Principal Stratification, With Application to a Needle Exchange Program. *J Am Stat Assoc*. 2004;99(465):239–249.

97. Frangakis CE, Brookmeyer RS, Varadham R, Safaeian M, Vlahov D, Strathdee SA. Methodology for evaluating a partially controlled longitudinal treatment using principal stratification, with application to a needle exchange Program. *J Am Stat Assoc*. 2004;99(465):239–249.

98. Barnard J, Frangakis CE, Hill J, Rubin DB. School choice in NY City: A Bayesian analysis of an imperfect randomized experiment. In: Gatsonis C, Kass RE, Carlin BP, et al., eds. *Case studies in Bayesian statistics*. Vol V. New York: Springer; 2002:3–98.

99. Muthén BO, Jo B, Brown CH. Comment on the Barnard, Frangakis, Hill & Rubin article, Principal stratification approach to broken randomized experiments: a case study of school choice vouchers in New York City. *J. Am. Stat Assoc*. 2003;98(462):311–314.

100. Frangakis CE, Rubin DB, Frangakis CE, Rubin DB. Principal stratification in causal inference. *Biometrics*. 2002;58(1):21–29.

101. Frangakis CE, Varadham R. Systematizing the evaluation of partially controlled studies using principal stratification: from theory to practice *Statistica Sinica*. 2004;14:945–947.

102. Jin H, Rubin DB. Principal stratification for causal inference with extended partial compliance. *J Am Stat Assoc*. 2008;103(481):101–111.

103. Rubin DB. Direct and indirect causal effects via potential outcomes. *Scand. J. Stat.* 2004;31(2):161–170.

104. Angrist JD, Imbens GW, Rubin DB. Identification of causal effects using instrumental variables. *J Am Stat Assoc.* 1996;91(434):444–455.

105. Asparouhov T, Muthén BO. Multilevel mixture models. In: Hancock GR, Samuelsen KM, eds. *Advances in latent variable mixture models.* Charlotte, NC: Information Age Publishing, Inc.; 2008: 27–51.

106. Muthen B. Latent varaible mixture modeling. In: Marcoulides GA, Schumacker RE, eds. *Advanced structural equational modling: New development nd techniques.* Hillsdale, NJ: Lawrence Earlbaum Associates; 2000: 1–33.

107. Muthén BO. Second-generation structural equation modeling with a combination of categorical and continuous latent variables: New opportunities for latent class/latent growth modeling. In: Collins LM, Sayer A, eds. *New Methods for the Analysis of Change.* Washington, D.C.: APA; 2001:291–322.

108. Muthén BO. Statistical and Substantive Checking In Growth Mixture Modeling: Comment on Bauer and Curran. *Psychological Methods.* 2003;8(3):369–377.

109. Muthen B. Latent variable modeling of longitudinal and multilevel data. *Soiol Methodo.* 2005;27:453–480.

110. Muthén B. Latent variable modeling of longitudinal and multilevel data. *Sociol Methodol.* 1997;27:453–480.

111. Muthén B, Brown CH. Estimating drug effects in the presence of placebo response: causal inference using growth mixture modeling. *Stat Med.* 2009;28(27):3363–3395.

112. Guo J. *Extending the principal stratification methods to multi-level randomized trials* [Doctoral Dissertation]. Tampa, FL: Epidemiology and Biostatistics, University of South Florida; 2010.

113. Brown CH, Indurkhya A, Kellam SG. Power calculations for data missing by design with application to a follow-up study of exposure and attention. *J Am Stat. Assoc.* 2000;95:383–395.

114. Czaja SJ, Valente TW, Nair SN, Villamar JA, Brown CH. Characterizing implementation strategies using a systems engineering survey and interview tool: a comparison across 10 prevention programs for drug abuse and HIV sexual risk behavior. *Implement Sci.* 2016;11(1):70.

115. Kossisakoff A, Sweet WN. *Systems engineering principles and practice.* Hoboken, NJ: John Wiley & Sons Inc.; 2003.

116. Czaja SJ, Nair SN. Human factors engineering and systems design. In: Salvendy G, ed. *Handbook of human factors and ergonomics.* 3rd ed. Hoboken, NJ: John Wiley & Sons Inc; 2006: 32–49.

117. Schulz R, Belle SH, Czaja SJ, Gitlin LN, Wisniewski SR, Ory MG. Introduction to the special section on Resources for Enhancing Alzheimer's Caregiver Health (REACH). *Psychol Aging.* 2003;18(3):357–360.

118. Saaty TL. The analytic hierarchy process in conflict management. *Int J Conflict Manage.* 1990;1(1):47–68.

119. Czaja SJ, Schulz R, Lee CC, Belle SH. A methodology for describing and decomposing complex psychosocial and behavioral interventions. *Psychol Aging.* 2003;18(3):385–395.

120. Rabiner LR. A tutorial on hidden Markov models and selected applications in speech recognition. *Proceedings of the IEEE.* 1989;77(2):257–286.

121. Deerwester S, Dumais ST, Furnas GW, Landauer TK, Harshman R. Indexing by latent semantic analysis. *J Am Soc Inform Sci.* 1990;41(6):391–407.

122. Hofmann T. Probabilistic latent semantic indexing. Proceedings of the 22nd annual international ACM SIGIR conference on Research and development in information retrieval; 1999; Berkeley, California, United States.

123. Li T, Zhu S, Ogihara M. Hierarchical document classification using automatically generated hierarchy. *J Intell Inf Syst.* 2007;29(2):211–230.

124. Li T, Zhu S, Ogihara M. Text categorization via generalized discriminant analysis. *Inform Process Manag.* 2008;44(5):1684–1697.

125. Larzelere RE, Daly DL, Davis JL, Chmelka MB, Handwerk ML. Outcome evaluation of girls and boys town's family home program. *Educ Treat Child.* 2004;27(2):130–150.

126. Dodge K, Sherrill M. *Deviant peer group effects in youth mental health interventions.* New York, Guilford. 2006.

127. Ryan J, Marshall J, Herz D, Hernandez P. Juvenile delinquency in child welfare: Investigating group home effects. *Child Youth Serv Rev.* 2008;30(9):1088–1099.

128. Wulczyn F, Orlebeke B, Melamid E. Measuring contract agency performance with administrative data. *Child Welfare.* 2000;79(5):457–474.

129. Chamberlain P, Leve L, DeGarmo D. Multidimensional treatment foster care for girls in the juvenile justice system: 2-year follow-up of a randomized clinical trial. *J Consult Clin Psychol.* 2007;75(1):187.

130. Eddy J, Bridges Whaley R, Chamberlain P. The prevention of violent behavior by chronic and serious male juvenile offenders. *J Emot Behav Disord.* 2004;12(1):2.

131. U.S. Department of Education, Office of Special Educational Research and Improvement, Office of Reform Assistance and Dissemination. *Safe, Disciplined, and Drug-Free Schools Programs.* Washington, DC; 2001.

132. U.S. Department of Health and Human Services, ed *Youth violence: A report of the Surgeon General.* Rockville, MD: U.S. Department of Health and Human Services, Centers for Disease Control and Prevention, National Center for Injury Prevention and Control; Substance Abuse and Mental Health Services Administration, Center for Mental Health Services; and National Institutes of Health, National Institute of Mental Health; 2001.

133. U.S. Department of Health and Human Services, ed. *Mental health: A report of the Surgeon General.* Rockville, MD: U.S. Department of Health and Human Services, Substance Abuse and Mental Health Services Administration, Center for Mental Health Services, National Institutes of Health, National Institute of Mental Health; 1999.

134. Aos S, Phipps P, Barnoski R, Leib R, eds. *The comparative costs and benefits of programs to reduce crime, 4.0.* Olympia, WA: Washington State Institute for Public Policy; 1999.

135. Rogers E. *Diffusion of innovations.* New York: Free Press; 1995.

136. Sosna T, Marsenich L. *Community development team model: Supporting the model adherent implementation of programs and practices.* Sacramento, CA: California Institute for Mental Health;2006.

137. Kalbfleisch JD, Prentice RL. *The statistical analysis of failure time data.* 2nd ed. New York: Wiley; 2002.

138. Liang K-Y, Zeger SL. Longitudinal data analysis using generalized estimating equations. *Biometrika.* 1986;73(1):13–22.

139. Zeger SL, Liang KY, Albert PS. Models for longitudinal data: a generalized estimating equation approach.[erratum appears in Biometrics 1989 Mar;45(1):347]. *Biometrics.* 1988;44(4):1049–1060.

140. Pulver AE, Liang K-y, Brown C, Wolyniec PS, et al. Risk factors in schizophrenia: season of birth, gender, and familial risk. *Br J Psychiatry.* 1992;160:65–71.

141. Palinkas L, Fuentes D, Holloway I, Wu Q, Chamberlain P. Social Networks and Implementation of Evidence-Based Practices in Public Youth-Serving Systems. Sunbelt XXX, International Network for Social Network Analysis Conference; July 3, 2010, 2010; Riva del Garda, Italy.

142. Chamberlain P, Brown CH, Saldana L, et al. Engaging and recruiting counties in an experiment on implementing evidence-based practice in California. *Adm Policy Ment Health.* 2008;35(4):250–260.

14

Measurement Issues in Dissemination and Implementation Research

CARA C. LEWIS, ENOLA K. PROCTOR, AND ROSS C. BROWNSON

INTRODUCTION

New fields are often beset with measurement challenges given the dearth of measures and psychometric studies, inconsistent and evolving use of constructs, underdeveloped theories, and isolated research teams.[1] In 2013 the National Institutes of Health acknowledged the issues threatening dissemination and implementation (D&I) research in health and held a 2-day working meeting on measurement and reporting standards.[2] Twenty-three leaders of large-scale initiatives were charged with establishing the current state of the field and articulating a research agenda.[2,3] Building from this meeting, this chapter provides an overview of work to date that attempts to advance D&I measurement.

The language of D&I is highly varied, as even these key processes (dissemination and implementation) may be described as diffusion, translation, and numerous other terms; indeed McKibbon et al.[4] identified 100 different terms with which to refer to D&I. The chapter follows the definitions of D&I offered by Rabin and colleagues[5] in chapter 2. Dissemination is an active approach of spreading evidence-based interventions (EBIs) to target audiences via determined channels using planned strategies. Implementation is the process of putting to use, or integrating EBIs within a specific setting.

The constructs for D&I measurement derive from conceptual models. The framework of D&I reflected in Figure 14.1 makes a number of key distinctions that carry implications for conceptualizing and measuring implementation processes and outcomes. First, the model distinguishes between the EBI being introduced and the *dissemination strategies* for spreading information about them and *implementation strategies* for putting those programs into place in usual settings of prevention or care. For more information on

D&I strategies and how they are measured, please see chapter 15. Grimshaw et al.[6] reported that meta-analyses of the effectiveness of implementation strategies have been thwarted by measurement issues, notably lack of detailed information about outcomes, use of widely varying constructs, reliance on dichotomous rather than continuous measures, and unit of analysis errors.[7] Second, these D&I *strategies* are different from their *outcomes*, which in turn need to be distinguished according to their several types. Dissemination and implementation outcomes serve as intermediate outcomes, or the proximal effects that are presumed to contribute to more distal outcomes, such as changes in service systems, in consumer health, behavior change, and larger population health. Service system outcomes reflect the six quality improvement aims set out in the Crossing the Quality Chasm reports: the extent to which services are safe, effective, patient-centered, timely, efficient, and equitable.[8,9] D&I outcomes along with service system outcomes are viewed as contributing to individual and population health outcomes.[10]

Clearly the progress of D&I science *and* practice requires the development of reliable, valid, and pragmatic measures of contexts and outcomes. Psychometrically and pragmatically strong D&I context and outcome measures will enable empirical testing of the success of efforts to disseminate and implement new interventions, identification of D&I mechanisms of change (moderators and mediators), and pave the way for comparative effectiveness research on D&I strategies. Moreover, measures have the potential to provide actionable information for tailoring D&I strategies to the context. Unfortunately, measurement issues undermine this potential. The current literature reflects a wide array of constructs that are used when discussing D&I processes and

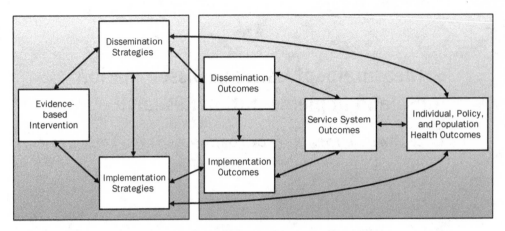

FIGURE 14.1 A framework for dissemination and implementation.

outcomes, terms that are often used inconsistently, reflecting issues of homonymy (i.e., measures that purportedly assess the same construct but do so with substantively different items), synonymy (i.e., measures that have similar items that purportedly assess different constructs), and instability (i.e., items in a measure that shift or are modified over time in an unpredictable manner). When these constructs have been studied, they are measured in different ways—ranging from qualitative, quantitative survey, and record archival[7,11]—but often without any reporting of their measurement properties or rigor. What follows is an overview of the current state of D&I context and outcome measurement.

CURRENT STATE OF D&I MEASUREMENT: CONTEXTUAL FACTORS

Theories, models, and frameworks derive the D&I constructs and their definitions for process evaluation. Tabak and colleagues[12] identified over 60 such models in their 2012 review, some with overlapping or redundant constructs and others with distinct constructs for evaluation. Content validity measurement issues such as homonymy, synonymy, and instability arise due to diversity in operationalization of D&I constructs across models.[13] Systematic reviews of D&I measures can summarize the psychometric quality of measures, such as their content validity. Seven systematic reviews of contextual factors have been conducted in the past decade;[14–20] see Rabin et al.[2] for a summary of these studies and related resources.

Three of these reviews focused on single constructs (i.e., fidelity and clinician behavior;[14,15] organizational readiness to change),[16] one on

five key organization-level constructs (i.e., leadership, vision, managerial relations, climate, and absorptive capacity),[17] and three on numerous constructs depicted in an established D&I model (i.e., Framework for Effective Implementation;[18] Consolidated Framework for Implementation Research;[19] Theoretical Framework for 27 Predictors of Adoption).[20] Unfortunately, only two studies evaluated measures' content validity and found that 56% and 58.14% of the measures, respectively, had established content validity evidence,[15,16] indicating that nearly half of the included measures had not ensured that the items represented all facets of a known construct. More common was that these studies reported broadly on psychometric strength of the measures, as in the Chor et al.[20] review wherein they simply stated "yes" or "no" with respect to whether a measure had demonstrated reliability or validity. Two cross-cutting findings emerged from these reviews: (1) the majority of measures are not psychometrically strong or they have never been tested for their psychometric quality and (2) measures are typically used only in a single study. These findings suggest that the majority of D&I studies are reporting on measures that may not be assessing their intended construct, all facets of the known construct, and may not operate consistently within and across studies. Accordingly, D&I reports on contextual factors should be interpreted with caution until more work is done to establish the psychometric properties of measures.

CURRENT STATE OF D&I MEASUREMENT: OUTCOMES

Dissemination outcomes are defined here as the effects of dissemination strategies, that is, the consequences of targeted distribution of information and intervention materials to a specific public health or clinical practice audience. Similarly, implementation outcomes are defined as the effects of deliberate and purposive actions to implement new interventions. D&I outcomes are proximal reflections of their respective processes, and thus serve as intermediate outcomes in larger efforts to improve the service system and ultimately individual or population health.[7] Distinguishing D&I effectiveness from program or intervention effectiveness is critical. When efforts to transport new programs, or the information about them, from laboratory settings to community health and mental health venues fail—as they often do (2/3 of efforts fail)[21]—we must be able to determine if failure occurred because the intervention was ineffective in the new setting (intervention failure), or if a good intervention was conveyed and deployed incorrectly (dissemination/implementation failure).

Table 14.1 provides a taxonomy of D&I outcomes. For each outcome, the table (a) nominates a level of analysis, (b) identifies the theoretical basis to the construct from literature, (c) offers different terms that are used for the construct in the literature, (d) suggests the point or stage within D&I processes at which the outcome may be most salient, (e) indicates whether the outcome is appropriate for latent variable conceptualization, and (f) lists the types of existing measures for the construct. Level of analysis is an important consideration because it has implications for the measure's target (stakeholder e.g., provider, middle manager, administrator), language (e.g., intended to capture individual perspective versus that of the larger group), and analysis (e.g., aggregated to reflect a group or organization). The theoretical basis should delineate the interrelations among constructs and inform its definition to ensure that item development reflects the content of what the construct is and is not (i.e., to establish construct and content validity). Different terms are offered but it remains an empirical question whether these terms are actually synonyms or reflective of unique constructs worthy of evaluation.

Of the 60+ theories, frameworks, and models, few indicate when in an implementation process each outcome is most relevant for measurement. That is, D&I outcomes are likely to differ in importance across phases. For example, feasibility may be most important once organizations and providers try new interventions. Later, it may be

a "moot point," once the intervention—initially considered novel or unknown—has become part of normal routine. However feasibility could once again become highly salient if resources or context changed. The literature suggests that studies usually capture measures of fidelity prior to, or during, initial implementation, while adoption is often assessed at 6,[22] 12,[23,24] or 18 months[25] after initial implementation. But most studies fail to specify a timeframe or are inconsistent in choice of a time point in the implementation process for measuring each implementation outcome. Clearer specification of the time frame chosen for measurement and the rationale for the choice is needed. The EPIS model—Exploration, Preparation, Implementation, Sustainment[26] is one of the few models that provides some guidance regarding the temporal relations of the D&I outcomes. Although a review of the EPIS model is beyond the scope of this chapter, we use it to illustrate where each D&I outcome would fall across the four stages to inform strategic assessment (see Table 14.1).

Finally, as can be seen in Table 14.1, many of the D&I outcomes can be inferred or measured in terms of expressed attitudes and opinions, intentions, or perspectives as is often the target of survey measurement methods. However, several of the D&I outcomes are not best conceptualized as latent variables and should instead be measured directly through observation (e.g., adoption), objective rating (e.g. fidelity), concrete information tracking (e.g., cost), or administrative data collection (e.g., penetration). As can be seen in Table 14.1, methods of measurement for each outcome do not always adhere to that which is most appropriate, as surveys tend to be the approach favored by researchers (despite likely issues of shared method variance undermining the accuracy of one's findings).

DISSEMINATION OUTCOMES

The literature on dissemination outcomes is sparse and scattered, reflecting no conceptual typology or list of dissemination outcomes, nor have there been any systematic reviews of dissemination outcome measures. Rabin and colleagues[27] reported that nearly half of all published reports of dissemination research in cancer fail to report any outcomes. However several constructs reflecting potential outcomes are mentioned in articles that discuss dissemination approaches, the most frequent of which is *change in attitude/*

TABLE 14.1 TAXONOMY OF DISSEMINATION AND IMPLEMENTATION (D & I) OUTCOMES

Dissemination and Implementation Outcome	Level of Analysis	Theoretical Basis	Other terms in the Literature	Salience by D & I Phase Informed by the EPIS Model[26]	Latent Variable* Y/N	Example Method of Measurement
Reach	Individual	RE-AIM	Participation	Exploration	N	Surveys Administrative data
Acceptability	Individual	Rogers: complexity and relative advantage Greenhalgh: user orientation	Satisfaction with the innovation System readiness	Primarily Exploration, Secondarily Implementation and Sustainment	Y	Survey Key informant interviews Administrative data
Appropriateness	Individual Organization Policy	Rogers: compatibility	Perceived fit Relevance Compatibility Suitability Usefulness Practicability	Primarily Exploration and Secondarily Preparation	Y	Surveys Key informant interviews Focus groups
Feasibility	Individual Organization Policy	Rogers: compatibility, trialability, observability	Actual fit or utility Suitability Practicability Community readiness	Primarily Exploration and Secondarily Preparation	Y	Surveys Administrative data
Adoption	Individual Organization Policy	Rogers: trialability, observability RE-AIM	Uptake Utilization Intention to try Use of the innovation Knowledge transfer	Preparation	N	Surveys Observation Key informant interviews Focus groups Administrative data
Fidelity	Individual	RE-AIM: part of implementation	Delivered as intended Adherence Integrity Quality of program delivery	Implementation and Sustainment	N	Observation Checklists Content analyses Self-report

Construct	Level	Theoretical basis	Indicators	Phase	Latent Variable	Data source
Cost	Individual Organization Policy	RE-AIM TCU Program Change Model: costs and resources	Marginal cost Cost effectiveness Cost benefit Economic evaluation	Primarily Exploration and Secondarily Implementation and Sustainment	N	Administrative data
Penetration	Organization Policy	RE-AIM necessary for reach	Spread Access to services Level of utilization	Primarily Implementation and Secondarily Sustainment	N	Surveys Case studies Key informant interviews
Sustainability	Organization Policy	Rogers: confirmation RE-AIM: maintenance	Maintenance Institutionalization Continuation Sustained use Standard of practice or care	Primarily Sustainment and Secondarily Exploration	Y	Surveys Case studies Record & policy reviews Key informant interviews

Note. Latent Variable refers to a variable that itself cannot be directly observed but can be inferred through measurable indicators.

behavior.[27] Other commonly referenced desired effects (outcomes) of dissemination include *awareness, receipt, acceptance*, and *use of information*.[28] Dingfelder & Mandell's[29] definition of dissemination strategies reflect such dissemination outcomes as *awareness of an innovation* and an *inclination to use* the innovation. Similarly, *intentions* emerged as one of the 14 domains delineated in the Theoretical Domains Framework,[30] a social psychology-informed listing of 84 constructs relevant to the kind of behavior change that occurs in implementation. The RE-AIM framework's constructs of *reach, adoption, implementation*, and *maintenance* are sometimes referenced as outcomes, although Rabin et al.[31] present them as mediators of the extent and speed of dissemination. Clearly, *reach* may reflect the breadth with which health information spreads, and thus serves as a key dissemination outcome.

IMPLEMENTATION OUTCOMES

The literature reflects at least eight conceptually distinct implementation outcomes—*acceptability, appropriateness, feasibility, adoption, fidelity, implementation cost, penetration*, and *sustainability*.[7,11] Proctor and colleagues[11] developed a taxonomy of implementation outcomes, offered conceptual definitions, and addressed their measurement challenges (see Table 14.1). *Acceptability* is the perception among implementation stakeholders that a given intervention or innovation is agreeable, palatable, or satisfactory. The referent of the implementation outcome "acceptability" (or the *"what" is acceptable*) may be a specific intervention, practice, technology, or service within a particular setting of care. Acceptability should be assessed based on the stakeholder's knowledge of or direct experience with various dimensions of the EBI to be implemented, such as its content, complexity, or comfort. Acceptability may be measured from the perspective of various stakeholders, such as administrators, payers, providers, and consumers, and acceptability is likely to be dynamic, changing with experience. Thus ratings of acceptability may be different when taken, for example, in the exploration phase and again in later stages of implementation.

Appropriateness is the perceived fit, relevance, or compatibility of the innovation or EBI for a given practice setting, provider, or consumer; and/or perceived fit of the innovation to address a particular issue or problem. "Appropriateness" is conceptually similar to "acceptability," and the literature reflects overlapping and sometimes inconsistent terms when discussing these constructs. Indeed, a series of laboratory and field studies recently revealed that although these terms are conceptually distinct, they are not meaningfully distinct in that rarely would it be the case that an intervention or innovation would be acceptable but not appropriate or vice versa.[32] More empirical work is needed to determine whether measurement of both acceptability and appropriateness is advantageous.

Feasibility is the extent to which a new program or policy can be successfully used or carried out within a given agency, in a particular setting, or in a certain population.[33] Typically, the concept of feasibility is invoked retrospectively as a potential explanation of an implementation's success or failure, as reflected in poor recruitment, retention, or participation rates. While feasibility is related to appropriateness, the two constructs are conceptually and meaningfully distinct. For example, a program may be appropriate for a service setting—in that it is compatible with the setting's mission or service mandate—but may not be feasible due to resource or training requirements.

Acceptability, appropriateness, and feasibility are predictors of adoption.[34] *Adoption* is the intention, initial decision, or action to try or employ an innovation or EBI.[31,35] Adoption also may be referred to as "uptake." Adoption could be measured from the perspective of provider or organization.

Incremental implementation cost is the additional expense of implementing an EBI. Chapter 6 on economic aspects of D&I provides a fuller exposition of this outcome, and details the ways in which implementation costs vary. Direct measures of implementation cost are essential for studies comparing the costs of implementing alternative interventions and of various implementation strategies.

Fidelity is the most common implementation outcome, defined as the degree to which an intervention was implemented as it was prescribed in the original protocol or as it was intended by the program developers.[31,36] Fidelity is typically measured by comparing the original EBI and the disseminated/implemented intervention in terms of (1) adherence to the program protocol, (2) dose or amount of program delivered, and (3) quality of program delivery. The literature identifies five implementation fidelity dimensions including adherence, quality of delivery, program component differentiation, exposure to the intervention, and participant responsiveness or involvement.[37,38] Provider fidelity is often of most interest, but there is evidence that providers are poor reporters of their intervention delivery, particularly when the intervention is new to them, whereas objectively rated measures of fidelity remain the gold standard.[39]

Penetration is defined as the integration of a practice within a service setting and its subsystems,[40] and is similar to Rabin et al.'s[31] notion of niche saturation. Stiles et al.[40] apply the concept of service penetration to service recipients (the number of eligible persons who use a service, divided by the total number of persons eligible for the service). Penetration also can be calculated in terms of the number of providers who deliver a given intervention divided by the total number of providers trained in or expected to deliver the service. From a service system perspective, the construct is also similar to "reach" in the RE-AIM framework.[41]

Sustainability is the extent to which a newly implemented intervention is maintained or institutionalized within a service setting's ongoing, stable operations. The literature reflects quite varied uses of the term "sustainability."[4,31,42-45] Rabin et al.,[31] emphasize the integration of a given program within an organization's culture through policies and practices, and distinguishes three stages that determine institutionalization: (1) passage (a single event such as transition from temporary to permanent funding), (2) cycle or routine (i.e., repetitive reinforcement of the importance of the EBI through including it into organizational or community procedures and behaviors, such as the annual budget and evaluation criteria), and (3) niche saturation (the extent to which an EBI is integrated into all subsystems of an organization). Thus the outcomes of "penetration" and "sustainability" may be related conceptually and empirically, in that higher penetration may contribute to long-term sustainability.

Lewis et al.[46] recently completed a systematic review of 104 implementation outcome measures identifying those fit for use in mental and behavioral health settings; no other systematic reviews of implementation outcome measures have yet been completed. They assessed each measure for evidence of: reliability (internal consistency), validity (structural and predictive), and pragmatic strength (norms, responsiveness, number of items). Only one measure had any evidence of all six rating criteria, with the remaining lacking information regarding the majority of these

critical psychometric and pragmatic properties (46% of measures lacked information for four of the six criteria). Scores were assigned to reflect the quality or strength of the psychometric evidence, with measures ranging in quality from 2 to 19.5, and a median of 8, of a total possible of 24 (i.e., 4-point scale across the criteria). The majority of measures assessed acceptability ($N = 50$), likely because of its longer history as a construct of interest in intervention development studies. Appropriateness, feasibility, cost, fidelity, and sustainability all had fewer than 10 associated measures. Review of the quality of these measures revealed that new measures of appropriateness, feasibility, and acceptability were needed, as the items of existing measures were not salvageable; this work is being carried out currently by the first author and her team.[19] Measures of adoption and sustainability are also in need of further development and psychometric testing. Conversely, excellent measures of fidelity exist, but they are traditionally intervention specific and so they were not included in the Lewis et al. review. Finally, cost and penetration are both assessed using formulas (i.e., through tracking of information) that are not appropriately subjected to a psychometric assessment, and it is unclear whether these formulas need revisions for optimization. Taken together, the measures used to assess implementation outcomes—the constructs we arguably care most about—require significant work (i.e., either initial development or psychometric testing).

Modeling Interrelationships Among D&I Outcomes

The literature has only begun to address the ways in which D&I outcomes are interrelated.[7,11] Dingfelder and Mandell's model[29] positions dissemination as a contributor to successful implementation outcome. Yet dissemination outcomes are likely interrelated in dynamic and complex ways, as are implementation outcomes.[47-50] For example, the perceived feasibility and implementation cost associated with an intervention will likely bear on ratings of the intervention's acceptability. Acceptability, in turn, will likely affect adoption, penetration, and sustainability. Similarly, consistent with Rogers' Diffusion of Innovations theory, the ability to adopt or adapt an innovation for local use may increase its acceptability.[51]

Important work needs to be done to model these interrelationships, and this work will likely inform definitions and thus shape our D&I language. For example, if two outcomes which we now define as distinct concepts are shown through research to always occur together, the empirical evidence would suggest that the concepts are really the same thing and should be combined, as is likely the case for acceptability and appropriateness. Similarly, if two of the outcomes are shown to have different empirical patterns, evidence would confirm their conceptual distinction. Refining the D&I contextual factors and outcomes taxonomy is critical to the advancement of the field.

MEASURING STAKEHOLDER PERSPECTIVES: CONTEXTUAL FACTORS AND OUTCOMES

Advancing methods to capture stakeholder perspectives is essential for D&I research.[52,53] A federal report, the "Road Ahead Report," calls for assessing the perspectives of multiple stakeholders, in order to improve the sustainability of EBIs in real-world care.[54] Successful D&I of EBIs depends largely on the fit of EBIs with the preferences and priorities of those who shape, deliver, and participate in care. Several groups of D&I stakeholders can be distinguished. *Community members* may include: (1) *health care consumers* who comprise the primary beneficiaries in the successful D&I of evidence-based health services and (2) the *whole population* in a community who benefits from dissemination of a population-level public health intervention (e.g., water fluoridation). Many dissemination efforts target health consumers directly, as in marketing campaigns designed to increase consumer demand for a particular program, drug, or service. *Families* comprise another group of D&I stakeholders, often sharing consumer desires for quality care and similarly affected by successful D&I. Service recipients and family members bring different perspectives to the evaluation of health care,[55] underscoring the importance of systematically assessing their perspectives on D&I of evidence-based health care.

Intervention developers constitute a third group of stakeholders. Many engage in D&I efforts, fueled by a desire that their interventions be used in real-world care and are then also known as intermediaries or purveyors. For example, many intervention developers (including nurse in-home visitation program developers)

have launched their own implementation "shops," many of which are proprietary. Many provide direct training, supervision, and consultation. Those who develop health policies, such as smoking bans, launch advertising campaigns, as do pharmaceutical firms, who also provide academic detailing aimed at changing provider prescribing behavior. Another set of stakeholders, *public health and health care advocates*, engage in similar efforts. Intervention developers and/or their marketing enterprises highly value the implementation outcomes of penetration, fidelity, and sustainability.

Many if not most D&I efforts target the *front line practitioners* who deliver health care and prevention services or *agency administrators*, through organizational implementation strategies. Health care providers themselves can serve important dissemination roles. For example, Kerner et al.[56] suggest that primary care physicians, dentists, and community health workers have high potential for exposing the broader public to evidence-based health promotion and disease prevention. Personnel in public health agencies have an obligation to survey the evidence carefully and decide when the science base is sufficient for widespread dissemination. Finally, *policymakers* at the local, regional, state, national, and international levels are an important audience for D&I efforts. These individuals are often faced with macro-level decisions on how to allocate the public resources for which they have been elected stewards. This often raises important dissemination issues related to balancing individual and social good or deciding on costs for implementing evidence-based policies.

A variety of established quantitative approaches for stakeholder preference assessment derive from medical decision-making and health services research[57,58] (standard gamble and time trade-off), psychophysics and psychology[59] (category rating and magnitude estimation), marketing[60] (conjoint analysis), cognitive anthropology[61] (cultural domain analysis and cultural consensus analysis), and sorting and ranking approaches common to multiple disciplines. Research is needed to test these methods for assessing the feasibility, acceptability, and validity of stakeholder perspectives using, for example, cognitive interviewing techniques such as "think aloud"[62] and quantitative measures of method performance. The Sawtooth Software "Conjoint Value Analysis" Web System software can be used for conjoint analysis. ANTHROPAC 4.98,[63] a menu-driven

DOS program, can be used to conduct metric and nonmetric multidimensional scaling and cluster analyses in exploratory analyses of stakeholder preference domains.

Salience of D&I Outcomes to Stakeholders: Pragmatic Measures

As noted, any effort to change care involves a range of stakeholders, including the intervention developers who design and test the intervention effectiveness, policymakers who design and pay for service, administrators who shape program direction, providers and supervisors, patients/clients/ consumers and their family members, and community members interested in health care. The success of efforts to implement EBIs may rest on their congruence with the preferences and priorities of those who shape, deliver, and participate in care. D&I outcomes may be differentially important to various stakeholders, just as the salience of clinical outcomes varies across stakeholders.[64] For example, implementation cost may be most important to policymakers and program directors, feasibility may be most important to direct service providers, and fidelity may be most important to intervention developers. To ensure applicability of implementation outcomes across a range of health care settings and to maximize their external validity, all stakeholder groups and priorities should be represented in this research.

Moreover, measures of D&I context, process, and outcomes should be pragmatic. Glasgow and Riley[65] describe pragmatic measures as those that measure constructs that are important to stakeholders, low burden, have broad applicability, are sensitive to change, and are actionable. Until pragmatic measures are prioritized, stakeholders will remain limited in terms of their ability to conduct implementations independently of researchers. Lewis and colleagues[19] are working to develop pragmatic rating criteria for D&I to inform measure development and evaluation. Their approach includes a synthesis of findings from a systematic literature review and stakeholder interviews followed by a concept mapping process to establish stakeholder-driven domains of relevance and a Delphi activity to uncover and come to consensus on stakeholder priorities. They will apply this set of pragmatic rating criteria along with a psychometric evidence-based assessment criteria to determine which measures of the Consolidated Framework for Implementation Research[66] (CFIR) and Implementation Outcomes[7,11] are both psychometrically strong and pragmatic, revealing a research agenda for the field.

CONCEPTUAL AND METHODOLOGIC CHALLENGES

Readers are invited to review a paper entitled, "Instrumentation Issues in Implementation Science" for an in-depth consideration of conceptual and methodologic challenges of D&I measurement;[67] a concise overview of key issues follows. Conceptualizing and measuring implementation outcomes will advance understanding of implementation processes, enhance efficiency in implementation research, and pave the way for studies of the comparative effectiveness of D&I strategies. Advancing the nominal and operational measurement of D&I outcomes requires work on several fronts. First, accurate measurement of D&I outcomes requires more consistent nominal definition, including the use of consistent terminology. Studies often use different labels for what appear to be the same construct, or use one term for the outcome's label or nominal definition but a different term for operationalizing or measuring the same construct. While language inconsistency is typical in most still-developing fields, implementation research may be particularly susceptible to this problem. No single discipline is "home" to D&I research. Studies are conducted across a broad range of disciplines, published in a scattered set of journals, and consequently are rarely cross-referenced.[7] The field now has the beginnings of a common language to characterize implementation outcomes, with much work to be done with dissemination outcomes. Continued progress is essential to our field's conceptual and empirical advancement. Those developing taxonomies serve to organize the key variables and frame research questions required to advance implementation science. Their measurement and empirical test helps specify the mechanisms and causal relations within D&I processes and advance a base of empirical evidence about successful D&I.

Measurement Approaches

The literature reflects a wide array of approaches for measuring implementation outcomes, ranging from qualitative to quantitative survey to record archival to administrative.[7,11] Examples of the often used measurement approaches for each implementation outcome are provided in Table 14.1. The preferred approach is (quantitative) survey, regardless of whether it is most appropriate. Unfortunately, much of the existing quantitative measurement has been "home-grown," often leading to this one-time use phenomenon, with virtually no work on the psychometric properties or measurement rigor. Importantly, as discussed in Martinez et al.,[67] these measurement approaches should be used strategically depending on the research question, design, context in which the study is being conducted, and the state of the measurement literature regarding the specific outcome(s) in question. Careful attention paid to selecting the measurement approach can help with the measure development and evaluation issues noted throughout this chapter.

Level of Analysis for Outcomes

Dissemination of health information and the implementation of new preventive practices involve change at multiple levels, ranging from the individual (health consumer, provider) to the organization, to the community and in policy.[7,68] Some outcomes, such as attitude change and acceptance may most appropriately be assessed at the individual level, while others, such as spread or penetration, may be more appropriate for aggregate analysis, such as at the level of the organization. Currently, very few studies reporting D&I outcomes specify the level at which measurement was taken. In one of the existing systematic reviews, Emmons et al.[17] found that the level of the measure and analysis did not always match. Specification and appropriate matching of the measure with its intended target is critical to advancing D&I theory.

Construct Validity

Construct validity is the degree to which a measure "behaves" in a way consistent with theoretical hypotheses[69] and is predictive of some external attribute (e.g., rate of smoking). Establishing construct validity for a measure begins in the development process by creating a nomological network that establishes the theoretical relations among constructs (e.g., antecedents, predicted outcomes).[19] Despite the existence of 60+ D&I models, there are few that delineate interrelations between constructs and outcomes, making construct validity difficult to test. Additionally, qualitative data, reflecting language used by various stakeholders as they think and talk about D&I processes, is important for validating outcome constructs. Through in-depth interviews, stakeholders' cognitive representations and mental models of outcomes can be analyzed using such methods as cultural domain analysis (CDA).[70,71]

Criterion-Related Validity

Criterion-related validity (sometimes considered a subset of construct validity) is the degree to which a measure is predictive of some "gold standard" measure of the same attribute,[63] as is the case for concurrent validity. Assessment of criterion validity is common in many areas of medical and public health research. For example, for concurrent validity, to gauge the accuracy of self-reported smoking behavior one might compare self-reported data with biochemical measures of cotinine (a nicotine breakdown product). However, in most areas of D&I research the gold standard does not exist to assess concurrent validity. Similarly, to assess accuracy of staff self-report of use of a new intervention, records might be audited for evidence of the intervention's delivery and supervisors might be queried. Currently, neither dissemination research nor implementation research adequately discusses or explores the validity of outcome measurement.

Perhaps of most interest to D&I researchers is the predictive validity component of criterion-related validity. As the term suggests, this is an evaluation to determine whether a D&I construct predicts an outcome that is measured at a later time interval. For example, one might explore whether organizational readiness to change predicts provider fidelity to an EBI post-deployment of an implementation strategy. Surprisingly, the minority of D&I measures are used to explore predictive validity. Of the seven systematic reviews of measures,[14-20] four reported specifically on predictive validity.[16-19] Weiner et al.'s[16] review of organizational readiness measures reported that 34.88% had been tested for predictive validity, 44.44% in the Emmons et al.[17] review of leadership measures, 51.61% of Chaudoir et al.'s[18] review of measures across five levels of analysis, and in Lewis et al.[19] only 17% of the 104 measures of implementation outcomes were tested for predictive validity.[46] It is unclear the reason for so few tests of predictive validity. One likely explanation is that studies are not designed to prospectively test the impact of determinants on implementation outcomes subsequent to an implementation intervention. The majority of the D&I literature to date simply characterizes barriers and facilitators at a single time point.

Using Implementation Outcomes to Model Success

Success in D&I is probably a function of a "portfolio" of factors, including the effectiveness of the intervention itself and the skillful use of D&I strategies.[7,11] For example, implementation strategies could be employed to increase provider acceptance, improve penetration, reduce implementation costs, and achieve sustainability of the intervention being implemented. It is important to conceptually and empirically address how various D&I outcomes contribute to success. For example, an EBI may be highly effective but it may be largely unknown to potential adopters; this poor dissemination outcome (low awareness) would undermine the likelihood of its implementation. This scenario may be modeled as follows:

$$Implementation\ success = function\ of\ effectiveness$$
$$(=high) + awareness(=low)$$

As another example, a program may be highly effective but only mildly acceptable and costly, making it difficult to sustain. The overall potential success of implementation in this case might be modeled as follows:

$$Implementation\ success = function\ of\ effectiveness$$
$$(=high) + acceptability(=moderate) + cost(high)$$
$$+ sustainability(low).$$

In a third situation, a given intervention might be only moderately effective but highly acceptable to stakeholders because current care is poor, the intervention is inexpensive, and current training protocols ensure high penetration through providers. This intervention's potential might be modeled in the following equation:

$$Implementation\ success = function\ of\ intervention$$
$$effectiveness(moderate) + acceptability(high)$$
$$+ potential\ to\ improve\ care(high)$$
$$+ penetration(high).$$

These examples suggest that successful change in public health and health delivery can be understood and modeled using the concepts of D&I

outcomes, thereby making decisions about what to implement more explicit and transparent. It is critical to specify these interrelations a priori so as to ensure psychometrically strong and pragmatic measures are available and administered at the appropriate time point in the implementation process (e.g., exploration, preparation, implementation, or sustainment).[26]

SUMMARY

The National Institutes of Health, the Agency for Healthcare Research and Quality, the CDC, and a number of private foundations have expressed the need for advancing the science of D&I. Interest in D&I research is present in many countries including the UK Centre for Reviews and Dissemination, the UK Medical Research Council, and the Canadian Institutes of Health Research. Improving health care requires not only effective programs and interventions, but also effective strategies to move them into community based settings of care. But before discrete strategies can be tested for effectiveness, comparative effectiveness, or cost effectiveness, context and outcome constructs must be identified and defined in such a way that enables their manipulation and measurement. Measurement is underdeveloped, with few psychometrically strong measures and very little attention paid to their pragmatic nature. A variety of tools are needed to capture health care access and quality, and no measurement issues are more pressing than those for D&I science.

ACKNOWLEDGEMENTS

Preparation of this chapter was supported by R01MH106510, P30MH068579 and UL1RR024992.

The authors acknowledge the following individuals, who contributed ideas or insights about measurement of dissemination and implementation outcomes: Graham Colditz, Lauren Gulbas, Curtis McMillen, Susan Pfefferle, Martha Shumway, and Bryan Weiner.

SUGGESTED READINGS AND WEBSITES

Readings

Dusenbury L, Brannigan R, Falco M, Hansen WB. A review of research on fidelity of implementation: implications for drug abuse prevention in school settings. *Health Educ Res.* 2003;18(2):237–256.

This article reviews the state of research on a key implementation outcome, fidelity. Of the implementation outcomes identified and discussed in this chapter, fidelity is that most frequently addressed in implementation trials and the one with the most advanced measurement work.

Glasgow RE, Vogt TM, Boles SM. Evaluating the public health impact of health promotion interventions: the RE-AIM framework. *Am J Public Health.*1999;89(9):1322–1327.

In this seminal article, Glasgow et al. evaluate public health interventions using the RE-AIM framework. The model's five dimensions (reach, efficacy, adoption, implementation, and maintenance) act together to determine a particular program's public health impact. The article also summarizes the model's strengths and limitations, and suggests that failure to evaluate on all five dimensions can result in wasted resources.

Lewis CC, Stanick CF, Martinez RG, et al. The Society for Implementation Research Collaboration Instrument Review Project: a methodology to promote rigorous evaluation. *Implement Sci.* 2015;10:2.

Martinez RG, Lewis CC, Weiner BJ. Instrumentation issues in implementation science. *Implement Sci.* 2014;9:118.

Lewis CC, Fischer S, Weiner BJ, Stanick C, Kim M, Martinez RG. Outcomes for implementation science: an enhanced systematic review of instruments using evidence-based rating criteria. *Implement Sci.* 2015;10:155.

Lewis CC, Weiner BJ, Stanick C, Fischer SM. Advancing implementation science through measure development and evaluation: a study protocol. *Implement Sci.* 2015;10:102.

Lewis and her team have contributed significant advancements to the D&I measurment literature through their enhanced systematic reviews of measures assessment constructs of the Consolidated Framework for Implementation Research and Implementation Outcomes. These four papers present results of an evidence based assessment of measures, identified issues and recommendations for the field, and a protocol describing their next steps.

Proctor E, Silmere H, Raghavan R, et al. Outcomes for implementation research: conceptual distinctions, measurement challenges, and research agenda. *Adm Policy Ment Health.* 2011;38(2):65–76.

Proctor et al. offer a groundbreaking summary of issues in the design and evaluation of implementation research, setting out a model that defines steps in the process and discusses a model for quantifying the benefits of program implementation. The ability to measure implementation outcomes leads to better understanding of the implementation process and improves efficiency.

Proctor E, Landsverk J, Aarons G, Chambers D, Glisson C, Mittman B. Implementation research in mental health services: an emerging science with conceptual, methodological, and training challenges. *Adm Policy Ment Health.* 2009;36(1):24–34.

The conceptual framework proposed in this artcile by Proctor et al. identifies the key components in implementaiton science—an evidence-based intervention or quality improvement to be implemented, an implementation strategy for putting the EBI into place in a new setting or health care context, and three types of outcomes that are conceptually related: implementaiton outcomes, service system outcomes, and health outcomes. Proctor et al. address the training needs for the D&I field, and offer a research agenda for advancing the field.

Rabin BA, Brownson RC, Kerner JF, & Glasgow RE. Methodologic challenges in disseminating evidence-based intervention to promote physical activity. *Am J Prev Med.* 2006; 31(4S): S24–S34.

This article addresses several of the methodological gaps in dissemination research. Through use of two scenarios (one at the population level and one at the clinical level), the authors illustrate a number of key approaches (i.e., issues of design, measures of outcomes and external validity, the balance between fidelity and adaptation to local settings, and the review and funding of dissemination science).

Rabin BA, Lewis CC, Norton WE, et al. Measurement resources for dissemination and implementation research in health. *Implement Sci.* 2016;11:42.

This article presents results from an environmental scan of published systematic reviews of D&I measures and publically available web resources. This work stemmed from the 2014 invited meeting sponsored by the National Institutes of Health that focused on advancing D&I measurement and reporting standards.

Selected Websites and Tools

Cancer Control P.L.A.N.E.T. http://cancercontrol-planet.cancer.gov/index.html.

Cancer Control P.L.A.N.E.T. acts as a portal to provide access to data and resources for designing, implementing and evaluating evidence-based cancer control programs. The site provides five steps (with links) for developing a comprehensive cancer control plan or program.

CDC BRFSS. https://www.cdc.gov/brfss/.

The BRFSS (Behavioral Risk Factor Surveillance System), an ongoing data collection program conducted in all states, the District of Columbia, and three US territories, and the world's largest telephone survey, tracks health risks in the United States. Information from the survey is used to improve the health of the American people. The CDC has developed a standard core questionnaire so that data can be compared across various strata.

CDC WONDER. http://wonder.cdc.gov.

CDC WONDER is an easy-to-use system that provides a single point of access to a wide variety of CDC reports, guidelines, and numeric public health data. It can be valuable in public health research, decision-making, priority setting, program evaluation, and resource allocation.

National Center for Health Statistics. http://www.cdc.gov/nchs/.

National Center for Health Statistics is the principal vital and health statistics agency for the US government. NCHS data systems include information on vital events as well as information on health status, lifestyle and exposure to unhealthy influences, the onset and diagnosis of illness and disability, and the use of health care. NCHS has two major types of data systems: systems based on populations, containing data collected through personal interviews or examinations (e.g., National Health Interview Survey and National Health and Nutrition Examination Survey), and systems based on records, containing data collected from vital and medical records. These data are used by policymakers in the US Congress and the administration, by medical researchers, and by others in the health community.

European Health for All database (HFA-DB). http://www.euro.who.int/en/data-and-evidence/databases/european-health-for-all-database-hfa-db.

The European Health for All Database provides statistics for demographic characteristics, health status, risk factors, health care resources and utilization, and health expenditures for the 53 countries in the WHO European Region.

https://obssr.od.nih.gov/scientific-initiatives/dissemination-and-implementation/.

This site provides information on NIH opportunities to support implementation and dissemination research, including research to advance measures of key constructs.

http://implementationscience.biomedcentral.com/.

Implementation Science is an open access, peer-reviewed online journal that aims to publish research relevant to the scientific study of methods to promote the uptake of research findings into routine health care in both clinical and policy contexts. The website provides links to articles, many of which address measurement issues in implementation research, as well as links to questionnaires for measuring key constructs in implementation research.

http://www.queri.research.va.gov/ciprs/.

Center for Implementation Practice and Research Support, The VA Center for Implementation Practice and Research Support (CIPRS) is a new QUERI resource center that aims to facilitate accelerated improvement in the quality and performance of the VA health care delivery system through enhanced VA implementation practice and research. CIPRS programs include education, technical assistance, and consultation to VA implementation practitioners and researchers, and development of implementation theory and methods. CIPRS also facilitates better linkages and partnerships between VA implementation researchers and VA clinical practice and policy leaders. CIPRS collaborates with CIDER, HERC, and VIReC in assessing and meeting the needs of the VA implementation community.

https://societyforimplementationresearchcollaboration.org/.

The Society for Implementation Research Collaboration (SIRC) is a free-standing society that grew out of an NIMH-funded R13 conference series grant led by principal investigator Kate Comtois. SIRC aims to advance rigorous methods and measurement for the evaluation and practice of D&I, primarily with respect to behavioral health. SIRC served as the springboard for the "Instrument Review Project," which includes a systematic review of measures pertaining to constructs of the CFIR[66] and the implementation outcomes framework[7,11] via an NIMH-funded R01 to principal investigator Cara Lewis.

https://www.gem-beta.org/Public/Home.aspx.

The Grid Enables Measures (GEM) Database represents a wiki platform dedicated to increasing access and harmonization of measures used in D&I.[72] GEM enables its users to add constructs and measures, contribute to and update measure metadata (e.g., psychometric quality), rate and comment on measures, access and share harmonized data, and access measures.

REFERENCES

1. Sallis JF, Owen N, Fotheringham MJ. Behavioral epidemiology: a systematic framework to classify phases of research on health promotion and disease prevention. *Ann Behav Med.* 2000;22(4):294–298.
2. Rabin BA, Lewis CC, Norton WE, et al. Measurement resources for dissemination and implementation research in health. *Implement Sci.* 2016;11:42.
3. Neta G, Glasgow RE, Carpenter CR, et al. A framework for enhancing the value of research for dissemination and implementation. *Am J Public Health.* 2015;105(1):49–57.
4. McKibbon KA, Lokker C, Wilczynski NL, et al. A cross-sectional study of the number and frequency of terms used to refer to knowledge translation in a body of health literature in 2006: a Tower of Babel? *Implement Sci.* 2010;5:16.
5. Rabin BA, Brownson RC. Developing the terminology for dissemination and implementation research in health In: Brownson RC, Colditz GA,

Proctor EK, eds. *Dissemination and implementation research in health: Translating science to practice.* 2nd ed. New York: Oxford University Press; 2017.

6. Grimshaw J, Eccles M, Thomas R, et al. Toward evidence-based quality improvement: evidence (and its limitations) of the effectiveness of guideline dissemination and implementation strategies 1966-1998. *J Gen Intern Med.* 2006;21 Suppl 2:S14–S20.

7. Proctor E, Landsverk J, Aarons G, Chambers D, Glisson C, Mittman B. Implementation research in mental health services: an emerging science with conceptual, methodological, and training challenges. *Adm Policy Ment Health.* 2009;36(1):24–34.

8. Institute of Medicine Committee on Quality of Health Care in America. *Crossing the quality chasm: A new health system for the 21st century.* Washington, DC: Institute of Medicine, National Academy Press; 2001.

9. Institute of Medicine Committee on Crossing the Quality Chasm. *Adaptation to mental health and addictive disorder: Improving the quality of health care for mental and substance-use conditions.* Washington, DC: Institute of Medicine, National Academies Press; 2006.

10. Brownson RC, Chriqui JF, Stamatakis KA. Understanding evidence-based public health policy. *Am J Public Health.* 2009;99(9):1576–1583.

11. Proctor E, Silmere H, Raghavan R, et al. Outcomes for implementation research: conceptual distinctions, measurement challenges, and research agenda. *Adm Policy Ment Health.* 2011;38(2):65–76.

12. Tabak RG, Khoong EC, Chambers DA, Brownson RC. Bridging research and practice: models for dissemination and implementation research. *Am J Prev Med.* 2012;43(3):337–350.

13. Gerring J. *Social science methodology: A criterial framework.* New York: Cambridge University Press; 2001.

14. Hrisos S, Eccles MP, Francis JJ, et al. Are there valid proxy measures of clinical behaviour? a systematic review. *Implement Sci.* 2009;4:37.

15. Ibrahim S, Sidani S. Fidelity of intervention implementation: a review of instruments. *Health.* 2015;7(12):1687–1695.

16. Weiner BJ, Amick H, Lee SY. Conceptualization and measurement of organizational readiness for change: a review of the literature in health services research and other fields. *Med Care Res Rev.* 2008;65(4):379–436.

17. Emmons KM, Weiner B, Fernandez ME, Tu SP. Systems antecedents for dissemination and implementation: a review and analysis of measures. *Health Educ Behav.* 2012;39(1):87–105.

18. Chaudoir SR, Dugan AG, Barr CH. Measuring factors affecting implementation of health innovations: a systematic review of structural, organizational, provider, patient, and innovation level measures. *Implement Sci.* 2013;8:22.

19. Lewis CC, Stanick CF, Martinez RG, et al. The Society for Implementation Research Collaboration Instrument Review Project: a methodology to promote rigorous evaluation. *Implement Sci.* 2015;10(2).

20. Chor KH, Wisdom JP, Olin SC, Hoagwood KE, Horwitz SM. Measures for predictors of innovation adoption. *Adm Policy Ment Health.* 2015;42(5):545–573.

21. Burnes B. Emergent change and planned change—competitors or allies?: the case of XYZ construction. *Int J Oper Prod Man.* 2004;24(9):886–902.

22. Waldorff FB, Steenstrup AP, Nielsen B, Rubak J, Bro F. Diffusion of an e-learning programme among Danish General Practitioners: a nationwide prospective survey. *BMC Fam Pract.* 2008;9:24.

23. Adily A, Westbrook J, Coiera E, Ward J. Use of on-line evidence databases by Australian public health practitioners. *Med Inform Internet Med.* 2004;29(2):127–136.

24. Fischer MA, Vogeli C, Stedman MR, Ferris TG, Weissman JS. Uptake of electronic prescribing in community-based practices. *J Gen Intern Med.* 2008;23(4):358–363.

25. Cooke M, Mattick RP, Walsh RA. Implementation of the "Fresh Start" smoking cessation programme to 23 antenatal clinics: a randomized controlled trial investigating two methods of dissemination. *Drug and Alcohol Review.* 2001;20(1):19–28.

26. Aarons GA, Hurlburt M, Horwitz SM. Advancing a conceptual model of evidence-based practice implementation in public service sectors. *Adm Policy Ment Health.* 2011;38(1):4–23.

27. Rabin BA, Glasgow RE, Kerner JF, Klump MP, Brownson RC. Dissemination and implementation research on community-based cancer prevention: a systematic review. *Am J Prev Med.* 2010;38(4):443–456.

28. Rabin BA, Brownson RC, Kerner JF, Glasgow RE. Methodologic challenges in disseminating evidence-based interventions to promote physical activity. *Am J Prev Med.* 2006;31(4 Suppl):S24–S34.

29. Dingfelder HE, Mandell DS. Bridging the research-to-practice gap in autism intervention: an application of diffusion of innovation theory. *J Autism Dev Disord.* 2011;41(5):597–609.

30. Cane J, O'Connor D, Michie S. Validation of the theoretical domains framework for use in behaviour change and implementation research. *Implement Sci.* 2012;7:37.

31. Rabin BA, Brownson RC, Haire-Joshu D, Kreuter MW, Weaver NL. A glossary for dissemination and implementation research in health. *J Public Health Manag Pract.* 2008;14(2):117–123.

32. Lewis CC. Advancing the Pragmatic Measures Construct and Three New Measures of Implementation Outcomes. 9th Annual Conference on the Science of Dissemination and Implementation in Health; 2016; Washington, DC.

33. Karsh BT. Beyond usability: designing effective technology implementation systems to promote patient safety. *Qual Saf Health Care.* 2004;13(5):388–394.

34. Lewis CC, Weiner BJ, Stanick C, Fischer SM. Advancing implementation science through measure development and evaluation: a study protocol. *Implement Sci.* 2015;10:102.

35. Rye CB, Kimberly JR. The adoption of innovations by provider organizations in health care. *Med Care Res Rev.* 2007;64(3):235–278.

36. Dusenbury L, Brannigan R, Falco M, Hansen WB. A review of research on fidelity of implementation: implications for drug abuse prevention in school settings. *Health Educ Res.* 2003;18(2):237–256.

37. Mihalic S. The importance of implementation fidelity. 2002; http://incredibleyears.com/wp-content/uploads/fidelity-importance.pdf.

38. Dane AV, Schneider BH. Program integrity in primary and early secondary prevention: are implementation effects out of control? *Clin Psychol Rev.* 1998;18(1):23–45.

39. Schoenwald SK, Garland AF, Chapman JE, Frazier SL, Sheidow AJ, Southam-Gerow MA. Toward the effective and efficient measurement of implementation fidelity. *Adm Policy Ment Health.* 2011;38(1):32–43.

40. Stiles PG, Boothroyd RA, Snyder K, Zong X. Service penetration by persons with severe mental illness: how should it be measured? *J Behav Health Serv Res.* 2002;29(2):198–207.

41. Glasgow RE. The RE-AIM model for planning, evaluation and reporting on implementation and dissemination research. NIH Conference on Building the Science of D & I in the Service of Public Health; 2007; Bethesda, MD.

42. Johnson K, Hays C, Center H, Daley C. Building capacity and sustainable prevention innovations: a sustainability planning model. *Eval Prog Plan.* 2004;27(2):135–149.

43. Turner KMT, Sanders MR. Dissemination of evidence-based parenting and family support strategies: learning from the Triple P—Positive Parenting Program system approach. *Aggress Violent Beh.* 2006;11(2):176–193.

44. Glasgow RE, Vogt TM, Boles SM. Evaluating the public health impact of health promotion interventions: the RE-AIM framework. *Am J Public Health.* 1999;89(9):1322–1327.

45. Goodman RM, McLeroy KR, Steckler AB, Hoyle RH. Development of level of institutionalization scales for health promotion programs. *Health Educ Q.* 1993;20(2):161–178.

46. Lewis CC, Fischer S, Weiner BJ, Stanick C, Kim M, Martinez RG. Outcomes for implementation science: an enhanced systematic review of instruments using evidence-based rating criteria. *Implement Sci.* 2015;10:155.

47. Woolf SH. The meaning of translational research and why it matters. *JAMA.* 2008;299(2):211–213.

48. Repenning NP. A simulation-based approach to understanding the dynamics of innovation implementation. *Organi Sci.* 2002;13(2):109–127.

49. Hovmand PS, Gillespie DF. Implementation of evidence-based practice and organizational performance. *J Behav Health Serv Res.* 2010;37(1):79–94.

50. Klein KJ, Knight AP. Innovation implementation. *Curr Direct Psychol Sci.* 2005;14(5):243–246.

51. Rogers EM. *Diffusion of innovations.* 4th ed. New York: The Free Press; 1995.

52. Chambers DA. Advancing the science of implementation: a workshop summary. *Adm Policy Ment Health.* 2008;35(1-2):3–10.

53. Kimberly J, Cook JM. Organizational measurement and the implementation of innovations in mental health services. *Adm Policy Ment Health.* 2008;35(1-2):11–20.

54. Council NAMH. *The road ahead: Research partnerships to transform services.* Bethesda, MD: National Institutes of Health, National Institute of Mental Health; 2006.

55. Coyne I, McNamara N, Healy M, Gower C, Sarkar M, McNicholas F. Adolescents' and parents' views of Child and Adolescent Mental Health Services (CAMHS) in Ireland. *J Psychiatr Ment Health Nurs.* 2015;22(8):561–569.

56. Kerner J, Rimer B, Emmons K. Introduction to the special section on dissemination: dissemination research and research dissemination: how can we close the gap? *Health Psychol.* 2005;24(5):443–446.

57. Lambooij MS, Hummel MJ. Differentiating innovation priorities among stakeholder in hospital care. *BMC Med Inform Decis Mak.* 2013;13:91.

58. Wahlster P, Goetghebeur M, Kriza C, Niederlander C, Kolominsky-Rabas P; National Leading-Edge Cluster Medical Technologies 'Medical Valley EMN. Balancing costs and benefits at different stages of medical innovation: a systematic review of Multi-criteria decision analysis (MCDA). *BMC Health Serv Res.* 2015;15:262.

59. Preston CC, Colman AM. Optimal number of response categories in rating scales: reliability, validity, discriminating power, and respondent preferences. *Acta Psychol (Amst)*. 2000;104(1):1–15.

60. Sándor Z, Wedel M. Heterogeneous conjoint choice designs. *J Marketing Res*. 2005;42(2):210–218.

61. Wierenga SJ, Kamsteeg FH, Simons RJ, Veenswijk M. Teachers making sense of result-oriented teams: a cognitive anthropological approach to educational change. *J Educ Change*. 2015;16(1):53–78.

62. Shumway M, Sentell T, Chouljian T, Tellier J, Rozewicz F, Okun M. Assessing preferences for schizophrenia outcomes: comprehension and decision strategies in three assessment methods. *Ment Health Serv Res*. 2003;5(3):121–135.

63. Palinkas LA. Nutritional interventions for treatment of seasonal affective disorder. *CNS Neurosci Ther*. 2010;16(1):3–5.

64. Shumway M, Saunders T, Shern D, et al. Preferences for schizophrenia treatment outcomes among public policy makers, consumers, families, and providers. *Psychiatr Serv*. 2003;54(8):1124–1128.

65. Glasgow RE, Riley WT. Pragmatic measures: what they are and why we need them. *Am J Prev Med*. 2013;45(2):237–243.

66. Damschroder LJ, Aron DC, Keith RE, Kirsh SR, Alexander JA, Lowery JC. Fostering implementation of health services research findings into practice: a consolidated framework for advancing implementation science. *Implement Sci*. 2009;4:50.

67. Martinez RG, Lewis CC, Weiner BJ. Instrumentation issues in implementation science. *Implement Sci*. 2014;9:118.

68. Raghavan R, Bright CL, Shadoin AL. Toward a policy ecology of implementation of evidence-based practices in public mental health settings. *Implement Sci*. 2008;3:26.

69. Frost MH, Reeve BB, Liepa AM, Stauffer JW, Hays RD, Mayo FDAP-ROCMG. What is sufficient evidence for the reliability and validity of patient-reported outcome measures? *Value Health*. 2007;10 Suppl 2:S94–S105.

70. Luke DA. *Multilevel modeling*. Thousand Oaks, CA: Sage; 2004.

71. *lme4: Linear mixed-effects models using S4 classes* [computer program]. Version R package version 0.99875-62007.

72. Rabin BA, Purcell P, Naveed S, et al. Advancing the application, quality and harmonization of implementation science measures. *Implement Sci*. 2012;7:119.

15

Implementation Strategies

JOANN E. KIRCHNER, THOMAS J. WALTZ, BYRON J. POWELL,
JEFFREY L. SMITH, AND ENOLA K. PROCTOR

INTRODUCTION

Persistent gaps in the quality of healthcare provided in routine care settings have led to the development and prioritization of implementation science. Core to this rapidly growing science is the recognition that evidence-based innovations must be complemented by evidence-based implementation strategies.[1] Throughout, this chapter uses the term "innovation" inclusively. In a clinical setting this may be a new clinical intervention. In a public health setting it may be a prevention program, or in a community setting a new model of service. In recognition of the need to build an evidence base for implementation, the identification, development, refinement, and testing of implementation strategies has been prioritized.[2–5] Our discussion is focused on implementation strategies, but note that there may be considerable overlap between strategies for implementation, de-implementation, and dissemination. The authors acknowledge that de-implementation and dissemination strategies may warrant their own emphasis elsewhere, including the development of taxonomies to describe the range of strategies available to de-implement or disseminate innovations (see chapter 2).

We define implementation strategies as methods to enhance the adoption, implementation, sustainment, and scale-up of an innovation.[6] We further differentiate discrete, multifaceted, and blended implementation strategies.[7;8] Discrete implementation strategies involve one action or process, such as educational meetings, reminders, or audit and feedback. More often, the challenges of effective implementation call for the use of multifaceted implementation strategies that combine two or more discrete strategies. Finally, blended strategies are comprised of multiple discrete strategies that are interwoven and packaged as protocolized or branded strategies. For example,

the Availability, Responsiveness, and Continuity (ARC) organizational implementation strategy and the Leadership and Organizational Change Intervention are two blended strategies that attempt to promote effective implementation by addressing organizational culture, climate, and leadership, respectively.[9–12]

The evidence-base for implementation strategies is developing, with an increasing number of rigorous studies testing the effectiveness of implementation strategies in community settings. Grimshaw et al. provide a helpful synthesis of the systematic reviews conducted by the Cochrane Collaboration's Effective Practice and Organization of Care (EPOC) group, including systematic reviews for educational meetings, audit and feedback, printed educational materials, local opinion leaders, and implementation strategies that are tailored to address identified barriers and facilitators.[13–18] In addition to the EPOC systematic reviews that review health, the Campbell Collaboration has recently formed a Knowledge Translation and Implementation review group in the hopes of generating more rigorous syntheses of the empirical literature.

Overall, the effect sizes for most implementation strategies are modest. Several factors limit our ability to understand how, when, where, and why implementation strategies are effective.[13] Chief among these factors is a lack of clear definition and reporting of implementation strategies, both of which limit replication in science and practice, and preclude our ability to determine which components of multifaceted and blended implementation strategies contribute to their effects.[18;19] In addition, there is a lack of clarity on which strategy or group of strategies should be applied given a specific innovation, setting context and recipients. Finally, little work has been done to assess and document fidelity to an implementation strategy as it is being delivered.[20] Described in the following is an effort to address the lack of definition of implementation strategies and to classify strategies to improve selection, processes through which one can select an implementation strategy, recommendations on how best to document an implementation strategy so that it can be replicated, efforts to develop and apply strategy fidelity tools, and an example of how to disseminate an implementation strategy once it has been shown to have effectiveness. The chapter concludes with recommendations for future research.

IMPLEMENTATION STRATEGIES—ADDRESSING THE LACK OF DEFINITION

Across the sciences, great benefits have been reaped from organizing the language used within an area of inquiry.[21] Replication, critical reviews, and syntheses of the literature—essential components of a maturing science—are grounded in the use and application of a lexicon for the area of inquiry. As areas of inquiry become more organized, reporting guidelines may emerge (e.g., CONSORT and PRISMA) that reflect scientific consensus for communication that can improve the replicability of findings. Even when key terms within a lexicon prove to be false starts, the organized approach they afford to an area of inquiry allows for them to be more systematically scrutinized.

Several taxonomies of implementation strategies have been developed, primarily in the context of scoping reviews of the literature by research teams.[7;22;23] While scoping reviews are an excellent place to start, creating an integrated compilation of discrete implementation strategies that represents the state of the field needs to reflect the experience and judgement of both researchers and practitioners who use these strategies under a variety of circumstances. The Expert Recommendations for Implementing Change (ERIC) project mobilized 71 of these stakeholders and utilized rigorous mixed-methods procedures to characterize expert consensus on an updated compilation of implementation strategies.[24]

The first aim of ERIC was to establish consensus for a common nomenclature for implementation strategy terms and their definitions. The panel consisted of 71 experts (90% with expertise in implementation, 45% with clinical practice experience, 35% with both) from North America (97% from the United States), the majority of whom were affiliated with the Veterans Health Administration (66%). A three-round modified-Delphi process was used whereby the first two rounds involved asynchronous web-based surveys. The first round presented the compilation of 68 discrete implementation strategies from Powell and colleagues.[7] Participants were able to provide feedback on the labels for the strategies, specify synonyms for the strategies, edit the definitions, propose alternate definitions, and propose new strategies (with definitions) to be added to the compilation. Respondent feedback from Round 1 was compiled for each strategy, new strategies were added to the compilation for feedback, and in Round 2 the experts had a second opportunity to comment on the updated compilation of strategies in the context of being presented with quantitative and qualitative summaries of Round 1 feedback for each strategy. These first two rounds identified that 69% of the strategies from the original compilation were not in need of revision.[7] The remaining strategies had one or more proposed alternate definitions and these were brought to vote in Round 3. This final round used a live, web-based polling platform and a live webinar to capture consensus in real time. Panelists were able to discuss strategy definition alternatives when the first round of voting failed to identify a consensus alternative. The definition for all strategies was determined by majority consensus resulting in a final compilation of 73 discrete implementation strategies.[8]

The strategies and definitions in Table 15.1 represent the first compilation of implementation strategies to reflect the consensus of both clinical and implementation experts. This compilation can be useful for improving the specification and reporting of implementation strategies used in a variety of prospective research trials, as well as to promote the consideration of a more comprehensive range of strategies in applied implementation efforts. These strategies may also be useful for retrospective research used to identify where the evidence base for strategies is clear, and areas where more research is needed. Hopefully this compilation will facilitate future research that provides a more thorough accounting of the strategies employed to support implementation, including those that may be endogenous to an organization (e.g., having an existing clinical reminder system). A discussion of the limitations of the ERIC compilation can be found in Powell et al.[8]

TABLE 15.1 ERIC STRATEGIES AND THEIR DEFINITIONS, BY CLUSTER

	Strategy (*Cluster*)	Definition
		Use evaluative and iterative strategies
4	Assess for readiness and identify barriers and facilitators.	Assess various aspects of an organization to determine its degree of readiness to implement, barriers that may impede implementation, and strengths that can be used in the implementation effort.
5	Audit and provide feedback.	Collect and summarize clinical performance data over a specified time period and give it to clinicians and administrators to monitor, evaluate, and modify provider behavior.
14	Conduct cyclical small tests of change.	Implement changes in a cyclical fashion using small tests of change before taking changes systemwide. Tests of change benefit from systematic measurement, and results of the tests of change are studied for insights on how to do better. This process continues serially over time, and refinement is added with each cycle.
18	Conduct local needs assessment	Collect and analyze data related to the need for the innovation.
23	Develop a formal implementation blueprint.	Develop a formal implementation blueprint that includes all goals and strategies. The blueprint should include the following; 1) aim/purpose of the implementation; 2) scope of the change (e.g, what organizational units are affected); 3) timeframe and milestones; and 4) appropriate performance/progress measures. Use and update this plan to guide the implementation effort over time
26	Develop and implement tools for quality monitoring.	Develop, test, and introduce into quality-monitoring systems the right input—the appropriate language, protocols, algorithms, standards, and measures (of processes, patient/consumer outcomes, and implementation outcomes) that are often specific to the innovation being implemented.
27	Develop and organize quality monitoring systems.	Develop and organize systems and procedures that monitor clinical processes and/or outcomes for the purpose of quality assurance and improvement.
46	Obtain and use patients/consumers and family feedback.	Develop strategies to increase patient/consumer and family feedback on the implementation effort.
56	Purposefully reexamine the implementation.	Monitor progress and adjust clinical practices and implementation strategies to continuously improve the quality of care.
61	Stage implementation scale up	Phase implementation efforts by starting with small pilots or demonstration projects and gradually move to a systemwide roll-out.
		Provide interactive assistance
8	Centralize technical assistance.	Develop and use a centralized system to deliver technical assistance focused on implementation issues.
33	Facilitation	A process of interactive problem solving and support that occurs in a context of a recognized need for improvement and a supportive interpersonal relationship

(continued)

TABLE 15.1 CONTINUED

	Strategy (*Cluster*)	Definition
53	Provide clinical supervision.	Provide clinicians with ongoing supervision focusing on the innovation. Provide training for clinical supervisors who will supervise clinicians who provide the innovation.
54	Provide local technical assistance.	Develop and use a system to deliver technical assistance focused on implementation issues using local personnel.
	Adapt and tailor to context	
51	Promote adaptability.	Identify the ways a clinical innovation can be tailored to meet local needs and clarify which elements of the innovation must be maintained to preserve fidelity.
63	Tailor strategies.	Tailor the implementation strategies to address barriers and leverage facilitators that were identified through earlier data collection.
67	Use data experts.	Involve, hire, and/or consult experts to inform management on the use of data generated by implementation efforts.
68	Use data warehousing techniques.	Integrate clinical records across facilities and organizations to facilitate implementation across systems.
	Develop stakeholder interrelationships	
6	Build a coalition.	Recruit and cultivate relationships with partners in the implementation effort.
7	Capture and share local knowledge.	Capture local knowledge from implementation sites on how implementers and clinicians made something work in their setting and then share it with other sites.
17	Conduct local consensus discussions.	Include local providers and other stakeholders in discussions that address whether the chosen problem is important and whether the clinical innovation to address it is appropriate.
24	Develop academic partnerships.	Partner with a university or academic unit for the purposes of shared training and bringing research skills to an implementation project.
25	Develop an implementation glossary.	Develop and distribute a list of terms describing the innovation, implementation, and stakeholders in the organizational change.
35	Identify and prepare champions.	Identify and prepare individuals who dedicate themselves to supporting, marketing, and driving through an implementation, overcoming indifference or resistance that the intervention may provoke in an organization.
36	Identify early adopters.	Identify early adopters at the local site to learn from their experiences with the practice innovation.
38	Inform local opinion leaders.	Inform providers identified by colleagues as opinion leaders or "educationally influential" about the clinical innovation in the hopes that they will influence colleagues to adopt it.
40	Involve executive boards.	Involve existing governing structures (e.g., boards of directors, medical staff boards of governance) in the implementation effort, including the review of data on implementation processes.
45	Model and simulate change.	Model or simulate the change that will be implemented prior to implementation.
47	Obtain formal commitments.	Obtain written commitments from key partners that state what they will do to implement the innovation.
48	Organize clinician implementation team meetings.	Develop and support teams of clinicians who are implementing the innovation and give them protected time to reflect on the implementation effort, share lessons learned, and support one another's learning.

52	Promote network weaving.	Identify and build on existing high-quality working relationships and networks within and outside the organization, organizational units, teams, etc. to promote information sharing, collaborative problem solving, and a shared vision/goal related to implementing the innovation.
57	Recruit, designate, and train for leadership.	Recruit, designate, and train leaders for the change effort.
64	Use advisory boards and workgroups.	Create and engage a formal group of multiple kinds of stakeholders to provide input and advice on implementation efforts and to elicit recommendations for improvements/
65	Use an implementation advisor.	Seek guidance from experts in implementation.
72	Visit other sites.	Visit sites where a similar implementation effort has been considered successful.

Train and educate stakeholders

15	Conduct educational meetings.	Hold meetings targeted toward different stakeholder groups (e.g., providers, administrators, other organizational stakeholders, and community, patient/consumer, and family stakeholders) to teach them about the clinical innovation.
16	Conduct educational outreach visits.	Have a trained person meet with providers in their practice settings to educate providers about the clinical innovation, with the intent of changing the provider's practice.
19	Conduct ongoing training.	Plan for and conduct training in the clinical innovation in an ongoing way.
20	Create a learning collaborative.	Facilitate the formation of groups of providers or provider organizations and foster a collaborative learning environment to improve implementation of the clinical innovation.
29	Develop educational materials.	Develop and format manuals, toolkits, and other supporting materials in ways that make it easier for stakeholders to learn about the innovation and for clinicians to learn how to deliver the clinical innovation.
31	Distribute educational materials.	Distribute educational materials (including guidelines, manuals, and toolkits) in person, by mail, and/or electronically.
43	Make training dynamic.	Vary the information delivery methods to cater to different learning styles and work contexts, and shape the training in the innovation to be interactive.
55	Provide ongoing consultation.	Provide ongoing consultation with one or more experts in the strategies used to support implementing the innovation.
60	Shadow other experts.	Provide ways for key individuals to directly observe experienced people engage with or use the targeted practice change/innovation.
71	Use train-the-trainer strategies.	Train designated clinicians or organizations to train others in the clinical innovation.
73	Work with educational institutions.	Encourage educational institutions to train clinicians in the innovation.

(continued)

TABLE 15.1 CONTINUED

Strategy (*Cluster*)	Definition
	Support clinicians
21	Create new clinical teams.	Change who serves on the clinical team, adding different disciplines and different skills to make it more likely that the clinical innovation is delivered (or is more successfully delivered).
30	Develop resource sharing agreements	Develop partnerships with organizations that have resources needed to implement the innovation.
32	Facilitate relay of clinical data to providers.	Provide as close to real-time data as possible about key measures of process/outcomes using integrated modes/channels of communication in a way that promotes use of the targeted innovation.
58	Remind clinicians.	Develop reminder systems designed to help clinicians to recall information and/or prompt them to use the clinical innovation.
59	Revise professional roles.	Shift and revise roles among professionals who provide care, and redesign job characteristics.
	Engage consumers
37	Increase demand.	Attempt to influence the market for the clinical innovation to increase competition intensity and to increase the maturity of the market for the clinical innovation.
39	Intervene with patients/consumers to enhance uptake and adherence.	Develop strategies with patients to encourage and problem solve around adherence.
41	Involve patients/consumers and family members.	Engage or include patients/consumers and families in the implementation effort.
50	Prepare patients/consumers to be active participants.	Prepare patients/consumers to be active in their care, to ask questions, and specifically to inquire about care guidelines, the evidence behind clinical decisions, or about available evidence-supported treatments.
69	Use mass media.	Use media to reach large numbers of people to spread the word about the clinical innovation.
	Utilize financial strategies
1	Access new funding.	Access new or existing money to facilitate the implementation.
2	Alter incentive/allowance structures.	Work to incentivize the adoption and implementation of the clinical innovation.
3	Alter patient/consumer fees.	Create fee structures where patients/consumers pay less for preferred treatments (the clinical innovation) and more for less-preferred treatments.
28	Develop disincentives.	Provide financial disincentives for failure to implement or use the clinical innovations.
34	Fund and contract for the clinical innovation.	Governments and other payers of services issue requests for proposals to deliver the innovation, use contracting processes to motivate providers to deliver the clinical innovation, and develop new funding formulas that make it more likely that providers will deliver the innovation.

42	Make billing easier.	Make it easier to bill for the clinical innovation.
49	Place innovation on fee for service lists/formularies.	Work to place the clinical innovation on lists of actions for which providers can be reimbursed (e.g., a drug is placed on a formulary, a procedure is now reimbursable).
66	Use capitated payments.	Pay providers or care systems a set amount per patient/consumer for delivering clinical care.
70	Use other payment schemes.	Introduce payment approaches (in a catch-all category).

Change infrastructure

9	Change accreditation or membership requirements.	Strive to alter accreditation standards so that they require or encourage use of the clinical innovation. Work to alter membership organization requirements so that those who want to affiliate with the organization are encouraged or required to use the clinical innovation.
10	Change liability laws.	Participate in liability reform efforts that make clinicians more willing to deliver the clinical innovation.
11	Change physical structure and equipment.	Evaluate current configurations and adapt, as needed, the physical structure and/or equipment (e.g., changing the layout of a room, adding equipment) to best accommodate the targeted innovation.
12	Change record systems.	Change records systems to allow better assessment of implementation or clinical outcomes.
13	Change service sites.	Change the location of clinical service sites to increase access.
22	Create or change credentialing and/or licensure standards.	Create an organization that certifies clinicians in the innovation or encourage an existing organization to do so. Change governmental professional certification or licensure requirements to include delivering the innovation. Work to alter continuing education requirements to shape professional practice toward the innovation.
44	Mandate change.	Have leadership declare the priority of the innovation and their determination to have it implemented.
62	Start a dissemination organization.	Identify or start a separate organization that is responsible for disseminating the clinical innovation. It could be a for-profit or non-profit organization.

CLASSIFYING IMPLEMENTATION STRATEGIES

The large number of discrete implementation strategies included in any compilation necessitates breaking them into categories, however tentative, in order to support their meaningful consideration. Ideally, a categorization scheme supports considering strategies that are similar in their action, function, or targets proximally to one another, otherwise potential similarities among strategies may be obscured in a large compilation. There is no consensus regarding how to best categorize strategies, and there are many examples of logical schemes for their organization.[25] For example, the Cochrane EPOC group organizes strategies by the domains of their targets: professional, organizational, regulatory, and financial.[22;23]

The ERIC project took a stakeholder participatory approach to implementation strategy categorization. This approach involved a particular form of group concept mapping, a mixed-methods procedure for engaging a stakeholders in a structured conceptualization process that facilitates the identification of categories within a collection of concepts.[26] To achieve this, 32 implementation and clinical experts completed a computerized sorting task where they sorted virtual cards representing each of the 73 implementation strategies into piles based on their view of their meaning or theme. The frequency in which the strategies were sorted together across all participants allowed for the interrelationships of the strategies to be visually represented using multidimensional scaling such that the relative distances between strategies reflects the relative frequency in which they were sorted together. Subsequently, hierarchical cluster analyses were conducted to identify groups of strategies that are most conceptually similar to one another given the frequency data. Figure 15.1 presents the nine clusters determined to be the best representation for categorizing the strategies in the ERIC compilation.[27]

Broad geographical themes can be identified when reviewing Figure 15.1. Clusters involving interpersonal interactions among key implementers and their supports extend from the lower right quadrant of the figure (i.e., *Train & educate stakeholders, Provide interactive assistance, Support clinicians,* and *Develop stakeholder interrelationships*). Nearly opposite from the clusters composing this theme is the *Engage consumers* cluster, which suggests that the interpersonal interactions focusing on consumers were viewed as relatively distinct from those involving professionals.

There are practical implications for classifying implementation strategies and characterizing their interrelationships. When selecting implementation strategies from a large compilation, it is useful for conceptually similar strategies to be proximal to one another. This not only decreases the cognitive burden of the task but also encourages careful consideration of similar strategies that may vary in their potential fit with the implementation context.

SELECTING AN IMPLEMENTATION STRATEGY

With 73 distinct implementation strategies available for consideration (see Table 15.1), researchers often find it overwhelming to contemplate which strategy, or collection of strategies, to deploy in a given effort to put a new innovation into practice. This task can prove much less daunting, however, when using an implementation science framework or theory to help guide the: (a) understanding of factors or determinants that may influence implementation, and (b) selection of implementation strategy (or strategies if multifaceted).[28;29] Although the value of using a theory or framework to guide implementation has been debated, proceeding without a theory base in implementation has produced mixed results.[28;30–33] Use of an implementation framework/theory allows one to: identify promising implementation strategies based on the framework/theory; identify or develop complementary improvement tools to support implementation; increase the probability for success in implementing the innovation or desired behavior change; and confirm or propose refinements to the framework/theory based on results, thereby contributing to an evolving evidence base for its value and applicability.[28]

Some implementation science frameworks propose a specific strategy as an integrated component. For example, the integrated "Promoting Action on Research Implementation in Health Services" (i-PARIHS) framework identifies use of "facilitation" strategies as the "active ingredient" for guiding individuals and clinical teams through change processes or contextual challenges to implementation.[34] Similarly, planned action or "process" models such as "Replicating Effective Programs" (REP) may be useful, as

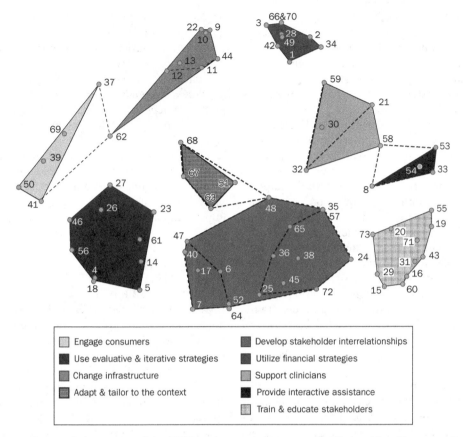

FIGURE 15.1 Point and cluster map of the ERIC implementation strategy compilation. Note: The map reflects the product of an expert panel (valid response n = 32) sorting 73 discrete implementation strategies into groupings by similarity, with each strategy being depicted by a dot and accompanied by a number supporting cross-referencing to the strategies enumerated in Table 15.1. Spatial distances reflect how frequently the strategies were sorted together as similar. In general, the closer two points are together, the more frequently those strategies were sorted together. Strategies distal from one another were infrequently, if at all, sorted together. These spatial relationships are relative to the sorting data obtained in this study, and distances do not reflect an absolute relationship (i.e., a 5-mm distance in the present map does not reflect the same relationship as a 5-mm distance on a map from a different data set). The legend provides the label for each of the nine clusters of strategies. Dotted lines within the Develop stakeholder inter-relationships cluster indicate how two separate clusters were merged into one large cluster due to conceptual similarity among their items. Dotted lines extending between other clusters archive the reassignment of strategies from their original cluster to a neighboring cluster to which there was a better conceptual fit (i.e., strategies #48, #58, and #62). (From Waltz et al., 2015.[27])

they specify a stepwise approach (strategy) to be taken within stages in the process of implementing research into practice.[35;36] Other frameworks such as the "Consolidated Framework for Implementation Research" (CFIR) are more agnostic in terms of proposing a *specific* implementation strategy, but include a domain that explicates broad processes of implementation effort (i.e., the "Process" domain), as well as four domains that identify various determinants that can serve as potential targets for implementation

strategies.[37] Frameworks can be inclusive of the impact implementation has on population health. For example, the Health Equity Impact Assessment (HEIA) is an overarching framework that can be used to identify unintended consequences of an intervention on service delivery or health impact for vulnerable groups within a care system.[38] The HEIA has an explicit health equity lens and a toolkit that has been developed to guide organizations in health equity evaluations and in implementing strategies to mitigate barriers to equitable care.[38] Overall, the different implementation frameworks sampled illustrate how frameworks can influence strategy selection for an implementation initiative. The selection of a particular framework should be done after careful consideration of the goals and scope of an initiative.

Selection and tailoring of an implementation strategy, whether guided by a framework/theory (as recommended above) or not, should also be informed by an assessment of the determinants of current practice within the targeted setting, including identification of implementation barriers and facilitators that may exist at the patient-, provider-, team-, clinic-, organizational-, and system-level. Formative evaluation, and more specifically *developmental* formative evaluation, is a rigorous assessment process typically involving collection of both qualitative and quantitative data to identify the determinants of current practice, barriers, and facilitators for a practice change or implementation of a given innovation, and stakeholder perspectives on feasibility of a proposed implementation strategy.[39] This type of assessment is sometimes referred to as a *needs assessment* or *organizational diagnosis* of factors to be considered and addressed in developing, tailoring, and operationalizing an implementation strategy. Facilitation strategies often include elements of formative evaluation as part of the facilitator's responsibilities;[39,40] similar processes are also included as early steps to be completed in numerous planned action models, including REP.[35,36] Assessment findings are used to tailor the implementation strategy and complementary improvement tools to the site's context and needs, taking into account other recommendations for strategies to be multifaceted (when appropriate), feasible, acceptable to stakeholders, trialable, readily adaptable, sustainable, and scalable for spread to similar settings if successful.[27,29] Table 15.2 provides an example of implementation strategies and tools developed and applied in a study to improve antipsychotic medication management for patients with schizophrenia, based on formative evaluation results.[28,41]

Note that the assessment processes described previously are often applied iteratively, where the implementation strategy and tools may be tailored or adapted multiple times during the course of a given project as needed to enhance fit to local context or to increase chances for achieving implementation or performance improvement goals. Accordingly, although the specification and operationalization of the implementation strategy/tools may vary by site (with documented rationale for variability), *the processes for tailoring and adapting the strategy to sites are uniform and replicable*. Indeed, innovative study designs such as "Multiphase Optimization Strategy Implementation Trials" (MOST) and "Sequential Multiple Assignment Randomized Implementation Trials" (SMART) structure adaptations to the implementation strategy at pre-planned intervals based on progress in achieving implementation or performance improvement goals.[42]

DOCUMENTING IMPLEMENTATION STRATEGIES

Implementation researchers and other stakeholders are not able to fully utilize the findings of studies focusing on implementation strategies because they are often inconsistently labeled and poorly described, are rarely justified theoretically, lack operational definitions or manuals to guide their use, and are part of "packaged" approaches whose specific elements are poorly understood. Implementation strategies cannot be used in practice or tested in research without a full description of their components and how they should be used. As with all intervention research, their descriptions must be precise enough to enable measurement and "reproducibility."

The study of implementation strategies should be approached in a similar fashion as evidence-based interventions, for strategies are in fact a type of intervention. Accordingly, their specification carries the same demands as treatment specification: If they are to be scientifically tested, communicated clearly in the literature, and accurately employed in actual healthcare practice, they must be specified both conceptually and operationally.[43]

The complexity of implementation strategies poses one of the greatest challenges to their clear description, operational definition, and measurement. Implementation strategies are inherently complex social interventions, as they address multifaceted and complicated processes within interpersonal, organizational, and community contexts.[29,44-46] Following is a suggested framework through which implementation strategies can be clearly documented.

TABLE 15.2 EXAMPLE OF USING THEORY TO GUIDE SELECTION
OF IMPLEMENTATION STRATEGIES AND TOOLS

Strategy/Tool	Rationale for Strategy/Tool Selection	Supporting Theory and/or Planning Model
Clinical Opinion Leader	Utilize influential local clinician leaders to inform other clinical staff about evidence-based antipsychotic medication management, model targeted prescribing behaviors, and motivate practice change.	Diffusion of Innovation, Social Cognitive Theory, Social Influence
External Facilitation	External facilitator maintains regular contact with clinical opinion leader at participating sites to assist with problem-solving and addressing challenges to intervention implementation as needed.	Promoting Action on Research Implementation in Health Services (PARIHS), Complexity Theory
Psychosis Guidelines Help File	Computerized resource with clinical pathway diagrams and flowcharts designed to enhance provider knowledge of guideline recommendations for treatment of schizophrenia (*addresses predisposing determinants of care*).	PRECEDE
Pocket Card on Antipsychotic Treatment for Schizophrenia	Brief, practical tool that allows clinicians to reference guideline recommendations for antipsychotic dosing and side effect monitoring as needed at the point of care (*enables appropriate care*).	PRECEDE
Pharmacy Order-Entry Reminder on Dose Recommendations for Antipsychotics	Computerized clinical reminder that provides guideline-recommended dose range on pharmacy order entry screen in electronic medical record when a physician prescribes an antipsychotic medication (*enables appropriate care*).	PRECEDE
Clinical Reminder on Olanzapine and Diabetes/High Lipids	Computerized clinical reminder that alerts physician when a patient is being treated with olanzapine and has also been identified as having diabetes mellitus and/or elevated lipids (conditions which may be worsened when olanzapine is used); reminder also offers potential clinical adjustments for physician consideration (*enables appropriate care*).	PRECEDE
Feedback Performance Report on Use of Antipsychotics	Monthly reports to provide ongoing feedback to clinical staff on performance related to dosing and monitoring side effects of antipsychotic medications (*reinforces adherence to guideline recommendations*).	PRECEDE

1. Name It

To be measured, an implementation strategy must first be named or labeled. Implementation stakeholders should be thoughtful as they name implementation strategies, preferably drawing upon the same terms as other researchers in the field when possible. When different terms are used (or created), they should be carefully distinguished from strategies that are already more established in the literature. It should be noted that naming may be more complicated with multifaceted and blended strategies.

2. Define it

A second step is to define the implementation strategy conceptually. A conceptual definition gives a general sense of what the strategy may involve, and allows the reader to more fully discern whether or not the current usage is consistent with other uses of the term represented in the literature. Using definitions from established taxonomies such as ERIC (described above) provides the basis for a common language.

3. Operationalize It

Strategies must be described clearly in a manner that ensures that they are discussed at a common level of granularity, are rateable across multiple dimensions, and are readily comparable. In a similar fashion, seven dimensions are proposed here that, if detailed adequately, would constitute the adequate operationalization of implementation strategies. The following sections address each of these dimensions.

The Actor

An "actor" is defined as a stakeholder who actually delivers the implementation strategy. A wide range of stakeholders can fill this function, as implementation strategies may be employed or enacted by payers, administrators, intervention developers, outside consultants, personnel within an organization charged with being 'implementers,' providers/clinicians/support staff, clients/patients/consumers, or community stakeholders.

The Action

Implementation strategies require dynamic verb statements that indicate actions, steps or processes, and sequences of behavior. Ideally, these actions are behaviorally defined a priori to allow comparison with what was actually done during the implementation process.

Action Target

The complexity of implementation strategies is also a function of where they are directed or the conceptual "targets" they attempt to impact. For example, strategies such as 'realigning payment incentives' target the policy context, while 'training' targets front line providers by increasing knowledge and skill, and "fidelity checklists" target the clarity of the intervention as well as the providers' understanding and ability to break down the intervention into more "doable" steps.

Temporality

The order or sequence of strategy use may be critical in some cases. For instance, Lyon et al.[47] suggest that strategies to boost providers' motivation to learn new treatments may need to precede other common implementation strategies such as training and supervision. Articles that report the use of strategies should include information about the stage or phase when the strategy was used.

Dose

Just as the intervention or treatment literature addresses the concept of dose, implementation strategies also can vary tremendously in dosage or intensity. Details about the dose or intensity of implementation strategies such as the amount of time spent with an external facilitator,[48] the time and intensity of training,[49] or the frequency of audit and feedback[15] should be designated a priori and reported.

The Implementation Outcome Affected

Strategies impact intermediate outcomes (i.e., acceptability, reach, adoption, appropriateness, feasibility, fidelity, cost, penetration, and sustainability) and contribute to more distal outcomes related to consumer health and service system functioning. Certain strategies may target one or more of these implementation outcomes (or other outcomes not identified in the Proctor et al. taxonomy).[50]

The Justification

Researchers should make efforts to provide justification or rationale for the strategies that they use to implement a given innovation.[29,51] Ideally, they should be selected because relevant theory,[33,52] empirical evidence,[13] and/or some pragmatic rationale (e.g., using a low-cost, low intensity intervention when theory and evidence for more intensive strategies is not compelling) suggest they may be appropriate to address the specific challenges posed by the implementation context.

Practical examples of reporting implementation strategies using the Proctor and colleagues guidelines are beginning to emerge.[50] For example, Bunger and colleagues used these guidelines to report the key components of a learning collaborative intended to increase the use of Trauma-Focused Cognitive Behavioral Therapy.[53] Similarly, Gold and colleagues use the guidelines to report a strategy to implement a diabetes quality improvement intervention within community health centers.[54] These examples demonstrate the utility of the reporting guidelines for enhancing the clarity of implementation strategies so that they can be replicated in research and practice. We note that additional guidelines to improve reporting implementation research exist, including the WIDER guidelines.[55-58] Table 15.3 details the original WIDER recommendations, along with supplementary recommendations outlined by Albrecht and colleagues.[55]

Colquhoun and colleagues have worked to develop a simplified framework that could be used to improve the reporting and design of implementation strategies. The core components of that framework include: (1) active ingredients (i.e., the defining characteristics of the implementation strategy), (2) causal mechanisms (i.e., the processes or mediators by which strategies exert change), (3) mode of delivery or practical application (i.e., the way an implementation strategy is applied (face-to-face, web-based), and (4) the intended target.[59] These guidelines will be updated and refined, and inevitably, new frameworks will emerge. However, our hope is that this type of guidance will lead to more careful reporting of implementation strategies so that we can begin to understand where, when, why, and how they are effective in improving implementation and clinical outcomes.

ASSESSING IMPLEMENTATION STRATEGY FIDELITY

To ensure appropriate application and spread of successful implementation strategies, it is important to develop and use tools and processes to measure and support fidelity to a given strategy's core components or elements. See chapter 16 for more detailed discussion on fidelity. In implementing evidence-based practices or other innovations, it is critical to give attention not only to documenting and assuring fidelity to the

---

TABLE 15.3 REPORTING IMPLEMENTATION STRATEGIES

WIDER Recommendations	Supplementary Recommendations
Detailed description of interventions in published papers	1) Characteristics of those delivering the intervention 2) Characteristics of the recipients 3) The setting 4) The mode of delivery 5) The intensity 6) The duration 7) Adherence/fidelity to delivery protocols 8) Detailed description of the intervention content provided for each study group
Clarification of assumed change process and design principles	1) The intervention development 2) The change techniques used in the intervention 3) The causal processes targeted by these change techniques
Access to intervention manuals/protocols	1) Submit protocols or manuals for publication to make these supplementary materials easily accessible (i.e., online).
Detailed description of active control conditions	1) Characteristics of those delivering the control 2) Characteristics of the recipients 3) The setting 4) The mode of delivery 5) The intensity 6) The duration 7) Adherence/fidelity to delivery protocols 8) Detailed description of the control content provided

innovation (i.e., ensuring that core components or processes involved with delivering the innovation are included or followed), but also to document and assess fidelity to core components of the *implementation strategy* to support its practical application and dissemination to other settings.[39] Despite calls to do so, this aspect of implementation science and practice is relatively underdeveloped and infrequently applied.[20]

A recent literature review assessing the extent and quality of documentation of fidelity to implementation strategies in 72 studies found that although 71% of the studies reported at least some details on the extent and/or quality of fidelity to the implementation strategy(ies) used, details were scarce or very limited for many of these studies.[20] Indeed, the authors did not find a single study that included a conceptual framework for fidelity, or even a fidelity definition. Clearly, this is an area that is ripe for research attention.

One example of developmental work in this area is a recent study to create and pilot a tool for assessing fidelity in use of implementation facilitation strategies to support use of evidence-based practices or other clinical innovations.[60] Implementation facilitation is a dynamic process of interactive problem solving and support to help clinical personnel implement and sustain a new program, process, or practice that occurs in the context of a recognized need for improvement and a supportive interpersonal relationship.[8;39;61] A number of studies have contributed to a growing evidence base in the literature for the impact of implementation facilitation strategies for promoting use of a new program or practice in healthcare settings.[62;63] A scoping literature review[64] of these studies was conducted to document and identify core components of facilitation through a rigorous consensus development process.[60] Scoping reviews aim to rapidly map the key concepts underpinning a research area and the main sources and types of evidence available, and can be undertaken as stand-alone projects in their own right, especially where an area is complex or has not previously been reviewed comprehensively.[65] Initial results from the review indicate that core components of implementation facilitation may include the following domains: *stakeholder engagement, relationship-building, assessment* (e.g., understanding context, identifying barriers/facilitators), *assisting with preparation/planning, providing education/training, performance monitoring* (e.g., monitoring adherence to implementation plan and clinical performance data (audit/feedback)), *problem-solving,* and *adapting/refining the implementation plan as needed to meet goals.* These results have been used to develop a prototype tool to assess implementation facilitation fidelity for ongoing testing and refinement.

ASSESSING OUTCOMES OF IMPLEMENTATION STRATEGIES: USE OF INNOVATIVE DESIGNS

Given that the majority of implementation strategies target provider- and organization-level change, the conduct of effectiveness studies can be challenging. At the very least they require large numbers of clinical settings, providers, community organizations, and other stakeholders. Prior chapters within this book have focused on implementation research design and measurement, therefore this section is used to describe the application of a particularly novel design that Kilbourne et al. have applied to assess the efficacy of three implementation strategies, the Adaptive Implementation of Effective Programs Trial (ADEPT). The protocol of this *pragmatic adaptive design* is available[66] Key factors associated with this innovative work are summarized as follows.

The ADEPT study, currently underway (NIH R-01MH099898-01), uses a SMART design to support an adaptive implementation strategy and compare three blended implementation strategies with increasing intensity of services. The first is Replicating Effective Programs (REP), a relatively low-intensity blended implementation strategy that focuses on toolkit development and marketing, provider training, and limited program assistance. The second is implementation facilitation using a facilitator who is external to the clinical setting and assists sites in implementing a clinical innovation, external facilitation (EF), and the third is the addition of a facilitator who is internal to the clinical organization to the existing external facilitator/internal facilitation (EF/IF).[62;67]

Of course as the intensity of the implementation strategy increases, there is an increase in cost and potential inability of an organization to apply this type of strategy throughout a system. In addition, not all sites may require the most intensive support. To address the questions of (1) who needs more intense levels of assistance and (2) does internal facilitation increase the uptake of a clinical innovation, Dr. Kilbourne and colleagues designed a program of study in which the implementation interventions are increased in intensity based on limited or lack of adoption of the innovation.

The evidence-based practice being implemented is Life Goals, a psychosocial treatment delivered to patients with mood disorders over six individualized or group sessions in 80 community-based primary care or mental health clinics.[68] Sites not responding to REP after 6 months following initiation of implementation are randomized to receive additional support from EF or EF/IF. Sites not responding to EF after another 6 months are randomized to continued EF or EF/IF. Figure 15.2 provides a schematic of this innovative design.

This type of design allows the assessment of whether an off-site EF alone versus the addition of a facilitator internal to the organization improves the uptake of the innovation. It also allows assessment of delaying the application of an internal facilitator on innovation uptake.

DISSEMINATION SUCCESSFUL IMPLEMENTATION STRATEGIES

Just as implementation science researchers have emphasized the need for study of the implementation of evidence-based *practices and innovations*, we must also turn our attention to the dissemination of evidence-based *implementation strategies*. To initiate lasting changes to care on a broad scale, policymakers and clinical managers must be capable of integrating implementation science knowledge and strategies into initiatives intended to foster adoption and spread of evidence-based practices or other innovations. As one might anticipate, just as there is a gap between evidence-based practices and their use in routine settings, there is likely a similar gap between evidence-based implementation strategies and *their* use in clinical or other organizational change processes.[69]

Kirchner et al have described the concept of implementation *practitioners* as those who increase the uptake of an EBP into practice by: (a) applying strategies and tools developed in implementation research and/or (b) working with those with implementation expertise to contextualize evidence-based implementation strategies and improve clinical processes.[70] Central to increasing the use of evidence-based implementation strategies by implementation practitioners is educating this key group about implementation science as well as processes through which

strategies with a documented evidence base can be transferred.

Several recent publications have focused on describing the foundations of implementation science, its methodology, and ways through which the knowledge gained by this field can be applied by policymakers and clinical managers (i.e., implementation practitioners).[70;71] These articles describe how both clinical quality improvement and educational objectives can be achieved by incorporating implementation strategies and products into practice. For example, the Accreditation Council for Graduate Medical Education (ACGME), in conjunction with the American Boards of Medical Specialties, identify six ACGME core competencies including practice-based learning and improvement and systems-based practice, both central components of implementation.[70;72]

Yet, as implementation scientists know quite well, education alone is rarely sufficient to effect meaningful or lasting change in clinical behavior. Therefore, an interactive approach to knowledge transfer is needed, with a dedicated focus on skill building. The Society for Implementation Research Collaboration (SIRC) encourages involvement of implementation practitioners, including, clinicians, managers, and policymakers, who participate in implementation or quality improvement activities. To support and incentivize such involvement, SIRC has established a stakeholder subgroup entitled the "EBP Champion Group," with presentations at SIRC meetings from this subgroup being highly encouraged and preferentially accepted. In addition, a recent review identified 11 training opportunities focusing on development of implementation science skills, from 1-day workshops to certificate courses.[73]

While the availability of training programs and resources noted earlier is certainly encouraging, an even more integrated approach for the transfer of implementation strategies to implementation practitioners may be warranted. One integrated approach for transferring knowledge and skills for a given implementation strategy would be through interactive training coupled with time-limited consultation with an expert or experienced practitioner of the strategy. For example, such processes have been applied in several initiatives focused on using implementation facilitation to support adoption of integrated primary care mental health clinics, measurement-based care for posttraumatic stress disorder,

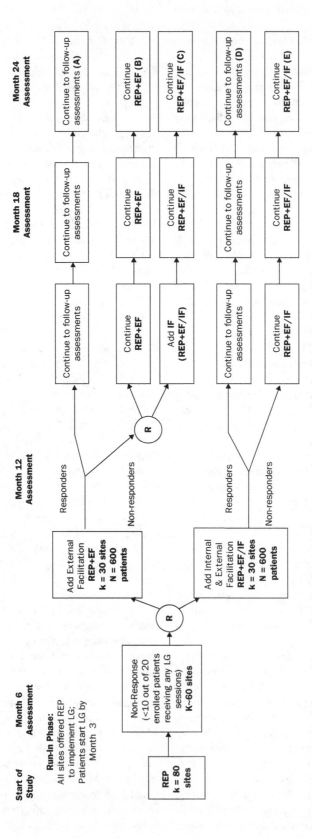

FIGURE 15.2 SMART trial design of REP combined with external (EF; REP +EF) and internal facilitation (IF, REP+ EF/IF).

and implementation of peer specialist services for behavioral health needs in primary care.[71;74] Finally, the implementation scientist may actually become part of the organization that is applying the evidence-based strategy. This is the model applied in the "warm handoff" of implementation facilitation from implementation researchers to the VA Office of Mental Health Operations and is described in our chapter's case study.

CASE STUDY: IMPLEMENTING AND DOCUMENTING IMPLEMENTATION STRATEGIES

The following uses a recent study conducted within the Department of Veteran Affairs (VA) to apply the concepts presented in this chapter. Occurring within a national VA initiative, the Blended Facilitation to Enhance Primary Care Mental Health (SDP 08-316) tested the effectiveness of an external/internal implementation facilitation strategy on the uptake of primary care mental health integration (PC-MHI) at sites identified by regional leadership as unable to implement the clinical innovation without assistance.

Addressing the Lack of Definition and Classifying Strategies

Within the ERIC taxonomy, facilitation is defined as "A process of interactive problem solving and support that occurs in a context of a recognized need for improvement and a supportive interpersonal relationship."[8] It is classified under the ERIC "Provide Interactive Assistance" Cluster (number 33 in Figure 15.1) and, not surprisingly, is grouped with providing local and centralized technical assistance as well as providing clinical supervision.[27]

Selecting an Implementation Strategy

Implementation facilitation was selected and operationalized based on the i-PARIHS (then named PARIHS) framework.[75] Implementation Facilitation is a multifaceted strategy that combines facilitation with multiple other discrete implementation strategies tailored to meet the needs of the local context. The implementation facilitation strategy combined an external expert with internal regional facilitators, who were inexperienced with implementation facilitation. The external facilitator provided mentoring to

transfer facilitation knowledge and skills to support future implementation initiatives.

Documenting the Implementation Strategy

To document how the implementation facilitation strategy was operationalized, the evaluation team conducted individual monthly debriefings with facilitators who described their activities, the rationale for them, and the results of their interventions, as well as the local context and stakeholders. A content analysis of the debriefing interviews revealed that across eight clinics, implementation facilitators applied over 50% of the discrete implementation strategies identified in the ERIC project.[76] The specific strategies used varied across settings, contextual factors, and the stakeholders with whom the facilitators were interacting. Additionally, implementation facilitators used structured spreadsheets to document types of activities they performed, the dates of the activities, stakeholders participating in the activities (if appropriate), and the amount of time activities required. This was provided to the evaluation team on a weekly basis.

Assessing Outcomes of Implementation Strategies

The mixed methods study used a multisite, quasi-experimental design with nonequivalent comparison groups. Eight PC clinics from two VA networks received implementation facilitation. These sites were compared with eight matched clinics in two matched networks that received national level support only, comprised primarily of education and national calls that provided technical support. The RE-AIM analytic framework guided the assessment of clinical and implementation outcomes and the PARIHS framework guided the analysis of variables influencing PC-MHI adoption. In addition to assessing reach, effectiveness, and adoption, the study assessed the quality of PC-MHI programs and their adherence to evidence, and the organizational costs of applying implementation facilitation, as well as how well programs and outcomes were sustained.

Disseminating Successful Implementation Strategies

Prior to the completion of data collection that would ultimately identify implementation facilitation as an evidence-based strategy, the VA Office of Mental Health Operations (OMHO) requested that study personnel develop a manual and training process to train OMHO personnel on the strategy. At the time, OMHO was charged with supporting sites in the implementation of mental health policy systemwide. To conduct this work, the lead investigator was supported at 20% to 30% effort by OMHO to train and mentor a team of technical assistant specialists who then worked at the regional and local level to improve uptake of VA Mental Health policy. Additionally, over the course of the study, the external expert facilitator transferred the implementation facilitation strategy to internal regional facilitators, one of whom accepted a position within OMHO and facilitated PC-MHI integration for that office.

FUTURE RESEARCH

While there has been substantial advancement in the establishment of a shared taxonomy and reporting processes for implementation strategies, there remain several areas for future work. First is the further development of designs and methods appropriate for evaluating implementation strategies. While many have called for the use of large implementation labs controlling for the context, recipient and innovation factors within these "labs" remain a challenge.[13] There is also a need for development and testing of innovative processes and tools to streamline assessment processes used to inform tailoring of implementation strategies and tools to site context in a timely manner, while also minimizing research and participant burden. As noted, there is a need for more work focused on assessing fidelity to the implementation strategy, in addition to the clinical innovation, for quality control and to help facilitate replication. In addition, there is a need for more research on strategies for ensuring long term sustainability, or "institutionalization," of clinical innovations within targeted settings once an active implementation strategy is concluded. Future studies should also address comparative effectiveness research on budget impact or cost efficiency of competing implementation strategies, to help inform policy makers on cost implications for adopting one strategy versus another. Finally, there is a need for the development of rigorous and tested methods to educate implementation practitioners on the use of evidence-based implementation strategies, thus insuring that we do not face a delay in putting the knowledge gained into the hands of those who need and will use it.

SUMMARY

As the field of implementation science moves beyond studying barriers to and facilitators of implementation to the comparative effectiveness of different strategies, it is essential that we create a common taxonomy to define the strategies that we study. Similarly, we must clearly document the implementation strategies that are applied, the factors that influence their selection, and any adaptation of the strategy during the course of implementation and sustainment of the innovation being implemented. By incorporating this type of rigor into our work we will be able to not only advance the science of implementation but also our ability to place evidence-based innovations into the hands of practitioners in a timely and efficient manner.

SUGGESTED READINGS AND WEBSITES

Readings

Kirchner JE, Ritchie MJ, Pitcock JA, Parker LE, Curran GM, Fortney JC. Outcomes of a partnered facilitation strategy to implement primary care–mental health. *J Gen Intern Med.* 2014;29(4):904–912.

This paper describes quantitative results from a quasi-experimental Type 3 Hybrid effectiveness-implementation study testing the impact of an implementation facilitation strategy to support establishment of integrated primary care–mental health clinics in the Veterans Health Administration. The implementation strategy applied in the study was based on the "Promoting Action on Research Implementation in Health Services" (PARIHS) framework, with selection of evaluation measures based on the RE-AIM model. This study served as the basis for the "Case Study" example described earlier in this chapter.

Powell BJ, Waltz TJ, Chinman MJ, et al. A refined compilation of implementation strategies: results from the Expert Recommendations for Implementing Change (ERIC) project. *Implement Sci.* 2015;10(1):1–14. doi: 10.1186/s13012-015-0209-1

This paper describes results from a highly rigorous expert consensus development process to provide clarity and consistency on terms and definitions for 73 discrete implementation strategies (see Table 15.1 in this chapter). Experts in implementation and clinical practice engaged in three rounds of a modified Delphi process to generate consensus on the implementation strategies and definitions.

Proctor E, Silmere H, Raghavan R, et al. Outcomes for implementation research: conceptual distinctions, measurement challenges, and research agenda. *Adm Policy Ment Health.* 2011;38(2):65–76. doi: 10.1007/s10488-010-0319-7

In this paper, the authors propose a working taxonomy of eight conceptually distinct implementation outcomes—acceptability, adoption, appropriateness, feasibility, fidelity, implementation cost, penetration, and sustainability—along with their nominal definitions that may help guide consideration and selection of measures to assess success of an implementation strategy.

Waltz TJ, Powell BJ, Matthieu MM, et. al. Use of concept mapping to characterize relationships among implementation strategies and assess their feasibility and importance: results from the Expert Recommendations for Implementing Change (ERIC) study. 2015; 10:109. *Implement Sci.* 2015;10:109. doi: 10.1186/s13012-015-0295-0

This paper describes use of concept mapping methodology to sort the 73 ERIC implementation strategies into similar groups (see Figure 15.1 in this chapter) and to rate each strategy's relative importance and feasibility for given practice change scenarios. Results from this study provided initial validation of the implementation strategies within the ERIC compilation as being conceptually distinct.

Sales A, Smith JL, Curran G, Kochevar L. Models, strategies and tools: the role of theory in implementing evidence-based findings into health care practice. *J Gen Intern Med.* 2006;1:S43–S49.

This paper proposes a systematic approach to using theory to guide the selection of implementation strategies, evaluating their effectiveness, and critically appraising the fit of the initially selected theory based on findings. A case example is provided for an implementation research project to improve antipsychotic medication management for patients with schizophrenia.

Stetler CB, Legro MW, Wallace CM, Bowman C, Guihan M, Hagedorn H, Kimmel B, Sharp ND, Smith JL. The role of formative evaluation in implementation research and the QUERI experience. *J Gen Intern Med.* 2006;21:S1–S8.

This paper describes the role of formative evaluation methods in informing selection of implementation strategies or tools to support use of evidence-based practices or other clinical innovations. Case examples are provided from multiple implementation research studies.

Selected Websites and Tools

The Quality Enhancement Research Initiative (QUERI). http://www.queri.research.va.gov/.

The Quality Enhancement Research Initiative (QUERI) is a quality improvement program that has become a central component of VA's commitment to improving the quality of Veterans' healthcare. This website includes access to the "QUERI Implementation Guide" that introduces approaches to doing research on implementation, as well as other tools that may be of use to implementation researchers.

Consolidated Framework for Implementation Research (CFIR). http://cfirguide.org/.

The CFIR provides a menu of constructs that can be used in a range of applications—as a practical guide for systematically assessing potential barriers and facilitators in preparation for implementing an innovation, to providing theory-based constructs for developing context-specific logic models or generalizable middle-range theories. This website includes sections on designing an implementation strategy or evaluation guided by CFIR.

Effective Practice and Organisation of Care (EPOC): EPOC Taxonomy. 2015. http://epoc.cochrane.org/epoc-taxonomy.

The Effective Practice and Organisation of Care (EPOC) Group is a Cochrane Review Group. The scope of the Cochrane EPOC group is to undertake systematic reviews of educational, behavioral, financial, regulatory, and organizational interventions designed to improve health professional practice and the organization of health care services.

REFERENCES

1. Grol R, Grimshaw J. Evidence-based implementation of evidence-based medicine. *Jt Comm J Qual Improv.* 1999;25:503–513.
2. Eccles MP, Armstrong D, Baker R, et al. An implementation research agenda. *Implement Sci.* 2009;4:18. doi: 10.1186/1748-5908-4-18
3. Newman K, Van Eerd D, Powell BJ, et al. Identifying priorities in knowledge translation from the perspective of trainees: results from an online survey. *Implement Sci.* 2015;10:92. doi: 10.1186/s13012-015-0282-5
4. Institute of Medicine. *Initial national priorities for comparative effectiveness research.* Washington, DC: The National Academies Press; 2009.
5. National Institutes of Health. Dissemination and implementation research in health (R01). 2016; http://grants.nih.gov/grants/guide/pa-files/PAR-16-238.html. Accessed March 2, 2017.
6. Proctor E, Powell B, McMillen J. Implementation strategies: recommendations for specifying and reporting. *Implement Sci.* 2013;8:139. doi: 10.1186/1748-5908-8-139
7. Powell BJ, McMillen JC, Proctor EK, et al. A compilation of strategies for implementing clinical innovations in health and mental health. *Med Care Res Rev.* 2012;69:123–157.

8. Powell BJ, Waltz TJ, Chinman MJ, et al. A refined compilation of implementation strategies: results from the Expert Recommendations for Implementing Change (ERIC) project. *Implement Sci.* 2015;10:21. doi: 10.1186/s13012-015-0209-1

9. Glisson C, Schoenwald SK, Hemmelgarn A, et al. Randomized trial of MST and ARC in a two-level EBT implementation strategy. *J Consult Clin Psychol.* 2010;78:537–550. doi: 10.1037/a0019160

10. Aarons GA, Ehrhart MG, Farahnak LR, Hurlburt MS. Leadership and Organizational Change for Implementation (LOCI): a randomized mixed method pilot study of a leadership and organization development intervention for evidence-based practice implementation. *Implement Sci.* 2015;10:11. doi: 10.1186/s13012-014-0192-y

11. Glisson C, Landsverk J, Schoenwald S, et al. Assessing the organizational social context (OSC) of mental health dervices: implications for research and practice. *Adm Policy Ment Health.* 2008;35:98–113.

12. Aarons GA, Ehrhart MG, Farahnak LR. The Implementation Leadership Scale (ILS): development of a brief measure of unit level implementation leadership. *Implement Sci.* 2014;9:45. doi: 10.1186/1748-5908-9-45

13. Grimshaw J, Eccles M, Lavis J, Hill S, Squires J. Knowledge translation of research findings. *Implement Sci.* 2012;7:50. doi: 10.1186/1748-5908-7-50

14. Forsetlund L, Bjørndal A, Rashidian A, et al. Continuing education meetings and workshops: effects on professional practice and health care outcomes. *Cochrane Database Syst Rev.* 2009. doi: 10.1002/14651858.CD003030.pub2

15. Ivers N, Jamtvedt G, Flottorp S, et al. Audit and feedback: effects on professional practice and healthcare outcomes. *Cochrane Database Syst Rev.* 2012. doi: 10.1002/14651858.CD00259.pub3

16. Farmer AP, Légaré F, Turcot L, et al. Printed educational materials: effects on professional practice and health care outcomes. *Cochrane Database Syst Rev.* 2011. doi: 10.1002/14651858.CD004398.pub2

17. Flodgren G, Parmelli E, Doumit G, et al. Local opinion leaders: effects on professional practice and health care outcomes. *Cochrane Database Syst Rev.* 2011. doi: 10.1002/14651858.CD000125.pub4

18. Baker R, Camosso-Stefinovic Janette, Gillies C, et al. Tailored interventions to address determinants of practice. *Cochrane Database Syst Rev.* 2015. doi: 10.1002/14651858.CD005470.pub3

19. Michie S, Fixsen D, Grimshaw JM, Eccles MP. Specifying and reporting complex behaviour change interventions: the need for a scientific method. *Implement Sci.* 2009;4:40. doi: 10.1186/1748-5908-4-40

20. Slaughter SE, Hill JN, Snelgrove-Clarke E. What is the extent and quality of documentation and reporting of fidelity to implementation strategies: a scoping review. *Implement Sci.* 2015;10:129. doi: 10.1186/s13012-015-0320-3

21. Yoon CK. *Naming Nature: The clash between instinct and science.* New York: W.W. Norton & Company; 2010.

22. Effective Practice and Organisation of Care (EPOC). EPOC Taxonomy. 2015; https://epoc.cochrane.org/epoc-taxonomy. Accessed March 6, 2017.

23. Mazza D, Bairstow P, Buchan H, et al. Refining a taxonomy for guideline implementation: results of an exercise in abstract classification. *Implement Sci.* 2013;8:32. doi: 10.1186/1748-5908-8-32

24. Waltz T, Powell B, Chinman M, et al. Expert recommendations for implementing change (ERIC): protocol for a mixed methods study. *Implement Sci.* 2014;9:39. doi: 10.1186/1748-5908-9-39

25. Grol R, Wensing M. Selection of strategies. In: Grol R, Wensing M, Eccles M, eds. *Improving patient care: The implementation of change in clinical practice.* London: Elsevier; 2005;122–134.

26. Kane M, Trochim WMK. *Concept mapping for planning and evaluation.* Thousand Oaks, CA: Sage; 2007.

27. Waltz TJ, Powell BJ, Matthieu MM, et al. Use of concept mapping to characterize relationships among implementation strategies and assess their feasibility and importance: results from the Expert Recommendations for Implementing Change (ERIC) study. *Implement Sci.* 2015;10:109. doi: 10.1186/s13012-015-0295-0

28. Sales A, Smith J, Curran G, Kochevar L. Models, strategies, and tools. Theory in implementing evidence-based findings into health care practice. *J Gen Intern Med.* 2006;21:S43–S49.

29. Mittman BS. Implementation science in health care. In: Brownson RC, Colditz GA, Proctor EK, eds. *Dissemination and implementation research in health: translating science to practice.* New York: Oxford University Press; 2012;400–418.

30. Bhattacharyya O, Reeves S, Garfinkel S, Zwarenstein M. Designing theoretically-informed implementation interventions: fine in theory, but evidence of effectiveness in practice is needed. *Implement Sci.* 2006;1:5. doi: 10.1186/1748-5908-1-1

31. Eccles M, Grimshaw J, Walker A, Johnston M, Pitts N. Changing the behavior of healthcare professionals: the use of theory in promoting the uptake of research findings. *J Clin Epidemiol.* 2005;58:107–112. doi: 10.1016/j.jclinepi.2004.09.002

32. Oxman AD, Fretheim A, Flottorp S. The OFF theory of research utilization. *J Clin Epidemiol*. 2005;58:113–116. doi: 10.1016/j.jclinepi.2004.10.002

33. The Improved Clinical Effectiveness through Behavioural Research Group (ICEBeRG). Designing theoretically-informed implementation interventions. *Implement Sci*. 2006;1:4. doi: 10.1186/1748-5908-1-4

34. Harvey G, Kitson A. PARIHS revisited: from heuristic to integrated framework for the successful implementation of knowledge into practice. *Implement Sci*. 2016;11:1–13. doi: 10.1186/s13012-016-0398-2

35. Kilbourne AM, Neumann MS, Pincus HA, Bauer MS, Stall R. Implementing evidence-based interventions in health care: application of the replicating effective programs framework. *Implement Sci*. 2007;2:42. doi: 10.1186/1748-5908-2-42

36. Going Lean in Health Care. IHI Innovation Series white paper. Cambridge, MA: Institute for Healthcare Improvement. 2005. www.IHI.org. Accessed March 6, 2017.

37. Damschroder LJ, Aron DC, Keith RE, Kirsh SR, Alexander JA, Lowery JC. Fostering implementation of health services research findings into practice: a consolidated framework for advancing implementation science. *Implement Sci*. 2009;4:50. doi: 10.1186/1748-5908-4-50

38. Ministry of Health and Long Term Care. *Health equity impact assessment (HEIA) workbook*. Toronto, ON: Author. 2012. http://www.health.gov.on.ca/en/pro/programs/heia/docs/workbook.pdf. Accessed March 6, 2017.

39. Stetler CB, Legro MW, Wallace CM, et al. The role of formative evaluation in implementation research and the QUERI experience. *J Gen Intern Med*. 2006;21:S1–S8.

40. Owen R, Drummond K, Viverito K, et al. Monitoring and managing metabolic effects of antipsychotics: a cluster randomized trial of an intervention combining evidence-based quality improvement and external facilitation. *Implement Sci*. 2013;8:120. doi: 10.1186/1748-5908-8-120

41. Curran GM, Thrush CR, Smith JL, Owen RR, Ritchie M, Chadwick D. Implementing research findings into practice using clinical opinion leaders: Barriers and lessons learned. *Jt Comm J Qual Patient Saf*. 2005;31:700–707.

42. Brown CH, Curran G, Palinkas LA et al. An overview of research and evaluation designs for dissemination and implementation. *Annu Rev Publ Health*. 2017;38:1–22.

43. Rosen A, Proctor E. Specifying the treatment process: the basis for effectiveness research. *J Soc Serv Res*. 1978;2:25–43. doi: 10.1300/J079v02n01_04

44. Alexander JA, Hearld LR. Methods and metrics challenges of delivery-system research. *Implement Sci*. 2012;7:15. doi: 10.1186/1748-5908-7-15

45. Craig P, Dieppe P, Macintyre S, Michie S, Nazareth I, Petticrew M. Developing and evaluating complex interventions: the new Medical Research Council guidance. *BMJ*. 2008;337:a1655. doi: 10.1136/bmj.a1655

46. May C. Towards a general theory of implementation. *Implement Sci*. 2013;8:18. doi: 10.1186/1748-5908-8-18

47. Lyon AR, Stirman SW, Kerns SEU, Bruns EJ. Developing the mental health workforce: review and application of training approaches from multiple disciplines. *Adm Policy Ment Health*. 2011;38:238–253. doi: 10.1007/s10488-010-0331-y

48. Kauth MR, Sullivan G, Blevins D, et al. Employing external facilitation to implement cognitive behavioral therapy in VA clinics: a pilot study. *Implement Sci*. 2010;5:75. doi: 10.1186/1748-5908-5-75

49. Herschell AD, Kolko DJ, Baumann BL, Davis AC. The role of therapist training in the implementation of psychosocial treatments: a review and critique with recommendations. *Clin Psychol Rev*. 2010;30:448–466. doi: 10.1016/j.cpr.2010.02.005

50. Proctor E, Silmere H, Raghavan R, et al. Outcomes for implementation research: conceptual distinctions, measurement challenges, and research agenda. *Adm Policy Ment Health*. 2011;38:65–76. doi: 10.1007/s10488-010-0319-7

51. Wensing M, Bosch M, Grol R. Selecting, tailoring, and implementing knowledge translation interventions. In: Straus S, Tetroe J, Graham ID, eds. *Knowledge translation in health care: Moving from evidence to practice*. Oxford: Wiley-Blackwell; 2009;94–113.

52. Grol RP, Bosch MC, Hulscher M, Eccles MP, Wensing M. Planning and studying improvement in patient care: the use of theoretical perspectives. *Milbank Q*. 2007;85:93–138.

53. Bunger AC, Hanson RF, Doogan NJ, Powell BJ, Cao Y, Dunn J. Can learning collaboratives support implementation by rewiring professional networks? *Adm Policy Ment Health*. 2016;43:79–92. doi: 10.1007/s10488-014-0621-x

54. Gold R, Bunce AE, Cohen DJ, et al. Reporting on the strategies needed to implement proven interventions: an example from a "real-world" cross-setting implementation study. *Mayo Clin Proc*. 2016;91:1074–1083. doi: 10.1016/j.mayocp.2016.03.014

55. Albrecht L, Archibald M, Arseneau D, Scott SD. Development of a checklist to assess the quality of reporting of knowledge

translation interventions using the Workgroup for Intervention Development and Evaluation Research (WIDER) recommendations. *Implement Sci.* 2013;8:52. doi: 10.1186/1748-5908-8-52

56. Workgroup for Intervention Development and Evaluation Research. WIDER recommendations to improve reporting of the content of behaviour change interventions. 2008; https://static-content. springer.com/esm/art%3A10.1186%2F1748-5908-7-70/MediaObjects/13012_2011_537_MOESM4_ESM.pdf. Accessed March 7, 2017.

57. Davidoff F, Batalden P, Stevens D, Ogrinc G, Mooney S; SQUIRE Development Group. Publication guidelines for improvement studies in health care: evolution of the SQUIRE project. *Ann Intern Med.* 2008;149:670–676. doi: 10.7326/0003-4819-149-9-200811040-00009

58. Pinnock H, Epiphaniou E, Sheikh A, et al. Developing standards for reporting implementation studies of complex interventions (StaRI): a systematic review and e-Delphi. *Implement Sci.* 2015;10:42. doi: 10.1186/s13012-015-0235-z

59. Colquhoun H, Leeman J, Michie S, et al. Towards a common terminology: a simplified framework of interventions to promote and integrate evidence into health practices, systems, and policies. *Implement Sci.* 2014;9:51. doi: 10.1186/1748-5908-9-51

60. Smith JL, Ritchie MJ, Kim B, Miller CJ, Chinman MJ, Kirchner JE. Scoping review to identify core components of implementation facilitation strategies (Manuscript in development). 2017.

61. Kirchner JE, Kearney LK, Ritchie MJ, Dollar KM, Swensen AB, Schohn M. Research & services partnerships: lessons learned through a national partnership between clinical leaders and researchers. *Psychiatr Serv.* 2014;65:577–579. doi: 10.1176/appi.ps.201400054

62. Kirchner JE, Ritchie MJ, Pitcock JA, Parker LE, Curran GM, Fortney JC. Outcomes of a partnered facilitation strategy to implement primary care-mental health. *J Gen Intern Med.* 2014;29(Suppl 4):904–912. doi: 10.1007/s11606-014-3027-2

63. Baskerville NB, Liddy C, Hogg W. Systematic review and meta-analysis of practice facilitation within primary care settings. *Ann Fam Med.* 2012;10:63–74.

64. Grant MJ, Booth A. A typology of reviews: an analysis of 14 review types and associated methodologies. *Health Info Libr J.* 2009;26:91–108. doi: 10.1111/j.1471-1842.2009.00848.x

65. Mays N, Roberts E, Popay J. Synthesising research evidence. In: Fulop N, Allen P, Clarke A, Black N, eds. *Studying the organisation and delivery of health services: Research methods.* London: Routledge; 2001;188–219.

66. Kilbourne AM, Almirall D, Eisenberg D, et al. Protocol: Adaptive Implementation of Effective Programs Trial (ADEPT): cluster randomized SMART trial comparing a standard versus enhanced implementation strategy to improve outcomes of a mood disorders program. *Implement Sci.* 2014;9:132. doi: 10.1186/s13012-014-0132-x

67. Kilbourne A, Abraham K, Goodrich D, et al. Cluster randomized adaptive implementation trial comparing a standard versus enhanced implementation intervention to improve uptake of an effective re-engagement program for patients with serious mental illness. *Implement Sci.* 2013;8:136. doi: 10.1186/1748-5908-8-136

68. Kilbourne AM, Post EP, Nossek A, Drill L, Cooley S, Bauer MS. Improving medical and psychiatric outcomes among individuals with bipolar disorder: a randomized controlled trial. *Psychiatr Serv.* 2008;59:760–768.

69. Ritchie MJ, Dollar KM, Kearney LK, Kirchner JE. Responding to needs of clinical operations partners: transferring implementation facilitation knowledge and skills. *Psychiatr Serv.* 2014;65:141–143. doi: 10.1176/appi.ps.201300468

70. Kirchner JE, Woodward EN, Smith JL, et al. Implementation science supports core clinical competencies: an overview and clinical example. *Prim Care Companion CNS Disord.* 2016;18(6). doi: 10.4088/PCC.16m02004

71. Bauer MS, Miller C, Kim B, et al. Partnering with health system operations leadership to develop a controlled implementation trial. *Implement Sci.* 2016;11:22. doi: 10.1186/s13012-016-0385-7

72. Kavic MS. Competency and the six core competencies. *JSLS.* 2002;6:95–97.

73. Proctor EK, Chambers DA. Training in dissemination and implementation research: a field-wide perspective. *Transl Behav Med.* 2016;1–12. doi:10.1007/s13142-016-0406-8

74. Rubenstein LV, Chaney EF, Ober S, et al. Using evidence-based quality improvement methods for translating depression collaborative care research into practice. *Fam Syst Health.* 2010;28:91–113.

75. Harvey G, Kitson A, (Eds.). *Implementing evidence-based practice in healthcare: A facilitation guide.* London: Routledge; 2015.

76. Ritchie M. Tailoring implementation strategies to context—extreme facilitation: helping challenged healthcare settings implement complex programs (S11). In: Proceedings of the 8th Annual Conference on the Science of Dissemination and Implementation. 14–15 December 2015. *Implement Sci.* 2016;11(Suppl 2):100. doi: 10.1186/s13012-016-0452-0

16

Fidelity and Its Relationship to Implementation Effectiveness, Adaptation, and Dissemination

JENNIFER D. ALLEN, RACHEL C. SHELTON, KAREN M. EMMONS, AND LAURA A. LINNAN

INTRODUCTION

Effective dissemination and implementation (D & I) of evidence-based interventions (EBIs) assumes that program strategies will be conducted with "fidelity." Fidelity has been defined as the "extent to which the intervention was delivered as planned. It represents the quality and integrity of the intervention as conceived by the developers."[1] More recently there has also been increased attention on fidelity as it relates to implementation strategies used to guide implementation of EBIs. Although not always specified, fidelity may relate to the underlying theory of an intervention, or specific strategies to implement the EBI or both.[2] Careful measurement of fidelity allows researchers and program implementers to fully appreciate whether outcomes of an intervention are related to the quality or extent of implementation or whether some other factors—unrelated to the intervention—may account for observed outcomes. In the case of interventions that do not achieve expected outcomes, fidelity is critical to understanding whether the failure of an intervention is attributable to poor or inadequate implementation (termed "Type III error")[3] or to intervention program theory failure, or some combination thereof. There is growing evidence that the fidelity with which an intervention is implemented is highly associated with success in achieving change in targeted outcomes.[4-7] Therefore, documenting and monitoring the fidelity-adaptation process is crucial for the successful D & I of interventions. In an era with considerable concern about reproducibility of scientific findings,[8,9] documenting and monitoring the fidelity-adaptation process is critical to ensure public health impact of D & I studies.

Foundational work on the topic of fidelity emerged originally from the fields of community psychology and education[10-15] and was typically addressed as part of process evaluation.[1] More recently, fidelity has received increased attention in both clinical health services and behavioral interventions.[2,16-20]

The purpose of this chapter is to discuss the importance of fidelity for D & I research, to propose a framework for considering factors that influence fidelity (including issues regarding adaptation), and to describe strategies for producing high fidelity in interventions. The chapter also shares an example of a community-based intervention and various attempts to assess fidelity, highlighting several key factors, processes, and challenges. It concludes by summarizing implications of fidelity and adaptation issues on intervention dissemination for practitioners, researchers, and policymakers. Our goal is to add conceptual clarity regarding fidelity across the study design spectrum.

Defining Fidelity

A variety of terms have been used interchangeably with fidelity in the literature, including "implementation fidelity,"[4,21-24] "treatment fidelity"[25-28] and "treatment integrity."[29,30] The looseness with which the term "fidelity" is used can lead to lack of clarity in terms of both conceptual and design parameters. This lack of clarity also makes measuring and/or monitoring fidelity a challenge. This chapter focuses on fidelity as it relates to the effective implementation of core intervention elements in the context of D & I research. "Core" intervention elements are those components of an intervention that were tested through rigorous research designs and linked with desired outcomes. These are considered fundamental to programmatic impact—directly responsible for intervention effects. They are the "essential ingredients" that represent the internal logic and underlying theory of the intervention.[13] As such, fidelity requires that core elements be implemented in the manner intended by program developers. In contrast to core elements, "adaptive" elements do not change the internal logic or core aspects of the intervention, such that their modification is not believed to alter the impact of the intervention.[13] In fact, such planned adaptations typically reflect cultural or contextual "translations" that are critical to successful D & I efforts in non-research settings. Adaptations that are *not planned* (e.g., spontaneously shortening or eliminating specific course activities while teaching due when running out of time) can affect fidelity to core components and potentially reduce the impact of an intervention.[31,32] Recently, there has been increased attention to the tradeoffs between fidelity and adaptation,[32–35] which are discussed later in this chapter.

The conceptualization of fidelity here is built on prior work[1,4,12,13] which has described five elements: adherence, dose, quality of delivery, participant responsiveness, and program differentiation. *Adherence* involves consideration of the intervention *dose* or *exposure*—the amount, frequency, and/or duration of intervention delivered. *Quality of delivery* reflects how well an intervention is implemented, both in terms of content and process. Quality is often assessed by comparing actual delivery with a standard, benchmark, or theoretical ideal.[4] *Participant responsiveness* is the extent to which the target audience engages with and accepts or is satisfied with the intervention. This is a concept analogous to the dose of "intervention received."[1] *Program differentiation* reflects the underlying mechanisms by which the intervention exerts its influence. It comprises the unique features and/or core elements of the intervention and the extent to which they are elucidated and described.[4] Some investigators urge that all five elements of fidelity be measured,[12] while others suggest that each of these elements may provide alternative means for assessment of fidelity.[4,23] In reality, it is often necessary to prioritize which elements will be measured. Decisions about the most relevant measures require consideration of the nature of the intervention and its objectives, as well as the personnel and resources available. Consistent with the authors' original approach[36] (Figure 16.1) and contemporary understanding of fidelity,[2,17,19] we also recognize that fidelity must be assessed within the larger context in which an intervention is situated, including social, political and environmental influences.

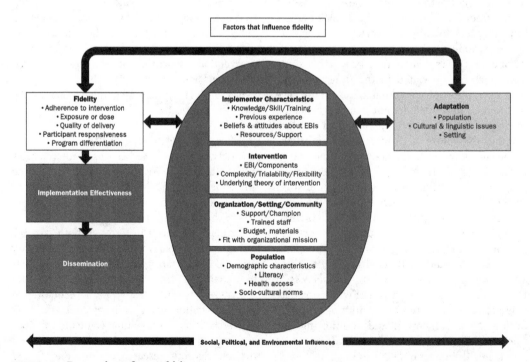

FIGURE 16.1 Factors that influence fidelity.

FIDELITY AS A RESEARCH DESIGN ELEMENT

Fidelity is an important consideration of research design planning for a number of reasons. Perhaps most obvious is fidelity's effects on validity.[16] *Internal validity* is adversely affected if an intervention is not administered as intended, as it becomes impossible to know if observed effects are due to the intervention or to external factors. In essence, if fidelity is not maintained, then internal validity is compromised and a true test of the intervention cannot be conducted. Described in detail in chapter 18, *external validity* is also impacted by fidelity, in that standardized implementation procedures are needed to ensure that an intervention can be replicated in other settings. If the intervention is effective but the procedures for implementing and/or adapting the intervention occur without attention to fidelity, there may be limits on its generalizability to other settings, populations, and/or health issues. A recent review of 72 implementation studies found that none reported a clear definition for fidelity and none used a conceptual framework related to fidelity to guide their assessments.[37]

Efforts to enhance one type of validity may result in a diminution of the other.[38,39] As more emphasis is placed on tightly controlling core intervention elements that may enhance internal validity, the intervention is likely to be more difficult to translate or adapt to diverse settings and populations. There is increasing recognition of this struggle between internal and external validity in study design.[38,39]

The intervention elements in efficacy studies are typically designed to maximize effects on primary outcomes, and thus may require considerable effort from individual participants, organizations, and study personnel. When dissemination is the goal, maintaining fidelity to such intensive, complex interventions can be extremely challenging. In a community-based setting such as a low-income/subsidized housing community, implementing a very complex intervention with high fidelity for one health issue may result in decreased attention to other health issues that are equally or more important for the health of the population.

Further, demanding fidelity to a protocol that may ultimately be offensive or impractical for a new group of participants or population subgroup may result in frustration, resentment, and ultimately, can ultimately lead to implementation and/or dissemination failure. Thus, it is critical to identify and monitor these core elements from the earliest phases of research and intervention design.[40] And consistent with principles of community-based participatory research, it may be helpful to engage with those who are likely to be the intended beneficiaries of the intervention to maximize effectiveness at the implementation, adaptation, and dissemination stages.[41,42]

Fidelity is also important by virtue of its impact on *effect size* and *statistical power*. The power to detect a difference between intervention and control/comparison groups in most study designs is a function of minimizing random variability and increasing intended variability between study groups.[16] If an intervention is not delivered as intended, particularly if there is more variability, less intervention dose delivered, or intended recipients do not engage with the intervention (low *participant responsiveness*), all of these factors are likely to reduce the potential effect size and diminish statistical power to detect differences between the groups.

A key consideration for implementation is to identify the minimal "dose" of the intervention that is required to produce desired change.[43] Monitoring fidelity allows one to estimate the impact of one or more "doses" of the intervention.[20] For example, it may be useful to determine whether outcomes were achieved when three of five core elements were delivered versus when all five core elements were delivered. Comparative effectiveness research designs may allow investigators to design studies that will help to evaluate these types of empirical questions.[44]

When fidelity is actively and accurately monitored, it is also possible to detect problems with intervention quality or deviations from the intervention protocol, to make mid-course corrections, and to provide encouragement, reward, or recognition for efforts produced. This type of feedback, when incorporated in the study design as a routine part of intervention delivery, is often underappreciated, but has been found to be a key part of maximizing participant engagement and contributing to effective implementation and dissemination efforts. For example, mid-course feedback on the quality and adherence to a worksite-based intervention protocol was provided to managers that increased both participation and ownership of the intervention in the Working Well Trial, which also resulted in increased fidelity.[45]

Beyond establishing a feedback loop between intervention practitioners and researchers during initial efficacy testing, improved communication between these parties within the context of D & I efforts could have a substantial impact on successful translation of research to practice. As discussed later, implementers should be involved in *"designing for fidelity,"* as they have experience and expertise about the types of interventions that may be acceptable, feasible, and effective for the communities with whom they work.

Finally, *assessment of fidelity* plays a key role in interpretation of study results. If significant intervention results are not found, knowing whether the intervention was delivered as intended makes it possible to eliminate variation in intervention delivery as a contributor to the findings. Particularly in the context of dissemination efforts, null outcomes from an EBI that was delivered with high fidelity to the underlying theory and to core implementation strategies would suggest that the intervention itself may not be addressing the key behavioral mediators or the most salient contextual factors facing the treatment settings and/or intervention participants. Such findings may suggest the need for a fundamental re-evaluation of the intervention theory or implementation effort, and/or the components of the evidence-based intervention if it was developed under ideal versus real-world settings.

FACTORS THAT INFLUENCE FIDELITY

Understanding factors that influence the fidelity with which interventions are implemented is vital to efforts to measure and maximize its occurrence. A growing body of literature documents factors that influence implementation processes.[46] The authors propose a schematic, as shown in Figure 16.1, which categorizes potential sources of influence on fidelity over the course of the planning, implementation, evaluation, and dissemination of interventions. The goal is to invite researchers and practitioners to consider these factors as designs and methods/measures are selected, and to help them anticipate potential unintended consequences (positive and negative) of the intervention by considering these broad range of influences upfront, before use of resources, time, or expertise are expended in ways that are not efficient or practical.

Four categories of influence and their interrelationships are depicted. First, *implementer characteristics* can impact ability to implement EBIs with fidelity. For example, a novice practitioner or researcher may have limited awareness about existing EBIs, and may be less able to anticipate and problem-solve implementation challenges. Thus, fidelity may be compromised when an implementer has inadequate skill, experience, training, or confidence, resulting in diminished amount, type, or quality of intervention delivered. Alternatively, highly experienced implementers may be more confident in their abilities to modify intervention elements, and therefore less likely to implement them in a manner consistent with original ideals. Implementation research of health education efforts in schools reveals great variability in implementation of "required" intervention curriculum based on school, teacher, and student characteristics that would not be apparent unless carefully documented.[47]

Second, *characteristics of the intervention* will influence fidelity. As discussed in chapter 17, factors such as intervention complexity, trial-ability, flexibility, and the extent to which one intervention provides a relative advantage over the current program/status quo, are all important influences on fidelity. These and other features were first described by Rogers in his seminal work on Diffusion of Innovations.[48] For example, highly complex interventions that have a large number of core elements are more difficult to implement than those with fewer, less complex elements. Furthermore, interventions that allow greater flexibility and are amenable to adaptation may be easier for practitioners to implement without omitting or changing core elements. Interventions that are adequately described for the purposes of replication are also more likely to be implemented (*program differentiation*). Similarly, those that are easily accessible to implementers, such as interventions posted on RTIPS (Research Tested Intervention Programs, a web site with evidence-based cancer prevention and control interventions),[49] may be more likely to be implemented with fidelity because of the clarity of the underlying theory of change, detailed description of core intervention elements, and/or access to materials provided. Further, the fit of the intervention components with workflow in the implementation setting is critical.[50]

Third, characteristics of the *organization or setting* in which the intervention is to be implemented or disseminated can have a substantial impact on fidelity. Organizational resources, including availability of trained staff, financial capital, as well as existence of a program "champion," exert a strong impact on the manner in which programs can be implemented.

For example, a study by Fagan and colleagues[51] examined adoption and implementation fidelity of science-based prevention programming in 24 communities; across conditions, the results indicated lower rates of implementation fidelity in the school-based compared with community-based programs. This is consistent with Dariotis and colleagues,[52] who found that schools had more challenges developing program champions and prioritizing prevention than community agencies. Organizational structure, communication channels, and decision-making processes such as the ability to make strategic decisions "on the front lines" can also affect implementation.[46] Weiner has noted that the "readiness" of a particular organization to adopt a new initiative can influence fidelity, implementation, and dissemination.[53]

Fourth, the *population* for whom the intervention is intended will impact fidelity. Differences across populations influence the relevance, impact and appropriateness of core or adaptive intervention elements. For example, demographics (age, gender, SES, education levels), sociocultural norms, and literacy levels can all influence *participant responsiveness* to the intervention and are all key population factors that are linked to the appropriateness and feasibility of implementing core elements. Such factors will require serious attention when adaptation and dissemination are considered. Several investigators[17,54] have eloquently discussed the tensions between fidelity and the necessary adaptations required so that cultural and ethical/moral issues that influence health equity and justice are considered. Adaptations for setting-specific issues and cultural considerations are considered in detail in chapter 17.

Maximizing the Fidelity–Adaptation Balance

Given that it can have a significant moderating effect on intervention impact, concerted efforts to maximize fidelity should be undertaken. We advocate efforts to maximize fidelity by attending to the four categories of influence described in Figure 16.1 (*implementer characteristics, characteristics of the intervention, organizational setting, and population*), which can all exert both independent and combined effects on fidelity and intervention adaptation. While methods to measure and maximize fidelity to core intervention elements have been discussed at length,[55] they are often inconsistently applied. This section begins

by discussing strategies to maximize fidelity. Then it identifies strategies for measuring and monitoring fidelity, so that it can be taken into consideration in analysis and interpretation of intervention effects, prior to widespread dissemination efforts.

As noted, efforts toward maintaining fidelity should begin with the initial process of intervention development. Despite tension created by the need to deliver the maximum dose of a highly intensive intervention so as to achieve significant change in primary outcomes, it is also necessary to consider whether such an approach could be scalable for widespread dissemination. *Designing for fidelity* refers both to the consideration of the extent to which tested intervention approaches could be applied in real-world settings, as well as providing adequate documentation of the theoretical basis, mediating and moderating factors, and description of activities so that they can be replicated. Not surprisingly, interventions described with a high degree of specificity are more easily and effectively implemented with fidelity than complex interventions that are insufficiently described.[4,13]

Implementing with fidelity entails putting mechanisms in place to assure that implementers have the knowledge, skills and resources required to deliver the intervention as planned (*quality of intervention delivery*). This can be accomplished in a number of ways, including providing standardized training for implementers, ensuring that implementers have the requisite knowledge and skills following training (e.g., pencil and paper test, return demonstration), and development of detailed implementation protocols or program manuals that clearly specify core intervention components and strategies.[4,16] Moreover, providing implementers with intervention scripts (e.g., for one-to-one or group interactions), standardized materials that help to ensure consistency of message delivery (e.g., flip charts, tip sheets, Q and A's), or checklists can also be useful. It is also important to anticipate the potential for "intervention drift," a phenomenon where either implementer skills or adherence to protocol diminishes over time.[16] Intervention drift can be counteracted by planning periodic booster training sessions, instituting quality control protocols that provide regular feedback to implementers, and providing problem-solving support targeted at potential reasons for drift.

Fidelity measures may be categorized as direct or indirect[18] (see Table 16.1). *Direct methods* are generally implemented by trained observers or

TABLE 16.1 DIRECT AND INDIRECT METHODS FOR ASSESSING AND MONITORING FIDELITY

	Advantages	Disadvantages
Direct		
Trained observers or independent auditors using checklists, rating scales	• Generally considered most accurate	• Observer variability possible; intensive training may be required. • More costly and labor intensive than indirect methods • In vivo observation may alter implementer behaviors • Observer may "miss" seeing subtle events. • Difficult to capture rare events • Not feasible for large-scale dissemination • May not be appropriate for some forms of intervention (e.g. counseling)
Audio or videotape	• May be as accurate as in vivo observation • Possible to establish interrater reliability; raters view same video or listen to same audio • Possible to review intervention delivery more than once • Can be used as tool for providing implementers with feedback about their performance • Less likely to impact implementer behaviors than direct observation	• Less costly than having an auditor present at intervention delivery • Potential to miss important non-verbal or contextual cues • Observer variability possible; intensive training may be required. • Video recording equipment is costly; audio equipment is less costly. • May be logistically difficult to bring equipment to setting of intervention delivery • Equipment malfunction may occur.
Indirect		
Data from implementers (e.g., intervention logs, diaries)	• Relatively inexpensive • Less time consuming • Can include implementer insights about factors that influenced fidelity, participant responsiveness	• Prone to bias, overreporting • Completion rates may be low. • Recall may be inaccurate, particularly if documentation doesn't occur immediately after intervention delivery.
Data collected from intervention participants (e.g., exit interviews, paper-and-pencil surveys, e-based communication (e.g., Twitter, Facebook)	• Enables assessment of participant responsiveness, perceived quality of delivery • Less costly and time consuming than direct methods	• Participants may want to reflect well on implementer; social desirability • Participants may not be able to recognize or distinguish between intervention components • Potential for low completion rates, depending on participant motivation

auditors. This method has traditionally been the gold standard for measuring fidelity, because independent observers are less prone to biased reporting.[13,18] Examples of direct assessment include in-person observation (e.g., completed with a checklist outlining key components), "shadowing" implementers (e.g., as in the case of one-to-one interventions), and audio- or video-taping intervention events for coding completion of key components at a later time. Advantages of direct observation include that they can yield highly accurate and valid data. Main disadvantages include cost and feasibility. Direct observation may be less feasible in large-scale dissemination initiatives. However, with carefully constructed sampling procedures, it may be feasible to do this on a limited basis[18] which may yield important insights. can be very fruitful.

Indirect measures often include self-reports by implementers, who may complete intervention logs, diaries, or checklists designed to document delivery of core elements, or may involve self-report by program participants. For example, participants may be asked about receipt of core intervention components and/or their level of satisfaction with the intervention (which may reflect *quality of delivery, participant responsiveness*). In-person data collection (e.g., interviews, focus groups) may be utilized, or participants may be asked to complete self-administered data collection forms (e.g., pencil-and-paper rating forms).[18] New technologies and social networking programs offer interesting options for quick feedback from participants via web-based, Facebook, texting, or Twitter.[56]

The main advantages of indirect methods are that they are generally less costly, time-consuming, and labor-intensive. Moreover, the collection of data from implementers or participants can provide helpful insights about the intervention (i.e., factors that influence fidelity, participant responsiveness) that would not otherwise be available. Disadvantages relate to the accuracy of data (i.e., potential for over-reporting, social desirability bias) and the possibility of missing data (e.g., either reports not completed or failure to document information about contextual or situational factors that may impact fidelity).

Considerations when selecting a data collection method should include cost, feasibility, efficiency, validity/reliability of data, reactivity, and ability to collect sufficient "samples" (i.e., intervention delivery) to accurately assess fidelity over time.[18] Additional considerations may include type of intervention delivery (e.g., in-person, telephone), characteristics and skill levels of implementers, as well as population characteristics (e.g., willingness to be observed).

Accurate measurement requires predefined, highly specific core intervention elements against which fidelity can be judged. Unfortunately, the level of specificity with which core intervention elements are described in the literature is rarely sufficient for this purpose.[57] Measurement instruments for assessing intervention-specific aspects of fidelity have been suggested;[22,24,58-60] however, a recent review of instruments designed to measure fidelity for behavioral interventions addressing addiction found that the majority did not establish psychometric properties.[61] Breitenstein and colleagues[18] further point out that intervention-specific instruments do not allow for standardization or cross-comparison of findings across studies and may hinder the ability to compare similar interventions sharing theoretical underpinnings and core components. They suggest that more general assessments of fidelity that can be utilized across interventions and settings may be more valuable in terms of advancing implementation and dissemination science.[18] Setting-specific fidelity measures and sample data collection instruments for interventions that take place in schools, worksites, and a variety of community-based settings have been summarized from several intervention studies by Linnan and Steckler.[1]

Monitoring fidelity during initial implementation, after adaptation, and prior to dissemination is essential. Monitoring should involve ongoing review of fidelity data from direct or indirect measurement and with a feedback loop ensuring that feedback is provided to those responsible for intervention delivery. If not undertaken, deviations or drift from protocol may go unnoticed until it is too late to make revisions or corrections. *Analyzing fidelity,* whereby data collected in the process of intervention implementation provides essential information about the extent to which the intervention was implemented as planned, can be valuable in the analysis of program effects. Berkel and colleagues clarify dimensions of implementation (facilitator and participant dimensions) and offer a thoughtful conceptual and measurement model for understanding interactions between fidelity and implementation, outcomes, and adaptation.[62] Lobb and colleagues measured the proportion of participants who received each set of core intervention components as planned, and then created a multi-item index of protocol completion to compute a "fidelity score."[63] Such an index can be included in analyses as an independent variable, to help explain unexpected findings or variability of intervention effects.[18] Clearly, more work is needed to identify methods and measures for assessing fidelity, and reporting on it in ways that will enhance implementation effectiveness and dissemination.[37]

BALANCING THE IMPORTANCE OF FIDELITY WITH NEED FOR ADAPTATION

Two prevailing views about the extent to which EBIs can be adapted for D&I studies have been described. One view is that complete fidelity, with strict adherence to intervention protocol, is required under all circumstances.[25,64] Indeed, in this view, successful replication is defined by not allowing modification of standardized content. As noted earlier, this approach maximizes the potential for internal validity, yet may reduce external validity. It may also reduce the opportunity to learn from the variability that is inherent in implementation across settings.[65] The other view taken is that "adaptation happens"; proponents of this view strongly discourage making major changes in "core components" and encourage documenting adaptations so that their impact can be better understood. Definitions and processes for adaptation are described in chapter 17. An overview of the issue of adaptation as it specifically relates to fidelity is provided here.

Balancing the need for *fidelity* while maintaining sufficient flexibility to accommodate differences across implementation settings, populations, and situational contexts, is a major challenge and a topic of recent increased discussion and study.[19,32,35,66,67] While high fidelity has been associated with positive program outcomes, it is common for changes to be made when evidence-based programs are implemented in real-world settings.[31,52,57] In fact, reviews of EBI implementation across a range of settings demonstrate that 40% to 80% of programs reported making adaptations to the original program.[32,57,68,69] There is growing recognition that adaptations are inevitable, particularly for interventions that are complex.[70,71]

Reasons for adaptations in uncontrolled settings are many and include limited time and resources, competing demands, difficulty engaging or retaining participants, desire to reach specific audiences, and efforts to enhance program fit.[31,32,72] Adaptation of EBIs may also occur in response to the complexity of characteristics of outer contexts (e.g., service systems) or inner contexts (e.g., organizations). With respect to the long-term sustainability of EBIs, it has also been proposed that some changes to interventions may be required in order to respond to real-world contexts that are dynamic and not static.[73,74-76] Contexts themselves may also need to adapt to facilitate program implementation (e.g., new partnerships, changes in organizational structure or culture).[77,78]

Some researchers have also argued that adaptation is necessary to respect the varied needs and priorities of communities, to enhance ownership and relevance for those implementing interventions, and encourage local buy-in.[66,79,80] In particular, there are many cases when cultural and linguistic adaptations are necessary. There is some evidence that suggests there may be positive effects of flexibility and adaptation on program outcomes and participant responsiveness, though there is inconsistency in how adaptation has been conceptualized and measured to date.[81-83] Chambers and colleagues propose that ongoing adaptation and continual learning and refinement of interventions is needed in multilevel interventions to enhance fit, and question the idea that interventions must be fully optimized prior to implementation.[73] Several researchers have also advanced the idea of adaptation as a phase bridging initial implementation with long-term sustainability, to help enhance the fit of the intervention with the context.[84,85] Taken together, these developments suggest that there is growing consideration that fidelity and adaptation may coexist, and that it is possible for a program's core components to be implemented with high fidelity while still making adaptations in response to or to enhance fit with local community needs or context. Still, proponents of the view that "adaptations happen" recognize that adaptations must not compromise the essence of the intervention, and major changes in core components are discouraged.

To date, the fidelity versus adaptation debate has been largely theoretical, and empirical findings have been somewhat mixed with respect to the impact of adaptation.[81,83,86-90] More empirical evidence is needed going forward to guide researchers and practitioners, to improve understanding of the impact of different types of adaptation on program outcomes, to determine the level of fidelity necessary to produce positive outcomes, and to assess under what conditions adaptations might enhance or impede program effectiveness and sustainability.

It will be important that adaptation is measured and examined distinctly from fidelity. To this end, several coding schemas have been proposed to study the full range of adaptations that can be made to interventions across settings.[32,91] Further, Chambers and Norton[92] have proposed multiple sources of intervention adaptation (e.g. service setting adaptation, target audience adaptation, mode of delivery adaptation, cultural adaptation) and propose the building of an "adaptome" data platform to systematically capture information about variations in the delivery of EBIs across populations and contexts.[92]

Fidelity should be monitored so that when adaptation occurs, every step is taken to document these changes and the effects they have on intervention impact over time. If adaptation occurs and no effort to assess fidelity of the adapted intervention is made, then it is entirely possible that initial intervention effectiveness may be compromised. In addition, the positive impact of adaptations may not be documented and therefore be non-replicable. While it would be ideal to measure all five elements of fidelity, consideration of available resources, the nature of intervention and issues of feasibility require consideration, as noted. At a minimum, adaptations should be observed, documented, and understood in order to enhance translation of EBIs into practice. When planning for adaptation, researchers and practitioners may find it useful to use one of the 12 adaptation frameworks that have recently been identified (e.g., ADAPT-ITT),[93] that typically include the following steps: assess community; understand the EBI; select EBI; consult experts; consult with stakeholders; decide what needs to be adapted; adapt the original program; train staff; test adapted materials; implement; and evaluate.[94] As noted earlier, the use of conceptual frameworks that address issue of fidelity and adaptation has been limited in the implementation literature, and deserves further attention.[37]

CASE EXAMPLE

Adaptation of Cosmetologist (Stylist) Training Workshops for Barbers Enrolled in the Trimming Risk in Men (TRIM) Research Study

Here, a case study is introduced from Linnan and colleagues' work that illustrates some of the challenges associated with measuring fidelity as part of implementation effectiveness, adaptation, and dissemination.

Background

Cancer-related disparities exist and African Americans suffer a disproportionately high incident and mortality burden for nearly all types of cancer nationally and in North Carolina. Interventions in beauty salons and barbershops take advantage of a setting where customers spend significant time at each visit, return often, focus on personal health and appearance, and develop a unique and trusted bond with the barber/stylist. The barbershop and beauty salons are a unique and historically cherished place that African Americans consider "safe havens," as well as places of trust and social exchange.[95,96]

Context

This example focuses on a training workshop for licensed cosmetologists that had been found to increase knowledge, self-efficacy, and intention to deliver key health messages to customers (e.g., eat at least five fruits/vegetables and get regular physical activity). The BEAUTY (Bringing Education and Understanding to You) intervention prompted changes in self-reported customer behavior immediately post-intervention and at a 12-month follow-up assessment.[97] Moving from this initial efficacy trial, we describe factors that influenced fidelity when we took the training workshop from BEAUTY and adapted it for use in Trimming Risk in Men (TRIM) with a new population (barbers), in a new setting (barbershops) and a new health topic (prostate/colorectal cancer screening).

Given the need for extensive adaptation, Linnan and colleagues employed a systematic approach starting with the messages/materials and training curriculum we had tested successfully with licensed stylists. We worked closely with members of the BEAUTY and Barbershop Advisory Board to develop the overall adaptation approach, following principles of social marketing to adapt the final stylist training workshop for barbers.[97a] Specifically, we conducted focus groups with African American men to assess their perceptions about health, cancer, and potential interest in getting health information in the barbershop. Next we interviewed barbershop owners and barbers to ascertain their interest in sharing health information generally, and specifically, information about how to make informed decisions about prostate and colorectal cancer screening. Finally, we conducted observations using established protocols[98] to better understand who initiates conversations between barbers/customers, and common topics of conversation in the shop. Building on these data and the findings of BEAUTY, we looked for intervention leverage points for the best way to introduce the messages during a typical barbershop visit. Once we gathered information from these sources, we developed a series of messages to start a conversation that could be delivered by barbers during a typical customer appointment in the barbershop. Two separate campaign messages and materials, as well as two separate barber training workshops were developed, implemented, and evaluated as part of the TRIM Study—one for colorectal cancer and one for prostate cancer.

To assess the effects of the adapted barber training workshop, we conducted a pilot workshop with barbers for each cancer target and measured changes in knowledge, self-efficacy and intention to deliver key messages to customers using pre/post-test training workshop evaluation forms.

Findings and Lessons Learned

During the process of collecting information to adapt the stylist training workshops for barbershops, core elements of the intervention were identified: (1) describing the role of the stylist/barber as a "natural helper" and wise adviser capable of promoting health among their customers; (2) dispelling myths and misconceptions; (3) learning the facts about cancer and cancer prevention; (4) reviewing key health messages/materials provided by the research team; (5) demonstrating how to introduce messages/materials by the research team; (6) role play activity with hypothetical customers, including feedback; and, (7) pre-post-test knowledge quiz.

Compared with pretest, posttest results indicated that participating barbers improved in all areas, including: increased knowledge; comfort in providing information; and self-confidence to give customers key messages and confidence of making an informed decision about getting the CRC/prostate cancer screening tests. In addition, 91% of participating barbers reported that they were extremely or very interested in attending future trainings. Thus, the transition from stylist training to barber training met an initial set of fidelity expectations by demonstrating the key desired outcomes.

A number of important lessons were learned about adapting the stylist workshops for the barbers/barbershops that have the potential for impacting fidelity, implementation effectiveness, and dissemination. Regarding *population issues*, it was learned that barbers (men) are different from stylists (women) in a number of important ways that influence intervention efforts. First, barbers spend less time with a customer in the chair, they are less likely to talk about personal issues with their customers, and are simply less likely to talk with a customer at all, compared with stylists. As a result, delivering health messages may be less likely during the barber-customer interaction in the chair. Barbers were more willing to direct a customer to a poster or other materials that might be strategically placed in the barbershop than to deliver the health message directly. Thus, the training and materials were modified to accommodate this difference. Lessons learned during adaptation addressed *setting* issues by recognizing that barbershops are very open, social places and offer less privacy between customer and barber than is typically found in beauty salons.[98] As a result, different strategies were developed to get barbers to deliver desired messages to their customers, such as display turnstile, business cards, and wrist bands for barbers to wear to prompt brief conversations and key health messages. And, a lesson learned about adapting to new *health* issues was that providing colorectal and prostate cancer information was far more sensitive than encouraging healthy eating or physical activity. To address this issue, a physician was included in the barber training workshops to answer all types of questions the barbers might have about this sensitive topic. This proved to be an excellent new addition to the training that barbers appreciated and helped remove barriers to initiating these conversations with their customers.

SUMMARY

There is substantial variability in the implementation of evidence-based interventions across the United States, which leads to inconsistent access to evidence-based prevention and treatment strategies at a population level.[99] Increased D & I of EBIs could result in significant public health gains. While the availability of EBIs is increasing, study of implementation, adaptation, and dissemination has only recently gained attention in public health. To date, less focus has been directed to the issue of fidelity. Consideration of fidelity is necessary to balance the need for internal and

TABLE 16.2 RECOMMENDATIONS TO ADVANCE RESEARCH AND PRACTICE IN THE AREA OF FIDELITY

Practitioners	Researchers	Policymakers/Funders/Journal Editors and Reviewers
• Be proactive in learning about available EBIs; know where to search for information about EBIs (e.g., [41, 66–69]). • Choose EBIs that are appropriate to specific audience, setting, implementer skills/knowledge, health issues, and available resources. • Contact researchers to gain access to information about core elements and what might be required for effective implementation, adaptation, and/or dissemination. • If adaptations are made, avoid modifying core elements. Consider one of the adaptation models and/or do what is necessary to understand your audience and setting so that adaptation is appropriate and done with fidelity prior to dissemination. • Partner with researchers and/or evaluators to provide input into how EBIs can be implemented in practice, and how barriers to implementation may be overcome.	• Design interventions with dissemination in mind—increased attention to external validity to enhance the ability of practitioners to implement interventions in "real world" settings. • Depict interventions with explicit logic models to enhance understanding of the intended process and outcomes. Be sure to clarify core versus adaptive elements. Be explicit about theory that guides the intervention and show key constructs/elements on the logic model. • Carefully measure and analyze fidelity. Consider undertaking component analysis or other post hoc analyses to examine impact of specific intervention elements. • Consider a conceptual framework for examination of factors that influence fidelity (see Figure 16.1) and integrate specific initiatives to maximize fidelity • Collect and summarize information and "lessons learned" from "first generation" implementers; provide to "second generation" implementers, and integrate their feedback on what is feasible and acceptable for implementation in the settings and for the populations with whom they work. • Package EBIs for implementation & dissemination. Provide access to intervention protocols to implementers; include sufficient detail so that activities can be replicated with fidelity. Develop and make available intervention protocols that maximize and measure fidelity. • Build a more robust literature on fidelity. Specifically address in key publications: Which factors in our conceptual model are most important in terms of ensuring and maintaining fidelity? What are the best methods for maximizing fidelity?	• Funders: Require assessment of and provide adequate funding for evaluation of fidelity in all phases of the research continuum. • Policymakers: Advocate for implementation of EBIs with emphasis on initial fidelity as well as allow for measuring/monitoring fidelity when EBIs are adapted for new health outcomes, settings, or populations. • Journal editors: Assess and report fidelity in guidelines for reporting of interventions (e.g., CONSORT).

external validity across the research continuum. There is also a need for a more robust literature to increase knowledge about sources of variability in fidelity, strategies for maximizing fidelity, and methods for measuring and analyzing fidelity.[100]

Like others[16,25], we echo recommendations for designing interventions with dissemination in mind, having a comprehensive plan for maximizing fidelity throughout intervention delivery, as well as a system for documenting what, how, and why adaptations are made. As discussed, there are a growing number of models designed to facilitate adaptation of EBIs while maintaining fidelity. It will be important to study the utility and feasibility of these models across different settings, populations and health issues, as well as the impact these adaptations have on program outcomes, including effectiveness and sustainability.

Ultimately, efforts to advance the science of D & I research with a particular focus on fidelity will require the involvement of researchers, practitioners, funders, and policymakers (Table 16.2). Researchers must lead the charge by: designing interventions that can be implemented with fidelity in practice settings, developing standardized methods and measures for assessing fidelity, evaluating strategies for maximizing fidelity, analyzing the impact of fidelity on program outcomes, making explicit the core elements in interventions, ensuring availability of appropriately "packaged" intervention materials, examining the efficacy of strategies for maximizing fidelity, and analyzing emerging models for EBI adaptation. In addition, further study of the impact of adaptive changes in implementation of EBIs is greatly needed.

Practitioners must be responsible for identifying available EBIs that are suitable for their populations and settings, and working with intended beneficiaries to make sure that the "fit" is acceptable/appropriate. They can make significant contributions to D & I research by communicating the challenges they encounter when delivering EBIs, the reasons for adaptation when this occurs, and for utilizing newly emerging models for adaptation that retain a focus on fidelity to core intervention elements. Such communication will help to build "practice-based evidence" that can advance both science and practice.

Policymakers can play a role in helping to create the infrastructure required for increased communication and exchange between researchers, practitioners, and intervention developers. Web-based technologies—listservs and databases

supported by NIH and/or CDC—could be a logical infrastructure home for this dialogue.

Funders can require attention to fidelity in research applications across the research continuum, and provide targeted funds for examination of the research questions that are needed to build a more robust literature in this field. Journal editors could require increased reporting of issues related to fidelity in publications (along the lines of CONSORT guidelines),[101] and reviewers could be asked to pay increased attention to fidelity in the manuscript review process.

ACKNOWLEDGEMENTS

This work was supported in part by cooperative agreements among the Centers for Disease Control and Prevention (CDC) and the National Cancer Institute (NCI) (Allen, U48-DP000064; Linnan U48DP000311); by the NCI (Linnan, R21-CA126373; Emmons, KO5-CA124415, RO1-CA126596, RO1-CA123228); by the American Cancer Society (Linnan, TURSG-02-190-01-PBP; Shelton, 124793-MRSG-13-152-01-CPPB).

SUGGESTED READINGS AND WEBSITES

Readings

Bellg, AJ, Borrelli B, Resnick B, Hecht J, Minicucci DS, Ory M, . . . Treatment Fidelity Workgroup of the, N. I. H. B. C. C. Enhancing treatment fidelity in health behavior change studies: best practices and recommendations from the NIH Behavior Change Consortium. *Health Psychol.* 2004;23(5):443–451. doi: 10.1037/0278-6133.23.5.443
This article describes a multisite initiative by the Treatment Fidelity Workgroup of the National Institutes of Health Behavior Change Consortium to conceptualize and address fidelity and its measurement. They offer recommendations for improving treatment fidelity, including strategies for monitoring and improving provider training, delivery and receipt of treatment, and enactment of treatment skills. Authors emphasize the need for funding agencies, reviewers, and journal editors to make treatment fidelity a standard component in reporting of health intervention research.

Berkel C, Mauricio AM, Schoenfelder E, Sandler IN. Putting the pieces together: an integrated model of program implementation. *Prev Sci.* 2011;12(1):23–33. doi: 10.1007/s11121-010-0186-1
This article presents a theoretical model of the relations between the dimensions of implementation and outcomes of prevention programs to help guide implementation research. The authors conceptualize the four dimensions of implementation to include behaviors of

program facilitators (fidelity, quality of delivery, and adaptation) and behaviors of participants (responsiveness), and present the evidence for these as predictors of program outcomes. The authors then propose a theoretical model through which the facilitator and participant implementation dimensions influence participant outcomes.

Bopp M, Saunders RP Lattimore D. The tug-of-war: fidelity versus adaptation throughout the health promotion program life cycle. *J Prim Prev.* 2013;34(3):193–207. doi: 10.1007/s10935-013-0299

This article describes the life cycle (phases) for research-based health promotion programs, the key factors that influence each phase, and issues related to the tension between fidelity and adaptation throughout the process. The authors discuss the importance of reconceptualizing intervention designs, engaging stakeholders, and monitoring fidelity and adaptation across all phases to facilitate implementation fidelity. Consideration is also given to the role of contextual factors in influencing implementation at each phase and the importance of developing a rigorous and flexible definition of implementation fidelity and completeness.

Breitenstein SM, Gross D, Garvey CA, Hill C, Fogg L, Resnick B. Implementation fidelity in community-based interventions. *Res Nurs Health.* 2010;33(2):164–173. doi: 10.1002/nur.20373

This article defines implementation fidelity, offers rationale for its importance in implementation science, describes data collection strategies and tools, and provides recommendations for advancing the study of implementation fidelity. Authors provide a comprehensive description of methods for measuring fidelity, including the advantages and limitations of each.

Carroll C, Patterson M, Wood S, Booth A, Rick J, Balain S. (2007). A conceptual framework for implementation fidelity. *Implement Sci.* 2007;2:40. doi: Artn 4010.1186/1748 5908-2-40

This article critically reviews literature on implementation fidelity (2002–2007) and presents a new framework for conceptualizing and evaluating fidelity. The authors define five elements of fidelity (adherence to intervention; exposure or dose; quality of delivery; participant responsiveness; and program differentiation) and suggest that two additional elements be included in the conceptualization of fidelity: intervention complexity and facilitation strategies.

Chambers D.A, Norton WE. The adaptome advancing the science of intervention adaptation. *Am J Prev Med.* 2016;51(4):S124–S131. doi: 10.1016/j.amepre.2016.05.011

This article discusses how the field has been limited by the notion that evidence generation must be complete prior to implementation, which sets up a dichotomy

between fidelity and adaptation and limits the science of adaptation to findings from RCTs of adapted interventions. The authors emphasize the need for advancement of strategies to study the science of adaptation in the context of implementation that would encourage opportunities for ongoing learning over time, and propose building an adaptome to serve as a common data platform to capture information about variations in EBI delivery across multiple populations and contexts.

Durlak JA, DuPre EP. (2008). Implementation matters: a review of research on the influence of implementation on program outcomes and the factors affecting implementation. *Am J Commun Psychol.* 2008;41(3-4):327–350. doi: 10.1007/s10464-008-9165-0

This review examines studies that assess the impact of implementation fidelity on program outcomes, and in addition, identifies factors that affect the implementation process. Authors describe the Interactive Systems Framework and argue that elements of this framework, including organizational capacity, training, and technical assistance are central to effective implementation.

Haynes A, Brennan S, Redman S, Williamson A, Gallego G, Butow P; CIPHER team (2016). Figuring out fidelity: a worked example of the methods used to identify, critique and revise the essential elements of a contextualised intervention in health policy agencies. *Implement Sci.* 2016;11:23. doi: 10.1186/s13012-016-0378-6

This article highlights challenges in conducting fidelity assessment of novel contextualized interventions, using a worked example to demonstrate how essential elements can be refined without compromising fidelity assessment. The authors discuss how they devised a method for critiquing the construct validity of their intervention's essential elements and modifying how they were articulated and measured, while using them as fidelity indicators. They also highlight how this theoretically and contextually informed process could be used or adapted for other contextualized interventions.

Klimes-Dougan B, August GJ, Lee C-YS., Realmuto GM., Bloomquist ML, Horowitz JL, Eisenberg TL. Practitioner and site characteristics that relate to fidelity of implementation: the Early Risers prevention program in a going-to-scale intervention trial. *Prof Psychol-Res Pr.* 2009;40(5):467.

This article discusses the translation of research to real-world practice settings, including how individual practitioner or organization characteristics can aid or impede effective implementation. The authors stress that a lack of fidelity to the original intervention can change the ultimate outcomes of prevention programs.

Linnan L, Steckler A. *Process evaluation for public health interventions and research.* San Francisco: Jossey-Bass; 2002.

This book provides a rationale and detailed description of how to plan and implement a comprehensive process evaluation effort for public health interventions that take place in a wide range of settings. A detailed overview chapter defines key terms of a process evaluation, and a process for undertaking the development of process evaluation. Chapters follow that provide detailed examples of process evaluation for worksite, school, and other community settings where sample data collection tools, key results, and lessons learned are offered. Additional chapters on process tracking data management systems and process evaluation for media campaigns are included which should benefit practitioners and researchers alike.

Perez D, Van der Stuyft P, Zabala MC, Castro M, Lefevre P. A modified theoretical framework to assess implementation fidelity of adaptive public health interventions. *Implement Sci.* 2016;11(1):91. doi: 10.1186/s13012-016-0457-8

This article suggests that classical fidelity dimensions and frameworks do not address the issue of how to adapt an intervention while maintaining its effectiveness. The authors suggest that fidelity and adaptation can coexist and that adaptations can have positive or negative impacts on program outcomes. The authors discuss adaptive interventions, and how an adequate fidelity-adaptation balance can be reached, and modify the Carroll et al.4 framework to facilitate a more comprehensive assessment of the implementation fidelity-adaptation balance.

Slaughter SE, Hill JN, Snelgrove-Clarke E. What is the extent and quality of documentation and reporting of fidelity to implementation strategies: a scoping review. *Implement Sci.* 2015;10:129. doi: 10.1186/s13012-015-0320-3

In this article, the authors conduct a scoping review and discuss the extent and quality of documentation and reporting of fidelity of implementation strategies that are used to implement evidence-informed interventions. The authors also identify the underreporting of fidelity of implementation strategies, and develop and test a simple checklist to assess the reporting of fidelity of implementation strategies.

Selected Websites and Tools

Using What Works: Adapting Evidence-Based Programs to Fit Your Needs. http://cancercontrol. cancer.gov/use_what_works/start.htm

This website provides a train-the-trainer course designed for health promoters and educators on the national, regional, State, and local levels. The goal is to instruct users on how to plan a health program using evidence-based programs (aka "research-tested programs") for cancer prevention and control.

U.S. Department of Health & Human Services: Agency for Healthcare Research and Quality Evidence-Based Practice. http://www.ahrq.gov/.

AHRQ aims to improve the delivery of clinical preventive health care by developing tools, resources, and materials to support health care organizations and engage the entire health care delivery system. The Research in Action syntheses section of the website provides an interpretation of findings from AHRQ-sponsored studies and demonstrates how results can be used in practice.

Research Tested Intervention Programs (RTIPS). http://rtips.cancer.gov/rtips/index.do

RTIPs is a searchable database of cancer control interventions and program materials and is designed to provide program planners and public health practitioners easy and immediate access to research-tested materials.

Substance Abuse and Mental Health Services Association's National Registry of Evidence-based Programs and Practices. http://nrepp.samhsa.gov/.

NREPP is an online registry of interventions and programs supporting mental health and substance abuse prevention and treatment. The site facilitates connections between intervention developers and members of the public so they can learn how to implement these intervention and program approaches in their communities.

The Cochrane Collaboration. Cochrane Reviews. http://www.cochrane.org/.

This site houses systematic reviews of research in human health care and health policy conducted by the Cochrane Collaboration, an international network established to assist health care providers, policymakers, patients, and their advocates make well-informed decisions about human health care by preparing, updating, and promoting the accessibility of evidence.

REFERENCES

1. Linnan L, Steckler A. *Process evaluation for public health interventions and research.* San Francisco: Jossey-Bass; 2002.
2. Haynes A, Brennan S, Redman S, et al. Figuring out fidelity: a worked example of the methods used to identify, critique and revise the essential elements of a contextualised intervention in health policy agencies. *Implement Sci.* 2016;11:23.
3. Dobson KS, Singer AR. Definitional and practical issues in the assessment of treatment integrity. *Clin Psychol-Sci Pr.* 2005;12(4):384–387.
4. Carroll C, Patterson M, Wood S, Booth A, Rick J, Balain S. A conceptual framework for implementation fidelity. *Implement Sci.* 2007;2:40.
5. Durlak JA, DuPre EP. Implementation matters: a review of research on the influence of implementation on program outcomes and the factors

affecting implementation. *Am J Commun Psychol.* 2008;41(3-4):327.

6. Eames C, Daley D, Hutchings J, et al. The Leader Observation Tool: a process skills treatment fidelity measure for the Incredible Years parenting programme. *Child Care Health Dev.* 2008;34(3):391–400.

7. Johnson-Kozlow M, Hovell MF, Rovniak LS, Sirikulvadhana L, Wahlgren DR, Zakarian JM. Fidelity issues in secondhand smoking interventions for children. *Nicotine Tob Res.* 2008;10(12):1677–1690.

8. National Institutes of Health. Reproducibility standards. (12/15/14). https://www.nih.gov/research-training/rigor-reproducibility/principles-guidelines-reporting-preclinical-research.

9. Collins FS, Tabak LA. Policy: NIH plans to enhance reproducibility. *Nature.* 2014;505(7485):612–613.

10. Bauman LJ, Stein RE, Ireys HT. Reinventing fidelity: the transfer of social technology among settings. *Am J Commun Psychol.* 1991;19(4):619–639.

11. Blakely CH, Mayer JP, Gottschalk RG, et al. The fidelity adaptation debate—implications for the implementation of public-sector social programs. *Am J Commun Psychol.* 1987;15(3):253–268.

12. Dane AV, Schneider BH. Program integrity in primary and early secondary prevention: are implementation effects out of control? *Clin Psychol Rev.* 1998;18(1):23–45.

13. Dusenbury L, Brannigan R, Falco M, Hansen WB. A review of research on fidelity of implementation: implications for drug abuse prevention in school settings. *Health Educ Res.* 2003;18(2):237–256.

14. Lichstein KL, Riedel BW, Grieve R. Fair tests of clinical trials: a treatment implementation model. *Adv Behav Res Ther.* 1994;16(1):1–29.

15. Moncher FJ, Prinz RJ. Treatment fidelity in outcome studies. *Clin Psychol Rev.* 1991;11(3):247–266.

16. Bellg AJ, Borrelli B, Resnick B, et al. Enhancing treatment fidelity in health behavior change studies: best practices and recommendations from the NIH Behavior Change Consortium. *Health Psychol.* 2004;23(5):443–451.

17. Bopp M, Saunders RP, Lattimore D. The tug-of-war: fidelity versus adaptation throughout the health promotion program life cycle. *J Prim Prev.* 2013;34(3):193–207.

18. Breitenstein SM, Gross D, Garvey CA, Hill C, Fogg L, Resnick B. Implementation fidelity in community-based interventions. *Res Nurs Health.* 2010;33(2):164–173.

19. Perez D, Van der Stuyft P, Zabala MC, Castro M, Lefevre P. A modified theoretical framework to assess implementation fidelity of adaptive public health interventions. *Implement Sci.* 2016;11(1):91.

20. Resnick B, Bellg AJ, Borrelli B, et al. Examples of implementation and evaluation of treatment fidelity in the BCC studies: where we are and where we need to go. *Ann Behav Med.* 2005;29 Suppl:46–54.

21. Byrnes HF, Miller BA, Aalborg AE, Plasencia AV, Keagy CD. Implementation fidelity in adolescent family-based prevention programs: relationship to family engagement. *Health Educ Res.* 2010;25(4):531–541.

22. Gingiss PM, Roberts-Gray C, Boerm M. Bridge-It: A system for predicting implementation fidelity for school-based tobacco prevention programs. *Prev Sci.* 2006;7(2):197–207.

23. Mihalic S. The importance of implementation fidelity. *Emot Behav Disord Youth.* 2004;4(4):83–105.

24. Rohrbach LA, Gunning M, Sun P, Sussman S. The project towards no drug abuse (TND) dissemination trial: implementation fidelity and immediate outcomes. *Prev Science.* 2010;11(1):77–88.

25. Cohen DJ, Crabtree BF, Etz RS, et al. Fidelity versus flexibility: translating evidence-based research into practice. *Am J Prev Med.* 2008;35(5 Suppl):S381–S389.

26. Eames C, Daley D, Hutchings J, et al. The Leader Observation Tool: a process skills treatment fidelity measure for the Incredible Years parenting programme. *Child Care Hlth Dev.* 2008;34(3):391–400.

27. Hogue A, Henderson CE, Dauber S, Barajas PC, Fried A, Liddle HA. Treatment adherence, competence, and outcome in individual and family therapy for adolescent behavior problems. *J Consult Clin Psychol.* 2008;76(4):544.

28. Spillane V, Byrne MC, Byrne M, Leathem CS, O'Malley M, Cupples ME. Monitoring treatment fidelity in a randomized controlled trial of a complex intervention. *J Adv Nurs.* 2007;60(3):343–352.

29. DiGennaro FD, Martens BK, McIntyre LL. Increasing treatment integrity through negative reinforcement: effects on teacher and student behavior. *School Psychol Rev.* 2005;34(2):220.

30. Burns MK, Peters R, Noell GH. Using performance feedback to enhance implementation fidelity of the problem-solving team process. *J Sch Psychol.* 2008;46(5):537–550.

31. Carvalho ML, Honeycutt S, Escoffery C, Glanz K, Sabbs D, Kegler MC. Balancing fidelity and adaptation: implementing evidence-based chronic disease prevention programs. *J Public Health Manag Pract.* 2013;19(4):348–356.

32. Moore JE, Bumbarger BK, Cooper BR. Examining adaptations of evidence-based programs in natural contexts. *J Prim Prev.* 2013;34(3):147–161.

33. Castro FG, Barrera M, Martinez CR. The cultural adaptation of prevention interventions: resolving tensions between fidelity and fit. *Prev Sci.* 2004;5(1):41–45.

34. Cohen DJ, Crabtree BF, Etz RS, et al. Fidelity versus flexibility: translating evidence-based research into practice. *Am J Prev Med.* 2008;35(5):S381–S389.

35. Morrison DM, Hoppe MJ, Gillmore MR, Kluver C, Higa D, Wells EA. Replicating an intervention: the tension between fidelity and adaptation. *Aids Educ Prev.* 2009;21(2):128–140.

36. Allen JD, Linnan LA, Emmons KM. Fidelity and adaptation of evidence-based intervention in public health. In: Brownson RC, Colditz, GA, Proctor EK, eds. *Dissemination and implementation research in health: Translating science to practice.* New York: Oxford University Press; 2012.

37. Slaughter SE, Hill JN, Snelgrove-Clarke E. What is the extent and quality of documentation and reporting of fidelity to implementation strategies: a scoping review. *Implement Sci.* 2015;10:129.

38. Glasgow RE. What types of evidence are most needed to advance behavioral medicine? *Ann Behav Med.* 2008;35(1):19–25.

39. Glasgow RE, Klesges LM, Dzewaltowski DA, Bull SS, Estabrooks P. The future of health behavior change research: what is needed to improve translation of research into health promotion practice? *Ann Behav Med.* 2004;27(1):3–12.

40. Kerner J, Rimer B, Emmons K. Introduction to the special section on dissemination: dissemination research and research dissemination: how can we close the gap? *Health Psychol.* 2005;24(5):443.

41. Cabassa LJ, Gomes AP, Meyreles Q, et al. Using the collaborative intervention planning framework to adapt a health-care manager intervention to a new population and provider group to improve the health of people with serious mental illness. *Implement Sci.* 2014;9:178.

42. Minkler M, Wallerstein N. *Community-based participatory research for health: From process to outcomes.* San Francisco: Jossey-Bass; 2011.

43. Brownson RC, Fielding JE, Maylahn CM. Evidence-based public health: a fundamental concept for public health practice. *Annu Rev Public Health.* 2009;30:175–201.

44. Horn SD, Gassaway J. Practice-based evidence study design for comparative effectiveness research. *Med Care.* 2007;45(10 Supl 2):S50–S57.

45. Linnan L, Thompson, B., & Kobetz, E. Process evaluation results from the Working Well Trial.

In: Steckler, A. and Linnan, L, eds. *Process evaluation in public health interventions and research.* San Francisco: Jossey Bass, Inc. 2002:155–183.

46. Greenhalgh T, Robert G, Macfarlane F, Bate P, Kyriakidou O. Diffusion of innovations in service organizations: systematic review and recommendations. *Milbank Q.* 2004;82(4):581–629.

47. Davis M, Baranowski T, Hughes M, Warnecke C, De Moor C, Mullis R. Using children as change agents to increase fruit and vegetable consumption among lower-income African American parents. *Process Eval Public Health Intervent Res.* 2002:249–267.

48. Rogers EF. Nature with water and the Spirit: a response to Rowan Williams. *Scot J Theology.* 2003;56(1):89–100.

49. Research Tested Intervention Programs. https://rtips.cancer.gov/rtips/index.do. Accessed 12/5/2016.

50. Grover V. Commentary: Implementing interventions: building a shared understanding of why. *New Dir Child Adolesc Dev.* 2016;2016(154):109–112.

51. Fagan AA, Arthur MW, Hanson K, Briney JS, Hawkins JD. Effects of Communities That Care on the adoption and implementation fidelity of evidence-based prevention programs in communities: results from a randomized controlled trial. *Prev Sci.* 2011;12(3):223–234.

52. Dariotis JK, Bumbarger BK, Duncan LG, Greenberg MT. How do implementation efforts relate to program adherence? Examining the role of organizational, implementer, and program factors. *J Community Psychol.* 2008;36(6):744–760.

53. Weiner BJ. A theory of organizational readiness for change. *Implement Sci.* 2009;4:67.

54. Kumanyika SK, Yancey AK. Physical activity and health equity: evolving the science. *Am J Health Promot.* 2009;23(6):S4–S7.

55. Backer TE. *Finding the balance: Program fidelity and adaptation in substance abuse prevention: A state-of-the-art review.* Rockville, MD: Center for Substance Abuse Prevention; 2001.

56. Lee CY, August GJ, Realmuto GM, Horowitz JL, Bloomquist ML, Klimes-Dougan B. Fidelity at a distance: assessing implementation fidelity of the Early Risers prevention program in a going-to-scale intervention trial. *Prev Sci.* 2008;9(3):215–229.

57. Fixsen DL, Naoom SF, Blase KA, Friedman M, Wallace F. Implementation Research: A Synthesis of the Literature. 2005; http://nirn.fpg.unc.edu/sites/nirn.fpg.unc.edu/files/resources/NIRN-MonographFull-01-2005.pdf.

58. Keith RE, Hopp FP, Subramanian U, Wiitala W, Lowery JC. Fidelity of implementation: development and testing of a measure. *Implement Sci.* 2010;5:99.

59. Nelson MC, Cordray DS, Hulleman CS, Darrow CL, Sommer EC. A procedure for assessing intervention fidelity in experiments testing educational and behavioral interventions. *J Behav Health Ser R.* 2012;39(4):374–396.

60. Teague GB, Mueser KT, Rapp CA. Advances in fidelity measurement for mental health services research: four measures. *Psychiat Serv.* 2012;63(8):765–771.

61. Baer JS, Ball SA, Campbell BK, Miele GM, Schoener EP, Tracy K. Training and fidelity monitoring of behavioral interventions in multisite addictions research. *Drug Alcohol Depend.* 2007;87(2-3):107–118.

62. Berkel C, Mauricio AM, Schoenfelder E, Sandler IN. Putting the pieces together: an integrated model of program implementation. *Prev Sci.* 2011;12(1):23–33.

63. Lobb R, Gonzalez Suarez E, Fay ME, et al. Implementation of a cancer prevention program for working class, multiethnic populations. *Prev Med.* 2004;38(6):766–776.

64. Elliott DS, Mihalic S. Issues in disseminating and replicating effective prevention programs. *Prev Sci.* 2004;5(1):47–53.

65. Balu R, Doolittle F. Commentary: Learning from variations in fidelity of implementation. *New Direct Child Adolesc Dev.* 2016;2016(154):105–108.

66. Castro FG, Barrera M, Jr., Martinez CR, Jr. The cultural adaptation of prevention interventions: resolving tensions between fidelity and fit. *Prev Sci.* 2004;5(1):41–45.

67. Wiltsey Stirman S, Kimberly J, Cook N, Calloway A, Castro F, Charns M. The sustainability of new programs and innovations: a review of the empirical literature and recommendations for future research. *Implement Sci.* 2012;7:17.

68. Durlak JA. Why program implementation is important. *J Prevent Intervent Community.* 1998;17(2):5–18.

69. Hallfors D, Godette D. Will the 'principles of effectiveness' improve prevention practice? Early findings from a diffusion study. *Health Educ Res.* 2002;17(4):461–470.

70. Botvin GJ. Advancing prevention science and practice: challenges, critical issues, and future directions. *Prev Sci.* 2004;5(1):69–72.

71. Ennett ST, Haws S, Ringwalt CL, et al. Evidence-based practice in school substance use prevention: fidelity of implementation under real-world conditions. *Health Educ Res.* 2011;26(2):361–371.

72. Hill LG, Maucione K, Hood BK. A focused approach to assessing program fidelity. *Prev Sci.* 2007;8(1):25–34.

73. Chambers DA, Glasgow RE, Stange KC. The dynamic sustainability framework: addressing the paradox of sustainment amid ongoing change. *Implement Sci.* 2013;8:117.

74. Aarons GA, Hurlburt M, Horwitz SM. Advancing a conceptual model of evidence-based practice implementation in public service sectors. *Adm Policy Ment Health.* 2011;38(1):4–23.

75. Damschroder LJ, Aron DC, Keith RE, Kirsh SR, Alexander JA, Lowery JC. Fostering implementation of health services research findings into practice: a consolidated framework for advancing implementation science. *Implementation Science.* 2009;4:50.

76. Lara M, Bryant-Stephens T, Damitz M, et al. Balancing "fidelity" and community context in the adaptation of asthma evidence-based interventions in the "real world." *Health Promotion Practice.* 2011;12(6_suppl_1):63S-72S.

77. Aarons GA, Hurlburt M, Horwitz SM. Advancing a conceptual model of evidence-based practice implementation in public service sectors. *Adm Policy Ment Hlth.* 2011;38(1):4–23.

78. Green AE, Aarons GA. A comparison of policy and direct practice stakeholder perceptions of factors affecting evidence-based practice implementation using concept mapping. *Implementation Science.* 2011;6:104.

79. Bernal G, Saez-Santiago E. Culturally centered psychosocial interventions. *J Community Psychol.* 2006;34(2):121–132.

80. Cabassa LJ, Baumann AA. A two-way street: bridging implementation science and cultural adaptations of mental health treatments. *Implement Sci.* 2013;8:90.

81. Kumpfer KL, Pinyuchon M, de Melo AT, Whiteside HO. Cultural adaptation process for international dissemination of the Strengthening Families Program. *Eval Health Prof.* 2008;31(2):226–239.

82. Marek LI, Brock DJ, Sullivan R. Cultural adaptations to a family life skills program: implementation in rural appalachia. *J Prim Prev.* 2006;27(2):113–133.

83. McGraw SA, Sellers DE, Stone EJ, et al. Using process data to explain outcomes. An illustration from the Child and Adolescent Trial for Cardiovascular Health (CATCH). *Eval Rev.* 1996;20(3):291–312.

84. Scheirer MA, Dearing JW. An agenda for research on the sustainability of public health programs. *Am J Public Health.* 2011;101(11):2059–2067.

85. Shediac-Rizkallah MC, Bone LR. Planning for the sustainability of community-based health programs: conceptual frameworks and future directions for research, practice and policy. *Health Educ Res.* 1998;13(1):87–108.

86. Galovski TE, Blain LM, Mott JM, Elwood L, Houle T. Manualized therapy for PTSD: flexing the structure of cognitive processing therapy. *J Consult Clin Psychol*. 2012;80(6):968–981.

87. Kalichman SC, Kelly JA, Hunter TL, Murphy DA, Tyler R. Culturally tailored HIV-AIDS risk-reduction messages targeted to African-American urban women: impact on risk sensitization and risk reduction. *J Consult Clin Psychol*. 1993;61(2):291–295.

88. Kennedy MG, Mizuno Y, Hoffman R, Baume C, Strand J. The effect of tailoring a model HIV prevention program for local adolescent target audiences. *AIDS Educ Prev*. 2000;12(3):225–238.

89. Levitt JT, Malta LS, Martin A, Davis L, Cloitre M. The flexible application of a manualized treatment for PTSD symptoms and functional impairment related to the 9/11 World Trade Center attack. *Behav Res Ther*. 2007;45(7):1419–1433.

90. Stanton B, Guo J, Cottrell L, et al. The complex business of adapting effective interventions to new populations: an urban to rural transfer. *J Adolesc Health*. 2005;37(2):163.

91. Stirman SW, Miller CJ, Toder K, Calloway A. Development of a framework and coding system for modifications and adaptations of evidence-based interventions. *Implementation Science*. 2013;8(1):65.

92. Chambers DA, Norton WE. The adaptome advancing the science of intervention adaptation. *Am J Prev Med*. 2016;51(4):S124–S131.

93. Wingood GM, DiClemente RJ. The Adapt-Itt model: A novel method of adapting evidence-based HIV interventions. *J Acquir Immune Defic Syndr*. 2008;47:S40–S46.

94. Escoffery C. A Scoping Study of Program Adaptation Frameworks for Evidence-Based Interventions. 9th Annual Conference on the Science of Dissemination and Implementation; Dec. 14, 2016.

95. Linnan LA, Ferguson YO. Beauty salons: a promising health promotion setting for reaching and promoting health among African American women. *Health Educ Behav*. 2007;34(3):517–530.

96. Linnan LA, Reiter PL, Duffy C, Hales D, Ward DS, Viera AJ. Assessing and promoting physical activity in African American barbershops: results of the FITStop pilot study. *Am J Mens Health*. 2011;5(1):38–46.

97. Linnan LA, Ferguson YO, Wasilewski Y, et al. Using community-based participatory research methods to reach women with health messages: results from the North Carolina BEAUTY and Health Pilot Project. *Health Promot Pract*. 2005;6(2):164–173.

97a. National Cancer Institute (2002). Making health communication programs work. U.S. Department of Health and Human Services. Accessed on 5/16/16 from https://www.cancer.gov/publications/health-communication/pink-book.pdf

98. Solomon FM, Linnan LA, Wasilewski Y, Lee AM, Katz ML, Yang J. Observational study in ten beauty salons: results informing development of the North Carolina BEAUTY and Health Project. *Health Educ Behav*. 2004;31(6):790–807.

99. Emmons K, Colditz, GA. Realizing the potential of cancer prevention—the role of implementation science. *N Engl J Med*. 2017:376:986–990.

100. Balu R, Doolittle F. Commentary: Learning from variations in fidelity of implementation. *New Dir Child Adolesc Dev*. 2016;2016(154):105–108.

101. Zwarenstein M, Treweek S, Gagnier JJ, et al. Improving the reporting of pragmatic trials: an extension of the CONSORT statement. *BMJ*. 2008;337:a2390.

17

Adaptation in Dissemination and Implementation Science

ANA A. BAUMANN, LEOPOLDO J. CABASSA,
AND SHANNON WILTSEY STIRMAN

INTRODUCTION

Over the past decade, the field of dissemination and implementation (D&I) science has moved from cross-sectional research to sophisticated evaluations of implementation strategies and theory-driven research on factors that predict successful implementation. Despite advances in research methods, we have not been able to answer the decades-old question of what works best for whom under what circumstances.[1] Investigators are still calling for increased action in promoting evidence-based interventions in usual care and for testing interventions and designs to optimize outcomes.[2,3] In light of the diversity of patient populations, providers, and service settings into which interventions are delivered, it is unlikely that the same program, techniques, and strategies can be implemented successfully in the exact same way across multiple contexts. Scholars from the fields of implementation science and cultural adaptation warn of the dangers of implementing evidence-based interventions without attending to the fit of the interventions to the context, in particular to the populations that are being served, the different providers who deliver these interventions, and the diversity of service settings that could benefit from these interventions.[4,5] In fact, numerous studies indicate the importance of matching the intervention with the population and context of interest, including attention to race, ethnicity, location, community norms, service settings, and organizational characteristics.[4,6,7]

This chapter draws from the cultural adaptation field and recent advances in D&I science to propose that scholars should carefully consider evaluating, documenting, and rigorously studying the adaptation process and outcomes. It uses the definition of cultural adaptation as "the systematic modification of an evidence-based intervention (EBI) to consider language, culture, and context in such a way that it is compatible with the client's cultural patterns meanings and values"[8] to refer to adaptations based on client cultural background. However, we suggest adaptations that go beyond cultural elements at the client level must also be considered, because adaptations can also be made by modifying interventions to fit provider characteristics, organizational contexts, and service settings (e.g., historical, political, and economic contexts). This broader conceptualization of adaptations provides us with a more thoughtful and deliberate alteration to the design and/or delivery of an intervention, with the goal of improving its fit and effectiveness in a given context.[9] Our assumption is that by clearly specifying and evaluating adaptation, we can increase the external validity of the intervention, its outcomes, and the implementation process.

This chapter first outlines why D&I science scholars should consider adaptation. Next, it describes when to adapt interventions, followed by outlining components scholars should consider adapting, how to adapt components that may require adapting, and how to evaluate the impact of adaptation. Finally, it provides the authors' recommendations for the D&I science field regarding adaptation of interventions.

WHY ADAPT

As Chambers and Norton[10] mention, the traditional path in science is to develop an intervention, test it, identify the discordance between the intervention and the context or the population, adapt the intervention, and then implement the intervention on a broader scale. However, evidence suggests that interventions that were previously adapted and tested are not being implemented in usual care, and interventions that are being implemented are not necessarily explicitly attending to the adaptation process.[5,11] The following text outlines the importance of attending to the process of adaptation and its impact on implementation, service, and consumer-level outcomes.

One of the main assumptions of the D&I field is that if an intervention has proved to be efficacious, the spread of such intervention would decrease the quality gap, reduce cost, or improve outcomes regardless of the setting where it is being implemented.[10,12–14] However, as Alegria and colleagues remind us, "One size does not fit all."[15] Implementation science acknowledges that an intervention is not implemented in a vacuum, and contextual factors at multiple levels (e.g., clients, providers, organizations, communities) influence its success.

There are at least three consequences to a "one size fits all," gold standard assumption. First, assuming that EBIs are the gold standard of interventions that will improve quality, cost, or outcomes once they are broadly disseminated and implemented overlooks the importance of contextual factors.[12] Consider, for example, parent interventions. We know that while parenting practices have some universal components, they are heavily culturally based and dependent on beliefs and orientations (e.g., the role of respect, of gender practices).[16,17] If an intervention developed for a group of parents (e.g., White Americans in urban settings in the United States) is delivered for a different group (e.g., Latino parents in rural setting in the United States) and engagement or outcomes are not promising, one needs to carefully examine whether the problem was with the implementation process, or rather with the mismatch between the intervention components and the population and context into which it was implemented.[12,18,19]

A second potential consequence related to the "gold standard assumption" and the emphasis on the assumption that any EBI is good for anyone in any context, is that it can hinder efforts to effectively address health care disparities. The Department of Health and Human Services defines health disparity as "a particular type of health difference that is closely linked with social, economic, and/or environmental disadvantage. Health disparities adversely affect groups of people who have systematically experienced greater obstacles to health based on their racial or ethnic

group."[20] While we have made some progress in the last 30 years, disparities in health and access to health care have yet to be eliminated.[21] Currently, non-White participants (e.g., African Americans, Latinos, Asian/Pacific Islanders, and Native Americans) are seriously underrepresented in studies in general, despite NIH's guidelines for the inclusion of racial and ethnic minorities in funded studies.[22] Specifically, the number of minority participants from the National Institute of Mental Health, the National Institute on Drug Abuse, and the National Institute on Alcohol Abuse and Alcoholism intervention studies are less than 20% of total participants.[3,23] Considering that at least 37% of the US population identifies as racial and ethnic minority,[24] the lack of inclusion of racial and ethnic diverse population in D&I studies is worrisome if we are to think about the external validity and appropriateness of these interventions for diverse population who are overrepresented in public systems (health, social service, criminal justice).[25] A similar argument can be made for participants with other characteristics, such as diverse socioeconomic status, disability, and/or gender identification.[26,27] One could argue that, only by developing a science grounded in a social-justice approach, we will be able to fully decrease the disparities gap.[28,29] We will only be able to eradicate health disparities if interventions are equally available to everyone, from the wealthiest to the most disadvantaged person in the United States.[30]

Often interventions have not been evaluated for a given population or context but there may be a pressing need to improve access to quality care. In such cases, interventions that are considered to be evidence based may represent the best option available. However, implementing an intervention that has not been tested in a particular population, culture or setting may not yield the desired outcomes.[31] More research and investments in services are needed to develop and test interventions across diverse populations, services settings, and communities so that we can evaluate which implementation strategies for which interventions can reduce health and mental health disparities.[32] Furthermore, the use of strategies to rapidly determine whether and how adaptations are necessary to promote optimal levels of engagement and outcomes are central to the implementation effort. Otherwise, a considerable amount of time could pass before a pattern of disappointing results becomes evident and more effective solutions are identified.[33]

A final, related consequence to a "gold standard" assumption is that while it is now demonstrated that adaptation frequently occurs when an intervention is transported from one setting to another,[6,34,35] assumptions are made about whether this is a positive or negative aspect of implementation. When adaptation is considered in D&I science, some have viewed it as a negative outcome that is inconsistent with fidelity[10,36] or emphasized the importance of attention to fidelity.[37] Others have suggested that adaptation is an essential aspect of implementation, without which interventions are unlikely to be successfully transported to routine settings.[38] However, there is limited empirical evidence regarding the impact of adaptations that occur in routine care, and the answer to the debate regarding whether adaptation is necessary or contraindicated is unlikely to be the same for every type of intervention, adaptation or context.[34]

Rather than making broad assumptions about adaptation, we argue that D&I scientists should engage in a careful evaluation of when, why, and how adaptation should occur by documenting and studying adaptation during the implementation process. As Rogers explained, an "innovation almost never fits perfectly in the organization in which it is being embedded."[35(p. 395)] Instead, implementation requires a process of mutual adaptation, in which both the practice innovation being implemented and the organizations and stakeholders involved in the implementation process must adjust to optimize fit.[28,36,37] When interventions are adapted with care, there is the potential for optimization of that intervention in the context in which it is delivered, but it also has the potential to produce undesired outcomes if undertaken in the absence of guidance from theory and research evidence.[34] However, adaptation processes are usually not documented and, consequently, not evaluated and understood.[5,10,11] This lack of attention has resulted in uncertainty regarding the types of adaptations that can maximize the success of implementation efforts and their impact on health.

Adaptation and Fidelity

When referring to adaptation of intervention, it is important to consider the relationship between adaptation and fidelity. As the authors from chapter 16 mention, much has been written about the tension between fidelity and adaptation of interventions.[10,38] The authors advocate here that attending to adaptation is important as

a *complement* to the assessment of fidelity, and not necessarily in conflict with fidelity.[34] Fidelity of an intervention is important because it predicts the interventions' intended outcomes.[39,40] Understanding which types of adaptations can occur without eroding the dose and fidelity to key intervention components (e.g., fidelity-consistent adaptations)[9] can provide guidance on how to optimize an intervention in a particular setting.[34] By monitoring the adaptation process, researchers can potentially improve the reach, engagement, effectiveness, and hopefully the sustainment of the interventions in usual care.[5,45] Fortunately, there is a developing literature that can provide guidance regarding when and how to make adaptations while evaluating their impact on the intervention outcomes.

WHEN TO ADAPT

It is our perspective that adaptations to EBIs should not be a separate or an additional step in the implementation process. Rather, adaptations could be considered both an implementation strategy and an implementation outcome. It can be considered an outcome in the same sense as fidelity and dosage,[42] as it is a complementary construct, and descriptive data on the nature and extent of adaptation are important to report. In addition some frameworks from the D&I science field support the idea of incorporating the adaptation process within the implementation of EBIs in new settings.[5] For example, the Dynamic Adaptation Process (DAP) model[42] specifies a process for identifying and incorporating adaptations at multiple levels throughout the phase of implementation to facilitate the adoption and use of EBIs in community settings.

Frameworks from the cultural adaptation field advocate for adaptations to occur as early as possible in the implementation process, when deciding which EBI to implement and in preparation for the new context and population.[4] For example, Lau's selective and directive cultural adaptation framework proposes a data-driven model, where adaptations are made when there is quantitative and/or qualitative evidence that: (a) the new population has distinctive and unique sociocultural context of risk and resilience that will require consideration or addition of new treatment elements to address these contextual issues, and/or (b) when the social validity of an intervention is compromised, thus limiting treatment engagement and the receipt of an adequate exposure to the treatment to achieve its intended effect.[43]

Similarly, Barrera and Castro[44] stipulate that adaptations are needed when qualitative and/or quantitative evidence indicates that two or more populations differ on: (a) treatment engagement dimensions (e.g., awareness of treatment, treatment completion); (b) the ability of the treatment to change mediating variables (action theory); and (c) the relationships between mediators and treatment outcomes (conceptual theory).[5]

WHAT TO ADAPT

Most interventions are multicomponent, and the contexts into which they are implemented will differ. Thus, many different forms of adaptations can occur. Understanding and documenting what these components are can facilitate better understanding of what types of adaptations yield the desired outcomes (e.g., engagement, adoption, improvements in health or functioning). Some work has been done to characterize adaptations made at the individual and population level. The cultural adaptation field has produced many frameworks aimed to guide the adaptation of content of the intervention. For example, Bernal and colleagues' Ecological Validity Model[8] was one of the first frameworks that outlined domains that one should consider to enhance cultural congruence between participants and the intervention: language, persons, metaphors, content, concepts, goals, methods, and contexts.[8] Other scholars have suggested surface-structure adaptations or deep-structure adaptations that can serve to maintain fidelity to the intervention model while making them more relevant and appealing to cultural groups.[45]

Recognizing the body of literature on cultural adaptation,[4] and with the intention of categorizing different types of interventions to facilitate the study of the nature and impact of adaptations, Stirman and colleagues developed a framework to document changes to programs and interventions that involve procedures delivered by individual practitioners or teams of practitioners,[30] illustrated and expanded in Figure 17.1. According to this framework, adaptations can occur at multiple levels and can be driven by different stakeholders. Identifying who initiated the adaptation (e.g., the provider, the organization, a coalition of stakeholders, the treatment developer, the clients or target population) is important, because it is possible that who decides which adaptations to make, and when and how adaptations are made, may have an impact on how effective they are. It is important to note that

recipients of the interventions are embedded in the coalition of stakeholders and have an important voice regarding the need for, and specific forms of adaptation. Contextual modifications are those that involve changes to the format (e.g., group vs. individual, telephone or web-based vs. in-person), setting (e.g., an intervention designed for an outpatient medical setting being delivered in a school or community setting), personnel who deliver the intervention (e.g., lay health worker instead of a mental health professional), or intervention recipients (e.g., an intervention originally developed for gay men being delivered to a transgender population). Adaptations to training may be made to facilitate implementation. Similarly, adaptations to the evaluation process may be needed when evaluation materials (e.g., surveys) are not feasible or are unlikely to be effective in a particular context. Content-level adaptations focus on the intervention itself. They can vary from very minor changes to an intervention that leave all major intervention principles or components intact (tailoring) to more significant adaptations such as removing or adding components or integrating other approaches into the intervention. Figure 17.1 describes different types of content-level adaptations. See Case Study #1 for an example of adaptations made to a trauma treatment intervention delivered in two low-income countries.

Rather than specifying cultural adaptation as a separate form of content-level adaptation, the expanded framework presented in this chapter suggests adding a code to indicate why a particular adaptation was made may be necessary. As illustrated in Figure 17.1, these reasons could include the appropriate cultural factors. This allows greater clarity about the types of cultural adaptations that are made, because they can vary from minor changes to language and terminology to removal, integration, or substitution of a different component, and can also vary in terms of the reasons that they are made. For example, if an adaptation was tailored so that examples and terminology would resonate more with a specific population, the content code would be "tailoring," and the [reason] specifier might be "recipient ethnicity" or "recipient religion." If tailoring were also necessary to adjust written materials to literacy level or to provide materials or exercises using mobile technology rather than paper, the corresponding code would be "tailoring" with a literacy specifier. An empirically driven process of refinement for these additions to the framework

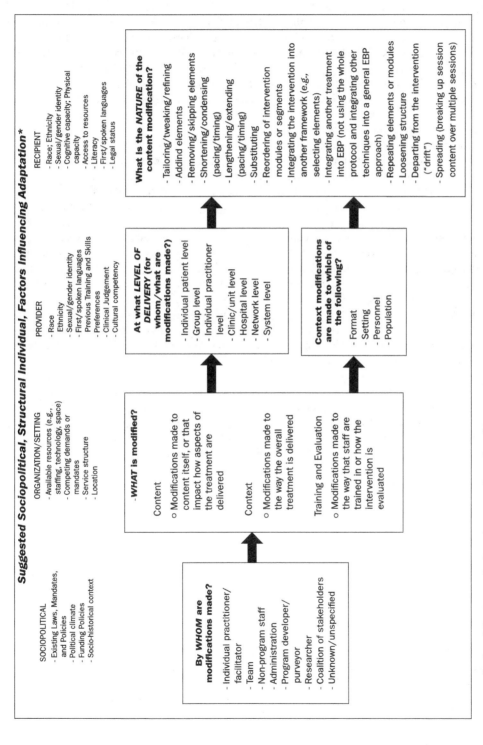

FIGURE 17.1 Framework of modifications and adaptations to evidence-based interventions.

(Adapted from Stirman, Miller, Toder & Calloway 2013.[34])

*Suggested individual, sociopolitical, and structural factors were not refined using the coding process used for the 2013 framework.

is still necessary, but, as the examples of potential specifiers in Figure 17.1 suggest, when identifying cultural adaptations and other reasons for adaptation, specificity is important. It is possible that some forms of, and reasons for, adaptation may result in increased engagement or sustainability of an intervention but poorer health outcomes, whereas others may yield similar or improved outcomes. For example, Stanton and colleagues,[50] with input from local stakeholders, adapted a sexual risk reduction intervention originally developed for an urban population to fit within the sociopolitical context and address the preferences of a rural population. This adaptation involved substituting a module on abstinence for the module on condom use that was originally part of the intervention. The adapted intervention was less effective than the original, suggesting that the condom use module may have been a core component of the intervention. However, other efforts to adapt sexual risk reduction interventions involved tailoring a video to match participant ethnicity and gender, and the level of effectiveness was not compromised.[51]

Some of the forms of adaptation described in the framework can be seen as enhancing or augmenting the intervention, while others may reduce or simplify it.[52] These adaptations can be further classified as fidelity consistent, and fidelity-inconsistent, depending on the components and requirements of the intervention itself.[9] Whether an adaptation is fidelity consistent or inconsistent can be determined based on theory or research that specifies core components for an intervention. However, in the context of exploring cultural adaptations, it is possible that new learning can occur about which aspects of an intervention are actually necessary to promote desired outcomes. The goal of such exploration would be to inform subsequent implementation efforts by specifying which aspects of the intervention are necessary to preserve desired outcomes, and how to adapt in a fidelity-consistent manner for a given population or setting.

CASE STUDY #1: ADAPTATION OF A TRAUMA TREATMENT FOR DELIVERY IN LOW-INCOME COUNTRIES: EXAMPLES OF WHAT TO ADAPT

An example of adapting cognitive processing therapy illustrates the application of a framework to characterize adaptations that have been made when implementing and testing the intervention, originally developed as a 12-session group intervention for survivors of assault or interpersonal violence in the United States, in low and middle income countries (Kurdistan and the Democratic Republic of Congo).[53,54] Lack of infrastructure necessitated changes to where, and by whom, the intervention was delivered. The Stirman et al.[34] framework would characterize adaptations at multiple levels. Two *contextual modifications* were made. Adaptations to personnel were necessary because there were no psychotherapists in these settings. Instead, trained lay health workers delivered the intervention. The *setting* also needed to be adapted, because mental health clinics were not in place. Treatment was delivered in participating villages or health clinics. *Content-level* adaptations included *tailoring* (simplifying jargon, removing written work, and/ or using pictorial or mnemonic cues as prompts instead of using written materials), *tailoring-cultural* (translating concepts to be culturally relevant), and *substituting-cultural* (*replacing of* a component that did not fit the cultural context).[54] Additionally, a component of the treatment was *removed* both to simplify the intervention due to *literacy* concerns and to fit the *cultural* context. The *training and supervision* process was also changed, with training workshops extended and supervision involving observation of groups by a trained supervisor. Adaptation of the *evaluation* strategy involved adapting the measures to use terminology that matched cultural descriptions of trauma symptoms and a shift from a likert-type scale to words and pictures that described symptom intensity, and verbal administration of measures. Results from the study in the Democratic Republic of Congo indicated that the treatment could be delivered successfully under very different conditions than that in which the original intervention had been designed, and it was more effective than an individual support condition, particularly at a 6-month follow-up.

How to Adapt

If adaptation is to be a planned, proactive data-driven process, rather than a reactive, idiosyncratic process, it should begin during the planning phase of an implementation effort. When considering the implementation of an intervention, cultural adaptation scholars suggest that one should carefully examine the following issues: (a) what evidence about the intervention is available (e.g., what information does the literature provide about the EBI?), (b) how different is the target population from the original population in the new setting (e.g., adults *vs.* teenagers), (c) what is the target domain of the intervention (e.g., changing parenting practices, improving coping skills, increasing self-management), and (d) what was the context of the original intervention (e.g., rural *vs.* urban). It is very likely that one or more of these variables will demand careful adaptation to fit the intervention to the new context.

Proactively specifying the nature of adaptations can facilitate better understanding of the elements of the intervention and/context that can be changed, and the elements that must be retained to achieve desired outcomes. Depending on the identified needs, content-level adaptations can be intended for an entire population or community, or they can be made for specific cohorts or individuals.[30] In some contexts, individual providers may also make decisions to adapt interventions for everyone that they serve due to perceptions of the intervention or beliefs that certain strategies will enhance outcomes or increase engagement, although evaluation is necessary to determine whether these beliefs are correct. There is no single, correct way to adapt all interventions.[4] However, to proactively plan an intervention, guidance from an adaptation framework is important.

Frameworks to Guide the Process of Adaptation

To complement the framework that describes what is adapted, and the implementation frameworks described in chapter 5, many cultural adaptation frameworks have been developed to guide the process of adaptation as it relates to modifying an existing intervention for a new cultural, racial, or ethnic group. Other scholars have provided in-depth reviews of the cultural adaptation models,[4,38] which in general recommend that the adaptations should (a) be informed by the expertise of stakeholders (e.g., researchers and community representatives) and with collaboration between treatment developer; (b) follow formative research methods to understand population needs and the context of practice; (c) be addressed with carefully pilot testing of fidelity; and (d) be formally evaluated with effectiveness trials.[4,5,38]

Some frameworks integrate both the "what" and the "how" of adaptation. These models include the Cultural Adaptation Process (CAP), which was developed to complement Bernal's EVM,[18,50] Barrera and Castro's framework,[41,44,51]

and the tailoring frameworks.[57,58] For example, CAP is influenced by Roger's diffusion of innovation approach.[35] Phase I involves the creation of collaborative approaches between different stakeholders: program developer, the scientist adapting the intervention, the practitioners, local policymakers, and those receiving the intervention. A needs assessment including literature review and focus group also take place in Phase I. Phase II consists of making the first iterations of adaptations and pilot testing the measures to be used on Phase III on a large trial. All Phases include feedback loops, and adaptations to the intervention may occur during the large trial.[18] A later iteration of the CAP framework has incorporated Aarons's DAP[42] and Forgatch's implementation[54] frameworks to describe the implementation process of the Parent Management Training-Oregon model in Mexico.[50] Case Study #2 describes another example of a model that defines the "what" and the "how" to adapt an existing health care manager intervention using the Collaborative Intervention Planning Framework.

In the D&I science field, Aarons' DAP framework[42] proposes similar steps in terms of the importance of involving stakeholders during the adaptation process. Within the DAP, decisions about the adaptation are made by an implementation resource team composed of multiple stakeholders (e.g., clinicians, researchers, administrators, clients, intervention developers). This team uses information from a careful assessment of system, organizational, provider, and client-level characteristics to negotiate system, organization, and intervention adaptations while maintaining core ingredients of the EBI. An important distinction between the cultural adaptation and this D&I science framework is that DAP considers adaptations beyond the EBI, such as modifications to the service context or the organization itself to facilitate implementation. In addition to choosing a framework to guide the adaptation process, it is important to follow recommended strategies for assessing whether the desired outcomes are achieved after adaptation occurs.[34]

CASE STUDY #2: THE COLLABORATIVE INTERVENTION PLANNING FRAMEWORK: MERGING THE WHAT WITH THE HOW TO ADAPT

Cabassa and colleagues developed the collaborative intervention planning framework (CIPF),[60] which blends principles of community-based participatory research (CBPR) and intervention mapping (IM) procedures to inform the adaptation of an existing health care manager intervention to a new client population (Latinos with serious mental illness) and provider group (social workers) to fit the context of a public outpatient mental health clinic in New York City.[55] This framework provides an example of how to combine cultural adaptations methods and D&I science.[56] In this framework, CBPR principles, such as capacity building and mutual trust, form the bedrock of the partnerships between stakeholders involved in the delivery of the intervention (e.g., social workers, primary care physicians, psychiatrists) and researchers through the creation of a community advisory board (CAB). IM, a systematic step-by-step approach that uses group activities, formative research, and visual tools (e.g., logic models) to develop, adapt, and implement interventions, is used to put this partnership into action and provides a roadmap for this collaborative approach.[62] The goals of CIPF are to bring the expertise of researchers, the wisdom of community members, and the clinical experience of service providers to systematically analyze the fit of each intervention component to the client population, provider groups, and local practice setting. The adaptation process followed by CIPF included fostering collaborations between CAB members and understanding the needs of the local population through a mixed-methods needs assessment, literature reviews, and group discussions to identify targets for adaptation and develop the adapted intervention. The application of IM procedures helped identify a series of cultural- and provider-level adaptations that enhanced the relevance, acceptability, feasibility, and cultural sensitivity of the health care manager intervention without compromising its core components.[60] CIPF represents one approach that can be used to involve stakeholders in the intervention adaptation process from the very beginning to enhance the transportability of interventions to new populations, providers and routine practice settings.

Evaluating the Impact of the Adaptation

The evaluation of the adapted intervention should be informed by the context and goals of the adaptation. When evaluating the implementation process, care should be taken when selecting the measures to be used. Measurement is still an area

that needs much attention in the implementation science field, as we are still developing and testing psychometric valid measures for several implementation outcomes.[63] Note the fact that silent in the discussion of measurements in the implementation field is the cultural context of such measures. This is a concern, as the lack of adjustments to cultural context may yield errors in measurement equivalence. For example, interventions may be adapted to improve their target outcomes, such as parenting practices.[64,65] When measuring client outcomes, data indicate that about 77% of one of the most common questionnaires to assess depression in children, the Children's Depression Inventory, are nonequivalent indicators of depression severity across White, Black, Latino, and Asian youth.[66] As such, if attention is not given to culture, assessment of depression symptoms in different racial/ethnic groups can be scored without any adjustment for group characteristics, yielding divergent findings due to measurement issues.[66] A similar concern could be related to the implementation outcomes, as these are very context-driven. Detailed description of the context and respondents is important as we work on the validation of measures for the implementation science field.

At other times, adaptations may be made to improve the implementation process (e.g., feasibility, acceptability, sustainability) or service outcomes (engagement, equity, satisfaction).[67] When doing so, it is important to understand the context when evaluating implementation outcomes. Consider fidelity of an intervention as an example. Chapter 16 provides information about the different types of fidelity measures. It is important to consider that measures of fidelity, which essentially evaluate and code interactions between people, can be subjective. As a case in point, studies in coding interactions between parents and children found that coders of different ethnicities and race than the parents viewed the interactions of parents and children differently compared with those with similar ethnicity and race, despite intensive trainings to reach reliability.[68–70] Assessing for adaptation and fidelity simultaneously might allow researchers to better characterize the content of the sessions and provide a shared language and understanding for how to code session elements when changes have occurred. Additionally, when possible, selecting measures that have been validated in the cultural context in which an intervention is implemented is particularly important in implementation science studies.

To address measurement issues and examine the effect of the adapted intervention and measures, the evaluation of adaptation in practice settings may occur through systematically monitoring client outcomes. In the literature, systematic measurement of client outcomes has been called progress monitoring, outcome monitoring, measurement-based care, or the use of feedback systems.[71] Data suggest that systematic monitoring results in improved client outcomes[72,73] and that, fortunately, providers have positive opinions about monitoring and feedback.[74] By systematically evaluating the effects of the adapted intervention on client outcomes, one can ensure that the adaptations are effective, and that the effective core components of the intervention are maintained.

The use of plan-do-study-act (PDSA) cycles, which include evaluation of the impact of adaptation[38] has been recommended to optimize outcomes in routine care contexts. This process allows ongoing examination of practice-level data to determine whether the adaptation is having the desired impact. For example, if cultural adaptations are made to the content of an intervention, practitioners could collect information on appointment attendance (engagement), satisfaction, symptoms, functioning, or behaviors that the intervention is intended to target. Ongoing evaluation of this nature allows real-time refinement of interventions through the PDSA process, and when combined with careful documentation of the nature of the adaptations that are made, it can be used to optimize outcomes in practice settings.[38]

While PDSA cycles can be used in routine care settings, evaluation in the context of implementation research may also be more comprehensive and on a larger scale. In most of the research on adaptation to date, the efficacy of the adapted intervention has been studied through randomized control trials (RCTs) comparing the adapted intervention to usual care.[75] Because RCTs are designed to control for contextual and patient-level differences, other types of designs have been proposed to test adaptation of interventions in routine care settings. Three of them are the Sequential Multiple Assignment Randomized Trial (SMART), the Multiphase Optimization Strategy (MOST), and the Usability and User-Centered Design (UCD) designs.

SMART designs, also called adaptive designs, can be defined as a sequence of decision rules that operationalize whether, how, or when and how (i.e., based on which measures) the dosage (i.e., frequency, duration and/or amount), type, or delivery of treatment are effective for those receiving the intervention.[76-78] The advantages of adaptive designs are that they use an empirical base to inform and test prescriptive approaches, and can be used to proactively augment, intensify, switch or diminish components of the intervention.[77,78] Participants are then re-randomized at decision points depending on their response to the adapted intervention, without compromising the integrity of the study. Adaptive designs can be important to improve efficiency from the perspective of multiple stakeholders by helping determine what constitutes the best dose, frequency, and under what condition the intervention needs to be modified.[78] In implementation studies, adaptive designs allow sites that are nonresponsive to the intervention to determine what is the added value of an adapted intervention and how long should any added component continue to improve the targeted outcomes. It is worth observing that the use of adaptive design has to be planned and used with accurately statistical hypothesis testing.[79]

Recently, the MOST framework has also emerged as an innovative methodological framework to support the scalability of interventions while testing the individual and combined effect of intervention components.[80] The framework has three phases: preparation, optimization, and evaluation. During the preparation phase, review of the empirical literature will assist researchers in developing a conceptual model of the problem, identifying strategies and conducting pilot work. The optimization phase is the important piece of this framework, whereby a pilot study is conducted to choose the best design to determine the effect of each component of the intervention. Finally, an evaluation is conducted to study the overall effect of the intervention. This process could be used to identify promising adaptations before conducting a full evaluation. Studies on smoking cessation using MOST framework have highlighted the importance of factorial designs to evaluate the relationship of different intervention components and their interactions with the outcomes.[81,82] A review by Collins et al. provides further examples of the use of MOST and SMART designs.[83]

Another approach, advocated by Lyon and Koerner,[84] is embedded in the UCD approach, which was developed in the human–computer interaction, industrial design, and cognitive psychology fields for developing, adapting, and testing interventions. The cornerstone of UCD is that adaptations are made considering what people will ultimately use, with the goals of (a) clearly identifying the end users (i.e., therapists delivering the intervention, patients receiving the intervention) and their needs, (b) prototyping the intervention with rapid iterations, (c) simplifying existing intervention parameters and procedures, and (d) exploring natural constraints to the implementation of the intervention.[84,85] The rapid prototyping of small modifications of the interventions allows for the exploration of ideas and solutions of different combinations of the intervention in microtrials prior to the large scale of the adapted intervention.[86] Recently, microtrials have been used as a method for testing parenting practices (e.g., praise) outside of the full trial to evaluate its discrete merit to parenting programs.[87,88]

In addition to providing needed information regarding the impact of adaptations, larger-scale research also allows exploration of the possibility that the factors that drive the need to adapt may moderate outcomes. For example, high levels of psychosocial stressors such as economic instability may require adaptation of a parenting intervention (e.g., adding modules on managing stress) and may in and of themselves impact parenting practices (e.g., harsh discipline). In treatments for depression and other disorders, in some populations, psychosocial stressors (e.g., unemployment, housing instability) can diminish treatment engagement and participation. Specific adaptations such as adding case management support to address these psychosocial stressors can enhance the outcome of these interventions in economically disadvantaged populations. The potential interrelationship between these factors should be taken into account when designing the methods and analysis. The timing of data collection and identification of adaptations should be carefully considered when planning for the evaluation of the study in order to establish temporal precedence of an adaptation and changes in symptoms, functioning, or other outcomes, and to facilitate analyses to explore mediation and moderation.

An alternative way of evaluating the effect of adaptation is to apply methodologies to aggregate evidence from different trials, allowing scholars to capitalize on large samples and evaluate what has worked for whom.[89] Coordinated trials of behavioral interventions have been conducted, in which the interventions are different but the targeted outcomes and population groups are similar, allowing the evaluation of different approaches and potential mechanisms of action. Examples consist of the Early Adult Reduction of weight thought Lifestyle intervention and interventions for overweight and obese pregnant women (the Lifestyle Interventions for Expectant Moms (LIFE-Moms) trials; details of these trials were described by Belle et al.[90] A key advantages of these trials that allows for the evaluation of different types of adaptation is the methodology: by choosing a framework to describe different components of the interventions, one can then link each component with the outcomes facilitating identification of the active intervention or adaptations that promote behavior change.[89,91] Other scholars have advocated for the use of dashboards to track outcomes metrics and support the evaluation of multiple trials.[10,92]

Finally, the use of qualitative methods should be strongly considered to supplement and enhance quantitative evaluation, both in research and practice contexts. Feedback from stakeholders can inform hypotheses about unexpected results or further adaptation that might be necessary.[93] Qualitative data can also provide information about whether the intent and goals of adaptation were met from the perspective of multiple stakeholders. More details about mixed method designs can be found on chapter 20.

SUMMARY

This chapter focused on adaptations in the context of D&I research and practice. Consistent with the existing literature, the authors recommend that adaptations be proactively and iteratively determined, strongly informed by a variety of stakeholders, and that efforts be made to carefully describe and document the nature of the adaptations and evaluate their impact on desired service, health, and implementation outcomes. While this chapter focused on adaptations to interventions and the context of practice, also note that adaptations may need to be made to implementation strategies. Only recently have scholars started to use adaptive designs to test implementation strategies.[95] Following the call by Proctor and colleagues[96] for further precision in defining and operationalizing implementation strategies, and based on evidence that scholars are not necessarily reporting what and how they are adapting the interventions,[11] scholars are urged to define and evaluate the adaptations that they are making not only to the interventions and context of practice but also to the implementation strategies.

It can be expected that in the coming years, more research findings on the impact of adaptations at multiple levels will become available, and that studies of the process of adaptation will elucidate best practices that maximize the likelihood of implementation success. Furthermore, development of methodologies to evaluate the impact of different types of adaptations will eventually provide guidance that can inform efforts to make appropriate adaptations to different forms of interventions and in different practice contexts.[10] Such advances can lead to more rapid and successful implementation of effective interventions in a manner that can fulfill the promise of EBIs for reducing health disparities. In short, the ability to successfully implement an intervention depends on the consistent alignment between the intervention and the realities of the system, including the timing of the implementation process.[97]

SUGGESTED READINGS AND WEBSITES

Readings

Chambers DA, Norton WE. The adaptome: advancing the science of intervention adaptation. *Am J Prev Med*. 2016;51(4):S124–S131. doi: 10.1016/j.amepre.2016.05.011

This paper presents a framework and research agenda to advance the science of adaption in the context of implementation. It introduces the idea of developing the adaptome, a data platform used to systematically capture and house information about the variations in the delivery of empirically-supported interventions and programs across multiple settings, populations, and communities and provide critical feedback to intervention developers as well as researchers and practitioners involved in implementation efforts.

Cabassa LJ, Baumann AA. A two-way street: Bridging implementation science and cultural adaptations of mental health treatments. *Implement Sci*. 2013;8:90. doi: 10.1186/1748-5908-8-90.

This paper discusses how implementation science and the field of cultural adaptation contribute valuable insights and methods on how empirically supported treatments and/or context can be customized to enhance implementation across routine practice settings and different populations. The development of a two-way street between the fields of implementation science and cultural adaptations of mental health treatments provides a critical avenue for transporting empirically supported treatments into practice and for reducing racial and ethnic disparities in mental health care.

Stirman SW, Miller CJ, Toder K, Calloway A. Development of a framework and coding system for modifications and adaptations of evidence-based interventions. *Implement Sci*. 2013;8. doi: 10.1186/1748-5908-8-65.

This paper describes the development and initial application of a framework for coding modifications and adaptations of evidence-based interventions. The framework was developed via a systematic review of the literature and initially tested by coding 32 published articles that described interventions implemented in routine practice settings. This coding system can be used to complement research on fidelity and help advance understanding of how intervention modifications impact their implementation.

Bernal G, Domenech Rodriguez MM. Cultural adaptation in context: Psychotherapy as a historical account of adaptations. In: Bernal & Domenech Rodriguez, ed. *Cultural adaptations: Tools for evidence-based practice with diverse populations*. Washington, DC: American Psychology Association Press; 2012:3–22.

This book describes the history of the cultural adaptation field, frameworks, and guidelines for cultural adaptation, including their applications in the field of health and mental health and a discussion about bridging the gap between research and practice from the perspective of the cultural adaptation field.

Selected Websites and Tools

https://pbrn.ahrq.gov/events/using-rapid-cycle-research-reach-goals-awareness-assessment-adaptation-acceleration-resource

This is a webinar supported by the Agency for Healthcare Research and Quality, delivered by Drs. Gustafson and Johnson. The webinar titled "Using rapid-cycle research to reach goals: Awareness, assessment, adaptation, acceleration—a resource document" describes methods for identifying problems and solving issues using a rapid cycle research

https://cancercontrol.cancer.gov/use_what_works/start.htm

This is a set of materials organized by the National Cancer Institute with four modules: (1) What do we mean by evidence-based?, (2) Needs Assessment, (3) Finding an evidence-based program, (4) Making the evidence-based program fit your needs: adaptation and your program summary, (5) Does it work? Module 4 contains an adaptation guideline and recommendations for pilot testing.

REFERENCES

1. Paul GL. Strategy of outcome research in psychotherapy. *J Consult Psychol*. 1967;31(2):109. http://dx.doi.org/10.1037/h0024436

2. National Institutes of Mental Health. *The National Institute of Mental Health Strategic Plan*; 2015.

http://www.nimh.nih.gov/about/strategic-plan-ning-reports/index.shtml

3. National Research Council and Institute of Medicine. *Preventing mental, emotional, and behavioral disorders among young people: progress and possibilities.* Washington, DC: The National Academies Press; 2009. http://www.nap.edu/catalog/12480/preventing-mental-emotional-and-behavioral-disorders-among-young-people-progress

4. Bernal G, Domenech Rodriguez MM. Cultural adaptation in context: Psychotherapy as a historical account of adaptations. In: Bernal & Domenech Rodriguez, ed. *Cultural adaptations: Tools for evidence-based practice with diverse populations.* Washington, DC: American Psychology Association Press; 2012:3–22.

5. Cabassa LJ, Baumann AA. A two-way street: Bridging implementation science and cultural adaptations of mental health treatments. *Implement Sci.* 2013;8:90. doi: 10.1186/1748-5908-8-90.

6. Aarons GA, Miller EA, Green AE, Perrott JA, Bradway, R. Adaptation happens: A qualitative case study of implementation of The Incredible Years evidence-based parent training programme in a residential substance abuse treatment. *J Child Serv.* 2012;4:233–245. doi: 10.1108/17466661211286463.

7. Graham PW, Kim MM, Clinton-Sherrod AM, et al. What is the role of culture, diversity, and community engagement in transdisciplinary translational science? *Transl Behav Med.* December 2015. doi: 10.1007/s13142-015-0368-2.

8. Bernal G, Bonilla J, Bellido C. Ecological validity and cultural sensitivity for outcome research: issues for the cultural adaptation and development of psychosocial treatments with Hispanics. *J Abnorm Child Psychol.* 1995;23(1):67–82. doi: 10.1007/BF01447045

9. Wiltsey Stirman S, A Gutner C, Crits-Christoph P, Edmunds J, Evans AC, Beidas RS. Relationships between clinician-level attributes and fidelity-consistent and fidelity-inconsistent modifications to an evidence-based psychotherapy. *Implement Sci.* 2015;10(1). doi: 10.1186/s13012-015-0308-z

10. Chambers DA, Norton WE. The adaptome: advancing the science of intervention adaptation. *Am J Prev Med.* 2016;51(4):S124–S131. doi: 10.1016/j.amepre.2016.05.011.

11. Baumann AA, Powell BJ, Kohl PL, et al. Cultural adaptation and implementation of evidence-based parent-training: a systematic review and critique of guiding evidence. *Child Youth Serv Rev.* 2015;53:113–120. doi: 10.1016/j.childyouth.2015.03.025.

12. Atkins M, Rusch D, Mehta TG, Lakind D. Future directions for dissemination and implementation science: aligning ecological theory and public health to close the research to practice gap. *J Clin Child Adolesc Psychol.* 2015;0:1–12. doi: 10.1080/15374416.2015.1050724.

13. Tanenbaum SJ. Evidence-Based Practice as mental health policy: three controversies and a caveat. *Health Aff (Millwood).* 2005;24(1):163–173. doi: 10.1377/hlthaff.24.1.163.

14. Raghavan R. The role of economic evaluation in dissemination and implementation research. *Dissem Implement Res Health Transl Sci Pract.* 2012:94–113.

15. Alegria M, Atkins M, Farmer E, Slaton E, Stelk W. One size does not fit all: taking diversity, culture and context seriously. *Adm Policy Ment Health.* 2010;37(1-2):48–60. doi: 10.1007/s10488-010-0283-2.

16. Donovick M, Rodríguez MMD. Parenting practices among first generation Spanish-speaking Latino families: a Spanish version of the Alabama Parenting Questionnaire. *Grad Stud J Psychol.* 2008;10:52–63.

17. Kotchick BA, Forehand R. Putting parenting in perspective: a discussion of the contextual factors that shape parenting practices. *J Child Fam Stud.* 2002;11(3):255–269. doi: 10.1023/A:1016863921662

18. Domenech Rodriguez MM, Baumann AA, Schwartz AL. Cultural adaptation of an evidence based intervention: from theory to practice in a Latino/a community context. *Am J Community Psychol.* 2011;47(1-2):170–186. doi: 10.1007/s10464-010-9371-4

19. Parra-Cardona JR, Bybee D, Sullivan CM, et al. Examining the impact of differential cultural adaptation with Latina/o immigrants exposed to adapted parent training interventions. *J Consult Clin Psychol.* 2017;85(1):58–71. doi: 10.1037/ccp0000160.

20. HHS. National Partnership for Action to End Health Disparities: Offices of Minority Health. https://minorityhealth.hhs.gov/npa/templates/browse.aspx?lvl=1&lvlid=34; 2011. Accessed December 27, 2016.

21. National Center for Health Statistics. *Health, United States, 2015: In Brief.* Hyattsville, M. D.: Health; 2016. https://www.cdc.gov/nchs/data/hus/hus15_inbrief.pdf. Accessed December 27, 2016.

22. Erves JC, Mayo-Gamble TL, Malin-Fair A, et al. Needs, Priorities, and recommendations for engaging underrepresented populations in clinical research: a community perspective. *J Community Health.* November 2016. doi: 10.1007/s10900-016-0279-2.

23. Santiago C DeCarlo, Miranda J. Progress in improving mental health services for racial-ethnic

minority groups: a ten-year perspective. *Psychiatr Serv.* 2014;65:180–185. http://dx.doi.org/10.1176/appi.ps.201200517

24. U.S. Census Bureau, Population Division. *Annual estimates of the resident population by sex, race, and hispanic origin for the United States, states, and counties: April 1, 2010 to July 1, 2014.* Washington, DC: Author; 2015.

25. Gatzke-Kopp LM. Diversity and representation: Key issues for psychophysiological science: diversity and representation. *Psychophysiology.* 2016;53(1):3–13. doi: 10.1111/psyp.12566.

26. Agran M, Spooner F, Singer GHS. Evidence-based practices. *Res Pract Pers Sev Disabil.* 2017;42(1):3–7. doi: 10.1177/1540796916685050

27. Wang M, Lam Y. Evidence-based practice in special education and cultural adaptations. *Res Pract Pers Sev Disabil.* 2017;42(1):53–61. doi: 10.1177/1540796916685872

28. Bastida EM, Tseng T-S, McKeever C, Jack L. Ethics and community-based participatory research: perspectives from the field. *Health Promot Pract.* 2010;11(1):16–20. doi: 10.1177/1524839909352841

29. Baumann AA, Domenech Rodriguez M, Parra-Cardona R. Community-based applied research with Latino immigrant families: informing practice and research according to ethical and social justice principles. *Fam Process.* 2011;50:132–148. doi: 10.1111/j.1545-5300.2011.01351.x

30. Hodge LM, Turner KMT. Sustained implementation of evidence-based programs in disadvantaged communities: a conceptual framework of supporting factors. *Am J Community Psychol.* 2016;58(1-2):192–210. doi: 10.1002/ajcp.12082

31. Aisenberg E. Evidence-based practice in mental health care to ethnic minority communities: has its practice fallen short of its evidence? *Soc Work.* 2008;53(4):297–306. https://doi.org/10.1093/sw/53.4.297

32. Cabassa LJ. Implementation Science: why it matters for the future of social work. *J Soc Work Educ.* 2016;52:S38–S50.

33. Weisz JR, Ng MY, Bearman SK. Odd Couple? Reenvisioning the relation between science and practice in the dissemination-implementation era. *Clin Psychol Sci.* 2014;2(1):58–74. doi: 10.1177/2167702613501307

34. Stirman SW, Miller CJ, Toder K, Calloway A. Development of a framework and coding system for modifications and adaptations of evidence-based interventions. *Implement Sci.* 2013;8. doi: 10.1186/1748-5908-8-65

35. Cook JM, Dinnen S, Thompson R, Ruzek J, Coyne JC, Schnurr PP. A Quantitative Test of an Implementation Framework in 38 VA Residential PTSD Programs. *Adm Policy Ment Health Ment Health Serv Res.* 2015;42(4):462–473. doi: 10.1007/s10488-014-0590-0.

36. Elliott DS, Mihalic S. Issues in disseminating and replicating effective prevention programs. *Prev Sci.* 2004;5(1):47–53. doi: 10.1023/B:PREV.0000013981.28071.52

37. Hogue A, Ozechowski TJ, Robbins MS, Waldron HB. Making fidelity an intramural game: localizing quality assurance procedures to promote sustainability of evidence-based practices in usual care. *Clin Psychol Sci Pract.* 2013;20(1):60–77. doi: 10.1111/cpsp.12023

38. Chambers DA, Glasgow RE, Stange KC. The dynamic sustainability framework: addressing the paradox of sustainment amid ongoing change. *Implement Sci.* 2013;(8):117–128. doi: 10.1186/1748-5908-8-117

39. Rogers E. *Diffusion of innovations.* 5th ed. New York: Free Press; 2003.

40. Damschroder LJ, Aron DC, Keith RE, Kirsh SR, Alexander JA, Lowery JC. Fostering implementation of health services research findings into practice: a consolidated framework for advancing implementation science. *Implement Sci.* 2009;4(1):50. doi: 10.1186/1748-5908-4-50

41. Palinkas LA, Soydan H. New horizons of translational research and research translation in social work. *Res Soc Work Pr.* 2012;22(1):85–92. https://doi.org/10.1177/1049731511408738

42. Ferrer-Wreder L, Sundell K, Mansoory S. Tinkering with perfection: theory development in the intervention cultural adaptation field. *Child Youth Care Forum.* 2012;41(2):149–171. doi: 10.1007/s10566-011-9162-6

43. Carroll M. Supervision: critical reflection for transformational learning (Part 2). *Clin Superv.* 2010;29(1):1–19. doi: 10.1080/07325221003730301

44. Forgatch MS, Patterson GR, DeGarmo DS. Evaluating fidelity: predictive validity for a measure of competent adherence to the Oregon model of parent management training. *Behav Ther.* 2006;36(1):3–13. http://dx.doi.org/10.1016/S0005-7894(05)80049-8

45. Barrera M, Berkel C, Castro FG. Directions for the advancement of culturally adapted preventive interventions: local adaptations, engagement, and sustainability. *Prev Sci.* September 2016. doi: 10.1007/s11121-016-0705-9

46. Aarons GA, Green AE, Palinkas LA, et al. Dynamic adaptation process to implement an evidence-based child maltreatment intervention. *Implement Sci.* 2012;7(1):32. doi: 10.1186/1748-5908-7-32

47. Lau AS. Making the case for selective and directed cultural adaptations of evidence-based treatments: examples from parent training. *Clin Psychol Sci Pract*. 2006;13(4):295–310. doi: 10.1111/j.1468-2850.2006.00042.x

48. Barrera M, Castro FG. A heuristic framework for the cultural adaptation of interventions. *Clin Psychol Sci Pr*. 2006;13(4):311–316. doi: 10.1111/j.1468-2850.2006.00043.x

49. Resnicow K, Baranowski T, Ahluwalia JS, Braithwaite RL. Cultural sensitivity in public health: defined and demystified. *Ethn Dis*. 1999;9(1):10–21.

50. Stanton B, Guo J, Cottrell L, et al. The complex business of adapting effective interventions to new populations: an urban to rural transfer. *J Adolesc Health*. 2005;37(2):163. doi: 10.1016/j.jadohealth.2004.10.005

51. Kalichman SC, Kelly JA, Hunter TL, Murphy DA, Tyler R. Culturally tailored HIV-AIDS risk-reduction messages targeted to African-American urban women: impact on risk sensitization and risk reduction. *J Consult Clin Psychol*. 1993;61(2):291–295. doi: 10.1037/0022-006X.61.2.291

52. Lau, A., Barnett, M., Stadnick, N., Saifan, D. Regan, J., Stirman, SW, Brookman-Frazee, L. Therapist report of adaptations to delivery of evidence-based practices within a system-driven reform of publicly-funded children's mental health services. J Consult Clin Psychol. 2017;85(7):664–675.

53. Bass JK, Annan J, McIvor Murray S, et al. Controlled trial of psychotherapy for Congolese survivors of sexual violence. *N Engl J Med*. 2013;368(23):2182–2191. doi: 10.1056/NEJMoa1211853

54. Kaysen D, Lindgren K, Zangana GAS, Murray L, Bass J, Bolton P. Adaptation of cognitive processing therapy for treatment of torture victims: experience in Kurdistan, Iraq. *Psychol Trauma Theory Res Pract Policy*. 2013;5(2):184–192. doi: 10.1037/a0026053

55. Baumann AA, Domenech Rodriguez MM, Amador Buenabad N, Forgatch MS. Parent Management Training-Oregon model (PMTO) in Mexico City: integrating cultural adaptation activities in an implementation model. *Clin Psychol Sci Pract*. 2014;21:32–47. doi: 10.1111/cpsp.12059

56. Barrera M, Castro FG, Strycker LA, Toobert DJ. Cultural adaptations of behavioral health interventions: a progress report. *J Consult Clin Psychol*. 2013;81(2):196–205. http://dx.doi.org/10.1037/a0027085

57. Kreuter MW, Haughton LT. Integrating culture into health information for African American women. *Am Behav Sci*. 2006;49(6):794–811. https://doi.org/10.1177/0002764205283801

58. Kreuter MW, Lukwago SN, Bucholtz DC, Clark EM, Sanders-Thompson V. Achieving cultural appropriateness in health promotion programs: targeted and tailored approaches. *Health Educ Behav*. 2003;30(2):133–146. doi: 10.1177/1090198102251021

59. Forgatch MS, Patterson GR, Gerwitz AH. Looking forward: the promise of widespread implementation of parent training programs. *Perspect Psychol Sci*. 2013;86:682–694. doi: 10.1177/1745691613503478

60. Cabassa LJ, Gomes AP, Meyreles Q, et al. Using the collaborative intervention planning framework to adapt a health-care manager intervention to a new population and provider group to improve the health of people with serious mental illness. *Implement Sci IS*. 2014;9:178. doi: 10.1186/s13012-014-0178-9

61. Cabassa LJ, Druss B, Wang Y, Lewis-Fernandez R. Collaborative planning approach to inform the implementation of a healthcare manager intervention for Hispanics with serious mental illness: a study protocol. *Implement Sci*. 2011;6:80. doi: 10.1186/1748-5908-6-80

62. Bartholomew LK, Parcel GS, Kok G, Gottlieb NH. *Intervention mapping: designing theory and evidencebased health promotion programs*. San Francisco: Jossey-Bass Publishers; 2006.

63. Rabin BA, Lewis CC, Norton WE, et al. Measurement resources for dissemination and implementation research in health. *Implement Sci*. 2016;11(1):1–9. doi: 10.1186/s13012-016-0401-y

64. Mejia A, Leijten P, Lachman JM, Parra-Cardona JR. Different strokes for different folks? contrasting approaches to cultural adaptation of parenting interventions. *Prev Sci*. June 2016. doi: 10.1007/s11121-016-0671-2

65. Parra Cardona JR, Domenech-Rodriguez M, Forgatch M, et al. Culturally adapting an evidence-based parenting intervention for latino immigrants: the need to integrate fidelity and cultural relevance. *Fam Process*. 2012;51(1):56–72. doi: 10.1111/j.1545-5300.2012.01386.x

66. Vaughn-Coaxum RA, Mair P, Weisz JR. Racial/ethnic differences in youth depression indicators: an item response theory analysis of symptoms reported by White, Black, Asian, and Latino Youths. *Clin Psychol Sci*. 2016;4(2):239–253. doi: 10.1177/2167702615591768

67. Proctor EK, Silmere H, Raghavan R, et al. Outcomes for implementation research: conceptual distinctions, measurement challenges, and research agenda. *Adm Policy Ment Health Ment Health Serv Res*. 2011;38:65–76. doi: 10.1007/s10488-010-0319-7

68. Costigan CL, Bardina P, Cauce AM, Kim GK, Latendresse SJ. Inter- and intra-group variability in perceptions of behavior among Asian Americans and European Americans. *Cultur Divers Ethnic Minor Psychol.* 2006;12(4):710–724. doi: 10.1037/1099-9809.12.4.710

69. Gonzales NA, Cauce AM, Mason CA. Interobserver agreement in the assessment of parental behavior and parent-adolescent conflict: African American mothers, daughters, and independent observers. *Child Dev.* 1996;67(4):1483–1498. doi: 10.1111/j.1467-8624.1996.tb01809.x

70. Yasui M, Dishion TJ. Direct observation of family management: validity and reliability as a function of coder ethnicity and training. *Behav Ther.* 2008;39(4):336–347. http://dx.doi.org/10.1016/j.beth.2007.10.001

71. Scott K, Lewis CC. Using measurement-based care to enhance any treatment. *Cogn Behav Pract.* 2015;22(1):49–59. http://dx.doi.org/10.1016/j.cbpra.2014.01.010

72. Fortney JC, Unützer J, Wrenn G, et al. A tipping point for measurement-based care. *Psychiatr Serv.* 2016:appi–ps. http://dx.doi.org/10.1176/appi.ps.201500439

73. Lambert MJ, Whipple JL, Vermeersch DA, et al. Enhancing psychotherapy outcomes via providing feedback on client progress: a replication. *Clin Psychol Psychother.* 2002;9(2):91–103. doi: 10.1002/cpp.324

74. Jensen-Doss A, Haimes EMB, Smith AM, et al. Monitoring treatment progress and providing feedback is viewed favorably but rarely used in practice. *Adm Policy Ment Health Ment Health Serv Res.* 2016. doi: 10.1007/s10488-016-0763-0

75. Bell EC, Marcus DK, Goodlad JK. Are the parts as good as the whole? A meta-analysis of component treatment studies. *J Consult Clin Psychol.* 2013;81(4):722–736. doi: 10.1037/a0033004

76. Almirall D, Chronis-Tuscano A. Adaptive interventions in child and adolescent mental health. *J Clin Child Adolesc Psychol.* 2016;45(4):383–395. doi: 10.1080/15374416.2016.1152555

77. Chow S-C, Chang M. Adaptive design methods in clinical trials—a review. *Orphanet J Rare Dis.* 2008;3(1):11. doi: 10.1186/1750-1172-3-11

78. Sherrill JT. Adaptive treatment strategies in youth mental health: a commentary on advantages, challenges, and potential directions. *J Clin Child Adolesc Psychol.* 2016;45(4):522–527. doi: 10.1080/15374416.2016.1169539

79. Chow S-C. Adaptive clinical trial design. *Annu Rev Med.* 2014;65(1):405–415. doi: 10.1146/annurev-med-092012-112310

80. Buscemi J, Janke EA, Kugler KC, et al. Increasing the public health impact of evidence-based interventions in behavioral medicine: new approaches and future directions. *J Behav Med.* 2017;40(1):203–213. doi: 10.1007/s10865-016-9773-3

81. Cook JW, Collins LM, Fiore MC, et al. Comparative effectiveness of motivation phase intervention components for use with smokers unwilling to quit: a factorial screening experiment: components for smokers unwilling to quit. *Addiction.* 2016;111(1):117–128. doi: 10.1111/add.13161

82. Schlam TR, Fiore MC, Smith SS, et al. Comparative effectiveness of intervention components for producing long-term abstinence from smoking: a factorial screening experiment: producing long-term abstinence from smoking. *Addiction.* 2016;111(1):142–155. doi: 10.1111/add.13153

83. Collins LM, Murphy SA, Strecher V. The Multiphase Optimization Strategy (MOST) and the Sequential Multiple Assignment Randomized Trial (SMART). *Am J Prev Med.* 2007;32(5):S112–S118. doi: 10.1016/j.amepre.2007.01.022

84. Lyon AR, Koerner K. User-centered design for psychosocial intervention development and implementation. *Clin Psychol Sci Pract.* 2016;23:180–200. doi: 10.1111/cpsp.12154

85. Courage C, Baxter K. *Understanding your users: A practical guide to user requirements methods, tools, and techniques.* San Francisco: Morgan Kaufmann Publishers Inc.; 2004.

86. Howe GW, Beach SRH, Brody GH. Microtrial methods for translating gene-environment dynamics into preventive interventions. *Prev Sci.* 2010;11(4):343–354. doi: 10.1007/s11121-010-0177-2

87. Leijten P, Dishion TJ, Thomaes S, Raaijmakers MA, Orobio de Castro B, Matthys W. Bringing parenting interventions back to the future: how randomized microtrials may benefit parenting intervention efficacy. *Clin Psychol Sci Pract.* 2015;22(1):47–57. doi: 10.1111/cpsp.12087

88. Leijten P, Thomaes S, Orobio de Castro B, Dishion TJ, Matthys W. What good is labeling what's good? A field experimental investigation of parental labeled praise and child compliance. *Behav Res Ther.* 2016;87:134–141. doi: 10.1016/j.brat.2016.09.008

89. Tate DF, Lytle LA, Sherwood NE, et al. Deconstructing interventions: approaches to studying behavior change techniques across obesity interventions. *Transl Behav Med.* 2016;6(2):236–243. doi: 10.1007/s13142-015-0369-1

90. Belle SH, Stevens J, Cella D, et al. Overview of the obesity intervention taxonomy and pooled analysis working group. *Transl Behav Med.* 2016;6(2):244–259. doi: 10.1007/s13142-015-0365-5

91. Bangdiwala SI, Bhargava A, O'Connor DP, et al. Statistical methodologies to pool across multiple intervention studies. *Transl Behav Med.* 2016;6(2):228–235. doi: 10.1007/s13142-016-0386-8

92. Rith-Najarian LR, Daleiden EL, Chorpita BF. Evidence-based decision making in youth mental health prevention. *Am J Prev Med.* 2016;51(4):S132–S139. doi: 10.1016/j.amepre.2016.05.018

93. Palinkas LA, Aarons GA, Horwitz S, Chamberlain P, Hurlburt M, Landsverk J. Mixed method designs in implementation research. *Adm Policy Ment Health Ment Health Serv Res.* 2011;38(1):44–53. doi: 10.1007/s10488-010-0314-z

94. Powell BJ, McMillen JC, Proctor EK, et al. A compilation of strategies for implementing clinical innovations in health and mental health. *Med Care Res Rev.* 2012;69(2):123–157. doi: 10.1177/1077558711430690

95. Kilbourne AM, Abraham KM, Goodrich DE, et al. Cluster randomized adaptive implementation trial comparing a standard versus enhanced implementation intervention to improve uptake of an effective re-engagement program for patients with serious mental illness. *Implement Sci.* 2013;8(1):1. doi: 10.1186/1748-5908-8-136

96. Proctor EK, Powell BJ, McMillen JC. Implementation strategies: recommendations for specifying and reporting. *Implement Sci.* 2013;8:139. doi: 10.1186/1748-5908-8-139.

97. Rubin RM, Hurford MO, Hadley T, Matlin S, Weaver S, Evans AC. Synchronizing watches: the challenge of aligning implementation science and public systems. *Adm Policy Ment Health Ment Health Serv Res.* 2016;43(6):1023–1028. doi: 10.1007/s10488-016-0759-9

18

Furthering Dissemination and Implementation Research

The Need for More Attention to External Validity

LAWRENCE W. GREEN AND MONA NASSER

INTRODUCTION

Channels and tools of dissemination have become ever more efficient (though not necessarily effective), accessible, and omnipresent in their indexing, distributing, and searching capacity. Practitioners seldom complain anymore that they can find nothing to read on their issue at hand, unless it is a truly emergent disease, condition, population, or setting. They complain, if at all, that the literature is overwhelmingly voluminous and often dubiously related to their own setting, problem, or population. They seem to be saying that they are drowning in information but starved for relevance. Increasingly, systematic reviews of public health interventions (e.g., the Guide to Community Preventive Services) provide an array of viable intervention options and synthesize the essence of numerous original studies and their relative strength of evidence. The problem may be less with disseminating systematic reviews than with relevance of the original research for health practice or policy. The authors heartily endorse the suggestion in another chapter in this book (chapter 11) that this problem could be addressed in part with the development of a system of channels linking the generation of original research (not just its synthesis) with the end-user practitioners,[1] and emphasizing "best processes" as much as "best practices."[2,3]

A related perspective of this chapter questions the assumption that greater rigor or scientific control increases the certainty that the studies available demonstrate that intervention X will cause the change in outcome Y when applied in other settings, populations, or circumstances.[4] Overriding the set of considerations of experimental design and statistical certainty of causality, or "internal validity," when it comes to adopting and applying an intervention with "proven" efficacy is whether it was proved under circumstances and in populations like those in which one would consider applying the intervention. Indeed, we may have fallen into a trap in our excessive use of the words proof, proved, or proven to apply to what are essentially probabilistic and conditional relationships between X and Y, limited in their generalizability to the narrow range of populations, settings, treatment conditions, and outcomes originally sampled and observed.[4]

With these considerations, D & I research will do well to consider supplementing and complementing these now established sources of evidence-based practices with more practice-based evidence.[3-6] Until practitioners and policymakers see more evidence that is generated in circumstances like their own, they will remain skeptical of the applicability, relevance, and fit of the evidence. Even greater perceived relevance would be gained if the practice-based research were generated through more participatory research processes, with more engagement of representative end-users in specification of the research questions, setting-specific systems and variables, and interpretation of the research findings.[6]

This chapter has as its main objective to examine ways to tilt this balance of emphasis for D & I research from studies with exquisite internal validity to a greater emphasis on external validity. It offers, as the essential core of the D & I research strategy to do this, an approach that (1) engages practitioners or policymakers more actively in the research process, and (2) asks not how can we get practitioners to adopt and implement evidence (with "fidelity" to the form of intervention in the original studies), but how can we study the adaptations and innovations that emerge from their attempts to do so, and what are the trade-offs between the original efficacy-tested forms of interventions and the adapted forms.

WHAT IS EXTERNAL VALIDITY?

Rothwell captured the problem most tersely and compellingly with his finding that "Lack of consideration of external validity is the most frequent criticism by clinicians of RCTs, systematic reviews, and guidelines"[7] Most of those clinicians might not have used the term "external validity" in expressing their criticism of the scientific literature on interventions, but for Rothwell it came down to that technical term in summarizing what the practitioners found lacking or problematic in the literature they were given to apply to their clinical practices. One hears this complaint at least as much, if not more, among public health professionals and policymakers, whose applications must be to even more diverse settings, populations, outcomes, and treatments:

1. Their treatments are usually more complex programs or policies rather than discrete, highly controlled interventions tested in most randomized trials.
2. Their populations more diverse insofar as they constitute a wider range of well and ill people, not just patients.
3. Their settings likely to have fewer resources and time to devote to the interventions and less training and supervision of intervention staff than in the experimental trials.

When we combine that perspective with the first perspective that dissemination is not the barrier to implementation, we are forced to consider whether more efficient dissemination of what practitioners find unusable is self-defeating.[8] We have cause for looking not so much down the science-to-practice pipeline at the failure of practitioners to take the final step to adoption and implementation, but rather up the pipeline at the production end of the science and the processes by which we vet the science through the pipeline. This chapter will acquaint the reader with the ways in which research is strengthened to meet the needs of scientists for internal validity and their peer review and systematic review processes, and the ways in which some of these processes undermine the external validity or relevance of

scientific results for the settings, populations, and circumstances in which they would be used.

Campbell and Stanley, in their classic work on *Experimental and Quasi-Experimental Designs for Research,*[9] distinguished internal validity from external validity, putting primary emphasis on internal validity as "the basic minimum without which any experiment is uninterpretable: Did in fact the experimental treatments make a difference in this specific experimental instance?" (p. 5). Campbell and Stanley go on to distinguish external validity as that which asks "To what populations, settings, treatment variables, and measurement variables can this effect be generalized?" (p. 5). They also acknowledge that "Both types of criteria are obviously important, even though . . . features increasing one may jeopardize the other" (p. 5). To be sure, one cannot expect much external validity without internal validity, and the plea in this chapter for more attention to external validity is not an appeal to sacrifice much internal validity to achieve it. But for applied health research, one must ask the "so what?" question if a study is airtight with its internal validity but has nowhere to go with its lack of external validity. The argument here is not to abandon the efficacy studies that establish internal validity, but to supplement them with more on-site, evaluative studies of the adaptation or substitution and implementation of components of the efficacy-tested interventions to make them fit local circumstances and to enhance their implementability.

External validity is one of two sources of generalizability of research. The other is *construct validity*. This is of more theoretical concern and refers to the degree to which the specific intervention, or the specific population sampled to study it, or the specific setting in which it was conducted, or the specific outcome measures, can be generalized to a more generic construction of any one of these concepts about the intervention, population, setting, or outcome.[10] It is a question of generalizing to the widest possible range of one or more of these elements of a study: types of people, types of settings, types of related outcomes measured, and types of intervention. For example, Egbert and colleagues[11] conducted a randomized controlled trial (RCT) in which the intervention patients were visited before their surgery by an anesthesiologist to explain what they should expect and what they could do postsurgically to minimize their symptoms and hasten their discharge. The reduction in hospital days before discharge was attributed to the rapport developed by the visit between a doctor and a patient. But the inference of that outcome might be generalizable to only some if any presurgical patient education delivered by any hospital staff member, or to any anesthesiologist visit to patients before surgery with a general anxiety-reducing or self-efficacy increasing message, or to the specific information imparted to the patient, which might have been by pamphlet or audio recording. Depending on further measurement of intermediate outcomes based on the theory used to develop the intervention, this study and its theory would have had stronger or weaker construct validity.

Constructs are the stuff of theorizing in that they describe an inference about cause and effect in a more general class of the objects or processes. The theory is confirmed or disconfirmed (not "proved" or disproved) by the study, and the theory is usually a highly generalized statement about the causal relationship or mechanism explaining the way treatment effects the outcome, with applicability across most if not all settings and populations. Insofar as theory development or testing is not the main purpose of this book, the focus here is on the other problem of generalizing from experimental studies—external validity.

External validity is concerned with whether a theoretical construct or an intervention based on it generalizes to most if not all units of people, treatments, observations, or settings. These are the four elements identified by Cronbach,[12] with the acronym "UTOS" of generalization: Units, Treatments, Outcomes, and Settings. External validity is concerned with whether a causal relationship can be expected to apply *across various (typical or representative) persons, settings, treatments, and outcomes*. It is the range of these that concerns external validity, and more so as the persons, settings, treatments, and outcomes of experiments become less representative of the "real-world" of the practitioners or policymakers who would apply the findings. As Cook and Campbell[13(p. 18)] have said, "Most experiments are highly localized and particularistic . . . but have general aspirations." If it were not the investigators of each experiment who aspired to generalization, the growing army of systematic review teams, meta-analytic reviewers, and "best practice" guideline producers seek to make the findings of multiple studies more generalizable by combining numerous cases of similar studies on the same class of treatment and outcome, but with variations in the units/populations, treatments, settings, and sometimes with different measures of the outcome.

SPECIFIC THREATS TO EXTERNAL VALIDITY

Mention was made of the classic distinction offered by Campbell and Stanley[9] among sources of invalidity in experiments. They identified eight threats to internal validity that can arise in the various generic evaluation designs, including three "pre-experimental" designs, three "true experimental" designs (p. 8), and eight "quasi-experimental" designs (pp. 40 & 56). For each of these 16 designs they also identify four threats to external validity that are either presented by the specific design or avoided by it. In a later edition Shadish, Cook, and Campbell[14] further divided the four threats into five.[14(pp. 86-93)] Here, paraphrased and highly condensed from Campbell and Stanley[13(pp. 16-22)] and from Shadish, Cook and Campbell[14(pp. 86-93)] are the threats to external validity, where X refers to the experimental intervention and its causal relationship to outcomes:

1. *Interaction of testing and X*: This refers to the ways in which a baseline or ongoing measurement ("testing" or observation before or during the experimental intervention) can cause the subjects of the experiment to be more prepared for, or more sensitive to, or more reactive to the intervention, and thus the results cannot be generalized to situations in which the intervention would not be accompanied by a pretest or other testing during the intervention. Physical exams, blood tests, written tests, interviews, questionnaires, and audio- or video-taping administered before or during an experimental intervention are usually sensitizing in ways that make generalization about the intervention invalid. This threat to validity could be especially biasing of results in dissemination or implementation studies insofar as the experimental subjects would be made more aware of the innovation to be adopted or implemented. With their focus on educational and social intervention evaluations, Campbell and his colleagues[14] would not have anticipated the extensive use made of pretests of many kinds in behavioral medicine, most of them sufficiently obtrusive, even invasive, as to surely

compromise the generalizability of results. Indeed, the demand by peer reviewers for baseline data to assure equivalence of experimental and control groups seems to have forgotten that equivalence of these groups was the main purpose of random assignment.

2. *Interaction of selection and X (interaction of units with the causal relationship)*: This threat to external validity refers to ways in which the sampling is not representative, screening might produce a further degradation of representativeness, and differential attrition or retention (especially between experimental and control groups) of subjects for the experiment or evaluation create a readiness or resistance to the intervention that biases the result toward or against the intervention. This has become a major concern with the increasingly controlled screening and selectivity of subjects for clinical studies seeking to minimize threats to internal validity by eliminating confounding factors associated with patients or subjects who have any complications (medical or social) that might interact with the relationship between X and the outcomes. This pursuit of homogeneity and simplicity of the profile of subjects makes for less complicated designs and statistical adjustments, but also makes the study results less generalizable. For an experiment requiring inconvenience for subjects or institutions in which they are to be found, the refusal of some to participate produces a biased sample of the universe of people or institutions to which one would want to generalize the results.

3. *Reactive arrangements (interaction of settings with the causal relationship)*: Besides testing, many of the other circumstances of experimentally controlled study settings and arrangements create a reactivity of subjects (and staff who would implement the intervention) that would not occur in normal circumstances to which the results are to be generalized. Informed consent requirements are just the beginning of a series of arrangements that produce either a "Hawthorne effect"

or an "I'm a guinea pig" response among subjects, a vigilance or a receptivity, a predisposition to behave as one assumes the researchers want one to behave. These reactive arrangements, combined with the preceding "interaction of selection with X" has led the authors to recommend that more of the scientific evaluation of innovations for D & I should be conducted within the routine and circumstances of normal, representative practice settings with representative practitioners as the deliverers of the X. More generally, an effect that is found in one setting might not generalize to other settings. Practice-based research helps but does not entirely solve this problem. The results will remain in need of further verification in other settings.

4. *Multiple-X interference (interaction of treatment variations with the causal relationship)*: This threat arises when the treatment cannot be replicated, cannot be adequately described, takes various forms with different personnel implementing them, or produce variations of effect with various combinations, dosages, or sequencing of the interventions. These situations arise with complex interventions, typical of public health or community interventions that pride themselves as having ecological robustness and systems thinking inherent in their construction. The ecological aspect means they recognize the necessity of intervening simultaneously at several levels of individual behavior, family or social norms and groups, organizations, and sometimes whole-community policy or environmental change. The systems aspect similarly recognizes that every system (e.g., a family or an organization) is a subsystem of another system, and that change in one will produce a feedback loop with adjustments and change in the other. Such interventions become more difficult to generalize in part because each of the components is interdependent with the others, and because they go quickly beyond the experimental control of the investigators who study them.

5. *Context-dependent mediation*: This added dimension of threats to external

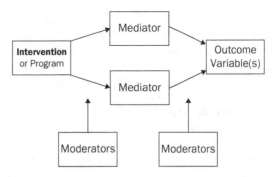

FIGURE 18.1 The place of mediating and moderating variables, the latter generally controlled rather than assessed in RCTs.

(Source: Green LW, Kreuter MW. *Health program planning: An educational and ecological approach.* 4th ed. New York: McGraw-Hill, 2005: 204.)

validity in Shadish et al.[14] acknowledges that studies of intervention effects seldom assume a direct relationship between interventions and outcomes, but rather mediated relationships. The mediating variables are transferring the effect of the intervention to the outcome, such as an educational intervention intended to affect behavior change through mediators of increased awareness of the action that is needed, knowledge of actions and how to take them, beliefs that the actions are important and effective, and possession of the ability and resources to take them. Each of these mediators may take on strength, depending on the context in which another set of variables, moderating variables, may influence the relationship between the intervention and the mediating variables and/or the relationship between the mediators and the outcomes, as shown in Figure 18.1. Moderators might be context-dependent variables such as the demographic and socioeconomic characteristics of the community or population in which the intervention is applied; the level of threat presented by the outcome in the community or population, and the availability of media to transmit the educational messages. If they are context dependent, the context in which the study of the intervention was conducted will determine how generalizable the results are to other contexts.

ALTERNATIVE WAYS TO GENERALIZE

Two ways in which studies can be made more generalizable are to assess them on two dimensions of external validity: (1) generalizability of alternative measures of the program or the outcomes and (2) generalizability to or across people, settings, and time.[13,14]

A much neglected and fruitful level of analysis to gain insight on external validity is on alternative or intermediate measures of the outcome, as in construct validity. This asks of a study whether the obtained results would occur if the program or the outcomes were measured in a different way, or the sampling design of the study had given it sufficient statistical power to detect significant differences between experimental and control groups on alternative outcomes. Studies that take multiple measures of the outcomes tend to do it based on a logic model for the program, with interventions shown to influence intermediate or mediating variables (such as behavioral or environmental changes), and from there to ultimate outcomes (such as health outcomes) as shown generically in 18.1. They tend to use the ultimate outcome, if possible, as the basis for setting a sample size sufficient to detect statistical differences between experimental and control groups. This sample size is often sufficient to assess the significance of differences on mediating variables as well (such as behavior change expected to lead to a health outcome), because the ultimate outcome has a lower probability of occurring than its determinants among the mediating variables within the time frame of most studies. But after publishing the main effects on the ultimate outcome, too many studies never get to the analysis or at least to the reporting of secondary analyses of effects on mediating variables. This is often because of space limitations and the preferences of journal editors.[15]

With D & I studies, the mediating and moderating variables have been extensively reviewed and catalogued by the late Everett Rogers over five editions of his book on *Diffusion of Innovations*.[16] The historical evolution of Rogers' theory is covered in chapter 3 of this text. The mediating and moderating variables can be summarized in the following adaptation showing the mediating variables in the arrows and the moderating variables in "prior conditions," the characteristics of the "decision-unit," and the characteristics of the "innovation" (Figure 18.2).

More attention in the studies of D & I to measuring each of these stages and their associated moderating variables would allow for greater interpretation of the generalizability of the study results, in addition to the ultimate outcome or end-point of interest.

The second form of external validity concerns generalizability across populations. This could be strengthened with systematic analyses of subgroups within a study or group of studies. This use of subgroup analysis within studies fell into disrepute especially after the vast and expensive NIH Multiple Risk-Factor Intervention Trial (MRFIT or Mister Fit) on cardiovascular risk reduction project of the 1970s obtained

disappointing aggregate results and the investigators set about examining subgroups within the study to see which groups benefitted or not, even though the average benefits were not statistically significant. An outcry arose from statisticians who objected to the subgroup analysis because the subgroups were not randomly assigned to the interventions. The technical truth in these objections obscures the waste of information when clear differences in outcomes between subgroups could lead to hypotheses, at least, and guides to practitioners at best on whether the results might apply to their population or subpopulations. It also denies the utility of the wide range of nonrandomized evaluations of programs and policies in real time and with situations that do not lend themselves to ethical or feasible random assignment. In short, applying this criterion to the legitimacy of subgroup analysis would eliminate from credibility all the literature based on quasi-experimental designs.[17-19] It would also preclude the closer inspection of results for subgroups of studies that were published with positive main effects comparing experimental and control groups. Examples are studies in which the significant main effects were examined further for comparison of the relative outcomes between low- and high-risk groups[20] and relative effects for different age groups.[21]

Another way in which past studies could serve more fruitfully to answer the applicability questions of practitioners and policymakers

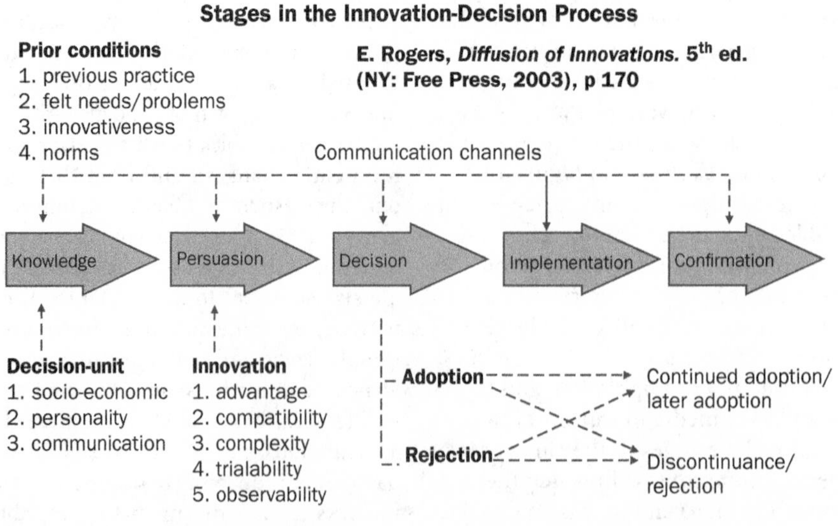

Stages in the Innovation-Decision Process

Prior conditions
1. previous practice
2. felt needs/problems
3. innovativeness
4. norms

E. Rogers, *Diffusion of Innovations*. 5th ed.
(NY: Free Press, 2003), p 170

Communication channels

Knowledge → Persuasion → Decision → Implementation → Confirmation

Decision-unit
1. socio-economic
2. personality
3. communication

Innovation
1. advantage
2. compatibility
3. complexity
4. trialability
5. observability

Adoption - - - - - - - → Continued adoption/later adoption

Rejection - - - - - - - → Discontinuance/rejection

FIGURE 18.2 Stages and influences in the innovation-decision-adoption-implementation-maintenance process.

(Source: Rogers E.[16])

that otherwise fail to get addressed in primary research is to ask what became of the people over a longer period than the primary studies were funded and originally planned to run. Often, such follow-up studies can be performed with death records, hospitalization records, school records, employee benefits or insurance claim records, primary care records in medical group plans such as Kaiser-Permanente, or linked medical records in the case of some jurisdictions in Canada, the United Kingdom, and other national health care systems. These systems preclude the necessity of pursuing the original study's subjects themselves, which is often too expensive or otherwise not feasible if many have died, or by informed consent limitations or other ethics rules. Examples of this are two other cases from the hypertension literature. One is the follow-up study by Morisky et al.[21] and Levine et al.[22,23] of the mortality in subjects of this randomized factorial design study on three hypertension control interventions. The original study showed reductions in blood pressure,[24,25] but the 5-year follow-up study was also able to show reductions in morbidity and mortality in the original study subjects who had been exposed to various combinations of the three interventions.[22]

A similar example of follow-up opportunities to answer practitioners' and policymakers' questions brings us back to the issue of subgroup analyses of the erstwhile MRFIT data, and follow-up opportunities that lie in such data sets when combined with other sources. Practitioners and policymakers are often challenged to defend their programs or proposed programs based on benefits beyond the specific disease it is intended to control. Hypertension is known to cause strokes and contributes to other cardiovascular diseases and deaths. Terry et al.[26] assessed the association of blood pressure with specific types of "accidental" death. They examined data from baseline interviews and 25 years of mortality follow-up (1973–1999) for 347,978 men screened for MRFIT, comparing associations of blood pressure with all external causes of death and individual causes. Men with stage 2 hypertension had nearly twice as many deaths from falls and nearly 1.5 times as many deaths from motor vehicle injuries.

The point of these examples is to illustrate ways to compensate for the absence of external validity in some studies, or to extend and squeeze some relevance and generalizability from them, where scientific concerns for internal validity has squeezed much of the relevance to practice

out of them. Until the priorities of research funding and publishing practices, and the demands of systematic reviews, all of which generally place a premium on internal validity at the expense of external validity, give greater attention to relevance of the research for practice and policy, these are ways to extract some relevance from them.

RELATED SOURCES AND SOLUTIONS OF THE EXTERNAL VALIDITY PROBLEM FOR D&I RESEARCH

Besides external validity in the strict sense defined earlier, many if not most of the research studies conducted with RCT designs that qualify them for systematic reviews and guidelines for evidence-based practice are conducted under such controlled (and often enriched) circumstances that they cannot be replicated or afforded in other settings or taken to scale in multiple, varied settings.

Two of the most prominent problems produced by excessive levels of control in RCTs relate to the inclusion and exclusion of units or subjects in the original studies. The studies are typically conducted in one setting, rather than in a random sample of settings. It is usually a setting over which the academic investigators have some control, such as clinics in the university's teaching hospital, or community settings in which the research grant provided funding for the interventions or evaluation such that the academic investigators could negotiate greater control over the training and supervision of those who would be the interventionists. The very act of agreeing to open the staff, patients, students, employees, or clients of an organization to the rigors of a controlled trial, especially a randomized controlled trial, makes that clinic, school, worksite, or other service-providing organization a special—possibly ungeneralizable—case. A remedy called "practical trials" has been proposed and now increasingly implemented to overcome this problem.[27] Practice-Based Research Networks have also developed standing arrangements for the experimental testing of new or routine practices in more natural medical, nursing and dental settings.[28] A growing emphasis on practice-based and participatory research among the Prevention Research Centers funded by the CDC has suggested ways to build greater reality testing and representativeness into multisite studies of D & I.[29]

Finally, a practice-based research emphasis on external validity with randomized trials can be pursued with systematic replication of trials in variable settings and populations. For example, after demonstrating the effectiveness of the Flu FOBT (fecal occult blood test kits distributed to general outpatients attending an influenza shot clinic) program in the San Francisco General Hospital, with significant increases in the use and submission of home fecal test specimens, and referrals for and completed colorectal exams in this underserved population,[30] the investigators replicated the trial (with appropriate adaptations) in a primary care clinic serving low-income Chinese Americans.[31] The repetition of positive results added to the external validity, but further replications in other settings and populations, each with appropriate adaptions to the organizational and population-specific needs, further strengthened the external validity and documented the types of adaptations needed in the varied settings and populations.[32]

The screening of subjects before random assignment to minimize confounding factors makes the samples of patients or subjects in most published studies further unrepresentative of the populations in which the interventions would be applied. They often eliminate patients, for example, who have multiple diagnoses or multiple risk factors. This exclusion is to minimize the confounding of the study results. Such homogenization of the study sample makes it unlike most of the patients or other populations to which one might wish to apply the treatment and to generalize the results. The problem of representativeness of the population sampled is compounded by the differential attrition or drop-out from experimental and control groups, especially when the experimental treatment requires effort or inconvenience from the subjects to the point that those who remain in the study to be measured at the end are not representative of the population enrolled, much less of other populations who might be enrolled under normal circumstances of care or prevention.

The homogeneity of the samples after screening and attrition adds another threat to external validity: most interventions in the "real world" will not be so restrictive in their responsiveness to the wider range of people eligible for, needing, or interested in the intervention, and the greater heterogeneity produced in the real-life samples changes the nature of the required intervention processes, forms, duration, or intensity. If a study of interventions to increase hypertension self-management, for example, eliminates from the study all the hypertension patients who also have diabetes, the results will not apply to the many hypertension patients in most clinical settings who have those two comorbidities.

The term "randomized controlled trials" refers neither to the random *sampling* of the population of units or people, nor to the random *sampling* of settings, but to the use of random *assignment* of units or subjects within the cooperating units or settings to experimental and control groups. This distinction between random sampling and random assignment is not lost on practitioners who often look first to the setting and population of the study to decide whether it is relevant to their own practice. When they look for more detail on the setting and population, or if satisfied with those as relevant, more detail on the description of the intervention, they are often disappointed to find too little detail to make an informed decision on whether the intervention and its results apply to their setting, population, and resources. Health science journals and their editors have tended, when print space limits are exceeded, to require cuts in some details of description of the intervention.

Many of the problems described are compounded when the interventions are complex, multilevel, and comprehensive and have other features known to be important to effective community- or population-level programs.[33] We can summarize these and other departures of the RCT circumstances in producing evidence for *population health interventions*, from the types of evidence needed in practice, in Table 18.1. The left column lists the widely acknowledged practice-based conditions that produce effective interventions (more likely programs and policies combined to produce a comprehensive set of synergistic interventions), and a matched list in the right column indicates what randomized controlled trials demand and produce. The conditions that produced the great public health successes with tobacco control in the last third of the 20th century, for example, were demonstrated with systematic evaluations of the statewide, comprehensive programs of California and Massachusetts. These states were not randomized, but their experience confirmed much of what was becoming the cumulative, practice-based wisdom of public health programs addressing the complex issues of lifestyle and social factors influencing population health. The nine characteristics of "Best Practices for Comprehensive Tobacco Control Programs" were compiled by the CDC

TABLE 18.1 THE IMPERATIVES OF POPULATION
HEALTH VS. RCT RULES OF EVIDENCE

The Imperatives of Population Health vs.
RCT Rules of Evidence

What We Know is Needed	What RCTs Often Seek & Test
• Comprehensive	• Isolation of independent variable
• Ecological	• Randomizable experimental units
• Upstream determinants	• Focus on proximal determinants
• Multi-sectoral intervention	• Intervention controlled
• Participatory	• Blinded, double-blinded . . .
• Adapted to cultures,	• Tests based on averages. Results
• contexts	• Standardized for everyone
• Tailored to individuals	• "Fidelity" to the tested form
• Professional discretion	• Protocol controlled
• Social justice	• Informed consent

from these states and others to produce a document by this name.[34]

But even at the clinical and other organizational levels of intervention, more comprehensive, ecological, upstream, multisectoral, participatory, culturally adapted, individually tailored, professionally guided, and socially just programs and interventions are generally found to be more effective, but difficult, and sometimes impossible, to evaluate using the strict criteria of RCTs.

HOW THE NEGLECT OF EXTERNAL VALIDITY RELATES TO D&I PRACTICE

The places and populations seen in diffusion theory and in D & I practice as hardest to reach, late adopters, and underserved, are often the ones underrepresented in much of the intervention research providing "evidence-based practices." The local decision-makers, program planners, and practitioners who would be expected as first-line adopters of the evidence find the undigested original research publications to have too little detail on the interventions (because of journal publication practices) to apply them systematically, much less to replicate them with "fidelity."[35] As Rothwell pointed out, ". . . researchers, funding agencies, ethics committees, the pharmaceutical industry, medical journals, and governmental regulators alike all neglect external validity, leaving clinicians to make judgments . . . [R]eporting of the determinants of external validity in trial publications and systematic reviews is usually inadequate."[7(p. 93)]

When described with greater detail on the intervention, the local would-be adopters find the studies often lacking in relevance or applicability to their population, patients, or practitioners, or to their local circumstances, resources, capabilities, or culture. They also find too little information on the numbers or proportion of eligible people who were or could be reached—not just how effective was the intervention with those who *were* reached and who agreed to participate in the study. They also find too little information on how acceptable the intervention is or was to the organization that must adopt it, and to the practitioners in that organization who must implement it, and how well it was maintained after adoption.

In an attempt to address these problems of reporting of original experimental studies in professional and scientific journals, a set of criteria based on the RE-AIM model (see chapter 16) were proposed [36] and a group of editors and associate editors of 13 leading professional health journals was convened to review the criteria and to consider possible ways to incorporate them into their guidelines to authors or peer review processes for their journal.[15] One, *Annals of Behavioral Medicine*, added referral to the methodology article[36] in its manuscript preparation guidelines for authors. Several indicated plans to increase their website pages to accommodate richer description of interventions. There is hope, then, that the publishing end of the pipeline is beginning to give increased attention to the need for authors of published articles to give greater description to the interventions and the methods for readers to judge the relevance and applicability of the findings of research for their actual practice population, setting, and interventions (Box 18.1).

Before publication, however, is the funding and conduct of the research. The journal editors the authors convened noted that unless the funding priorities and peer review of research grant applications provide for more attention to external validity in funded research, there would be little point in expecting the journals or their authors to report more on it. Priorities for federal funding have turned notably in the direction of greater attention to participatory research,[30] which should be expected to increase the relevance of the research to the needs of communities, practitioners, and policymakers (see chapter 10). The Robert Wood Johnson Foundation made community-based participatory research a requirement of its Clinical Scholars Program.[33] The CDC made community-based participatory research a central expectation of funding for its Prevention Research Centers, which also put an emphasis on making the research more practice based.[34]

Finally, there is the point downstream from publication in the research-to-practice pipeline where evidence from multiple individual studies are indexed, compiled, systematically reviewed, and recommendations derived for "evidence-based practice" guidelines for practitioners, program planners, and policymakers. These guidelines become the justification or requirement for funding of programs, thereby limiting funding to those interventions that can be shown to have this source justification. The systematic reviews have a history of development and institutionalization in the tradition of evidence-based medicine, which places its emphasis on internal validity, based on the *strength* of evidence. It less often reports data to judge the *weight* of evidence across settings, populations, and times that would bear on the applicability of the results of the systematic reviews.[36]

REGRESSION, CONSTRUCT VALIDITY AND EXTERNAL VALIDITY IN SYSTEMATIC REVIEWS OF HEALTH INTERVENTIONS

Systematic reviews provide a way of bringing together what is known from research using explicit and accountable methods.[37] A systematic approach toward considering construct validity and external validity can enhance the applicability of the systematic reviews in the later steps

of the research-to-practice pipeline. One such approach is to use more regression analysis with meta-analytic techniques in systematic reviews to understand and explain the heterogeneity in effects across subsets of the data. These could be especially informative in knowing where and with whom the effects are variously effective, rather than the usual point estimates that imply fixed effects of the interventions. This could address some of the external validity concerns and needs of practitioners and policymakers by adding a multistudy dimension to the subgroup analyses of individual studies, discussed elsewhere in this chapter, but often the multiple studies required for a metaregression analysis are not available. Even when they are, Hauck et al. "recommend that the primary analyses adjust for important prognostic covariates . . . to come as close as possible to the clinically most relevant subject-specific measure of treatment effect. Additional benefits would be . . . improved external validity. The latter is particularly relevant to meta-analyses."[38]

Construct Validity

The existing theoretical frameworks on the inference between cause and effect can help systematic reviewers in defining the purpose and the eligibility criteria of studies for the review. Besides quantitative studies, qualitative studies can help in defining how and why participants' characteristics or contextual factors can influence effectiveness and how broad or narrow the question should be.[39] For example, the Agency for Healthcare Research and Quality uses an "analytical framework" in their comparative effectiveness research program to provide an overview of the clinical concepts underlying the health topic.[40] Similarly, the Community Preventive Services Task Force develops a detailed logic model or "logic framework" to guide each systematic review and updates of previous reviews. These logic models identify the presumed sequence of determinants, interventions, and mediating and moderating variables, while distinguishing the connecting arrows between each pair of these according to whether that causal link was included in the review or not.[41] An example of such a logic model used to develop the review and published with the Task Force recommendations is shown in Figure 18.3.[42]

External Validity

As with primary research studies, systematic reviewers are presumed to have evaluated in their

BOX 18.1
GUIDELINES FOR CONDUCT AND REPORTING OF TRIALS TO ASSURE GREATER ATTENTION TO EXTERNAL VALIDITY

1. SETTINGS AND POPULATIONS

A. Participation: Are there analyses of the participation rate among potential (a) settings, (b) delivery staff, and (c) patients (consumers)?

B. Target audience: Is the intended target audience stated for adoption (at the intended settings such as worksites, medical offices, etc.) and application (at the individual level)?

C. Representativeness—Settings: Are comparisons made of the similarity of settings in a study to the intended target audience of program settings—or to those settings that decline to participate?

D. Representativenes—Individuals: Are analyses conducted of the similarity and differences between patients, consumers, or other subjects who participate versus either those who decline, or the intended target audience?

2. PROGRAM OR POLICY IMPLEMENTATION AND ADAPTATION

A. Consistent implementation: Are data presented on level and quality of implementation of different program components?

B. Staff expertise: Are data presented on the level of training or experience required to deliver the program or quality of implementation by different types of staff?

C. Program adaptation: Is information reported on the extent to which different settings modified or adapted the program to fit their setting?

D. Mechanisms: Are data reported on the process(es) or mediating variables through which the program or policy achieved its effects?

3. OUTCOMES FOR DECISION-MAKING

A. Significance: Are outcomes reported in a way that can be compared with either clinical guidelines or public health goals?

B. Adverse consequences: Do the outcomes reported include quality of life or potential negative outcomes?

C. Moderators: Are there any analyses of moderator effects—including of different subgroups of participants and types of intervention staff—to assess robustness versus specificity of effects?

D. Sensitivity: Are there any sensitivity analyses to assess dose-response effects, threshold level, or point of diminishing returns on the resources expended?

E. Costs: Are data on the costs presented? If so, are standard economic or accounting methods used to fully account for costs, including volunteer time?

4. TIME: MAINTENANCE AND INSTITUTIONALIZATION

A. Long-term effects: Are data reported on longer term effects, at least 12 months following treatment?

B. Institutionalization: Are data reported on the sustainability (or reinvention or evolution) of program implementation at least 12 months after the formal evaluation?

C. Attrition: Are data on attrition by condition reported, and are analyses conducted of the representativeness of those who drop out?

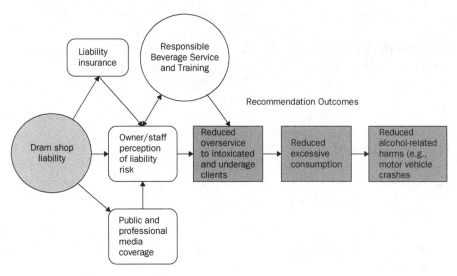

FIGURE 18.3 A logic model showing the variables included in a systematic review.

(Source: Task Force on Community Preventive Services.[42])

recommendations whether the causal relation from intervention to outcome is generalizable to different units, treatments, outcomes, and settings (UTOS). Currently no universal approach exists to deal with it, but reviewers can adjust in their review to achieve this:

1. *Using external validity tools to evaluate the conduct and reporting of the included research studies in a systematic review:* External validity tools can help reviewers assess the extent to which these UTOS dimensions are considered in the included primary trials and how it might affect the recommendation based on the synthesis of the trials. Tools vary from single question as part of a quality assessment tool or reporting checklist[42] to a validated comprehensive checklist for evaluating external validity of trials.[36] For example, Klesges et al. applied the Glasgow & Green tool[36] for external validity in a review of studies of childhood obesity prevention, examining dimensions of reach and representativeness, implementation and adaptation, outcomes of decision-making, and maintenance and institutionalization.[43] Depending on the question of the review, reviewers might also decide to develop a specific external validity tool for the research question of the review.[44]

2. *Differentiating pragmatic and explanatory trials:* Randomized trials can be differentiated as efficacy versus effectiveness trials or explanatory versus pragmatic trials. These refer to conducting trials under ideal testing environments and circumstances (efficacy or explanatory trials) versus conducting trials under usual situations. Although studies not purely one or another, reviewers could determine the position of the trial in the pragmatic-explanatory continuum in comparison with each other.[45]

3. *Exploring heterogeneity across population, setting, treatment variations, and outcomes:* Systematic reviews provide an opportunity to investigate the effectiveness of the intervention across different populations, contexts, treatment variations, and outcomes. Subgroup analyses[46] and metaregression are two quantitative methods to explore the heterogeneity across different groups; however, they have pitfalls and need to be carefully interpreted.

Individual-patient data meta-analysis can be an asset in exploring the interaction between interventions and patient-level characteristics. A Cochrane systematic review evaluating home safety education and provision of safety equipment for injury prevention accessed individual patient data for certain research studies and thereby could estimate not only a total summarized effect but also variations in the intervention effect across social variables, child age, gender, ethnic groups, single parent family, and measures of deprivation.[47,48]

Reviewers could also investigate the effect of intervention across different levels of disadvantage in groups and can inform programs aiming to reduce health inequalities. Disadvantaged groups can be identified, depending on the question of the review, by place of residence, race or ethnicity, occupation, gender, religion, education, socioeconomic position and social capital, sexual orientation, disability, or age.[49–51]

4. *Mediating factors in the interaction between intervention–outcome (context-dependent mediation and moderators).* Reviewers could identify and report potential contextual moderators and mediating factors on the causal relationship of intervention to outcomes, provide a framework on how they can change the intervention, and finally provide research evidence about such context and modifying factors.[52] For example, a Cochrane systematic review on the effect of pharmaceutical pricing and purchasing policies on drug use, health care utilization, health outcomes, and costs also listed a summary of factors that could affect reference pricing, like equivalence of the drug, incentives, and drug availability, and provide available evidence or a rational for them.[53–55]

SUMMARY

This chapter has raised questions about the reliability of much "evidence-based practice" disseminated from the original studies and systematic reviews of those studies, insofar as they were often conducted and reviewed with inadequate attention to external validity. Important issues are raised for D & I researchers. Indeed, the pressure on investigators to provide for increasingly rigorous controls on threats to internal validity, and to exclude studies that fall below standards for internal validity, has made many such sources of evidence more suspect in their external validity and less credible to the practitioners or policymakers who would adopt them. Dissemination of such evidence as "best practices" for application "with fidelity" in wide-ranging settings, populations, and circumstances may imply that local discretion and professional judgment in adapting such interventions should be suppressed. Greater attention is needed to ways to incorporate considerations of external validity into studies and in systematic reviews of studies to produce more generalizable evidence, and greater attention to practice-based evidence that can complement the more formal evidence-based practices in the process of implementing and evaluating the dissemination and implementation process.

SUGGESTED READINGS AND WEBSITES

Readings

Higgins JPT, Green S, eds. *Cochrane handbook for systematic reviews of interventions Version 5.1.0* (updated March 2011). The Cochrane Collaboration, 2011. Available from http://training.cochrane.org/handbook.
The method guide of the Cochrane Collaboration on how to synthesize data from primary trials in systematic reviews, it includes methods to deal with heterogeneity.

Lavis JN, Oxman AD, Souza NM, Lewin S, Gruen RL, Fretheim A. SUPPORT Tools for evidence-informed health policymaking (STP) 9: assessing the applicability of the findings of a systematic review. *Health Res Policy Syst.* 2009;7 Suppl 1:S9.
The article is part of a series of articles to help people responsible for making decisions about health policies and provide a guide on assessing the applicability of the findings of a systematic review to a specific setting.

Schünemann HJ, Fretheim A, Oxman AD. Improving the use of research evidence in guideline development: 13. Applicability, transferability and adaptation. *Health Res Policy Syst.* 2006;4:25.
A background paper on applicability, transferability and adaptation of guidelines for the World Health Organization (WHO) advisory committee on Health research.

Thorpe KE, Zwarenstein M, Oxman AD, Treweek S, Furberg CD, Altman DG, Tunis S, Bergel E, Harvey I, Magid DJ, Chalkidou K. A pragmatic-explanatory continuum indicator summary (PRECIS): a tool to help trial designers. *CMAJ.* 2009;180(10):E47–E57.
A tool to determine the extent to which a clinical trial is pragmatic or explanatory.

Tugwell P, Petticrew M, Kristjansson E, Welch V, Ueffing E, Waters E, Bonnefoy J, Morgan A, Doohan E, Kelly MP. Assessing equity in systematic reviews: realising the recommendations of the Commission on Social Determinants of Health. *BMJ.* 2010;341:c4739. doi: 10.1136/bmj.c4739

Guidance on assessing equity for users and authors of systematic reviews of interventions.

Welch V, Tugwell P, Petticrew M, de Montigny J, Ueffing E, Kristjansson B, McGowan J, Benkhalti Jandu M, Wells GA, Brand K, Smylie J. How effects on health equity are assessed in systematic reviews of interventions. *Cochrane Database Syst Rev.* 20108;12:MR000028.

A systematic review of methods to assess effects of health equity ins systematic reviews of effectiveness of health care interventions.

West SL, Gartlehner G, Mansfield AJ, et al. Comparative effectiveness review methods: Clinical heterogeneity. In: *Agency for Healthcare Research and Quality. comparative effectiveness review methods: Clinical heterogeneity.* Posted 09/28/2010. Rockville, MD. Available at http://effectivehealthcare.ahrq.gov/.

Summary and review of the current methods for addressing clinical heterogeneity in systematic reviews and comparative effectiveness research

Selected Websites and Tools

Cancer Control P.L.A.N.E.T. http://cancercontrolplanet.cancer.gov/index.html.

Cancer Control P.L.A.N.E.T. acts as a portal to provide access to data and resources for designing, implementing and evaluating evidence-based cancer control programs. The site provides five steps (with links) for developing a comprehensive cancer control plan or program.

Task Force on Community Preventive Services. http://www.thecommunityguide.org.

The Community Guide provides a repository of the 200 + systematic reviews conducted by the Task Force, an independent, interdisciplinary group with staff support by the Centers for Disease Control and Prevention. Each review gives attention to the "applicability" of the conclusions beyond the study populations and settings in which the original studies were conducted.

Cochrane Collaboration. http://www.cochrane.org/.

The Cochrane Collaboration prepares Cochrane Reviews and aims to update them regularly with the latest scientific evidence. Members of the organization (mostly volunteers) work together to assess evidence to help people make decisions about health care practices and policies. Some people read the health care literature to find reports of randomized controlled trials; others find such reports by searching electronic databases; others prepare and update Cochrane Reviews based on the evidence found in these trials; others work to improve the methods used in Cochrane Reviews; and others provide a vitally important consumer perspective.

RE-AIM. http://www.RE-AIM.org.

The acronym refers to Reach, Effectiveness, Adoption, Implementation, and Maintenance, all important dimensions in the consideration of D & I research and in the external validity or applicability of research results in original studies for the alternative settings and circumstances in which they might be applied.

REFERENCES

1. Minkler M, Salvatore AL, Chang C. Participatory approaches for study design and analysis in dissemination and implementation research. In Brownson RC, Colditz GA, Proctor EK, eds). *Dissemination and implementation research in health: Translating science to practice.* 2nd ed. New York: Oxford University Press, 2018.

2. Mercer SL, MacDonald G, Green LW. Participatory research and evaluation: from best practices for all states to achievable practices within each state in the context of the Master Settlement Agreement. *Health Promot Pract.* 2004;5(3 Suppl):167s-178s.

3. Green LW. From research to "best practices" in other settings and populations. *Am J Health Behav.* 2001;25(3):165–178.

4. Green LW. Public health asks of systems science: to advance our evidence-based practice, can you help us get more practice-based evidence? *Am J Public Health.* 2006;96(3):406–409.

5. Green LW, Ottoson JM, Garcia C, Hiatt RA. Diffusion theory and knowledge dissemination, utilization, and integration in public health. *Ann Rev Public Health.* 2009;30:151–174.

6. Ammerman A, Smith TW, Calancie L. Practice-based evidence in public health: improving reach, relevance, and results. *Ann Rev Public Health.* 2014;35:47–63.

7. Rothwell PM. External validity of randomised controlled trials: "to whom do the results of this trial apply?". *Lancet.* 2005;365(9453):82–93.

8. Ottoson J, Hawe PE. Knowledge utilization, diffusion, implementation, transfer, and translation: implications for evaluation. new directions in evaluation. *New Directions for Evaluation Winter.* 2009;124:7–20.

9. Campbell D, Stanley J. *Experimental and quasi-experimental designs for research.* Chicago: Rand McNally; 1963.

10. Cronbach L, Ambron S, Dornbusch S, et al. *Toward reform of program evaluation.* San Francisco: Jossey-Bass; 1980.

11. Egbert LD, Battit GE, Welch CE, Bartlett MK. Reduction of postoperative pain by encouragement and education of patients. A study of doctor-patient rapport. *N Engl J Med.* 1964;270:825–827.

12. Cronbach L. *Designing evaluations of educational and social programs.* San Francisco: Jossey-Bass; 1982.

13. Cook T, Campbell D. *Quasi-experimentation, design and analysis issues for field settings.* Chicago: Rand McNally; 1979.

14. Shadish W, Cook T, Campbell D. *Experimental and quasi-experimental designs for generalized causal inference.* Boston: Houghton Mifflin Co; 2002.

15. Green LW, Glasgow RE, Atkins D, Stange K. Making evidence from research more relevant, useful, and actionable in policy, program planning, and practice: slips "twixt cup and lip." *Am J Prev Med.* 2009;37(6 Suppl 1):S187–S191.

16. Rogers E. *Diffusion of innovations.* 5th ed. New York: Free Press; 2003.

17. Mercer SL, DeVinney BJ, Fine LJ, Green LW, Dougherty D. Study designs for effectiveness and translation research: identifying trade-offs. *Am J Prev Med.* 2007;33(2):139–154.

18. Sanson-Fisher RW, Bonevski B, Green LW, D'Este C. Limitations of the randomized controlled trial in evaluating population-based health interventions. *Am J Prev Med.* 2007;33(2):155–161.

19. Hawkins NG, Sanson-Fisher RW, Shakeshaft A, D'Este C, Green LW. The multiple baseline design for evaluating population-based research. *Am J Prev Med.* 2007;33(2):162–168.

20. Morisky DE, Levine DM, Green LW, et al. The relative impact of health education for low- and high-risk patients with hypertension. *Prev Med.* 1980;9(4):550–558.

21. Morisky DE, Levine DM, Green LW, Smith CR. Health education program effects on the management of hypertension in the elderly. *Arch Intern Med.* 1982;142(10):1835–1838.

22. Morisky DE, Levine DM, Green LW, Shapiro S, Russell RP, Smith CR. Five-year blood pressure control and mortality following health education for hypertensive patients. *Am J Public Health.* 1983;73(2):153–162.

23. Levine DM, Green LW, Morisky D. Effect of a structured health education program on reducing morbidity and mortality from high blood pressure. *Bibl Cardiol.* 1987(42):8–16.

24. Levine DM, Green LW, Deeds SG, Chwalow J, Russell RP, Finlay J. Health education for hypertensive patients. *JAMA.* 1979;241(16):1700–1703.

25. Green LW, Levine DM, Wolle J, Deeds S. Development of randomized patient education experiments with urban poor hypertensives. *Patient Couns Health Educ.* 1979;1(3):106–111.

26. Terry PD, Abramson JL, Neaton JD. Blood pressure and risk of death from external causes among men screened for the Multiple Risk Factor Intervention Trial. *Am J Epidemiol.* 2007;165(3):294–301.

27. Tunis SR, Stryer DB, Clancy CM. Practical clinical trials: increasing the value of clinical research for decision making in clinical and health policy. *JAMA.* 2003;290(12):1624–1632.

28. Green LA, Hickner J. A short history of primary care practice-based research networks: from concept to essential research laboratories. *J Am Board Fam Med: JABFM.* 2006;19(1):1–10.

29. Katz DL, Murimi M, Gonzalez A, Njike V, Green LW. From controlled trial to community adoption: the multisite translational community trial. *Am J Public Health.* 2011;101(8):e17–e27.

30. Potter MB, Walsh JME, Yu TM, Gildengorin G, Green LW, McPhee SJ. The effectiveness of the FLU–FOBT program in primary care: a randomized trial. *Am J Prev Med.* 2011;41(1): 9–16.

31. Potter MB, Yu A, Yu TM, Gildengorin G, Yu AY, Chan K, McPhee SJ, Green LW, Walsh J. Adaptation of the FLU-FOBT program for a primary care clinic serving a low-income Chinese-American community: new evidence of effectiveness. *J Health Care Poor Underserved,* 2011;22(1):284–295.

32. Walsh JME, Gildengorin G, Green LW, Jenkins J, Potter M. The FLU-FOBT Program in community clinics: durable benefits of a randomized controlled trial. *Health Educ Res.* 2012; 27(5):886–894.

33. Armstrong K, Green L, Hayward R, Rosenthal M, Wells KE. Bridging clinical scholarship and community scholarship: new directions for the Robert Wood Johnson Foundation's Clinical Scholars Program. *Am J Prev Med (Special Issue).* 2009;37(6S1):S187–S191.

34. Centers for Disease Control and Prevention. *Best practices for comprehensive tobacco control programs.* Atlanta, GA: U.S. Department of Health and Human Services, Centers for Disease Control and Prevention, National Center for Chronic Disease Prevention and Health Promotion, Office on Smoking and Health; 1999.

35. Cohen DJ, Crabtree BF, Etz RS, et al. Fidelity versus flexibility: translating evidence-based research into practice. *Am J Prev Med.* 2008;35(5 Suppl):S381–S389.

36. Green LW, Glasgow RE. Evaluating the relevance, generalization, and applicability of research: issues in external validation and translation methodology. *Eval Health Prof.* 2006;29(1):126–153.

37. Gough D, Thomas J, Oliver S. Clarifying differences between review designs and methods. *Syst Rev.* 2012;1:28.

38. Hauck WW, Anderson S, Marcus SM. Should we adjust for covariates in nonlinear regression analyses of randomized trials? *Control Clin Trials.* 1998;19(3):249–256.

39. Harris J. Using qualitative research to develop robust effectiveness questions and protocols for Cochrane systematic reviews. In: Noyes J, Booth A,

Hannes K, Harden A, Harris J, Lewin S, Lockwood C, eds. *Supplementary guidance for inclusion of qualitative research in Cochrane systematic reviews of interventions. Version 1* (updated August 2011). Cochrane Collaboration Qualitative Methods Group; 2011. http://methods.cochrane.org/qi/supplemental-handbook-guidance

40. Helfand M, Balshem H. AHRQ series paper 2: principles for developing guidance: AHRQ and the effective health-care program. *J Clin Epidemiol.* 2010;63(5):484–490.

41. Zaza S, PA. B, Harris K. *The guide to community preventive servies: What works to promote health?.* New York: Oxford University Press; 2005.

42. Task Force on Community Preventive Services. Recommendations for reducing excessive alcohol consumption and alcohol-related harms by limiting alcohol outlet density. *Am J Prev Med.* 2009;37(6):570–571.

43. Klesges LM, Dzewaltowski DA, Glasgow RE. Review of external validity reporting in childhood obesity prevention research. *Am J Prev Med.* 2008;34(3):216–223.

44. Haraldsson BG, Gross AR, Myers CD, et al. Massage for mechanical neck disorders. *Cochrane Database Syst Rev.* 2006(3):Cd004871.

45. Thorpe KE, Zwarenstein M, Oxman AD, et al. A pragmatic-explanatory continuum indicator summary (PRECIS): a tool to help trial designers. *J Clin Epidemiol.* 2009;62(5):464–475.

46. Sun X, Briel M, Busse JW, et al. Subgroup Analysis of Trials Is Rarely Easy (SATIRE): a study protocol for a systematic review to characterize the analysis, reporting, and claim of subgroup effects in randomized trials. *Trials.* 2009;10:101.

47. Stewart L, Tierney J, Clarke M. Reviews of individual patient data. In: Higgins J, Green S, eds. *Cochrane handbook for systematic reviews of interventions Version 5.0.1* (updated September 2008). The Cochrane Collaboration; 2008. Available from www.cochrane-handbook.org2008.

48. Kendrick D, Young B, Mason-Jones AJ, et al. Home safety education and provision of safety equipment for injury prevention (Review). *Evid Based Child Health.* 2013;8(3):761–939.

49. Berkey CS, Hoaglin DC, Mosteller F, Colditz GA. A random-effects regression model for meta-analysis. *Stat Med.* 1995;14(4):395–411.

50. Armstrong R, Waters E, Doyle J. Reviews in health promotion and public health. In: Higgins J, Green S, eds. *Cochrane handbook for systematic reviews of interventions Version 5.0.1* (updated September 2008). The Cochrane Collaboration, 2008. Available from http://www.cochrane.org/resources/handbook.

51. Kavanagh J, Oliver S, Lorenc T. *Reflections on developing and using PROGRESS-Plus.* Equity Update 2. Available from http://equity.cochrane.org/Files/Equity_Update_Vol2_Issue1.pdf2008.

52. Fisher EB. The importance of context in understanding behavior and promoting health. *Ann Behav Med.* 2008;35(1):3–18.

53. Acosta A, Ciapponi A, Aaserud M, et al. Pharmaceutical policies: effects of reference pricing, other pricing, and purchasing policies. *Cochrane Database Syst Rev.* 2014(10):Cd005979.

54. Lavis JN, Oxman AD, Souza NM, Lewin S, Gruen RL, Fretheim A. SUPPORT Tools for evidence-informed health Policymaking (STP) 9: assessing the applicability of the findings of a systematic review. *Health Res Policy Syst.* 2009;7 Suppl 1:S9.

55. Schünemann H, Oxman A, Vist G, et al. Chapter 12: Interpreting results and drawing conclusions. . In: Higgins J, Green S, eds. *Cochrane Handbook for Systematic Reviews of Interventions Version 5.0.1 (updated September 2008).* The Cochrane Collaboration, 2008. Available from www.cochrane-handbook.org2008.

19

Evaluation Approaches for Dissemination and Implementation Research

BRIDGET GAGLIO AND RUSSELL E. GLASGOW

INTRODUCTION

This chapter focuses on evaluation approaches to assessing dissemination and implementation science (D&I) research. An important take-home point is that evaluation should be considered an ongoing process, rather than a one-time, post hoc activity. Like planning for dissemination, best results are obtained by an integrated series of evaluation activities stretching from initial needs assessment to formative evaluation, ongoing process evaluation, and finally summative evaluation, all of which are interactive and provide feedback to key stakeholders and decision-makers. There is moderate overlap between this chapter and others on related topics, particularly the ones on models and frameworks for D&I research (chapter 5), external validity (chapter 18), and mixed methods evaluation (chapter 20). After a brief overview of the scope of evaluation activities relevant to D&I, the predominant evaluation approaches as well as emerging methods are reviewed, including their unique foci and contributions, followed by a case study. The chapter concludes with a summary of the status of current research/practice and future directions in D&I-related evaluation and suggested readings and selected websites and tools.

THE ROLE OF EVALUATION IN DISSEMINATION AND IMPLEMENTATION SCIENCE

Evaluation is defined in authoritative papers and texts as the systematic collection of information about the activities, characteristics, and results of programs to make judgments about the program, improve or further develop program effectiveness, inform decisions about future programming, and/or increase understanding.[1,2] Evaluation research is a multidisciplinary field, has its own professional organization (American Evaluation Association) and journals (*American Journal of Evaluation and Research Evaluation*), and includes a broad range of conceptual models, frameworks, perspectives, and measurement approaches. Importantly, evaluation research includes multimethod approaches, which can be used to inform program planning, iteratively assess progress and guide adaptations, and comprehensively assess program outcomes. This chapter is limited in scope and focuses on evaluation methods and approaches most relevant to D&I science. It first reviews key D&I evaluation issues and how evaluation has been used in D&I research, and then discusses key evaluation models and frameworks that have guided D&I research.

In contrast to more standard program evaluation[3–5] and effectiveness evaluations, D&I research focuses on issues related to the wide scale adoption, implementation, and generalizability of program and policy impacts. Although there is overlap and not a clear boundary between effectiveness outcomes research, quality improvement research,[6] and D&I evaluations,[7] the purposes of these types of evaluations are different. Instead of focusing on the results of an intervention in a specific setting when an intervention is evaluated under well-controlled conditions,[8] or rapid improvement when developing new innovations,[6] D&I evaluation seeks to understand implementation processes, identify contextual influences, and assess external validity[8,9] (see chapter 18). Implementation outcomes are also different than those in efficacy, effectiveness, and often quality improvement research, which are often focused on a single primary outcome. Implementation research, in contrast, is focused on outcomes including acceptability, adoption, appropriateness, costs, feasibility, fidelity, penetration, and sustainability[10] or, stated differently, on the

RE-AIM dimensions of reach, effectiveness across subgroups (including unintended outcomes), adoption, implementation (including costs and adaptations), and maintenance.[11,12] In summary, the ultimate goal of D&I evaluation (although usually not possible to answer in a given study) is to determine "What interventions (programs or policies) and what components of these interventions, conducted under what conditions and in what settings, conducted by which agents, is effective in producing which outcomes, for which populations (and subgroups), how much does it cost, and how does it come about?."[13,14]

Planning and Program/ Policy Design

Evaluation approaches, usually termed formative or evaluability assessments,[9,15] have been productively used to design interventions that will be robust across different settings and over time. A frequent mantra in D&I research, although seldom practiced in detail, is that it is never too early to design for dissemination (and evaluate potential and actual implementation). More recently, such planning has also come to focus on planning for sustainability or program.[16] Evaluation models and tools such as Diffusion of Innovations,[17] PRECEDE-PROCEED,[18] RE-AIM,[19] or system dynamics modeling[20] can be used with stakeholders and implementation staff to do a priori estimates of impacts on different D&I outcomes and help plan interventions to maximize their reach, effectiveness, and sustainability.[21,22] More iterative approaches to evaluate program implementation and initial effects during program or policy delivery can also be used, but with the exception of informal, nonsystematic assessments in quality improvement methods such as the Plan, Do, Study, Act cycle efforts,[23,24] there have been few reports of iterative use of D&I evaluation models. Hopefully within the next 5 years, there will be a sufficient literature on such iterative approaches to conduct reviews of their use and derive lessons learned from such applications.

Application of D&I models and evaluation methods during the course of an intervention bring up another important evaluation issue. Such applications can inform program adjustments or modifications to enhance impact and to decrease the likelihood that possible "negative results" are not due to insufficient implementation or fidelity.[25,26] Fidelity issues are discussed in greater detail in chapter 16. Here, the chapter briefly describes a rapidly evolving area of

evaluation termed adaptation research.[27,28] The genesis for this area of evaluation is the universal experience that in real-world applications, interventions are never delivered in the same way that they have been in efficacy or effectiveness studies conducted in optimal settings and under tightly controlled conditions.[29]

Some of these adaptations are undoubtedly not advisable, for example, if they result in failure to deliver essential effective components of a program or policy. However, some adaptations are increasingly being found to be useful, and maybe even necessary for successful application in different settings.[28,30] In particular, adaptations to make programs culturally appropriate, feasible to conduct in low resource settings, and compatible with existing workflow are likely to be important. Paradoxically and somewhat provocatively, recent conceptual approaches have suggested that adaption to changing context may be necessary and should be encouraged to produce or even exceed prior effectiveness study outcomes, and to produce sustainable interventions in a rapidly changing health care environment.[28,31]

Pragmatic and Comparative Effectiveness Evaluations

Pragmatic[13,32] and realist[33] approaches to evaluation have become more common over the past several years. These approaches focus on questions relevant to D&I such as the conditions under which different results can be obtained, and address generalizability concerns related to reach and breadth of effects, especially among subgroups (e.g., low income or minority participants).[34] Pragmatic and realist approaches have also been part of comparative effectiveness research (CER) evaluations.[35,36] In the prior version of this text, Glasgow and Steiner[37] discussed D&I-based approaches to comparative effectiveness research that are termed "CER-T" or CER that can translate.

D&I evaluation approaches have also been prominently featured in pragmatic trials, especially those supported by the Patient-Centered Outcomes Research Institute www.pcori.org and some National Institutes of Health (NIH) programs (e.g. NIH Collaboratory www.nihcollaboratory.org; National Institute of Diabetes and Digestive and Kidney Diseases www.niddk.nih.gov; National Heart, Lung, and Blood Institute www.nhlbi.nih.gov).[38] Pragmatic investigations are concerned with the conduct of studies under more representative conditions rather than ideal or efficacy conditions. Tools and evaluation methods have been developed to help plan, guide, and evaluate pragmatic studies.[32,39,40] In addition to effectiveness and heterogeneity of effects, these approaches are also concerned with issues of costs and relative impact of different, real-world approaches and their feasibility under different conditions and in different settings. Most prominent among these, and widely used especially in Canada and the United Kingdom, is the PRagmatic Explanatory Continuum Indicator Summary (PRECIS) and its revision, termed PRECIS-2.[39,40] The PRECIS-2 tool and approach focuses on 9 domains (previously 10 in the original PRECIS model) on which a proposed or delivered intervention can be rated according to its degree of pragmatism. This model is discussed in greater detail later in this chapter.

Related reporting standards for implementation research have been published recently by Pinnock et al.[41] Called the Standardized Reporting Implementation studies (StaRI) statement, these recommendations resulted from a systematic review and multistage e-Delphi process involving international experts in D&I to identify the most important types of data to report in D&I studies. This international effort builds on both the CONSORT and other reporting criteria for traditional outcomes research, and earlier recommendations for reporting on contextual and external validity issues.[42] The 27 items in StaRI are intended to promote standard, transparent, and accurate reporting to describe implementation strategies and the effectiveness of the intervention on key implementation outcomes. The annotated bibliography at the end of this chapter provides further description, but in brief the StaRI criteria include reporting on context and contextual changes, process, cost, representativeness, fidelity, and adaptation that apply across a broad range of research designs.

Finally, discussion of pragmatic research should address the issue of the practicality of use of evaluation methods. Many D&I assessments, and especially those often cited as exemplary evaluations (see Case Study later in chapter) are very comprehensive and detailed. This is appropriate and necessary for definitive or large-scale investigations, or where detailed knowledge of outcomes will determine public policies or substantial investment of scarce resources. However, there is also a need for "pragmatic measures"[13,43-45] that are more feasible, widely applicable, and can be acted on to produce more rapid results.

EVALUATION APPROACHES

Many interventions found to be effective in health services research studies fail to translate into meaningful patient care or public health outcomes, or across different contexts.[46] Complex interventions are increasingly used in the health service and public health practice, but they pose a number of evaluation challenges.[47] A key question in evaluating complex interventions is about practical effectiveness, whether the intervention works in everyday practice, in which case it is important to understand the whole range of effects, how they vary among recipients of the intervention, across sites, over time, and causes of variation.[48] Barriers to implementation arise at multiple levels of health care delivery: the patient; the provider team or group; the organizational; and policy levels.[49,50] Formative, process, and mixed-methods evaluations are useful to assess the extent to which implementation is effective in a specific context, to optimize intervention benefits, prolong sustainability of the intervention in the context, and inform dissemination into other contexts.[51,52] There is an increased use of theoretical and conceptual approaches to provide a better understanding and explanation of how and why dissemination and implementation succeeds or fails.[53,54] While this chapter does not provide an exhaustive list (see chapter 5), the following is a summary of several key evaluation approaches and frameworks that have been proven to be practical in guiding and evaluating translation of research findings (see Table 19.1). Summarized here are conceptual approaches that have been developed and used primarily to help evaluate programs, rather than others that are designed to categorize and understand interventions such as the Consolidated Framework for Implementation Research, the Promotion Action on Research Implementation in Health Services, or Reflecting Effective Programs.[55-57] Some of the approaches are intended to help guide both the development and evaluation of the intervention, some to address dissemination and implementation endeavors; and others are solely for evaluation.

PRECEDE-PROCEED Model

PRECEDE is an acronym for *p*redisposing, *r*einforcing, and *e*nabling *c*onstructs in *e*ducational/ecological *d*iagnosis and *e*valuation. PROCEED is an acronym for *p*olicy, *r*egulatory, and *o*rganizational *c*onstructs in *e*ducation and *e*nvironmental *d*evelopment. The PRECEDE-PROCEED Model is one of the most comprehensive and cohesive

TABLE 19.1 SUMMARY OF SELECTED EVALUATION APPROACHES FOR DISSEMINATION AND IMPLEMENTATION RESEARCH

Evaluation Approach	Acronym	Emphasis on Planning, Evaluation or both	Summary and Key Features	Key Recommended References
PRECEDE-PROCEED Model	PRECEDE-PROCEED	Planning and Evaluation	Links intervention planning and evaluation into one integrated framework. Comprehensive model emphasizing a multidisciplinary approach to assessing the multiple factors that impact and influence health. Eight phase model: 1. Social assessment—identifying the ultimate desired goal or result 2. Epidemiological assessment—identifying the genetics, behavioral, and/or environmental indicators that may contribute to or interact with overall desired goal or result 3. Educational and ecological assessment—identifying predisposing, reinforcing, and enabling factors that can effect the behaviors, genetic, and environmental indicators identified in prior phase 4. Identifying the administrative and policy factors that influence what can be implemented 5. Implementation—conducting the intervention 6. Process evaluation—determines the extent to which the program components were implemented as planned 7. Impact evaluation—how well the intended audiences were reached 8. Outcome evaluation—determines the effect of the program on the overall goal or result as well as quality-of-life indicators	Green and Kreuter.[18] www.lgreen.net
Reach, Effectiveness, Adoption, Implementation, and Maintenance Framework	RE-AIM	Planning and Evaluation	Emphasizes five dimensions that together determine public health impact. Places equal emphasis on external and internal validity. Evaluates results at both the setting/contextual and individual levels. *Reach* is the absolute number, proportion, and representativeness of individuals who are willing to participate in a given initiative. *Effectiveness* is the impact of an intervention on outcomes, including potential negative effects, quality of life, and economic outcomes. *Adoption* is the absolute number, proportion, and representativeness of settings and intervention agents who are willing to initiate a program. *Implementation* refers to the intervention agents' fidelity to the various elements of an intervention's protocol. This includes consistency of delivery as intended, adaptations made, and the time and cost of the intervention. *Maintenance* is the extent to which a program or policy becomes institutionalized or part of the routine organizational practices and policies. At the individual level, it is defined as the long-term effects of a program on outcomes six or more months after the most recent intervention contact.	Glasgow et al.[19] www.re-aim.org

Name	Abbreviation	Category	Description	Reference
Practical, Robust Implementation and Sustainability Model	PRISM	Planning and Evaluation	PRISM helps to identify factors needed to successfully implement research in practice settings and to measure success. This framework looks at how intervention design, external environment, organizational characteristics, and the intended population influence intervention effectiveness when implementing evidence-based practices. PRISM expands RE-AIM by adding increased focus on multi-level contextual factors. PRISM was developed using several models: Diffusion of Innovations, the Chronic Care Model, the Model for Improvement and the RE-AIM framework.	Feldstein and Glasgow.[66]
Pragmatic-Explanatory Continuum Indicator Summary	PRECIS/ PRECIS-2	Planning	PRECIS-2 has 9 domains, each of which is intended to help trialists think about the consequences of that design decision for applicability of the results of their trial. 1. Eligibility 2. Recruitment 3. Setting 4. Organization 5. Flexibility: delivery 6. Flexibility: adherence 7. Follow-up 8. Primary outcome 9. Primary analysis	Loudon et al.[39]
Evaluability Assessment	n/a	Planning	Evaluability assessment is a pre-evaluation activity designed to maximize the chances that any subsequent evaluation of programs, practices, or policies will result in useful information. Consists of six steps: 1. Involving the intended users of evaluation information 2. Clarifying the intended program 3. Exploring program reality 4. Reaching agreement on needed changes in activities or goals 5. Exploring alternative evaluation designs 6. agreeing on evaluation priorities and intended uses of information	Leviton et al.[9]
Medical Research Council Guidance for Assessing Complex Interventions	n/a	Planning and Evaluation	This framework for process evaluation emphasizes three themes: implementation, mechanisms, and context. The focus is for a systematic approach to designing and conducting process evaluations. While each process evaluation will be different, the framework provides guidance in thinking through some of the common decisions that need to be addressed when developing a process evaluation. Recommendations are provided for: 1. Planning a process evaluation 2. Designing and conducting a process evaluation 3. Analysis of process data, and integration of process and outcome data 4. Reporting findings	Moore et al.[47].

models in that it combines the causal assessment and the intervention planning and evaluation into one overarching framework.[18,58,59] The goals of the model are to explain health-related behaviors and environments, and to design and evaluate the interventions needed to influence both the behaviors and the social and contextual conditions that influence them and their consequences. Due to the flexibility and scalability of this classic model, it has been extensively applied and tested in a wide variety of settings, especially for public health programs, and policies.[60-62]

The PRECEDE-PROCEED model has two main components. The first component, PRECEDE, consists of four phases aimed at generating information. The original PRECEDE model was developed in the 1970s and has probably been more widely used than any other model to plan and evaluate public health interventions (http://lgreen.net). This part of the model recognizes the need for assessment prior to intervention planning. The phases of PRECEDE consist of:

1. Social assessment—identifying the ultimate desired goal or result
2. Epidemiological assessment—identifying the genetics, behavioral, and/or environmental indicators that may contribute to or interact with overall desired goal or result
3. Educational and ecological assessment—identifying predisposing, reinforcing, and enabling factors that can affect the behaviors, genetic, and environmental indicators identified in prior phases
4. Identifying the administrative and policy factors that influence what can be implemented

This is followed by the second component of the model, PROCEED, which was added in the early 1990s. It highlights the importance of environmental, contextual, and genetic factors (added later in 2005) as determinants of health and health inequities. PROCEED consists of four additional phases that focus on the actual implementation of the intervention and careful evaluation of it. The phases in this part of the model consist of:

5. Implementation—conducting the intervention
6. Process evaluation—determines the extent to which the program components were implemented as planned

7. Impact evaluation—how well the intended audiences were reached
8. Outcome evaluation—determines the effect of the program on the overall goal or result that was proposed in phase 1, as well as quality-of-life indicators[18]

The PRECEDE-PROCEED model provides a structured framework to apply health behavior theories at all levels. Moreover, the model stresses a multidisciplinary approach and evaluation of the multitude of factors that impact health and well-being.

RE-AIM Framework

The RE-AIM Framework, which is an acronym for Reach, Effectiveness, Adoption, Implementation, and Maintenance, is almost 20 years old. The first RE-AIM publication was in 1999.[19] The model grew out of the need for reporting on key issues related to implementation, replication, generalizability, and population impact of much of the health promotion and health care research literature. RE-AIM was developed partially as a response to the primary focus on internal validity of research conducted under optimal efficacy conditions and a neglect of emphasis on external validity necessary for application in complex, real-world settings.[63] The problem was not that this type of research was being conducted, but that it was and is still often considered the only type of valid research and the "gold standard" for reviews, decision-making, and guideline development. Although intended for and useful at all stages of research from planning through evaluation and reporting, RE-AIM has been most widely used for dissemination and implementation evaluation.[11,64]

The dimensions of the multilevel framework are defined as follows.[11,12,65] *Reach* is the absolute number, proportion, and representativeness of individuals who are willing to participate in a given initiative. *Effectiveness* is the impact of an intervention on outcomes, including potential negative effects, heterogeneity of intervention effects, quality of life, and economic outcomes. *Adoption* is the absolute number, proportion, and representativeness of (a) settings and (b) intervention agents who are willing to initiate a program. *Implementation* refers to the intervention agents' fidelity to and adaptation of the various elements of an intervention's protocol. This includes consistency of delivery as intended and the time and costs of the intervention. *Maintenance* at the setting level is the extent to which a program or policy becomes institutionalized or part of the routine organizational practices and policies. At the individual level, it is defined as the long-term effects of a program on outcomes 6 or more months after the most recent intervention contact.

As this framework has continued to evolve over time, there are several issues that are commonly misinterpreted about RE-AIM.[11,12] These issues are:

1. Confusing the definitions of reach and adoption. Reach is used for reporting representativeness of *individual* participants, whereas adoption is used for reporting representativeness of *settings* and intervention *staff*.
2. RE-AIM addresses issues at both the individual level (reach and effectiveness) and the setting/staff level (adoption and implementation). The maintenance dimension has components on both levels.
3. Cost is important in the RE-AIM model. It is considered under the implementation dimension, as cost is one of the key questions decision-makers have when considering practical issues such as who can implement a program, what resources are required, etc.
4. Consistency (or lack of consistency) of results is important at each level. Thus, RE-AIM is concerned not only with overall mean results, but also with impacts on subgroups related to health disparities, by different implementation staff, and in different settings.

Additional resources related to using the RE-AIM framework can be found at www.re-aim.org.

Practical, Robust, Implementation and Sustainability Model

The Practical, Robust, Implementation and Sustainability Model (PRISM) is an extension of RE-AIM that was developed to help identify and assess contextual factors and influences needed to successfully implement research in practice settings and to measure success.[66] This framework looks at how intervention design, external environment, organizational characteristics, and the intended population influence intervention effectiveness when implementing evidence-based practices.[66] PRISM was developed using several models: Diffusion of Innovations, the Chronic Care Model, the Model for Improvement and the RE-AIM framework. As can be seen in Figure 19.1, PRISM focuses on multilevel contextual factors related to a program and relies upon RE-AIM dimensions to evaluate program effects. The PRISM model integrates existing concepts relevant to translating research into practice to conceptualize, implement, and evaluate evidence-based programs and policies. It has recently been used to understand multilevel stakeholder perspectives related to a colon cancer screening program.[67]

PRagmatic-Explanatory Continuum Indicator Summary

Although technically not an evaluation framework, the PRECIS model is a valuable approach to help planning and evaluation.[39,40,68] The PRECIS tool was originally developed in 2008 to assist researchers in designing trials by identifying and quantifying research study characteristics that differentiate pragmatic and explanatory (i.e., efficacy) trials.[40] A pragmatic trial attempts to answer the question—does this intervention work under usual conditions; whereas an explanatory trial addresses the question—does this intervention work under ideal conditions? The PRECIS tool originally evaluated studies along 10 domains identified as being critical to distinguishing pragmatic trials from explanatory trials. The domains were: (1) participant eligibility criteria, (2) flexibility of experimental intervention, (3) experimental intervention—practitioner expertise, (4) flexibility of the comparison intervention, (5) comparison intervention—practitioner expertise, 6) follow-up intensity, (7) primary trial outcome, (8) participant compliance with "prescribed" intervention, (9) practitioner adherence to study protocol, and (10) analysis of the primary outcome.

The tool was revised in 2015; PRECIS-2 has nine domains including three new ones.[39] The domains of the new tool are: (1) eligibility, (2) recruitment, (3) setting, (4) organization, (5) flexibility: delivery, (6) flexibility: adherence, (7) follow-up, (8) primary outcome, and (9) primary analysis. The scale for all domains ranges from 1 (very explanatory) to 5 (very pragmatic). Recently the PRECIS and PRECIS-2 have been used to conduct literature reviews and demonstrate the level of and variability in pragmatic interventions studies.[32,69,70]

The PRECIS results are summarized in the form of a "spoke and wheel plot," where the

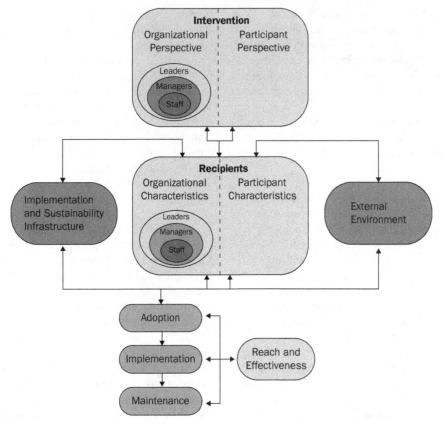

FIGURE 19.1 The Practical, Robust, Implementation, and Sustainability Model (PRISM). (From Feldstein and Glasgow.⁶⁶)

explanatory end of the continuum is the hub and the pragmatic end is the outside edge. Each spoke is labeled with a domain. Each domain is then marked along the range of the spoke to indicate how pragmatic versus explanatory the trial is on that dimension. The dots are then connected to create a visual representation of where a trial falls along the pragmatic-explanatory continuum (Figure 19.2). The main purpose of PRECIS is to determine the degree to which study design decisions align with the trial's stated purpose, and thus was originally intended to be used at the design stage; however, it has also been applied in variety of ways in an attempt to expand its utility to evaluate studies post completion, including use in systematic reviews.[68,71] PRECIS-2 is still intended primarily to be used to help consider design decisions that are consistent with the purpose of the trial and the usefulness of the future results to the intended audience. By using PRECIS-2 to consider applicability at the design stage, the intent is that the results of the trial will likely be more useful to their intended users than they otherwise would have been.[39]

EVALUABILITY ASSESSMENT

Evaluability assessment was developed in the late 1970s in response to the challenge of dealing with programs that were inappropriate or premature for evaluation.[9] This assessment method consists of six steps to be conducted prior to investing in a large-scale project: (1) involving the intended users of evaluation information, (2) clarifying the intended program, (3) exploring program reality, (4) reaching agreement on needed changes in activities or goals, (5) exploring alternative evaluation designs, and (6) agreeing on evaluation priorities and intended uses of information. This model is participatory in that it involves stakeholders using an iterative process to create a logic model that represents the expectations, goals, and rationale for the project.[9] Once the logic model is completed, a plausibility assessment is

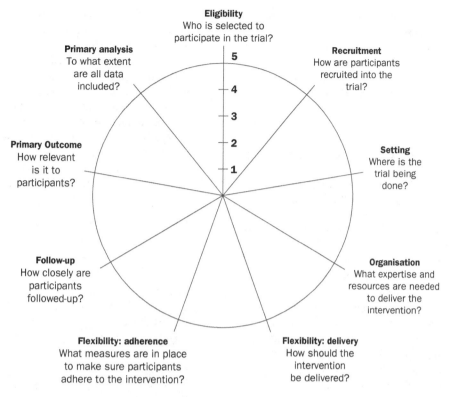

FIGURE 19.2 Pragmatic-Explanatory Continuum Indicator Summary (PRECIS-2). (From Loudon K., et al.[39])

conducted. This involves assessment on whether outcomes are achievable given the context of the project, timeframe, resource availability and allocation, and implementation efforts of the project. Plausibility analysis lays the groundwork for the formal evaluation. While evaluability assessment has its roots in the core functions of public health, it is now being used in translating research into practice. As evidence-based programs are being implemented, evaluability assessment can test assumptions about the program being tested in a new context and setting. This method can guide adaptations to real-world conditions or raise a warning early on that constraints are too great for implementation.[9]

Medical Research Council Guidance for Assessing Complex Interventions

The Medical Research Council of the United Kingdom has produced periodic guidance from panels of experts on the design and evaluation of complex interventions.[72] Recently they have updated and expanded this guidance to include the process evaluation of complex interventions.[47] This is especially relevant to D&I science, since the vast majority of interventions evaluated in D&I are complex. The new MRC guidance (https://www.mrc.ac.uk/documents/pdf/mrc-phsrn-process-evaluation-guidance-final/) focuses on transparent reporting on the three core issues of implementation, mechanisms, and context. Guidance is provided on these factors as they pertain to the planning, design and conduct, analysis, and reporting stages of research. It does not provide a rigidly defined checklist; the diversity of the interventions evaluated by health researchers, and the uncertainties posed by them, means that not all process evaluations will look the same. However, it offers guidance in thinking through some of the common decisions that will need to be addressed when developing a process evaluation. The key recommendations include:

Planning a Process Evaluation

- Carefully define the parameters of relationships with all stakeholders

involved in intervention development and implementation.
- Ensure there is sufficient expertise and experience among research team.
- Decide the degree of separation or integration between process and outcome evaluation teams.

Design and Conduct

- Clearly describe the intervention and clarify causal assumptions (in relation to how it will be implemented, and the mechanisms through which it will produce change, in a specific context).
- Identify key uncertainties and systematically select the most important questions to address.
- Select a combination of methods appropriate to the research questions including consideration of collecting data at multiple time points to capture change over time. Figure 19.3 highlights commonly used data collection and analysis methods for process evaluation.

Analysis

- Provide descriptive quantitative information on fidelity, dose, and reach.
- Consider more detailed modelling of variations between participants or sites in terms of factors such as fidelity or reach.
- Integrate quantitative process data into outcome datasets to examine whether effects differ by implementation or prespecified contextual moderators, and test hypothesized mediators.
- Collect and analyze qualitative data iteratively so that themes that emerge in early interviews can be explored in later ones.
- Ensure that quantitative and qualitative analyses build upon one another.
- Where possible, initially analyze and report process data before trial outcomes are known to avoid biased interpretation.
- Transparently report whether process data are being used to generate hypotheses or for post hoc explanation.

Reporting

- Identify existing reporting guidance specific to the methods adopted.
- Report the logic model or intervention theory and clarify how it was used to guide selection of research questions and methods.
- Disseminate findings to policy and practice stakeholders.
- If multiple journal articles are published from the same process evaluation, ensure that each article makes clear its context within the evaluation as a whole.[47]

In summary, while each evaluation framework and model has its unique strengths and limitations, the evaluation approaches for D&I tend to emphasize several common themes.[73,74] First, implementation is heavily dependent on context, and one needs to understand and be sensitive to

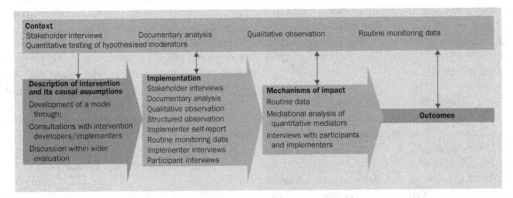

FIGURE 19.3 Commonly used data collection and analysis methods for process evaluation.
(From Moore GF et al.[47])

local conditions, history, and resources. Second, as discussed in more detail in chapter 16 on fidelity-adaptation, quality of implementation is a frequent challenge, and programs are almost never implemented exactly as they were designed or tested in efficacy studies.[75] Third, both implementation and dissemination are complex multilevel undertakings, not easily explained by simplistic models or appropriately evaluated by reductionistic designs. Finally, traditional evaluation and research methods tend to ignore or undervalue the importance of several D&I factors such as reach and engagement of the target audience in partnership research;[64] the need to operationalize and provide practical assessments of setting, delivery staff, organizational and individual factors and their interactions;[73,76] issues of cost and economic outcomes;[77] and external validity.[42] The important point is not to argue about the minor differences among approaches or to say which one is "best," but rather to have program developers and evaluators select a framework, or combination of frameworks, that fits their question and needs and then use the framework(s) consistently to evaluate results—including collecting data on factors hypothesized by the model to produce outcomes.

CASE STUDY

Table 19.2 illustrates the example of how RE-AIM was used to evaluate an application of the Body and Soul healthy eating program, as well as how it was reported in the peer review literature. Allicock et al.[78] reported on all aspects of the RE-AIM model using a mixed methods approach. They reported reasonably good reach (32%) among a high-risk population, and that 19 of the 40 black churches approached participated in the program. Such measures of adoption among potential settings is an important and seldom reported feature in research reports.[11] Implementation of core elements of the program was good, although adaptations and costs were not reported. The program produced modest but significant improvements in fruit and vegetable consumption relative to a randomized control set of churches, and six of the eight churches in the Body and Soul program intended to continue the program.

COLLECTING EVALUATION INFORMATION

Qualitative Methods in Evaluation

Qualitative evaluation methods are an essential part of the tools that evaluators can draw upon

(see chapter 20). Certain questions, problems, and purposes are more fitting with qualitative methods than with others, and these approaches can almost always be used to help understand and explain quantitative findings. Qualitative methods can be used in evaluation work to provide detail and context to the interpretation of statistical data.[79] Qualitative approaches to evaluation are themselves diverse. They can range from formative studies to outcome evaluation, process studies, implementation evaluation, program comparisons, documenting development over time, investigating system change, and conducting "post-mortem" exams to explore unanticipated results.[80,81] Qualitative evaluations often rely on a handful of data collection methods. These methods include focus groups, case studies, in-depth interviews, and observational field notes. Integrating qualitative methods with more traditional quantitative evaluation methods lends depth and clarity to understanding outcomes.

In D&I research, mixed method designs have been increasingly used to understand and overcome barriers to implementation. More recently, they have been used in the design and implementation of strategies to facilitate the implementation of evidence based practices.[82] Mixed method designs focus on collecting, analyzing, and merging both quantitative and qualitative data into one or more studies. The central premise of these designs is that the use of quantitative and qualitative approaches in combination provides a better understanding of research issues than either approach alone.[83,84] In mixed method evaluation designs, qualitative methods are used to explore and obtain depth of understanding as to the reasons for success or failure to implement evidence-based practice or to identify strategies for facilitating implementation, while quantitative methods are used to test and confirm hypotheses based on an existing conceptual model and obtain breadth of understanding of predictors of successful implementation.[83,4] The use of mixed methods in D&I science is discussed in greater detail in chapter 20.

Assessing Costs in D&I

Information on cost issues is often the primary consideration in whether a potential program or policy will be adopted. Information on costs, anticipated during planning stages, actually experienced during implementation, and projected during dissemination phases, is an important aspect of evaluation. However, costs are one of

TABLE 19.2 CASE STUDY—EXAMPLE OF APPLYING THE RE-AIM FRAMEWORK TO EVALUATE A HEALTHY EATING PROGRAM IN BLACK CHURCHES

	RE-AIM Dimension	Application
Promoting fruit and vegetable consumption among members of Black churches, Michigan and North Carolina, 2008-2010. Allicock et al.[78]	REACH—The absolute number, proportion, and representativeness of individuals who are willing to participate in a given initiative	Data for the number of active congregants aged 50 years or older were available for 6 churches and totaled 730. Only 302 congregants completed the baseline and follow-up surveys. Overall reach (proportion of eligible congregants who participated in the full study) was estimated at 32% (231/730). Study participants were: • Mainly women (71%) • Married or partnered (51.5%) • Had some college education or a college degree (71%) • Had annual household incomes of less than $50,000
	EFFECTIVENESS—The impact of an intervention on outcomes, including potential negative effects, heterogeneity of intervention effects, quality of life, and economic outcomes	Baseline mean fruit and vegetable consumption for participants (n = 302) was 4.07 servings per day. Servings per day at follow-up was higher (mean, + 0.14 servings; standard deviation [SD], 3.79; P = .63), but this increase was not significant.
	ADOPTION—The absolute number, proportion, and representativeness of a) settings and b) intervention agents who are willing to initiate a program.	Contacted 40 churches in Michigan and North Carolina. • 14 declined or did not respond • 26 expressed interest; 7 did not meet eligibility criteria. Nineteen churches enrolled. • 10 churches were randomized to a colon cancer screening intervention • 9 churches were randomized to Body and Soul. One church withdrew from the study after baseline survey completion because of organizational changes.
	IMPLEMENTATION—The intervention agents' fidelity to and adaptation of the various elements of an intervention's protocol.	Through pastor and coordinator interviews, all churches reported pastoral support; • 4 churches made environmental changes • 6 churches conducted at least 1 or 2 educational activities (2 reported 3–5 activities). The overall intervention period varied from 9 to 17 months depending on church personnel changes, the coordinator's availability, and other events in the church taking priority over study activities.

(continued)

TABLE 19.2 CONTINUED

RE-AIM Dimension	Application
MAINTENANCE—At the setting level is the extent to which a program or policy becomes institutionalized or part of the routine organizational practices and policies. At the individual level, it is defined as the long-term effects of a program on outcomes 6 or more months after the most recent intervention contact.—*Example only reported at setting level.*	At follow-up, 6 coordinators reported intentions to continue the program, but 1 stipulated that extra staff would be needed to do so. The 2 churches that had no plans for continuing cited low interest of congregants, competing church programs, and lack of personnel.

the least often captured components of evaluation.[64,77,85] Costs and related issues such as cost-effectiveness, cost–benefit, and return on investment are seldom reported in evaluations of behavioral or D&I interventions. Chapter 6 by Ramesh Raghavan presents an overview of how D&I science can be evaluated from an economic point of view. It begins with a brief review of economic concepts followed by a discussion of cost and outcome estimation from a D&I perspective. Here, costs are discussed primarily from the perspective of smaller potential adopting organizations and staff (e.g. schools, clinics, worksites, local communities) or patients/families.

Primary challenges to including cost information in evaluations are (a) the time-consuming, intrusive, and ironically, costly procedures often involved in assessing costs;[77] (b) the need to involve economists, accountants or other professionals; and (c) the costs and interdisciplinary collaboration issues associated with economic evaluations. There have been recent efforts to reduce the burden associated with assessing costs, for example, only doing time sampling at different points during an intervention instead of continuously,[86] but these are beyond the scope of this chapter. The primary issue that is raised here is understanding costs from the perspective of the adopting organizations and individuals such as employers, health care clinics or providers, or patients and families.

The perspective and concerns of these stakeholders is often different than that most often reported in economic reports[87] and differ across different stakeholders. As in other areas of D&I, understanding what implementing partners and potential adoptees value and the types of costs they are most concerned about is central to conducting relevant economic evaluations likely to be useful to consumers. For example, rather than formal business or societal definitions of "return on investment," health care clinics and patients/families are often primarily concerned about time involved, burden, and degree of disruption in usual workflows or daily patterns (as well as opportunity costs, although often not articulated as such).

SUMMARY

Considerable progress has been made in evaluation of D&I science and research; however, we are still lacking knowledge in several key areas. The complexity, inherently multilevel and contextual nature of D&I science, and the always (sometimes rapidly) changing environment present ongoing challenges.[31,74] Given these challenges, evaluation of D&I efforts need more adapted, novel, refined, and sophisticated approaches to evaluation and especially, more pragmatic measures.[13,43]

Since the first edition of this book, we have seen increased focus and emphasis on D&I from a variety of organizations. The National Institute for Health Research, funded by the United Kingdom's Department of Health, has a dissemination center that aims to put research evidence at the heart of decisions made by clinicians, commissioners, and patients in the National Health Service. The Canadian Institutes for Health Research, the major federal agency responsible for funding health research in Canada, is dedicated to translation of health knowledge from the research setting into real-world applications. The National Health and Medical Research Council in Australia aims to accelerate the transfer of research into policy and practice through targeted funding announcements and the establishment of the Research Translation Faculty. In the United States, many of the leading agencies of health research have funding announcements that focus on evaluating and/or refining strategies to disseminate and implement evidence-based practices into public health, clinical practice, and community settings.

As evaluation of D&I science continues to evolve, several new areas must be considered. Engaging patients, stakeholders, and communities in research continues to gain momentum and popularity in pragmatic, real-world studies; however, evaluation of engagement and its impact on study outcomes as well as impact on dissemination and implementation efforts needs further attention. Future work will need to consider if understanding context is enough to capture the impact of engagement on dissemination and implementation efforts, or if existing models and frameworks will need to be revised to account for this change to how research is conducted. Genomic methods[88] and precision medicine[89] applications continue to progress. Evaluation of precision medicine applications will be challenging but needs to be undertaken to assess outcomes, and importantly, unintended consequences. Evaluations of multilevel interventions will continue to challenge the field not only because of the complexity of the interventions themselves but their interactions and how they change over time. How this is reported in a transparent manner needs to continue to be a priority for the field.

We hope that the next revision of this chapter will be able to more conclusively answer the key, ultimate use question mentioned early in this chapter of "What interventions (programs or policies) and what components of these interventions, conducted under what conditions and in what settings, conducted by which agents, is

effective in producing which outcomes, for which populations (and subgroups), how much does it cost, and how does it come about?"

SUGGESTED READINGS AND WEBSITES

Readings

Moore G.F., Audrey S., Barker M., Bond L., et al. Process evaluation of complex interventions: Medical Research Council guidance. *BMJ*. 2015;350:h1258.

This article presents a framework for process evaluation focused on three themes: implementation, mechanisms, and context. It argues for a systematic approach to designing and conducting process evaluations, drawing on clear descriptions of intervention theory and identification of key process questions.

Pinnock H., Barwick M., Carpenter C.R., Eldridge S., Grandes G., et al. Standards for reporting implementation studies (StaRI) statement. *BMJ*. 2017;356:i6795.

This article presents a 27-item checklist to prompt researchers to describe both the implementation strategy and the effectiveness of the intervention being implemented. The checklist applies to a broad range of research methodologies employed in implementation science.

Gaglio B., Shoup J.A., Glasgow R.E. The RE-AIM framework: a systematic review of use over time. *AJPH*. 2013;103(6):e38–e46.

This article describe criteria for reporting on various dimensions of the RE-AIM framework' reviews the empirical published literature to describe the application, consistency of use, and reporting on RE-AIM dimensions over time; highlights lessons learned from applying RE-AIM; and makes recommendations for future applications.

Glasgow R.E. and Riley W.T. Pragmatic measures: what they are why we need them. *Am J Prev Med*. 2013;45(2):234–243.

This article proposes necessary and recommended criteria for pragmatic measures, provides examples of projects to develop and identify such measures, addresses potential concerns about these recommendations, and identifies areas for future research and application.

Loudon K., Treweek S., Sullivan F., Donnan P., Thorpe K.E., Zwarenstein M. The PRECIS-2 tool: designing trials that are fit for purpose. *BMJ*. 2015;350:h2147.

This article gives guidance on how to use an improved, validated version, PRECIS-2, which has been developed with the help of over 80 international trialists, clinicians, and policymakers. Keeping the original simple wheel format, PRECIS-2 now has nine domains scored from 1 (very explanatory) to 5 (very pragmatic) to facilitate domain discussion and consensus.

Proctor E.K., Silmere H., Raghavan R., Hovmand P., et al. Outcomes for implementation research: conceptual distinctions, measurement challenges, and research agenda. *Adm Policy Ment Health.* 2011;38(2):65–76.

This article proposes a heuristic, working "taxonomy" of eight conceptually distinct implementation outcomes—acceptability, adoption, appropriateness, feasibility, fidelity, implementation cost, penetration, and sustainability—along with their nominal definitions. A two-pronged agenda is proposed for research on implementation outcomes. Conceptualizing and measuring implementation outcomes will advance understanding of implementation processes, enhance efficiency in implementation research, and pave the way for studies of the comparative effectiveness of implementation strategies.

Websites and Tools

Better Evaluation—Sharing Information to Improve Evaluation. http://betterevaluation.org/en

An international collaboration to improve evaluation practice and theory by sharing and generating information about options (methods or processes) and approaches.

PRECEDE-PROCEED model for health planning and evaluation. http://www.lgreen.net

This is a resource that provides full citation of references that use the PRECEDE-PROCEED model. Many of the references have direct links to Medline or PubMed abstracts.

RE-AIM website. www.re-aim.org

The RE-AIM website provides an explanation of and resources for those wanting to apply the RE-AIM framework.

Making Research Matter. http://www.makeresearch-matter.org/

The mission of the Make Research Matter website is to give researchers the tools they need to increase the dissemination and implementation potential of their products.

Grid-Enable Measures Database (GEM). https://www.gem-beta.org/Public/MeasureList.aspx?cat=2&viewall=false&scont=35

Provides a compendium of measures considered for inclusion in a battery of pragmatic measures for use in primary care settings, and includes information on length, psychometric characteristics, sensitivity to change, and other criteria.

Quality Enhancement Research Initiative (QUERI)— U.S. Department of Veterans Affairs. http://www.queri.research.va.gov/

The overall mission of QUERI is to improve the health of Veterans by supporting the more rapid implementation of effective clinical practices into routine care.

University of Colorado Department of Family Medicine—Evaluation Hub. http://cufamilymedicine.org/evaluation_hub/

This site provides a variety of practical resources for helping low resource settings and especially primary care organizations to understand basics of program evaluation and for pragmatic assessment of unfunded programs.

REFERENCES

1. Patton MQ. *Utilization-focused evaluation.* 4th ed. London: Sage Publications; 2008.
2. Trochim WM, Rubio DM, Thomas VG, Evaluation Key Function Committee of the CC. Evaluation guidelines for the Clinical and Translational Science Awards (CTSAs). *Clin Transl Sci.* 2013;6(4):303–309.
3. Wholey JS, PHatry HP, Newcomer KE, eds. *Handbook of practical program evaluation.* 3rd ed. San Francisco: Jossey-Bass; 2010.
4. Yarbrough DB, Shulha LM, Hopson RK, Caruthers FA, eds. *The program evaluation standards: A guide for evaluators and evaluation users.* 3rd ed. Thousand Oaks, CA: Sage Publications; 2011.
5. American Evaluation Association. American Evaluation Association Guiding Principles for Evaluators. July 2004; http://www.eval.org/p/cm/ld/fid=51. Accessed December 20, 2016.
6. Ogrinc G, Davies L, Goodman D, Batalden P, Davidoff F, Stevens D. SQUIRE 2.0 (Standards for QUality Improvement Reporting Excellence): revised publication guidelines from a detailed consensus process. *BMJ Qual Safety.* 2016;25(12):986–992.
7. Curran GM, Bauer M, Mittman B, Pyne JM, Stetler C. Effectiveness-implementation hybrid designs: combining elements of clinical effectiveness and implementation research to enhance public health impact. *Med Care.* 2012;50(3):217–226.
8. Shadish WR, Cook TD, Campbell DT. *Experimental and quasi-experimental designs for generalized causal inference.* Boston: Houghton Mifflin Company; 2002.
9. Leviton LC, Khan LK, Rog D, Dawkins N, Cotton D. Evaluability assessment to improve public health policies, programs, and practices. *Annu Rev Public Health.* 2010;31:213–233.
10. Proctor EK, Silmere H, Raghavan R, et al. Outcomes for implementation research: conceptual distinctions, measurement challenges, and research agenda. *Adm Policy Ment Health.* 2011;38(2):65–76.
11. Gaglio B, Shoup JA, Glasgow RE. The RE-AIM framework: a systematic review of use over time. *Am J Public Health.* 2013;103(6):e38–e46.

12. Kessler RS, Purcell EP, Glasgow RE, Klesges LM, Benkeser RM, Peek CJ. What does it mean to "employ" the RE-AIM model? *Eval Health Prof.* 2013;36(1):44–66.

13. Glasgow RE. What does it mean to be pragmatic? Pragmatic methods, measures, and models to facilitate research translation. *Health Educ Behav.* 2013;40(3):257–265.

14. Paul GL. Behavior modification research: Design and tactics. In: Franks CM, ed. *Behavior therapy: Appraisal and status.* New York: McGraw-Hill; 1969:26–62.

15. Trevisan MS, Walser TM. *Evaluability assessment: Improving evaluation quality and use.* Thousand Oaks, CA: Sage Publications; 2014.

16. Calhoun A, Mainor A, Moreland-Russell S, Maier RC, Brossart L, Luke DA. Using the Program Sustainability Assessment Tool to assess and plan for sustainability. *Prev Chronic Dis.* 2014;11:130185.

17. Rogers EM. *Diffusion of innovations.* 5th ed. New York: Free Press; 2003.

18. Green LW, Kreuter MW. *Health program planning: An educational and ecological approach.* 4th ed. New York: McGraw-Hill; 2005.

19. Glasgow RE, Vogt TM, Boles SM. Evaluating the public health impact of health promotion interventions: the RE-AIM framework. *Am J Public Health.* 1999;89(9):1322-1327.

20. Hovmand PS. *Community-based system dynamics.* New York: Springer; 2014.

21. Klesges LM, Estabrooks PA, Dzewaltowski DA, Bull SS, Glasgow RE. Beginning with the application in mind: designing and planning health behavior change interventions to enhance dissemination. *Ann Behav Med.* 2005;29 Suppl:66–75.

22. RE-AIM website. RE-AIM Self-rating Quiz Tool. http://re-aim.org/resources-and-tools/self-rating-quiz/. Accessed December 21, 2016.

23. Institute for Healthcare Improvement. Plan-Do-Study-Act (PDSA) Worksheet. http://www.ihi.org/resources/Pages/Tools/PlanDoStudyActWorksheet.aspx. Accessed December 21, 2016.

24. Langley GL, Moen R, Nolan KM, Nolan TW, Norman CL, Provost LP. *The improvement guide: A practical approach to enhancing organizational performance.* 2nd ed. San Francisco: Jossey-Bass; 2009.

25. JaKa MM, Haapala JL, Trapl ES, et al. Reporting of treatment fidelity in behavioural paediatric obesity intervention trials: a systematic review. *Obes Rev.* 2016;17(12):1287–1300.

26. Breitenstein SM, Gross D, Garvey CA, Hill C, Fogg L, Resnick B. Implementation fidelity in community-based interventions. *Res Nur Health.* 2010;33(2):164–173.

27. Stirman SW, Miller CJ, Toder K, Calloway A. Development of a framework and coding system for modifications and adaptations of evidence-based interventions. *Implement Sci:* 2013;8:65.

28. Chambers DA, Norton WE. The adaptome: advancing the science of intervention adaptation. *Am J Prevent Med.* 2016;51(4 Suppl 2):S124–S131.

29. Glasgow RE, Emmons KM. How can we increase translation of research into practice? Types of evidence needed. *Annu Rev Public Health.* 2007;28:413–433.

30. Castro FG, Barrera M, Jr., Holleran Steiker LK. Issues and challenges in the design of culturally adapted evidence-based interventions. *Annual review of clinical psychology.* 2010;6:213–239.

31. Chambers DA, Glasgow RE, Stange KC. The dynamic sustainability framework: addressing the paradox of sustainment amid ongoing change. *Implementation science: IS.* 2013;8:117.

32. Gaglio B, Phillips SM, Heurtin-Roberts S, Sanchez MA, Glasgow RE. How pragmatic is it? Lessons learned using PRECIS and RE-AIM for determining pragmatic characteristics of research. *Implementation science: IS.* 2014;9:96.

33. Pawson R, Tilley N. *Realistic evaluation.* Thousand Oaks, CA: Sage Publications; 1997.

34. Bennett GG, Glasgow RE. The delivery of public health interventions via the Internet: actualizing their potential. *Annu Rev Public Health.* 2009;30:273–292.

35. Chalkidou K, Tunis S, Whicher D, Fowler R, Zwarenstein M. The role for pragmatic randomized controlled trials (pRCTs) in comparative effectiveness research. *Clinical trials.* 2012;9(4):436–446.

36. Kairalla JA, Coffey CS, Thomann MA, Shorr RI, Muller KE. Adaptive designs for comparative effectiveness research trials. *Clinical research and regulatory affairs.* 2015;32(1):36–44.

37. Glasgow RE, Steiner JF. Comparative effectiveness research to accelerate translation: Recommendatiosn for an emerging field of science. In: Brownson RC, Colditz G, Proctor EK, eds. *Dissemination and implementation research in health.* New York, NY: Oxford University Press; 2012:72–93.

38. Glasgow RE, Vinson C, Chambers D, Khoury MJ, Kaplan RM, Hunter C. National Institutes of Health approaches to dissemination and implementation science: current and future directions. *Am J Public Health.* 2012;102(7):1274–1281.

39. Loudon K, Treweek S, Sullivan F, Donnan P, Thorpe KE, Zwarenstein M. The PRECIS-2 tool: designing trials that are fit for purpose. *BMJ.* 2015;350:h2147.

40. Thorpe KE, Zwarenstein M, Oxman AD, et al. A pragmatic-explanatory continuum indicator

summary (PRECIS): a tool to help trial designers. *J Clin Epidemiol.* 2009;62(5):464–475.

41. Pinnock H, Barwick M, Carpenter CR, et al. Standards for Reporting Implementation Studies (StaRI) Statement. *BMJ.* 2017;356:i6795.

42. Green LW, Glasgow RE. Evaluating the relevance, generalization, and applicability of research: issues in external validation and translation methodology. *Eval Health Prof.* 2006;29(1):126–153.

43. Glasgow RE, Riley WT. Pragmatic measures: what they are and why we need them. *Am J Prevent Med.* 2013;45(2):237–243.

44. Rabin BA, Purcell EP, Glasgow RE. Harmonizing measures for implementation science using crowd-sourcing. *Clin Med Res.* 2013;11(3):158.

45. Toobert DJ, Hampson SE, Glasgow RE. The summary of diabetes self-care activities measure: results from 7 studies and a revised scale. *Diabetes Care.* 2000;23(7):943–950.

46. Glasgow RE, Lichtenstein E, Marcus AC. Why don't we see more translation of health promotion research to practice? Rethinking the efficacy-to-effectiveness transition. *Am J Public Health.* 2003;93(8):1261–1267.

47. Moore GF, Audrey S, Barker M, et al. Process evaluation of complex interventions: medical Research Council guidance. *BMJ.* 2015;350:h1258.

48. Craig P, Dieppe P, Macintyre S, Michie S, Nazareth I, Petticrew M. *Developing and evaluating complex interventions: New guidance.* London: Medical Research Council; 2006.

49. McLeroy KR, Bibeau D, Steckler A, Glanz K. An ecological perspective on health promotion programs. *Health Educ Q.* 1988;15(4):351–377.

50. Purtle J, Brownson RC, Proctor EK. Infusing science into politics and policy: the importance of legislators as an audience in mental health policy dissemination research. *Admin Policy Ment Health.* 2017;44(2):160–163.

51. Baquero B, Linnan L, Laraia BA, Ayala GX. Process evaluation of a food marketing and environmental change intervention in Tiendas that serve Latino immigrants in North Carolina. *Health Promot Pract.* 2014;15(6):839–848.

52. Bamberger M, Rao V, Woolcock M. Using mixed methods in monitoring and evaluation: Experiences from international development evaluation. In: Tashakkori A, Teddlie C, eds. *Sage handbook of mixed methods in social and behavioral research.* 2nd ed. Thousand Oaks, CA: Sage Publications; 2010:613–642.

53. Tabak RG, Khoong EC, Chambers DA, Brownson RC. Bridging research and practice: models for dissemination and implementation research. *Am J Prevent Med.* 2012;43(3):337–350.

54. Nilsen P. Making sense of implementation theories, models and frameworks. *Implement Sci.* 2015;10:53.

55. Damschroder LJ, Aron DC, Keith RE, Kirsh SR, Alexander JA, Lowery JC. Fostering implementation of health services research findings into practice: a consolidated framework for advancing implementation science. *Implement Sci.* 2009;4:50.

56. Harvey G, Kitson A. PARIHS revisited: from heuristic to integrated framework for the successful implementation of knowledge into practice. *Implement Sci.* 2016;11:33.

57. Kilbourne AM, Neumann MS, Pincus HA, Bauer MS, Stall R. Implementing evidence-based interventions in health care: application of the replicating effective programs framework. *Implement Sci.* 2007;2:42.

58. Bartholomew-Eldredge LK, Markham CM, Ruiter RAC, Fernandez ME, Kok G, Parcel GS. *Planning health promotion programs: An intervention mapping approach.* 4th ed. San Francisco: Jossey-Bass; 2016.

59. Gielen AC, McDonald EM, Gary TL, Bone LR. Using the PRECEDE-PROCEED model to apply health behavior theories. In: Glanz K, Rimer BK, Viswanath K, eds. *Health behavior and health education: Theory, research, and practice.* San Francisco: Jossey-Bass; 2008:407–433.

60. Weir C, McLeskey N, Brunker C, Brooks D, Supiano MA. The role of information technology in translating educational interventions into practice: an analysis using the PRECEDE/PROCEED model. *J Am Med Inform Assoc.* 2011;18(6):827–834.

61. Tramm R, McCarthy A, Yates P. Using the Precede-Proceed Model of Health Program Planning in breast cancer nursing research. *J Adv Nurs.* 2012;68(8):1870–1880.

62. Pocetta G, Votino A, Biribanti A, Rossi A. Recording non communicable chronic diseases at risk behaviours in general practice. a qualitative study using the PRECEDE-PROCEED Model. *Ann Ig.* 2015;27(3):554–561.

63. Kessler R, Glasgow RE. A proposal to speed translation of healthcare research into practice: dramatic change is needed. *Am J Prevent Med.* 2011;40(6):637–644.

64. Harden SM, Gaglio B, Shoup JA, et al. Fidelity to and comparative results across behavioral interventions evaluated through the RE-AIM framework: a systematic review. *Syst Rev.* 2015;4:155.

65. RE-AIM website. www.re-aim.org. Accessed December 21, 2016.

66. Feldstein AC, Glasgow RE. A practical, robust implementation and sustainability model (PRISM)

for integrating research findings into practice. *Jt Comm J Qual Patient Safe.* 2008;34(4):228–243.

67. Liles EG, Schneider JL, Feldstein AC, et al. Implementation challenges and successes of a population-based colorectal cancer screening program: a qualitative study of stakeholder perspectives. *Implementat Sci.* 2015;10:41.

68. Glasgow RE, Gaglio B, Bennett G, et al. Applying the PRECIS criteria to describe three effectiveness trials of weight loss in obese patients with comorbid conditions. *Health Serv Res.* 2012;47(3 Pt 1):1051–1067.

69. Johnson KE, Tachibana C, Coronado GD, et al. A guide to research partnerships for pragmatic clinical trials. *BMJ.* 2014;349:g6826.

70. Sanchez MA, Rabin BA, Gaglio B, et al. A systematic review of eHealth cancer prevention and control interventions: new technology, same methods and designs? *Transl Behav Med.* 2013;3(4):392–401.

71. Koppenaal T, Linmans J, Knottnerus JA, Spigt M. Pragmatic vs. explanatory: an adaptation of the PRECIS tool helps to judge the applicability of systematic reviews for daily practice. *J Clin Epidemiol.* 2011;64(10):1095–1101.

72. Craig P, Dieppe P, Macintyre S, et al. Developing and evaluating complex interventions: the new Medical Research Council guidance. *BMJ.* 2008;337:a1655.

73. Neta G, Glasgow RE, Carpenter CR, et al. A framework for enhancing the value of research for dissemination and implementation. *Am J Public Health.* 2015;105(1):49–57.

74. Rabin BA, Lewis CC, Norton WE, et al. Measurement resources for dissemination and implementation research in health. *Implement Sci.* 2016;11:42.

75. Harden SM, McEwan D, Sylvester BD, et al. Understanding for whom, under what conditions, and how group-based physical activity interventions are successful: a realist review. *BMC Public Health.* 2015;15:958.

76. Brimhall KC, Fenwick K, Farahnak LR, Hurlburt MS, Roesch SC, Aarons GA. Leadership, organizational climate, and perceived burden of evidence-based practice in mental health services. *AdminPolicy Ment Health.* 2016;43(5):629–639.

77. Ritzwoller DP, Sukhanova A, Gaglio B, Glasgow RE. Costing behavioral interventions: a practical guide to enhance translation. *Ann Behav Med.* 2009;37(2):218–227.

78. Allicock M, Johnson LS, Leone L, et al. Promoting fruit and vegetable consumption among members of black churches, Michigan and North Carolina, 2008-2010. *Prev Chronic Dis.* 2013;10:E33.

79. Patton MQ. *Qualitative research & evaluation methods: Integrating theory and practice.* 4th ed. Thousand Oaks, CA: Sage; 2015.

80. Webster LA, Ekers D, Chew-Graham CA. Feasibility of training practice nurses to deliver a psychosocial intervention within a collaborative care framework for people with depression and long-term conditions. *BMC Nurs.* 2016;15:71.

81. Huntink E, Wensing M, Timmers IM, van Lieshout J. Process evaluation of a tailored intervention programme of cardiovascular risk management in general practices. *Implement Sci.* 2016;11(1):164.

82. Proctor EK, Landsverk J, Aarons G, Chambers D, Glisson C, Mittman B. Implementation research in mental health services: an emerging science with conceptual, methodological, and training challenges. *Admin Policy Ment Health.* 2009;36(1):24–34.

83. Creswell JW, Clark VLP. *Designing and conducting mixed methods research.* 2nd ed. Thousand Oaks, CA: Sage; 2011.

84. Teddlie C, Tashakkori A. *Foundations of mixed methods research: Integrating quantitative and qualitative approaches in the social and behavioral sciences.* Thousand Oaks, CA: Sage; 2009.

85. Ritzwoller DP, Toobert D, Sukhanova A, Glasgow RE. Economic analysis of the Mediterranean Lifestyle Program for postmenopausal women with diabetes. *Diabetes Educ.* 2006;32(5):761–769.

86. Krist AH, Cifuentes M, Dodoo MS, Green LA. Measuring primary care expenses. *J Am Board Fam Med.* 2010;23(3):376–383.

87. Neumann PJ, Sanders GD, Russell LB, Siegel JE, Ganiats TG, eds. *Cost-effectiveness in health and medicine.* 2nd ed. Oxford: Oxford University Press; 2017.

88. Khoury MJ, Clauser SB, Freedman AN, et al. Population sciences, translational research, and the opportunities and challenges for genomics to reduce the burden of cancer in the 21st century. *Cancer Epidemiol Biomarkers Prev.* 2011;20(10):2105–2114.

89. Collins FS, Varmus H. A new initiative on precision medicine. *N Engl J Med.* 2015;372(9):793–795

Mixed Methods Evaluation in Dissemination and Implementation Science

LAWRENCE A. PALINKAS AND BRITTANY RHOADES COOPER

INTRODUCTION

Mixed methods is a methodology that focuses on collecting, analyzing, and mixing both quantitative and qualitative data in a single study or multiphased study. Its central premise is that the use of quantitative and qualitative approaches in combination provides a better understanding of research problems than either approach alone.[1] Although there is some debate as to whether one approach must, of necessity, assume the dominant role and the other approach a supplementary role in a research project,[1-3] there is general agreement that the critical feature of mixed methods is the integration of quantitative and qualitative methods; conducting one or more qualitative studies and one or more quantitative studies in the same project without integrating the methods or the results (i.e., engaging in "parallel play") is not mixed methods per se,[4-6] but is perhaps better described as a multimethod design. In a mixed method design, each set of methods plays an important role in achieving the overall goals of the project and is enhanced in value and outcome by its ability to offset the weaknesses inherent in the other set and by its "engagement" with the other set of methods. Consequently, mixed methods represent both a model of and a model for transdisciplinary research.[7]

In the past decade, mixed methods have come to play a critical role in the field of dissemination and implementation (D&I) science. A recent study found that 69% of 67 D&I research grants funded by the National Cancer Institute between fiscal years 2010 and 2012 planned to use both qualitative and quantitative methods.[8] This role has emerged from both necessity and opportunity. Similar to the use of hybrid designs in which evidence-based practice effectiveness and implementation are addressed simultaneously,[9] mixed methods are often used to simultaneously answer confirmatory and exploratory research questions, and therefore verify and generate theory in the same study.[3,4] As D&I science is a relatively "new" discipline, generating theory has been accorded the highest priority.[10] Some of the theories, frameworks, and models that have been developed explicitly call for the use of both quantitative and qualitative methods due to the complexity of the subject matter, the importance of understanding both general principles and specific context, and the need to acquire depth as well as breadth of understanding of D&I.[11,12] Further,

"empirical research is needed to study how and the extent to which implementation theories, models and frameworks contribute to more effective implementation and under what contextual conditions or circumstances they apply (and do not apply). It is also important to explore how the current theoretical approaches can be further developed to better address implementation challenges. Hence, both inductive construction of theory and deductive application of theory are needed."[13(p. 9)]

In D&I science, mixed methods are most commonly used to identify barriers and facilitators to successful implementation, but may also be used as a tool for developing strategies and conceptual models of implementation and sustainment, monitoring the implementation process, and enhancing the likelihood of successful implementation and sustainment. Qualitative methods are generally used inductively to examine the context and process of implementation with depth of understanding, while quantitative methods are commonly used deductively to examine the content and outcomes of implementation with breadth of understanding. Following the examples of nursing,[14,15] evaluation,[3,16] public health,[17,18] health services,[19-21] education,[22] and the social and behavioral sciences,[4,23] there are several typologies and guidelines for the use of mixed methods designs in D&I science.[24-27]

The aims of this chapter are to: (1) provide a brief overview as to the structure, function, and process of mixed methods; (2) describe what quantitative and qualitative methods can and cannot do within the context of D&I science; and (3) provide examples of what mixed methods can accomplish in implementation science.

CHARACTERISTICS OF MIXED METHODS DESIGNS

Structure

Mixed method designs in D&I research can be categorized in terms of their structure, function, and process.[24-27] Quantitative and qualitative methods may be used simultaneously or sequentially, with one method viewed as dominant or primary and the other as secondary,[2] although equal weight can be given to both methods.[1,3] A review of published studies of D&I found that most studies involved the simultaneous use of quantitative and qualitative methods, and most used quantitative methods as the primary or dominant method and qualitative methods as the secondary or subordinate method.[24] However, a little less than half of the studies used balanced designs in which quantitative and qualitative methods were used simultaneously and given equal weight. For instance, Whitley and colleagues[28] documented the process of implementation of an illness management and recovery program for people with severe mental illness in community mental health settings using qualitative data to assess perceived barriers and facilitators of implementation and quantitative data to assess implementation performance based on assessments of fidelity to the practice model, with no overriding priority assigned to either aim. Some studies gave equal weight to qualitative and quantitative data for the purpose of evaluating fidelity and implementation barriers/facilitators even though the collection of qualitative data to assess implementation was viewed as secondary to the overall goal of evaluating the effectiveness of an intervention.[29-31]

Function

In D&I research, mixed methods have been used to achieve one or more of five different functions (Table 20.1). First, qualitative and quantitative methods may be used sequentially or

simultaneously to answer the same question. This is known as convergence. There are two specific forms of convergence: triangulation and transformation. Triangulation involves the use of one type of data to validate or confirm conclusions reached from analysis of the other type of data. Swain and colleagues[32] used triangulation to identify commonalities and disparities between quantitative data obtained from closed-ended questions and qualitative data obtained from open-ended questions of a survey administered to 49 participants, each participant representing a distinct practice site. Aarons and colleagues[33] compared findings obtained from analyses of quantitative and qualitative data to assess convergence of assessments of feasibility, acceptability, and utility of a leadership implementation intervention. Transformation involves the sequential quantification of qualitative data or the use of qualitative techniques to transform quantitative data. The technique of concept mapping,[34] used by Aarons and colleagues,[35] where qualitative data elicited from focus groups are "quantitized" using multidimensional scaling and hierarchical cluster analysis to identify stakeholder perceptions of barriers and facilitators of implementing evidence-based practices in community mental health settings, is an example of transformation. In another illustration, Watts and colleagues[36] conducted semistructured interviews with staff at participating clinics using the Promoting Action on Research Implementation in Health Services (PARiHS)[37] framework to develop overarching questions in a study of the implementation of evidence-based psychotherapies for PTSD in VA specialty clinics. Transcripts of these interviews were coded by domain and element of the PARiHS framework, and a scoring rubric was used to transform each element of the framework into a numeric value. Damschroder and Lowery[38] embedded the constructs of the Consolidated Framework for Implementation Research[11] in semistructured interviews and then assigned numerical ratings that reflected their valence (positive or negative influence) and their magnitude or strength. Qualitative comparative analysis[39] is another form of mixed method that "can be used to (1) analyze small to medium number of cases (i.e., 10 to 50) when traditional statistical methods are not possible, (2) examine complex combinations of explanatory factors associated with translation or implementation "success," and (3) combine quantitative and qualitative data using a unified and systemic analytical approach."[5 (p.201)]

TABLE 20.1 FUNCTIONS OF MIXED METHOD DESIGNS

Design type	Purpose
Convergence	• Corroboration of findings (data + interpretation) generated through quantitative methods with findings generated through qualitative designs (Triangulation) • Conversion of one type of data into another (Quantitizing/qualitizing)
Complementarity	• Findings generated through qualitative methods answer exploratory questions while findings generated through quantitative methods answer confirmatory questions. • Qualitative methods provide depth of understanding to complement breadth of understanding afforded by quantitative methods • Qualitative methods used to study process and context and quantitative methods to study outcomes
Expansion	• Findings from a qualitative study used to expand the depth of understanding of issues addressed in a quantitative study • Findings from a quantitative study used to expand the breadth of understanding of issues addressed in a qualitative study.
Exploratory/Development	• Findings from a qualitative study used to develop questions or items for a quantitative survey or instrument, develop or modify a conceptual framework used to generate hypotheses for quantitative analyses, or develop an intervention or program that can be evaluated quantitatively
Sampling	• Use of one set of methods to identify participants who will provide data using the other set of methods (e.g., purposeful sampling of research participants for semistructured interviews based on information collected from a quantitative survey; random sampling of a subpopulation of participants identified from interviews or participant observation as being of particular interest

Second, quantitative and qualitative methods may be used to answer related questions for the purpose of evaluation or elaboration. This is known as complementarity. In evaluative designs, quantitative data are used to evaluate outcomes while qualitative data are used to evaluate process. In elaborative designs, qualitative methods are used to provide depth of understanding and quantitative methods are used to provide breadth of understanding. This includes studies that present descriptive quantitative data on subjects, and studies that used qualitative data to focus on beliefs and perspectives. Gilburt et al.[40] used mixed methods to achieve complementarity in their evaluation of implementation of a recovery-oriented practice through training across a system of mental health services, using a quantitative audit of care plans in a random sample of 700 patients to assess change in core plan topics and in responsibility of action and semi-structured interviews with team leaders to explore understanding of recovery, implementation within the service and the wider system,

and perceived impact of the training on individual practice and that of the team.

Third, one method may be used in sequence to answer questions raised by the other method. This is known as expansion or explanation. Kramer and Burns[41] used data from qualitative interviews with providers as part of a summative evaluation to understand the factors contributing to partial or full implementation of a CBT for depressed adolescents in two publically funded mental health care settings. Brunette and colleagues[42] used qualitative data collected from interviews and ethnographic observations to elucidate barriers and facilitators to implementation of integrated dual disorders treatment and explain differences in treatment fidelity across the study sites. Duffy and colleagues[43] used the qualitative data obtained from a smaller number of nurse interviews to further explain the more close-ended, but more generalizable, patient and nurse surveys and EMR data that were obtained from larger numbers of participants.

Fourth, one set of methods may be used to answer questions that will enable use of the other method to answer other questions. This is known as development. In implementation research, there are three distinct forms of development: instrument development, conceptual development, and intervention development or adaptation. Zazzali and colleagues[44] connected qualitative data collected from semistructured interviews with 15 program administrators to the development of a conceptual model of implementation of Functional Family Therapy that could then be tested using quantitative methods. Blasinsky et al.[45] used qualitative data obtained from semistructured interviews to develop a rating scale to construct predictors of program outcomes and sustainability of a collaborative care intervention to assist older adults suffering from major depression or dysthymia. Sales and colleagues[46] describe a protocol for using quantitative outcomes data and qualitative data on implementation barriers and facilitators to design feedback reports for staff as an strategy for implementing goals of care conversations with veterans in VA long-term care settings.

Finally, there is the sequential use of one method to identify a sample of participants for use of the other method. This is known as sampling. Aarons and Palinkas[47] purposively sampled 15 case managers selected to represent those having the most positive and those having the most negative views of the Safe Care® home-based intervention based on results of a web-based quantitative survey asking about the perceived value and usefulness of Safe Care®. Woltmann

et al[48] used qualitative data obtained through interviews with staff, clinic directors, and consultant trainers to create categories of staff turnover and designations of positive, negative, and mixed influence of turnover on implementation outcomes. These categories were then quantitatively compared with implementation outcomes via simple tabulations of fidelity and penetration means for each category.

Process

The process of integrating quantitative and qualitative data occurs in three forms, merging the data, connecting the data, and embedding the data (Figure 20.1).[1] In implementation research, merging the data occurs when qualitative and quantitative data are brought together in the analysis phase to answer the same question through triangulation or related questions through complementarity.[24,27] Connecting the data occurs when the analysis of one dataset leads to (and thereby connects to) the need for the other dataset, such as when quantitative results lead to the subsequent collection and analysis of qualitative data (i.e., expansion) or when qualitative results are used to build to the subsequent collection and analysis of quantitative data (e.g., development). Embedding the data occurs when qualitative or mixed method studies of treatment or implementation process or context are embedded within larger quantitative studies of treatment or implementation outcome for the purpose of complementarity, convergence, or expansion. In general, quantitative and qualitative data are merged when the two sets of data

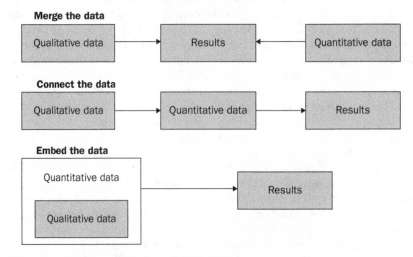

FIGURE 20.1 Three ways of mixing quantitative and qualitative data.

are used to provide answers to the same questions, connected when they are used to provided answers to related questions sequentially, and embedded when they are used to provide answers to related questions simultaneously. In describing a protocol for an implementation science study of HIV-related stigma in communities and health settings within a large, pragmatic cluster-randomized trial of a universal testing and treatment intervention for HIV prevention in Zambia and South Africa, Hargreaves and colleagues[49] propose to collect quantitative data on indicators of HIV-related stigma from large probability samples of community members, health workers, and people living with HIV, and qualitative data including in-depth interviews and observations from members of these same groups. These data will be used to accomplish three specific aims: (1) compare HIV-related stigma measures between study arms; (2) link data on stigma to measures of intervention implementation; and (3) explore changes in the dominant drivers and manifestations of stigma in study communities and the health system.

Operation

An illustration of how and why quantitative and qualitative methods are mixed can be found in a randomized cluster trial study protocol of an intervention model, Implementing School Nursing Strategies to Reduce LGBTQ Adolescent Suicide.[50] Mixed methods will be used to examine individual, school, and community factors influencing both implementation process and youth outcomes. A cluster randomized controlled trial will quantitatively assess whether LGBTQ students and their peers in Reduce LGBTQ Adolescent Suicide (RLAS) intervention schools report reductions in suicidality, depression, substance use, bullying, and truancy related to safety concerns compared with those in usual care schools. Implementation progress and fidelity for each evidence-based (EB) strategy in RLAS intervention schools will be measured using a modified version of the Stages of Implementation Completion checklist.[51] During the implementation and sustainment phases, annual focus groups will be conducted with the RLAS intervention schools to document their experiences identifying and advancing adaptation supports to facilitate use of EB strategies and their perceptions of the Dynamic Adaptation Process.[52]

"Data will be merged by the following: (a) linking qualitative and quantitative databases;

and (b) embedding one within the other so that each play a supporting role for the other. Results of each data set will be placed side-by-side to examine: (1) convergence—do interview data concur with New Mexico Youth Risk and Resilience Survey data regarding the impact of the intervention on suicide risk among LGBTQ students?; (2) expansion – can web-based survey data that suggest a disempowering school climate be explained by qualitative interview data?; and (3) complementarity – do the qualitative results describe contextual factors that reflect the variability represented by confidence intervals or variance estimates in statistical analyses of "bullying on school grounds" and "fear-based bullying"?[50 (p. 8)]

The protocol for examining individual and organizational factors that affect implementation of interventions for children with autism in public schools described by Locke and colleagues[53] is also explicit in the structure, function, and process of the mixed-method design. Researchers will employ a sequential (QUAN → QUAL) design, giving equal weight to the two sets of methods, beginning with a quantitative assessment of individual (e.g., attitudes of EBIs) and organizational (e.g., culture and climate, leadership) characteristics as predictors of implementation and sustainment of autism interventions, followed by qualitative methods to understand the appropriateness and fit of four autism EBIs within the school context, and principals' and teachers' experiences and perspectives regarding the implementation process in a subset of classrooms that are either high or low performing based on their fidelity data. The function of the design is evaluative and elaborative complementarity (quantitative data to assess outcomes and qualitative data to assess implementation process), and the process is connecting the two data sets so that the qualitative data builds upon the findings of the quantitative data.

WHAT QUANTITATIVE METHODS CAN AND CANNOT DO IN IMPLEMENTATION SCIENCE

"Quantitative research is a mode of inquiry used often for deductive research, when the goal is to test theories or hypotheses, gather descriptive

information, or examine relationships among variables. These variables are measured and yield numeric data that can be analyzed statistically. Quantitative data have the potential to provide measurable evidence, to help to establish (probable) cause and effect, to yield efficient data collection procedures, to create the possibility of replication and generalization to a population, to facilitate the comparison of groups, and to provide insight into a breadth of experience."[20 (pp. 4–5)]

Quantitative methods have specific characteristics that affect the role they play in D&I research. As the name implies, quantitative methods focus on the *quantity* of phenomenon being studied, mostly through the analysis of numeric data to determine statistical significance of the associations between constructs or the differences across groups.[20,21] Given the recent explosion of conceptual models and frameworks proposed to explain the characteristics of and processes by which successful D&I occur,[13,54] quantitative methods are often used deductively to test assertions and confirm hypotheses based on existing conceptual frameworks and models.

Many of these frameworks and models describe implementation in terms of key stages or processes.[55] One reason to use quantitative methods is to quantify or characterize these stages and processes. For example, recent studies have used finite mixture modeling to identify and characterize subgroups with distinct patterns of intervention participant attendance across time[56] and implementation quality.[57,58] McIntosh and colleagues[56] found four distinct patterns of implementation in a large sample of schools implementing a schoolwide positive behavioral support framework across 5 years: Sustainers (schools likely to meet fidelity criterion all 5 years), Slow Starters (schools with inconsistent fidelity across the first 3 years, but higher likelihood of meeting fidelity criterion in years 4 and 5), Late Abandoners (schools likely to meet fidelity criterion in first 3 years and unlikely in years 4 and 5), and Rapid Abandoners (schools likely to meet fidelity criterion during the first year, followed by rapid decline across the remaining 4 years). Quantitative methods were also used

in these studies to examine predictors of the identified patterns[56,58] and to determine how the patterns related to other implementation and intervention outcomes.[57]

Implementation frameworks and models also posit the community, organizational, and intervention factors associated with successful implementation[11] and/or the links between aspects of implementation and participant outcomes.[59] Therefore, quantitative methods are also used to test hypotheses related to predictors of successful implementation[38,60–63] and to quantify implementation barriers and facilitators.[64] In a cross-sectional study, Shapiro et al[64] surveyed 174 mental health service providers who were trained within the last 2 years to implement Triple P, an evidence-based parenting intervention. They used logistical and linear regression analysis to determine whether provider attributes, perceived barriers and facilitators to program use, and attitudes toward use of evidence-based practice predicted providers' self-reported use of the intervention following initial training. Aarons and colleagues[60] also used quantitative methods to survey service providers about the factors predictive of continued use of a parenting intervention. The authors used ordinal regression analyses to determine how different types of administration leadership (e.g., transformational, transactional, passive-avoidant) within the inner and outer context of the intervention were associated with the organizations' level of program sustainment (full, partial, or nonsustainment).

The theoretically based assertions about how different aspects of implementation lead to intervention outcomes can also be tested using quantitative methods[57,58,65,66] Goncy et al.[66] examined the relative impact of teachers' instructional adherence, procedural adherence, and quality of delivery of a classroom-based bullying prevention program on students' responsiveness to the intervention. These variables were quantitatively assessed through 288 observations of 44 teachers' implementation of the program over 2 years. The authors used multilevel models, which accounted for clustering of multiple observations for the same teacher across time and controlled for important covariates (e.g., school, intervention year, number of years teacher had experience with intervention), to determine whether the different aspects of adherence and quality of delivery were significantly associated with student responsiveness above and beyond other confounds. In a study by Berkel et al.,[65] several fidelity scores were devised to determine how fidelity-specificity was related to participant outcomes in an evidence-based family intervention for rural African American youth and their caregivers. Fidelity was operationalized as total number of fidelity items completed, divided by total possible and multiplied by 100 to produce a percentage of content delivered. The authors conducted a series of three regression analyses, with fidelity scores predicting change in youth racial socialization—each analysis was designed to examine fidelity's impact at increasing degrees of specificity for the targeted outcome: average fidelity across all sessions, average fidelity for the session on racial socialization, and average fidelity for the activity in that session on racial socialization.

Another goal of D&I science is to develop and evaluate discrete strategies aimed at effectively moving evidence-based health interventions into routine use in routine care settings.[67–70] Quantitative methods, especially within the context of randomized controlled designs, are used to determine the impact implementation strategies have on measureable implementation (e.g., adoption, fidelity, sustainability) and intervention outcomes (e.g., participant health outcomes).[71] For example, Atkins and colleagues[72] designed a study to test the impact of using peer-identified teachers (i.e., key opinion leaders) for disseminating information on educational and mental health best practices for students with attention-deficit/hyper-activity disorder (ADHD). Schools were randomly assigned to one of two conditions: key opinion leader plus mental health consultants or mental health consultants only. Mixed effect regression models were used to determine whether teacher-reported use of the ADHD best practices varied by condition, and whether these differences could be explained by the support teachers received from the key opinion leader in their school. In another randomized controlled trial, Lochman and colleagues[73] designed a study to test the impact of two different training models (high intensity vs. normal intensity) for school counselors implementing Coping Power, an evidence-based aggression prevention program. Fifty-seven school counselors were randomly assigned to one of three conditions: high intensity (basic training plus ongoing, individualized monitoring, technical assistance and feedback), normal intensity (basic training only), or a comparison condition (no training). They used hierarchical linear modeling to compare the changes in student behavioral outcomes in schools where

counselors received high, normal, or no training, to determine whether training intensity made a difference for intervention outcomes.

Glisson et al.[74] also conducted a randomized controlled trial to test the added benefit of combining an intervention strategy with an existing evidence-based treatment (Multisystemic Therapy, MST). In this case, the implementation strategy being tested was ARC (availability, responsiveness, and continuity), an organizational intervention designed to improve community-based mental health service delivery by developing social networks with key community stakeholders, and identifying and removing service barriers. They used a 2 × 2 factorial design to first randomly assign counties to ARC, the organizational intervention, and then randomly assigned delinquent youth within those counties to receive MST, the evidence-based treatment, or not. This resulted in four conditions: MST plus ARC, MST only, ARC only, or control. The researchers used multilevel, mixed effect regression analyses to compare youth behavioral and service outcomes (i.e., out-of-home placements) across all four conditions. They also examined if MST fidelity levels significantly varied across the two conditions implementing MST in an attempt to determine if the effects of ARC could be explained by improvements in MST fidelity.

Another reason quantitative methods are used in D&I science is for summarizing quantitative findings across multiple studies in systematic reviews and meta-analyses.[70,75–79] These reviews are often used to determine the degree to which specific types of implementation strategies or interventions are effective across studies and settings.[70,76,77,79] For example, Powell and colleagues[70] conducted a systematic review of 11 studies testing the effectiveness of implementation strategies for facilitating the delivery of evidence-based mental health treatments. They used vote counting to determine the proportion of studies that found statistically significant positive results of the strategy on implementation or clinical outcomes. Meta-analysis uses more formalized quantitative techniques to summarize quantitative findings across studies. For example, Webb and colleagues[79] identified 85 randomized controlled trial studies (N = 42,236 participants) testing the effectiveness of Internet-based health behavior change interventions. They used Hedges g (the difference between treatment and control means, divided by the pooled standard deviation) to determine the effect size for each intervention and then computed a weighted average effect size across all interventions on participants' health behavior. Systematic reviews and meta-analyses are also helpful in determining how similar or different results are across studies and synthesizing findings related to specific implementation frameworks and models[75,78]

As illustrated in the studies described, quantitative methods play an important role in D&I science. However, if used in isolation, they are likely to hinder the field's advancement due to several important limitations. Some of these limitations are driven by the fact that quantitative methods are only as good as the research designs, measures, and statistical analyses available to D&I researchers.[80] For example, quantitative methods rely on existing survey instruments and the validity (or lack thereof) of those instruments.[81,82] Therefore, quantitative methods are not useful for identifying new barriers/facilitators or exploring new constructs related to successful implementation if they are not included in existing measures or models. Similarly, quantitative methods are not well suited to provide explanations for novel or null findings—as they also are not represented in the hypotheses being tested, based on existing conceptual frameworks and models.

Quantitative methods emphasize breadth and generalizability of findings, and therefore they are also limited in their ability to provide depth of understanding for how and why implementation varies across different circumstances and settings.[65,83] This is especially true when the subgroup of interest is small.[64,66,84] Few quantitative methods are well suited to examine quantitative phenomenon with low variability or in small samples. For example, contrary to their theory-based hypotheses, Shapiro et al.[64] found no significant associations between the perceived barriers/facilitators for program use and number of families served by the intervention. They hypothesized that this null finding may be in part due to lack of variability in the number of families served across providers (the majority served fewer than 10 families in the past year). However, they also pointed out that a small number of providers (N = 4) used the program with a very high number of families (more than 100 families in the past year). Because of the size of this subgroup, they were unable to statistically examine what facilitated this high level of program use. Fortunately, as discussed in the following section, many of the limitations associated with quantitative methods can be addressed with qualitative methods.

WHAT QUALITATIVE METHODS CAN AND CANNOT DO IN IMPLEMENTATION SCIENCE

"A salient strength of qualitative research is its focus on the contexts and meaning of human lives and experiences for the purpose of inductive or theory-development-driven research. It is a systematic and rigorous form of inquiry that uses methods of data collection such as in-depth interviews, ethnographic observation, and review of documents. Qualitative data help researchers understand processes, especially those that emerge over time, provide detailed information about setting or context, and emphasize the voices of participants through quotes. Qualitative methods facilitate the collection of data when measures do not exist and provide a depth of understanding of concepts."[20(p. 4)]

As with quantitative methods, there are certain things that can and cannot be done with qualitative methods in D&I science. One of the most frequently cited reasons for using qualitative methods in implementation research is to understand barriers and facilitators to implementation[29–31,42,46,85,86] and sustainment.[45,87] While the findings of these studies point to several commonly occurring barriers and facilitators, thus increasing the generalizability of these qualitative findings, other studies have highlighted barriers and facilitators that are context or setting specific. For instance, in using data from focus groups and individual semistructured interviews, Fox and colleagues[88] ascertained barriers and facilitators of implementing an evidence-based quality improvement intervention that have been identified in settings with other interventions (e.g., scheduling trainings for busy providers) and barriers and facilitators that were specific to both the setting and the intervention (e.g., audio-visual equipment that sometimes failed, space not being optimal at some sites, and complexities inherent in adapting a training initially developed for individual completion to a group setting).

Another reason for using qualitative methods is to document implementation processes. Patton argues for the use of qualitative methods for implementation evaluation because such evaluation "requires case data rich with the details of program content and context. Because it is impossible to anticipate in advance how programs will adapt to local conditions, needs, and interests, it is impossible to anticipate what standardized quantiles could be used to capture the essence of each program's implementation. Under these evaluation conditions, a strategy of naturalistic inquiry is particularly appropriate."[3(p. 162)] Aarons and Palinkas[47] collected qualitative data through annual interviews and focus groups to assess the process of implementation of Safe Care®, an intervention designed to reduce child neglect and out-of-home placements of neglected children into foster care. Lessard et al.[89] used semistructured interviews with implementation facilitators to understand their role and the dynamics of facilitations between facilitators, family medicine groups, and other change actors. Hoagwood and colleagues[90] used a case study of an individual child to describe the process of implementation of an evidence-based, trauma-focused, cognitive-behavioral therapy for treatment of symptoms of PTSD in children living in New York City in the aftermath of the World Trade Center attack on September 11, 2001. Related to an understanding of process is the use of qualitative methods to evaluate implementation success by identifying and explaining which aspects of the program are working or not working, for whom and in what circumstances[91] and to understand how interventions are sustained.[45,87,92] As Albright et al. observe, "qualitative approaches are also useful when seeking to understand why evidence-based practices were successfully or unsuccessfully implemented, or when seeking strategies for facilitating implementation."[26(p. 202)]

Qualitative methods are used in implementation research to confirm or validate quantitative analyses through the technique of triangulation or convergence. In a pragmatic study comparing a nurse-administered tobacco tactics intervention to usual care, Duffy and colleagues[43] collected and analyzed quantitative data from recruitment logs, chart audits, and surveys administered to study participants, as well as qualitative data collected from structured interviews. "The qualitative results were triangulated with quantitative results, which involved cross-verifying the same information from different sources, in this case comparing patient data, nurse survey and interview data, and EMR data."[53(p. 5)] Use of qualitative methods to confirm or validate quantitative analyses is especially important in implementation research because the unit of analysis is the organization at which implementation occurs, resulting in sample sizes that are often too small to provide adequate statistical power.[24,26] Saldana[92] is using qualitative data to increase understanding of how behavior in agencies implementing evidence-based practices, as defined by the quantitative Stages of Implementation Completion (SIC) measure, relates to on-the-ground decision-making. In this instance, qualitative data is used to determine extent of convergence between reliable patterns of behaviors and particular patterns of SIC scores, "thereby helping to unpack the potential for SIC scores to serve as a proxy for less easily observed phenomenon."[9 (p. 8)]

Qualitative methods are also well suited to understanding the context in which implementation occurs. "Understanding the context under which interventions work and how different ways of implementing an intervention lead to successful outcomes are required for "T3" (i.e., D&I of evidence-based interventions) and "T4" translations (i.e., policy development to encourage evidence-based intervention use among various stakeholders"[5(p. 201)]

Qualitative methods can also be used to develop and establish construct validity of quantitative implementation outcome measures. According to Proctor and colleagues, "Qualitative data, reflecting language used by various stakeholders as they think and talk about implementation processes, is important for validating implementation outcome constructs."[71(p. 71)] Martinez and colleagues[94] recommend the use of mixed methods for addressing the instrumentation issue in implementation science of choosing the most appropriate evaluation method and approach.

In each of these instances, qualitative methods are used to elicit the perspectives of implementation stakeholders, including administrators, providers, and patients/clients.[24,26] As Proctor and colleagues observe,

> "Any effort to implement change in care involves a range of stakeholders, including the treatment developers who design and test the effectiveness of ESTs, policy makers who design and pay for the service, administrators who shape program direction, providers and

supervisors, patients/clients/consumers and their family members, and interested community members and advocates. The success of efforts to implement evidence-based treatment may rest on their congruence with the preferences and priorities of those who shape, deliver, and participate in care."[71(p. 72)]

Elsey and colleagues[95] used semistructured interviews with providers and patients to understand patient and health worker knowledge about tobacco and patients' motivation to quit to inform the design of a cessation intervention. Kane and colleagues[5] also conducted interviews with providers to assess perspectives on feasibility and acceptability of new guidelines.

While qualitative methods have important roles to play in the scientific endeavor that extends from identification of a phenomenon to active intervention, they are also limited in certain respects. For instance, while qualitative methods are often used to generate hypotheses related to D&I, they are rarely used for hypothesis testing. Some researchers have argued that qualitative data can be used to test hypotheses.[4,96] Deductive approaches to analyzing the content of qualitative data where themes are identified a priori can be viewed as one form of hypothesis testing. Colon-Emeric et al.[87] analyzed interview transcripts using framework analysis of a priori concepts, combined with inductive analyses. Sommerbakk and colleagues[97] used a combination of thematic analysis using an inductive approach and theoretical thematic approach, applying codes to Grol & Wensing's[98] multilevel model of barriers and facilitators. Still other studies have relied on theoretical models to inform use of qualitative methods in mixed method implementation studies. Elsey and colleagues[65] used Normalization Process Theory[99] to understand barriers and facilitators to implementation of a tobacco cessation intervention in primary care settings in Nepal. However, other researchers have noted that qualitative methods are better suited to inductively generating hypotheses than deductively testing them.[100] Still others take a "pragmatic approach," arguing that inductive and deductive techniques can be employed in the same study in an iterative fashion. As Patton observes,

"The extent to which a qualitative study is inductive or deductive varies along a continuum. As evaluation fieldwork begins, an evaluator may be open to whatever emerges from the data, a discovery, or inductive approach. Then, as the inquiry reveals patterns and major dimensions of interest, the evaluator will begin to focus on verifying and elucidating what appears to be emerging – a more deductively oriented approach to data collection and analysis."[3(p. 253)]

Second, qualitative methods are generally not used to produce generalizable findings due to the lack of samples that are selected at random from a larger population and of insufficient size to provide adequate power for statistical analysis. Occasionally, efforts are made to insure that the information gained from one sample or study is "transferable" to another sample or setting, which is not the same as claiming that the findings obtained from a sample of a population is "generalizable" to other members of the population not sampled.[100] However, although some forms of purposive sampling are designed to identify a range of variation in participant or organizational characteristics and behavior,[101] such methods are not designed to eliminate known or unknown potential sources of bias that may limit generalizability. Nevertheless, as Padgett asserts, findings can have generalizability and resonance without being "generalizable" in a statistical sense bas on how the sample was selected." [100 (p. 183)]

Third, when quantifying and analyzing qualitative data using statistical methods, caution must be exercised in adhering to the assumption associated with the conduct of such analyses. It must be remembered that despite their numerical form, findings from the analysis quantitized qualitative data are primarily exploratory and descriptive.

CASE STUDY

Background

Several models of research translation have been proposed over the years (see Tabak et al.[102] and Damschroder et al.[11] for a reviews). Many of these models consider sustainment to be the final stage of the process of implementation,[103,104] but the factors that predict sustainment are not well understood.[10,105] In part, this may be attributed to a lack of consensus as to what constitutes sustainment and how to measure it. There are no uniform or agreed upon criteria for determining whether something has been sustained or not.[106] This may be due to the fact that what is to be sustained differs from one program to the next. For instance, with respect to the community coalitions supporting drug and suicide prevention activities, some definitions of sustainment focus on the coalition itself while others focus on the activities and impacts of the coalition.[106] Furthermore, with few exceptions,[107–109] most studies reporting positive results have focused on earlier stages of implementation progress (exploration, adoption, routine use) and not on sustainment. In addition to uncertainty as to how to define sustainment, there is a lack of consensus as to how to measure it.

Palinkas and colleagues[92] describe a protocol for the development and evaluation of a system of measuring sustainment of US Substance Abuse and Mental Health Services Administration (SAMHSA)-supported prevention programs that target substance abuse prevention at the state or single community level, suicide prevention, and prevention of aggressive/ disruptive behavior in elementary schools. An examination of all four grant programs simultaneously provides an opportunity to determine what is meant by the term "sustainment" and identify and support both the *unique* contextual requirements for improving sustainability for each program as well as for developing a *generalizable* framework comprised of core components of sustainment across diverse prevention approaches.

Context

The mixed method design is sequential, giving priority to the development of the quantitative measurement system (qual → QUAN) through convergence (comparing qualitative and quantitative data and quantisizing qualitative data) and development (using qualitative data to develop a quantitative measure) by merging and connecting the data. In the first phase of the study, researchers interviewed 45 representatives of 10 grantees within four SAMHSA programs (Strategic Prevention Framework—State Initiative Grants, Sober Truth on Preventing Underage Drinking [STOP-Act], Garrett Lee Smith Suicide Prevention Program, and Prevention Practices in Schools). Data collection consisted of a semistructured interview to identify experiences with implementation and sustainment barriers and facilitators, a free listing exercise to elicit participant conceptions of the word "sustainment" and what it will take to sustain their programs; and a checklist of elements of the Consolidated Framework for Implementation Research to identify which are important for sustainment. Semistructured interview data were analyzed using a grounded theory approach[110] of coding, consensus, co-occurrence and comparison.[111] Coding was conducted by five members of the research team using the cloud-based Dedoose qualitative software. Comparisons of coding of the same transcripts by each team member revealed an average of 91.25% agreement across three levels of codes. Individual codes were then used to construct larger themes. Frequency counts and rank ordering of items obtained by the free list exercise were used to identify the salience of what is meant by sustainment/sustainability, program elements to be sustained, and requirements for sustainment. The procedure of constant comparison was used to identify meaningful clusters of items representing similar constructs. Implementation domains perceived to be relevant to sustainment were quantified by calculating the percent of informants citing the domain as high or very high in importance and a mean domain score (0 = not important, 1 = yes/no, 2 = important, 3 = very important). The lists of sustainment constructs obtained from the three sets of qualitative data were then compared side by side to identify those constructs appearing in more then one data set.

In the second phase of this project, these results along with an assessment on SAMHSA data collection systems will be used to develop a flexible measurement system, with both general and specific components, that can bring precision to monitoring sustainment of infrastructure, activities, and outcomes for each prevention approach.[92] In the third phase, the sustainment measurement system will be administered to all current and recently grantees funded by the four SAMHSA programs to quantitatively evaluate its utility in monitoring progress and improving the likelihood of sustainment. This project is intended to improve sustainment of the supporting prevention infrastructure, activities, and outcomes that are funded by federal, state, community, and foundation sources.

Lessons Learned

Four elements for measurement were identified by all three data sets collected in Phase I of the project (ongoing coalitions, collaborations, and networks; infrastructure and capacity to support sustainment; ongoing evaluation of performance and outcomes; and availability of funding and resources), and five elements were identified by two of three data sets (community need, community buy-in and support, leadership, presence of a champion, and evidence of positive outcomes). Some differences in construct priorities were also observed across programs, including norms; values and guiding principles of organizations; pressure from other states, tribes, or communities; perception of the current situation as needing change; knowledge and beliefs about the program; coalitions; collaboration and networking; and community specific activities that grantees wished to see sustained.[112]

FUTURE DIRECTIONS IN MIXED METHODS

As with any field of inquiry, scientific advancements often dictate or capitalize on advancements in methodology. This principle also applies to the use of mixed methods in D&I science. One potential focus of innovation in mixed methods lies in the development of a comprehensive understanding of implementation that links process to outcomes and both process and outcomes to context. Understanding the process of D&I is believed to be critical to understanding its outcome,[26] but new causal models linking the two may require broader application of specific mixed methods such as qualitative comparative analysis.[5] While qualitative methods are appropriately used to gain an in-depth understanding of the context in which D&I occurs, some generalization of process and outcomes is necessary to achieve a level of understanding that extends beyond merely a collection of unique experiences and circumstances. Further efforts are required to identify the "sweet spot" that exists between the generalizable and the specific characteristics of D&I processes and outcomes.

A second focus of mixed methods innovation is the identification of new strategies to support implementation of innovative evidence-based programs and practices.[70] For instance, Palinkas and colleagues[113,114] examined the role of social networks in scaling up evidence-based practices in county-level service systems in California and Ohio. Analysis of quantitative data of social networks found an association between the size and structure of social networks of child welfare, mental health, and juvenile justice systems leaders and stage of implementation of an evidence-based practice for treatment of behavioral health problems experienced by youth in foster care. Social networks were constructed using quantitative data collected from a web-based survey and qualitative data collected from semistructured interviews.[115] A complementary analysis

of semistructured interview data also revealed that collaborations between organizations were viewed by systems leaders as critical to implementing EBPs because they provided opportunities to exchange information and advice regarding specific EBPs and to pool resources, especially in small, rural counties where agencies have limited resources on their own.[116] Three sets of collaboration characteristics were identified: (1) characteristics of the collaboration itself, including focus (within or across counties), formality and frequency; (2) characteristics of the external environment, including availability of funding, county size, existence of clients in need of the services provided by each agency, and government mandates; and (3) characteristics of participating organizations, including a common language, common recognition of the problem to be addressed, common goals and values, a buy-in and commitment to innovation and change, policies and procedures designed to ensure accountability, existence of interpersonal relationships and social networks, an individual who could serve as a broker or advocate for the EBP, leadership that was supportive of the implementation, and participants possessing qualities of honesty, credibility, trust, and respect for others.

Another implementation strategy identified by mixed methods is the use of research evidence. Analysis of qualitative data obtained from semistructured interviews and a focus group with child welfare, mental health, and juvenile justice systems leaders informed the development of the quantitative Structured Interview for Evidence Use (SIEU)[117] The scale was then used to assess use of research evidence was collected from 151 directors and senior administrators of child welfare, mental health, and juvenile justice systems in 36 California and 9 Ohio counties participating in an RCT of the use of community development teams (CDTs) to scale up implementation of Treatment Foster Care Oregon (formerly known as Multidimensional Treatment Foster Care) over a 3-year period (2010–2012). Separate multivariate models were used to assess independent effects of evidence acquisition (input), evaluation (process), application (output), and total engagement (SIEU Total) on two measures of EBP implementation: highest stage reached and proportion of activities completed at preimplementation, implementation, and sustainment phases. Stage of implementation and proportion of activities completed in the implementation and sustainment phases were independently associated with acquisition of evidence and total engagement in use of research evidence. Participation in CDTs was significantly associated with acquisition and total engagement in evidence use.[118]

SUMMARY

In reviewing the rapidly growing literature on the use of mixed methods to address important issues confronting the science of D&I, we conclude with two observations. The first observation is that mixed methods reflect an iterative process of data collection and analysis that involves both inductive and deductive approaches to understanding complex phenomena. As such, researchers may be forced to alter or abandon a priori strategies for data collection and analysis. How these activities actually occur may bear little resemblance to how they were imagined to occur when the grant application was prepared and submitted. This is especially true during the exploratory phases of a multiphase project, where determining the most appropriate means for collecting and analyzing data may lead to some form of methodological trial and error.

Second, this chapter began with the observation that using mixed methods is more than parallel play involving separate quantitative and qualitative studies. One of the implications of the defining characteristic that the methods must somehow be integrated is that the standards for insuring the rigor and appropriateness of each method when conducted as part of a mixed method strategy may not be the same as the standards when conducted independently. In a mixed method design, it is conceivable if not necessarily desirable that qualitative data may be analyzed quantitatively despite their failure to adhere to the assumptions of sufficient sample size, normality, and generalizability required for use of statistical tests. Such a practice may run counter to the disciplinary traditions of both quantitative and qualitative methodologists. The point here is that mixed methods represent both naturalistic inquiry and experimentation. The nature of D&I requires innovation in use of both quantitative and qualitative methods, and not every innovation will be successful.

Both the iterative nature of D&I science and the likely debate and compromises involved in selection and application of quantitative and qualitative methods in a mixed method design demand attention on the part of the investigators to document and detail the rationale for the selection of methods and the process and outcomes

of their use. Without such documentation, the strengths and weaknesses of mixed method designs will be as context specific with limited generalizability and utility as the phenomena of D&I to which these methods are applied.

ACKNOWLEDGMENTS

Support for this chapter was provided by the following grant funded by the National Institute on Drug Abuse: R34 DA037516-01A1 and 2P30 DA 027828-06.

SUGGESTED READINGS AND WEBSITES

Readings

Aarons GA, Fettes DL, Sommerfeld DH, Palinkas LA. Mixed methods for implementation research: application to evidence-based practice implementation and staff turnover in community-based organizations providing child welfare services. *Child Maltreat*. 2012;17:67–79.

This article applies the typology for mixed method studies developed by Palinkas and colleagues to examining factors impacting staff retention during an evidence-based intervention implementation in a statewide child welfare system. The authors integrate qualitative data with previously published quantitative analyses of job autonomy and staff turnover in order to illustrate the utility of mixed method approaches in providing a more comprehensive understanding of opportunities and challenges in implementation research.

Albright K, Gechter K, Kempe A. Importance of mixed methods in pragmatic trials and dissemination and implementation research. *Acad Pediatr*. 2013;13:400–407.

This article discusses a number of dimensions of mixed methods research, utilizing at least one qualitative method and at least one quantitative method, that may be helpful when designing projects or preparing grant proposals for conducting pragmatic trials and dissemination and implementation research.

Creswell JW, Klassen AC, Plano Clark VL, Smith KC for the Office of Behavioral and Social Sciences Research. *Best practices for mixed methods research in the health sciences*. August 2011. National Institutes of Health.

This report was commissioned by the NIH Office of Behavioral and Social Science Research to serve as a resource that would provide guidance to NIH investigators on how to rigorously develop and evaluate mixed methods research applications. The report summarizes the nature and design of mixed methods research; teamwork, infrastructure, resources, and training for mixed methods research, incorporating mixed methods research in research, fellowship, career, training, and center grant applications; and criteria for reviewing mixed methods applications.

Cresswell JW, Plano Clark VL. *Designing and conducting mixed method research*. 2nd ed. Thousand Oaks, CA: Sage, 2011.

This is perhaps the most often cited textbook on the use of mixed method designs. The purpose of the book is to provide an introduction to mixed methods research, to discuss the steps involved in designing and conducting this form of inquiry, and, within these steps, to focus on four types of mixed methods designs. The book targets advanced graduate students as well as researchers at all levels from diverse disciplines who are designing mixed method studies.

Palinkas LA, Aarons GA, Horwitz SM, Chamberlain P, Hurlburt, M., Landsverk J. Mixed method designs in implementation research. *Adm Policy in Ment Health.* 2011;38:44–53.

This paper describes the application of mixed method designs in implementation research in 22 mental health services research studies published in peer-reviewed journals over the last 5 years. The authors' analyses revealed 7 different structural arrangements of qualitative and quantitative methods, 5 different functions of mixed methods, and 3 different ways of linking quantitative and qualitative data together. Complexity of design was associated with number of aims or objectives, study context, and phase of implementation examined. The findings provide suggestions for the use of mixed method designs in implementation research.

Websites and Tools

Journal of Mixed Methods Research. http://journals.sagepub.com/home/mmr

The Journal of Mixed Methods Research (JMMR) is an innovative, quarterly, interdisciplinary, international publication that focuses on empirical, methodological, and theoretical articles about mixed methods research across the social, behavioral, health, and human sciences. The scope includes delineating where mixed methods research may be used most effectively, illuminating design and procedure issues, and determining the logistics of conducting mixed methods research.

Web-Based Certificate Program in Mixed Methods Research.https://ssw.umich.edu/offices/continuing-education/certificate-courses/mixed-methods-research

The Certificate in Mixed Methods Research is designed for researchers and practitioners in social work, nursing, psychology, public health, anthropology, political science, sociology, education, and other applied fields who are interested in: ways to integrate qualitative and quantitative research methods and data,

commonly used qualitative and quantitative data collection methods and procedures, popular data analysis techniques used in the applied professions, and effective approaches to research conducted in practice settings

Mixed Methods Research Training Program for the Health Sciences. http://www.jhsph.edu/academics/training-programs/mixed-methods-training-program-for-the-health-sciences/

The Mixed Methods Research Training Program for the Health Sciences is funded by the National Institutes of Health through the Office of Behavioral and Social Science Research (OBSSR), and is the only program of its kind in the United States. The program fulfills a national need for training in mixed methods and is a natural next step following the publication of the OBSSR "Best Practices for Mixed Methods Research in the Health Sciences"

Center for Qualitative and Mixed Methods. http://www.rand.org/capabilities/methods-centers/qualitative-and-mixed-methods.html

The RAND Center for Qualitative and Mixed Methods (C-QAMM) develops and promotes tools for generating empirically based insights through iterative, exploratory data collection and analysis.

REFERENCES

1. Cresswell JW, Plano Clark VL. *Designing and conducting mixed method research*. 2nd ed. Thousand Oaks, CA: Sage; 2011.
2. Morse JM, Niehaus L. *Mixed method design: Principles and procedures*. Walnut Creek, CA: Left Coast Press; 2009.
3. Patton MQ. *Qualitative research and evaluation methods*. 3rd ed. Thousand Oaks, CA: Sage; 2002.
4. Teddlie C, Tashakkori A. Major issues and controversies in the use of mixed methods in the social and behavioral sciences. In: Tashakkori A, Teddlie C, eds. *Handbook of mixed methods in the social and behavioral sciences*. Thousand Oaks, CA: Sage; 2003:3–50.
5. Kane H, Lewis MA, Williams PA, Kahwati LC. Using qualitative comparative analysis to understand and quantify translation and implementation. *Translational Behav Med.* 2014;4:201–208.
6. Stange K, Crabtree BF, Miller WL. Publishing multimethod research. *Ann Fam Med.* 2006;4:292–294.
7. Palinkas LA, Soydan H. *Translation and implementation of evidence based practice*. New York: Oxford University Press; 2012.
8. Neta G, Sanchez MA, Chambers DA et al. Implementation science in cancer prevention and control: a decade of grant funding by the National Cancer Institute and future directions. *Implement Sci.* 2015;10:4.

9. Curran GM, Bauer M, Mittman B, Pyne JM, Stetler C. Effectiveness-implementation hybrid designs: combining elements of clinical effectiveness and implementation research to enhance public health impact. *Med Care*. 2012;50(3):217–226.

10. Proctor EK, Landsverk J, Aarons G, Chambers D, Glisson C, Mittman B. Implementation research in mental health services: an emerging science with conceptual, methodological and training challenges. *Adm Policy Ment Health*. 2009;36:24–34.

11. Damschroder LJ, Aron DC, Keith RE, Kirsh SR, Alexander JA, Lowery JC. Fostering implementation of health services research findings into practice: a consolidated framework for advancing implementation science. *Implement Sci*. 2009;4:50.

12. Demakis JG, McQueen L, Kizer KW, Fuessner JR. Quality Enhancement Research Initiative (QUERI): a collaboration between research and clinical practice. *Med Care*. 2000; 38:17–25.

13. Nilsen P. Making sense of implementation theories, models and frameworks. *Implement Sci*. 2015;10:53.

14. Morse JM. Approaches to qualitative-quantitative methodological triangulation. *Nurs Res*. 1991;40:120–123.

15. Sandelowski M. Combining qualitative and quantitative sampling, data collection, and analysis techniques in mixed method studies. *Res Nurs Health*. 2000;23:246–255.

16. Greene JC, Caracelli VJ, Graham WF. Toward a conceptual framework for mixed method evaluation designs. *Educ Eval Policy Analysis*. 1989;11:255–274.

17. Morgan DL. Practical strategies for combining qualitative and quantitative methods: applications to health research. *Qual Health Res*. 1998; 8:262–276.

18. Steckler A, McLeroy KR, Goodman RM, et al Toward integrating qualitative and quantitative methods: an introduction. *Health Educ Q*. 1992;19:1–8.

19. Cresswell JW, Fetters MD, Ivankova NV. Designing a mixed methods study in primary care. *Ann Fam Med*. 2004; 2:7–12.

20. Creswell JW, Klassen AC, Plano Clark VL, Smith KC for the Office of Behavioral and Social Sciences Research. *Best practices for mixed methods research in the health sciences*. August 2011. National Institutes of Health. https://obssr.od.nih.gov/wp-content/uploads/2016/02/Best_Practices_for_Mixed_Methods_Research.pdf

21. Curry L, Nunez-Smith M. *Mixed methods in health services research: A practical primer*. Thousand Oaks, CA: Sage Publications; 2015.

22. Cresswell JW. Mixed method research: introduction and application. In: Cizek GJ, ed. *Handbook of educational policy*. San Diego: Academic Press; 1999:455–472.

23. Waszak C, Sines MC. Mixed methods in psychological research. In: Tashakkori A., Teddlie C., eds. *Handbook of mixed methods in the social and behavioral sciences*. Thousand Oaks, CA: Sage; 2003:3–50.

24. Palinkas LA, Aarons GA, Horwitz SM, Chamberlain P, Hurlburt, M., Landsverk J. Mixed method designs in implementation research. *Adm Policy Ment Health*. 2011;38:44–53.

25. Aarons GA, Fettes DL, Sommerfeld DH, Palinkas LA. Mixed methods for implementation research: application to evidence-based practice implementation and staff turnover in community-based organizations providing child welfare services. *Child Maltreat*. 2012;17:67–79.

26. Albright K, Gechter K, Kempe A. Importance of mixed methods in pragmatic trials and dissemination and implementation research. *Acad Pediatr*. 2013;13:400–407.

27. Palinkas LA. Qualitative and mixed methods in mental health services and implementation research. *J Clin Child Adolesc Psychology*. 2014;43:851–861.

28. Whitley R, Gingerich S, Lutz WJ, Mueser KT. Implementing the illness management and recovery program in community mental health settings: facilitators and barriers. *Psychiatr Serv*. 2009;60:202–209.

29. Marshall T, Rapp CA, Becker DR, Bond GR. Key factors for implementing supported employment. *Psychiatr Serv*. 2008;59:886–892.

30. Marty D, Rapp C, McHugo G, Whitley R. Factors influencing consumer outcome monitoring in implementation of evidence-based practices: results from the National EBP Implementation Project. *Adm Policy Ment Health*. 2008;35:204–211.

31. Rapp CA, Etzel-Wise D, Marty, D, et al. Barriers to evidence-based practice implementation: results of a qualitative study. *Community Ment Health J*. 2010;46(2):112–118.

32. Swain K, Whitley R, McHugo GJ, Drake RE. The sustainability of evidence-based practices in routine mental health agencies. *Community Ment Health J*. 2010;46(2):119–129.

33. Aarons GA, Ehrhart MG, Farahnak LR, Hurlburt MS. Leadership and organizational change for implementation (LOCI): a randomized mixed method pilot study of a leadership and organization development intervention for evidence-based practice implementation. *Implement Sci*. 2015;10:11.

34. Trochim WM. An introduction to concept mapping for planning and evaluation. *Eval Prog Plan*. 1989;12:1–16.

35. Aarons GA, Wells R, Zagursky K, Fettes DL, Palinkas LA. Implementing evidence-based practice in community mental health agencies: multiple stakeholder perspectives. *Am J Public Health.* 2009;99(11), 2087–2095.

36. Watts BV, Shiner B, Zubkoff L, Carpenter-Song E, Ronconi JM, Coldwell CM. Implementation of evidence-based psychotherapies for posttraumatic stress disorder in VA specialty clinics. *Psychiatr Serv.* 2014; 65(5):648–653.

37. Kitson A, Harvey G, McCormack B. Enabling the implementation of evidence based practice: a conceptual framework. *Qual Health Care.* 1998;7:149–158.

38. Damschroder L, Lowery JC. Evaluation of a large-scale weight management program using the consolidated framework for implementation research (CFIR). *Implement Sci.* 2013;8:51.

39. Ragin CC. *Redesigning social inquiry: Fuzzy sets and beyond.* Chicago: University of Chicago Press; 2009.

40. Gilburt H, Slade M, Bird V, Oduola S, Craig TK. Promoting recovery-oriented practice in mental health services: a quasi-experimental mixed-methods study. *BMC Psychiatry.* 2013;13:167.

41. Kramer TF, Burns BJ. Implementing cognitive behavioral therapy in the real world: a case study of two mental health centers. *Implement Sci.* 2008;3:14.

42. Brunette MF, Asher D, Whitley R, et al. Implementation of integrated dual disorders treatment: a qualitative analysis of facilitators and barriers. *Psychiatr Serv.* 2008;59:989–995.

43. Duffy SA, Ronis DL, Ewing LA, et al. Implementation of the Tobacco Tactics intervention versus usual care in Trinity Health community hospitals. *Implement Sci.* 2016;11:147.

44. Zazzali JL, Sherbourne C, Hoagwood KE, Greene D, Bigley MF, Sexton TL. The adoption and implementation of an evidence based practice in child and family mental health services organizations: a pilot study of functional family therapy in New York State. *Adm Policy Mental Health.* 2008;35:38–49.

45. Blasinsky M, Goldman HH. Unützer J. Project IMPACT: a report on barriers and facilitators to sustainability. *Adm Policy Mental Health.* 2006;33:718–729.

46. Sales AE, Ersek M, Intrator OK, et al. Implementing goals of care conversations with veterans in VA long-term care setting: a mixed methods protocol. *Implement Sci.* 2016;11:132.

47. Aarons GA, Palinkas LA. Implementation of evidence-based practice in child welfare: service provider perspectives. *Adm Policy Ment Health.* 2007;34:411–419.

48. Woltmann EM, Whitley R, McHugo GJ., et al. The role of staff turnover in the implementation of evidence-based practices in health care. *Psychiatr Serv.* 2008;59:732–737.

49. Hargreaves JR, Stangl A, Bond V, et al. HIV-related stigma and universal testing for HIV prevention and care: design of an implementation science evaluation nested in the HPTN 071 (PopART) cluster-randomized trial in Zambia and South Africa. *Health Policy Plan.* 2016;31:1342–1354.

50. Willging CE, Green AE, Ramos MM. Implementing school nursing strategies to reduce LGBTQ adolescent suicide: a randomized cluster trial study protocol. *Implement Sci.* 2016;11:145.

51. Chamberlain P, Brown CH, Saldana L. Observational measure of implementation progress in community-based settings: the stages of implementation completion (SIC). *Implement Sci.* 2011;6:116.

52. Aarons GA, Green AE, Palinkas LA, et al. Dynamic adaptation process to implement an evidence-based child maltreatment intervention. *Implement Sci.* 2012;7:32

53. Locke J, Beidas RS, Marcus S, et al. A mixed methods study of individual and organizational factors that affect implementation of interventions for children with autism in public schools. *Implement Sci.* 2016;11:135.

54. Tabak RG, Khoong EC, Chambers D, Brownson RC. Models in dissemination and implementation research: useful tools in public health services and systems research. *Am J Prev Med.* 2012;43(3):337–350.

55. Aarons GA, Hurlburt M, Horwitz SM. Advancing a conceptual model of evidence-based practice implementation in public service sectors. *Adm Policy Ment Health.* 2011;38(1):4–23.

56. Mauricio AM, Tein JY, Gonzales NA, Millsap RE, Dumka LE, Berkel C. Participation patterns among Mexican-American parents enrolled in a universal intervention and their association with child externalizing outcomes. *Am J Community Psychol.* 2014;54(3-4):370–383.

57. Low S, Smolkowski K, Cook C. What constitutes high-quality implementation of SEL programs? A latent class analysis of Second Step-Implementation. *Prev Sci.* 2016;17(8):981–991.

58. Mcintosh K, Mercer SH, Nese RNT, Ghemraoui A. Identifying and predicting distinct patterns of implementation in a school-wide behavior support framework speed and patterns of implementation. *Prev Sci.* 2016:992–1001.

59. Berkel C, Mauricio AM, Schoenfelder E, Sandler IN. Putting the pieces together: an integrated model of program implementation. *Prev Sci.* 2011;12(1):23–33.

60. Aarons GA, Green AE, Trott E, et al. The roles of system and organizational leadership in

system-wide evidence-based intervention sustainment: a mixed-method study. *Adm Policy Ment Health*. 2016;43(6):991–1008.

61. Welsh JA, Chilenski SM, Johnson L, Greenberg MT, Spoth RL. Pathways to sustainability: 8-Year follow-up from the PROSPER project. *J Prim Prev*. 2016;37(3):263–286.

62. Green AE, Trott E, Willging CE, Finn NK, Ehrhart MG, Aarons GA. The role of collaborations in sustaining an evidence-based intervention to reduce child neglect. *Child Abus Negl*. 2016;53:4–16.

63. Hunter SB, Han B, Slaughter ME, Godley SH, Garner BR. Associations between implementation characteristics and evidence-based practice sustainment: a study of the Adolescent Community Reinforcement Approach. *Implement Sci*. 2015;10:173.

64. Shapiro CJ, Prinz RJ, Sanders MR. Sustaining use of an evidence-based parenting intervention: practitioner perspectives. *J Child Fam Stud*. 2015;24:1615–1624.

65. Berkel C, Murry VM, Roulston KJ, Brody GH. Understanding the art and science of implementation in the SAAF efficacy trial. *Health Educ*. 2013;113(4):297–323.

66. Goncy EA, Sutherland KS, Farrell AD, Sullivan TN, Doyle ST. Measuring teacher implementation in delivery of a bullying prevention program: the impact of instructional and procedural adherence and competence on student responsiveness. *Prev Sci*. 2015;16(3):440–450.

67. Azocar F, Cuffel B, Goldman W, McCarter L. The impact of evidence-based guideline dissemination for the assessment and treatment of major depression in a managed behavioral health care organization. *J Behav Health Serv Res*. 2003;30:109–118.

68. Beidas RS, Kendall PC. Training therapists in evidence-based practice: a critical review of studies from a systems-contextual perspective. *Clin Psychol Sci Pract*. 2010;17(1):1–30.

69. Kilbourne AM, Abraham KM, Goodrich DE, et al. Cluster randomized adaptive implementation trial comparing a standard versus enhanced implementation intervention to improve uptake of an effective re-engagement program for patients with serious mental illness. *Implement Sci*. 2013;8:136.

70. Powell BJ, Proctor EK, Glass JE. A systematic review of strategies for implementing empirically supported mental health interventions. *Res Soc Work Pract*. 2014;24(2):192–212.

71. Proctor E, Silmere H, Raghavan R, et al. Outcomes for implementation research: conceptual distinctions, measurement challenges, and research agenda. *Adm Policy Ment Health*. 2011;38(2):65–76.

72. Atkins MS, Frazier SL, Leathers SJ, et al. Teacher key opinion leaders and mental health

consultation in low-income urban schools. *J Consult Clin Psychol*. 2008;76(5):905–908.

73. Lochman JE, Boxmeyer C, Powell N, Qu L, Wells K, Windle M. Dissemination of the Coping Power program: importance of intensity of counselor training. *J Consult Clin Psychol*. 2009;77(3):397–409.

74. Glisson C, Schoenwald SK, Hemmelgarn A, et al. Randomized trial of MST and ARC in a two-level evidence-based treatment implementation strategy. *J Consult Clin Psychol*. 2010;78(4):537–550.

75. Kirk MA, Kelley C, Yankey N, Birken SA, Abadie B, Damschroder L. A systematic review of the use of the Consolidated Framework for Implementation Research. *Implement Sci*. 2016;11(1):72.

76. Yost J, Ganann R, Thompson D, et al. The effectiveness of knowledge translation interventions for promoting evidence-informed decision-making among nurses in tertiary care: a systematic review and meta-analysis. *Implement Sci*. 2015;10(1):98.

77. Grudniewicz A, Kealy R, Rodseth RN, Hamid J, Rudoler D, Straus SE. What is the effectiveness of printed educational materials on primary care physician knowledge, behaviour, and patient outcomes: a systematic review and meta-analyses. *Implement Sci*. 2015;10:164.

78. Davies P, Walker A, Grimshaw J. A systematic review of the use of theory in the design of guideline dissemination and implementation strategies and interpretation of the results of rigorous evaluations. *Implement Sci*. 2010;5:14.

79. Webb TL, Joseph J, Yardley L, Michie S. Using the internet to promote health behavior change: a systematic review and meta-analysis of the impact of theoretical basis, use of behavior change techniques, and mode of delivery on efficacy. *J Med Internet Res*. 2010;12:1–18.

80. Brown CH, Curran G, Palinkas LA, et al. An overview of research and evaluation for dissemination and implementation. *Annu Rev Public Health*. 2017;38(March):1–48.

81. Chaudoir SR, Dugan AG, Barr CH. Measuring factors affecting implementation of health innovations: a systematic review of structural, organizational, provider, patient, and innovation level measures. *Implement Sci*. 2013;8:22.

82. Lewis CC, Stanick CF, Martinez RG, et al. The Society for Implementation Research Collaboration Instrument Review Project: a methodology to promote rigorous evaluation. *Implement Sci*. 2015;10:2.

83. Gibbs DA, Krieger KE, Cutbush SL, Clinton-Sherrod AM, Miller S. Implementer-initiated adaptation of evidence-based interventions: kids remember the blue wig. *Health Educ Res*. 2016;31(3):405–415.

84. Brownson RC, Allen P, Jacob RR, et al. Understanding mis-implementation in public health practice. *Am J Prev Med.* 2015;48(5):543–551.

85. Cohen DJ, Balasubramanian BA, Gordon L, et al. A national evaluation of a dissemination and implementation initiative to enhance primary care practice capacity and improve cardiovascular disease care: the ESCALATES study protocol. *Implement Sci.* 2016;11:86.

86. Kozica SL, Lombard CB, Harrison CL, Teede HJ. Evaluation of a large healthy lifestyle program: informing program implementation and scale-up in the prevention of obesity. *Implement Sci.* 2016;11:151.

87. Colon-Emeric C, Toles M, Cary Jr. MP, et al. Sustaining complex interventions in long-term care: a qualitative study of direct care staff and managers. *Implement Sci.* 2016;11:94.

88. Fox AB, Hamilton AB, Frayne SN, et al. Effectiveness of an evidence-based quality improvement approach to cultural competence training: The Veterans Affairs "Caring for Women Veterans" program. *J Continuing Educ Health Professions.* 2016;36:96–103.

89. Lessard S, Bareil C, Lalonde L, et al. External facilitators and interprofessional facilitation teams: a qualitative study of their roles in supporting practice change. *Implement Sci.* 2016;11:97.

90. Hoagwood KE, Vogel JM, Levitt JM, D'Amico PJ, Paisner WI, Kaplan SJ. Implementing an evidence-based trauma treatment in a state system after September 11: the CATS Project. *J Am Acad Child Adolesc Psychiatry.* 2007;46(6):773–779.

91. McHugh S, Tracey ML, Riordan F, O.Neill K, Mays N, Kearney PM. Evaluating the implementation of a national clinical programme for diabetes to standardize and improve services: a realist evaluation protocol. *Implement Sci.* 2016;11:07.

92. Palinkas LA, Spear SE, Mendon SJ, et al. Measuring sustainment of prevention programs and initiatives: a study protocol. *Implement Sci.* 2016;11:95.

93. Saldana L. The states of implementation completion for evidence-based practice: protocol for a mixed methods study. *Implement Sci.* 2014;9:43.

94. Martinez RG, Lewis CC, Weiner BJ. Instrumentation issues in implementation science. *Implement Sci.* 2014;9:118.

95. Elsey H, Khanal S, Manandhar S, et al. Understanding implementation and feasibility of tobacco cessation in routine primary care in Nepal: a mixed methods study. *Implement Sci.* 2016;11:104.

96. Miles MB, Huberman AM. *Qualitative data analysis: An expanded sourcebook.* 2nd ed. Thousand Oaks, CA: Sage; 1994.

97. Sommerbakk R, Haugen DF, Tjora A, Kaasa S, Hjermstad MJ. Barriers to and facilitators for implementing quality improvements in palliative care—results for a qualitative interview study in Norway. *BMC Palliat Care.* 2016; 15:61.

98. Grol R, Wensing M. What drives change? Barriers to and incentives for achieving evidence-based practice. *Med J Aust.* 2004;180(6 Suppl):S57–60.

99. May C, Finch T. Implementation, embedding and integration: an outline of normalization process theory. *Sociology.* 2009;43:535–554.

100. Padgett DK. *Qualitative methods in social work research.* 2nd ed. Los Angeles, CA: Sage; 2008.

101. Palinkas LA, Horwitz SM, Green CA, Wisdom JP, Duan N, Hoagwood KE. Purposeful sampling for qualitative data collection and analysis in mixed method implementation research. *Adm Policy Ment Health.* 2015;42:533–544.

102. Tabak RG, Khoong EC, Chambers DA, Brownson RC. Bridging research and practice: models for dissemination and implementation research. *Am J Prev Med.* 2012;43(3):337–350.

103. Aarons GA, Hurlburt M, Horwitz SM. Advancing a conceptual model of evidence-based practice implementation in public service sectors. *Adm Policy Ment Health.* 2011;38:4–23.

104. Greenhalgh T, Robert G, Macfarlane F, Bate P, Kyriakidou O. Diffusion of innovations in service organizations: systematic review and recommendations. *Milbank Q.* 2004; 82(4):581–629.

105. Chambers DA, Glasgow RE, Stange KC. The dynamic sustainability framework: addressing the paradox of sustainment amid ongoing change. *Implement Sci.* 2013;8:117.

106. Benz J, Infante A, Oppenheimer C, Scherer H, Wilson W. *Developing a conceptual framework to assess the sustainability of community coalitions post-federal funding.* Chicago: National Opinion Research Center; 2011.

107. Feinberg ME, Bontempo DE, Greenberg MT. Predictors and level of sustainability of community prevention coalitions. *Am J Prev Med.* 2008; 34(6):495–501.

108. Gloppen KM, Arthur MW, Hawkins JD, Shapiro VB. Sustainability of the Communities That Care prevention system by coalitions participating in the Community Youth Development Study. *J Adolesc Health.* 2012; 51(3):259–264.

109. Rhew IC, Brown EC, Hawkins JD, Briney JS. Sustained effects of the Communities That Care system on prevention service system transformation. *Am J Public Health.* 2013; 103(3):529–535.

110. Glaser BG, Strauss AL. *The discovery of grounded theory: Strategies for qualitative research.* New York: Aldine de Gruyter, 1967

111. Willms DG, Best JA, Taylor DW, et al. A systematic approach for using qualitative methods in primary prevention research. *Med Anthro Q.* 1990;4(4), 391–409.

112. Palinkas LA, Spear S, Mendon S, Villamar J, Brown CH. Definition and Prediction of Sustainment of Prevention Programs and Initiatives. Presented at the 9th Conference on the Science of Dissemination and Implementation, Washington DC, December 14, 2016.

113. Palinkas LA, Holloway IW, Rice E, Fuentes D, Wu Q, Chamberlain, P. Social networks and implementation of evidence-based practices in youth-serving systems: a mixed methods study. *Implement Sci.* 2011;6:113.

114. Palinkas LA, Holloway IW, Rice E, Brown CH, Valente T, Chamberlain P. Influence network linkages across treatment conditions in a randomized controlled trial of two implementation strategies for scaling up evidence-based practices in public youth-serving systems. *Implement Sci.* 2013;8:133.

115. Rice ER, Holloway, IW, Barman-Adhikari A, Fuentes D, Brown CH, Palinkas LA. A mixed methods approach to network data collection. *Field Methods.* 2014;26(3):252–268.

116. Palinkas LA, Fuentes D, Garcia AR, Finno M, Holloway IW, Chamberlain P. Inter-organizational collaboration in the implementation of evidence-based practices among agencies serving abused and neglected youth. *Adm Policy Ment Health.* 2014;41:74–85.

117. Palinkas LA, Garcia AR, Aarons GA, et al. Measuring use of research evidence in child-serving systems: the Structured Interview for Evidence Use (SIEU). *Res Soc Work Pract.* 2016;26(5):550–564.

118. Palinkas LA, Brown CH, Saldana L, Chamberlain P. Association between inter-organizational consensus on use of research evidence and stage of implementation of an evidence-based practice. *Implement Sci.* 2015;10(Suppl 1):A20.

21

Dissemination and Implementation Research in Community and Public Health Settings

CYNTHIA A. VINSON, KATHERINE A. STAMATAKIS, AND JON F. KERNER

INTRODUCTION

Dissemination and implementation (D&I) research in community and public health settings holds great promise for widespread improvements in population health by closing the gap between scientific evidence and public health action. The goal of public health is centered on implementing preventive measures intended to decrease morbidity and mortality from a broad array of infections, chronic diseases, mental illness, abusive substances, and injuries. Public health action may take the form of programs and policies that intervene broadly at national levels or that specifically address regional or local issues.

Settings for public health are as diverse as the contexts in which public health-related action occurs. The Institute of Medicine report *The Future of Public Health* defined the concept of a public health system as "what we as a society do collectively to assure the conditions in which people can be healthy."[1] This definition expands the notion of public health outside of government agencies, to encompass other sectors and settings including the community at large, mass media and worksites, as well as more traditional public health agencies.[2,3] In addition, the transfer and integration of evidence-based interventions to communities occurs both through institutions and organizations and directly to community members, defining the two main groups of audiences. Given that both types of audiences may be found in community and public health settings, D&I strategies may range from those that target "implementers" (e.g., public health practitioners and policymakers) to interventions aimed at improving dissemination directly to "end-users" (e.g., members of the community). This heterogeneous mix of settings and levels can be viewed as comprising a linked system, albeit with varying degrees of integration across components, which

offers opportunities not only to strengthen the translation of scientific discoveries into practice settings, but equally important, for research to be informed by the needs and priorities of practitioners and policymakers.

While public health resources and infrastructure vary considerably both in developed and developing countries internationally, for the purpose of this chapter, the focus is on government public health systems in the United States, highlighting characteristics relevant for D&I research. Other settings relevant for public health described in detail in other chapters of this book include social services (chapter 22), health care delivery systems (chapter 23), schools (chapter 24), worksites (chapter 25), policymaking settings (chapter 26), and global settings (chapter 28).

In the United States, governmental public health agencies are considered the backbone of the public health system,[4] structured by laws, regulations, and organizational components, and driven by human, informational, and fiscal resources.[5] At the national level, public health agencies play an important role in setting the nation's agenda for public health (e.g., Healthy People objectives), securing funding, dispersing resources at state and local levels, and policymaking, although primary authority for public health in the United States resides at the state level.[5] The passage of the Patient Protection and Affordable Care Act (commonly referred to as the Affordable Care Act, or ACA, in short) in 2010 provided a legal foundation for widespread reform of the health care system, with an aim of near-universal health care coverage and provisions to strengthen primary care access, incentivize prevention, and increase integration between public health and health care (e.g., requirement for nonprofit hospitals to engage public health partners in community health planning).[6]

Dispersal of community health resources occurs through local agencies, including local public health departments and health care centers. The Health Center Program (also called Community Health Centers, supported by the Health Resources and Services Administration [HRSA]) funds Federally Qualified Health Centers (FQHC), FQHC "Look-Alikes" (FQHCLA), and outpatient health programs/facilities operated by tribal organizations focused on medically underserved populations and areas. In 2009, over 1,100 Health Center Program's operated more than 7,900 clinics (half in rural areas) and served almost 19 million patients.[7] By 2016, over 1,400 Health Center Program's were operating in over 9,800 clinic sites;[8] in 2015 alone, 430 new sites were funded. Local health departments (LHDs) implement community and public health programs and provide services directly or in partnership with other agencies and organizations, often serving as a bridge linking state and federal infrastructure and resources with local communities.[8] In addition, LHDs are organizations where population-based interventions often mix with health care provision in the same setting (i.e., as FQHCLA), with many agencies directly providing or contracting preventive health care services. There are almost 2,800 LHDs in the United States[9]

While there are a number of systematic reviews and compilations of evidence-based practices for community health promotion and disease prevention, such as the Guide to Community Preventive Services,[10] the demand for and readiness to implement and maintain evidence-based practice varies across settings. Furthermore, the potential efficacy of evidence-based practice designed and tested under ideal research conditions is likely to differ from the effectiveness when applied in real world practice. Dissemination and implementation research grounded in strong research-practice-policy linkages offers many opportunities to address these challenges.

This chapter discusses the evidence base, theories, and other important themes guiding current D&I research in community and public health settings, and provides some case examples that highlight gaps and opportunities for future work in this area. The chapter provides multiple examples from the field of cancer prevention and control. While this content area is featured, the principles apply to other areas of public health.

EVIDENCE-BASED PRACTICES FOR COMMUNITY AND PUBLIC HEALTH SETTINGS

A growing number of resources and tools have been developed to enhance the ease with which public health and clinical practitioners can find and use evidence-based programs and practices. These range from systematic reviews of public health intervention and policy approaches to IT tools to help practitioners find evidence-based resources for planning and implementation. Key research questions in D&I research revolve around examining how and to what extent practitioners are using these tools, identifying barriers, and testing the relative effectiveness of strategies for disseminating and integrating research into practice (e.g., Brownson et al.[11]).

Some of the tools designed for use by practitioners and policymakers are described in the following.

Guide to Community Preventive Services

In 1996, the US Department of Health and Human Services established the Task Force for Community Preventive Services to develop guidelines for evidence-based practice based on the systematic review of community-based health promotion and disease prevention interventions.[12] The Guide to Community Preventive Services[10] is an online resource for identifying interventions that have been evaluated, the intervention effect, the intervention aspects that users can identify as most appropriate for their respective communities, and the intervention cost and return on investment. Interventions are rated as "recommended," "recommended against," or "insufficient evidence," with those that are recommended also rated according to the strength of the evidence, as "strong" or "sufficient." The rigorous systematic review methods employed by the Task Force[13–15] are described straightforwardly on the website. Practitioners can browse the website by following links to various health topics, which are broken down further according to results of systematic reviews in specific areas of each topic. A newly designed website launched in 2016 has a new GuideCompass that allows users to customize the type of guidance they receive based on their role and what they want to accomplish, such as addressing specific health issues, preparing an organization for public health accreditation, developing a community health improvement plan, educating about evidence-based strategies, developing policies, programs, funding proposals, research, education, and for other general uses.

National Registry of Evidence-based Programs and Practices

In 1997, the Substance Abuse and Mental Health Services Administration (SAMHSA) launched the National Registry of Effective Prevention Programs (NREPP)[16] as a resource to help practitioners identify and implement substance abuse prevention programs. Under the initial NREPP program 1,100 programs were externally peer-reviewed and were identified as "model," "effective," or "promising" programs and made available online. Programs that were deemed as "model" programs were provided additional resources from SAMSHA to facilitate dissemination of the program by enhancing program materials and expanding program training. The NREPP site expanded to include mental health and substance abuse prevention and treatment interventions in 2004, and also modified the rating and review criteria they had been using.

The NREPP was updated in 2007 with the new name of National Registry of Evidence-based Programs and Practices. In 2015, NREPP went through an additional redesign and modification of their review process. New outcome ratings of "effective," "promising," "ineffective," and "inconclusive" are assigned based on rigorous peer review criteria. (Programs posted prior to 2015 redesign are being systematically re-reviewed and new ratings for these programs will be updated by 2018.) Practitioners can currently search over 425 programs online by keyword or set specific criteria (program type, age, outcome categories, race/ethnicity, special populations, gender, geographic locations, settings, implementation/dissemination (materials), or outcome rating). The new NREPP site also includes a learning center that includes resources to help with program planning, evaluation, and implementation[16]

Cancer Control P.L.A.N.E.T.

Launched in 2003, the Cancer Control P.L.A.N.E.T. (Plan, Link, Act, Network with Evidence-based Tools)[17] is a web portal designed to provide cancer control practitioners with access to data and evidence-based resources to assist in planning and implementation of evidence-based programs. The site was originally designed to help planners and public health practitioners walk through a process for identifying and adapting evidence-based cancer control plans and programs. The latest redesigned site is co-sponsored by the National Cancer Institute (NCI), Centers for Disease Control and Prevention (CDC), Agency for Healthcare Research and Quality (AHRQ), and the International Cancer Control Partnership. Practitioners can access state and county level cancer incidence, mortality, and prevalence data from the State Cancer Profiles website and create easy to understand jurisdiction-specific maps, graphs, and tables in seconds. Practitioners and researchers can connect and collaborate on Research to Reality, NCI's interactive community of practice. Access to research reviews are currently available from the Guide to Community Preventive Services and the U.S. Preventive Services Task Force. The Research-Tested Intervention Programs website described in the following provides access to more than 170 evidence-based interventions. The Reach, Effectiveness, Adoption, Implementation, Maintenance (RE-AIM) framework is available to assist practitioners with evaluation. Cancer control plans from the United States and 82 other countries are also available.

Research-tested Interventions Programs Website

In 2002, the NCI began developing the Research-tested Interventions Programs (RTIPs) website[18] to provide cancer control practitioners access to programs that had been conducted in peer-reviewed grant-funded studies, had positive outcomes published in peer-reviewed journals, and had materials that could be disseminated (by NCI or the developer) and adapted for use in community or clinical settings. NCI chose not to label programs as "model" or "effective" but rather provided sufficient information so that practitioners could make an informed decision about a program fit based on the level of evidence and the appropriateness for the specific community level of resources required for implementation. The NCI partnered with SAMHSA, modified the criteria from the NREPP program, and began posting programs on the RTIPs website in April 2003. Similar to the NREPP program, the RTIPs website evolved over time. The site currently contains over 180 programs in breast, cervical, and colorectal cancer screening, informed decision-making for cancer screening, human papilloma virus (HPV) vaccination, diet/nutrition, obesity physical activity, public health genomics, sun safety, survivorship/supportive care, and tobacco control, with a majority of the programs focused on community or public health settings. The eligibility criteria for posting programs on the site were modified in 2009 to allow programs that were not evaluated in a peer-reviewed, grant-funded, research project. However, all programs included must have had outcomes published in peer-reviewed journals and must have utilized an experimental or quasi-experimental evaluation design.[18]

High Impact HIV/AIDS Prevention Project

HIV prevention researchers and practitioners have been pioneers in dissemination and implementation of evidence-based interventions. Beginning in 1999, the CDC sponsored High Impact HIV/AIDS Prevention Project (HIP) (formerly known as DEBI) conducted a systematic review of evidence-based HIV prevention interventions and published a compendium of tested interventions that currently includes over 80 programs that have been proven effective in research studies, utilized experimental or quasi-experimental study design, and have materials packaged and ready for dissemination.[19] To enhance the dissemination process, the project staff provides training and technical assistance for the programs posted in the compendium, which is seen as essential for building the capacity of individuals, organizations, and communities.[20]

Center of Excellence for Training and Research Translation

A hybrid of research-tested and practice-tested interventions can be found at the Center of Excellence for Training and Research Translation site sponsored by the University of North Carolina-Chapel Hill in collaboration with one of the CDC's Prevention Research Centers.[21] Criteria for inclusion of an intervention on this site are similar to RTIPs and DEBI for research-tested interventions. Practice-tested interventions are included as a separate category, recognizing that varying levels of evidence exist and providing access to interventions that have been evaluated in practice but not tested in a formal research studies. Both the research-tested and practice-tested interventions and programs are reviewed based on the criteria from the RE-AIM framework as well as readiness for dissemination.[22]

D&I CHALLENGES IN COMMUNITY AND PUBLIC HEALTH SETTINGS

Infrastructure and Workforce Issues

Community and public health settings have the potential to play an important role in the widespread application of evidence-based programs and policies, although they vary greatly in size and resources, and in many areas, lack the capacity to implement a full array of public health services.[9] In the United States, state and local health departments are positioned to serve as a link between producers of research evidence (i.e., federal agencies and academia) and sources of tacit knowledge (e.g., local practitioners, community members),[23,24] by cultivating community advocacy and partnerships,[25] and adapting and developing programs and policies to the unique context of the organizations and communities that may influence their effective application over time.[26,27]

There is little systematic information on the functioning of public health systems. However, a number of studies have discussed a set of barriers that practitioners have identified as impeding the use of evidence-based practice in public health settings. These include both personal and institutional barriers, such as lack of time, inadequate funding, absence of cultural and managerial support (especially the absence of incentives),[28-32] and the perception of institutional priority for evidence-based practices and actual use of research to inform program adoption and implementation.[29,33] While some barriers, particularly personal barriers, may be overcome by improving training opportunities,[31] progress in dissemination research will be made by involving practitioners in all steps of the research process, from identifying barriers and setting priorities to designing strategies for improved D&I.[34,35] Similarly, nongovernmental organizations (NGO's) play a key role in promoting the utilization of public health services (e.g., screening), as well as advocating for public health policy change (e.g., increased tobacco excise taxes). The complex interrelationship between government, the private sector, and NGOs, and the different resources each sector can bring to bear to effect change, makes for a highly variable set of conditions within public health both over time and across jurisdictions.

Practice Implications/Fundamental Issues for Practitioners

Most government research funding agencies are mandated to share the information generated from the research they fund, and similarly NGOs who fund research also select research findings to communicate to the public and their donor populations. Historically, government research funding agencies have used three broad approaches to move science into practice: (1) communication and diffusion of research findings (e.g., conferences, publications, press releases), (2) dissemination campaigns to alter knowledge and behavior, and (3) demonstration projects that focus on scaling-up implementation of evidence-based programs (e.g., Body and Soul).[36,37] All three approaches share some characteristics in that funding for these efforts is usually time limited (constraining sustainability) and proportionately small compared with the major investments in the primary mission of these agencies (research), and the levels of agency support varies depending on the agency's annual budget. Application, practice, and service support agencies (e.g., Health Resources and Service Administration) often use similar diffusion and dissemination approaches. Given that the bulk of their funding supports service delivery, the proportion of the budget available to link science with service is also relatively small.[38]

Research results are most commonly communicated through the peer-reviewed publication of research findings. With respect to the communication of research results to the public, the news media are regularly contacted by research funding agencies to alert the public of new findings. As such, both the news media and the research community may be more focused on novelty rather than the public health or clinical significance of new scientific knowledge.

The high level of public and private investment in health research, in combination with the current funding emphasis on basic discovery research, creates an interesting information dissemination paradox. On the one hand, enormous amounts of information are being generated through research, published in thousands of discipline-specific journals and presented in hundreds of discipline-specific professional meeting venues. On the other hand, so much information is being pushed out through this passive process of information diffusion that a "signal-to-noise" ratio problem exists with respect to translating research into practice and policy.[38]

The massive and largely passive diffusion approach used in science may also raise unrealistic expectations in the practice community. Many individual research reports, while suggesting exciting new innovations that may lie ahead in the future, have little or no immediate application in practice. Thus, it may be difficult for the practice community to distinguish the signal about what is currently important to practice from the noise of what may or may not become important in the future.[39]

Over the years, a number of organizations began including a focus on utilizing evidence-based interventions as a condition of receiving funding. This is a shift from a focus on funding innovative interventions that may not yet be based on research evidence of efficacy or effectiveness. For example, in 2015, the CDC awarded six 5-year grants that focus on increasing the implementation of evidence-based cancer survivorship interventions to six organizations that participate in the National Comprehensive Cancer Control Programs.[40]

While it is often assumed that the demand for evidence-based health promotion and disease prevention interventions is high, many in the public health, clinical practice, and public policy communities do not hold with this assumption, albeit privately, and there are equal and often opposing forces to the dissemination and implementation of new knowledge gained from research. These include the mass of tacit knowledge gained from practice and policy experience,[41,42] as well as the complex service delivery and political policymaking contextual factors that constrain the acceptance, adaptation, and implementation of innovations based on research.[43] Thus, it has been posited that to close the gap between scientific discovery and service delivery, if we want more evidence-based practice, we need more practice-based evidence.[44]

Dissemination of research evidence about new approaches to promote health and prevent disease to public health practitioners should take into account (1) the level of training of most public health practitioners (e.g., masters or bachelors trained) for translating information into practical knowledge that can be applied in public health practice contexts, (2) the variation in resources in international, national, state/provincial, and local public health practice contexts that influence the implementation of public health interventions based on new health promotion information, and (3) the extent to which public health practitioners working in resource-limited practice contexts may or may not be amenable to change.

Ferlie and Dopson[45] argue that a shift to evidence-based practice in health, as an example of organizational change, is highly context dependent and not at all generic in nature. However, they also contend that there are core context factors that produce low-level patterning, if not predictive laws. So, for example, health care (and presumably health promotion) delivery contexts vary across time and place, so that D&I strategies that work in a country or at a time when there is universal access to health care (e.g., Canada), may not apply where universal access is not available (e.g., United States). They also note that there are significant differences in roles, provider relationships, and practices from one service sector to another, as well as different histories, cultures, and capabilities for learning and change across service sectors, all of which may be key modifiers of the impact of translating and implementing evidence-based interventions in practice. A key challenge for the emerging field of D&I research will be to develop reliable measures of these contextual factors and use them across service contexts to sort out the extent to which there are general principles for how contextual factors influence dissemination and implementation.[46]

In recent years, there has been a large-scale push for public health accreditation through a voluntary program launched nationally in 2011.[47] At the core of the program is the idea that benchmarking standards through the voluntary program offer a tool for public health departments to engage in continuous quality improvement.[48] In so doing, evidence-based practices, which are referenced in a number of accreditation standards and metrics, become better integrated in organizational functions and processes. In addition, the widespread rollout of the program provides an opportunity to examine dissemination and implementation-related research questions by characterizing variation across localities on a potentially national scale.[49]

OVERVIEW OF RESEARCH IN COMMUNITY AND PUBLIC HEALTH SETTINGS

Summary of Existing Research

While a large number of intervention studies exist that contribute to the evidence base for interventions applied in D&I research, there continue to be fewer studies in community and public health settings that are explicitly D&I research studies. Dissemination and implementation research focused in clinical settings continues to exceed research in community settings. Much of the research in community settings has been conducted in schools (subject of chapter 24), and other notable examples in government public health agencies, worksites, churches, and private sector settings (Figure 21.1).

Two studies have employed quasi-experimental or experimental designs to examine the impact of D&I strategies in government public

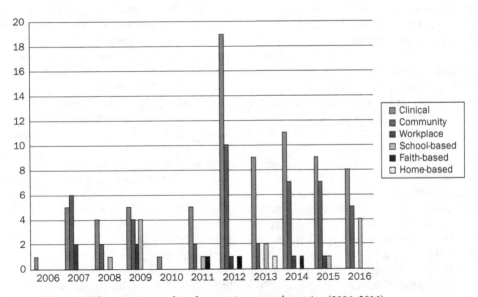

FIGURE 21.1 NIH funded dissemination and implementation grants by setting (2006–2016).

health agencies. Brownson et al.[33] studied the effect of providing workshops on guidelines (Community Guide) for evidence-based practice in physical activity promotion in state and local health departments in the United States, resulting in improvements in endpoints including awareness and adoption, though important differences at state and local levels were found. More recently, Dobbins et al.[50] employed a randomized-controlled trial to examine the relative impacts of various knowledge translation and exchange strategies to increase the use of evidence-informed healthy body weight programs and policies in a national sample of health departments in Canada. A treatment effect on the number of programs and policies was observed only for tailored, targeted messages (the other two strategies were providing a knowledge broker and online access to informational resources), with notable moderation by organizational culture. Future evaluation of funded D&I research studies should explore which implementation strategies are being funded and as results from these studies are published, which implementation strategies are shown to be effective (or ineffective).

Some D&I research has also been conducted in churches, worksites, and other private sector settings. An evaluation of a national dissemination campaign of the church-based Body & Soul intervention is currently underway (funded by NCI as part of their strategic dissemination initiative of research-tested intervention programs), with preliminary results indicating that repeated contact with knowledgeable staff has been key to early dissemination efforts.[37] Results from the Working Well Trial found that the maintenance of tobacco control activities in study worksites over time was related to the degree of institutionalization, which included the existence of assigned committees and budget allotments.[51] Research on dissemination and implementation of skin cancer interventions has been conducted in a number of private sector settings, including swimming pools and zoos.[52-54] With respect to the relative impact of various strategies, more intensive treatment did not always result in better outcomes; in some cases, more intensive, "enhanced" treatment groups exhibited better outcomes,[54] while in others, the less intensive (generic materials) treatments showed relatively better results.[50,53]

Research-tested interventions that are posted on several of the previously noted resources are not designed to be disseminated and require significant modifications to be ready for widespread use. Programs posted on the RTIPs website are not currently required to include information on core program components primarily because researchers do not test or report on this in outcome publications. However, implementation guides have been developed for programs posted on the site to assist users with maintaining fidelity to the original studied intervention. An evaluation of the Cancer Control P.L.A.N.E.T. site in 2007 found that more than 50% of users incorporated components of programs posted on the site into existing or developing programs.[55] A similar finding was found from a pilot project called Team-Up: Cancer Screening Saves Lives that was designed to encourage the use of research-tested interventions by creating partnerships in counties experiencing high cervical cancer mortality rates. The pilot was sponsored by NCI, the American Cancer Society, and the CDC, and an evaluation was conducted in 2008. The evaluation found that there were challenges among practitioners concerning what constituted an evidence-based program. Questions arose over whether a program had to be implemented with fidelity to be considered evidence-based and to what extent teams could modify tested interventions by using only certain components based on demographic and geographic characteristics of the women they were trying to reach. For complex, multicomponent interventions, partnerships often selected the components that they felt would be most appropriate for their audience and were affordable to implement.[56] A new user-review feature was added to the RTIPs website in late 2016 as a method for capturing real-world experiences using the research-tested interventions. A new comprehensive evaluation of the Cancer Control P.L.A.N.E.T. web portal and RTIPs website is being conducted in 2017 and results will be available in 2018.

Generating Evidence of What Works from D&I Research

In 2005, the National Institutes of Health initiated a trans-NIH funding opportunity focused on dissemination and implementation research, which was open to international investigators. The portfolio of NIH funded dissemination and implementation research grants has grown significantly. As of 2016, NIH had funded a total of 182 D&I grant. 66 of these projects have been funded in community and public health settings, three of which were in international settings, comprising 36% of the dissemination and implementation

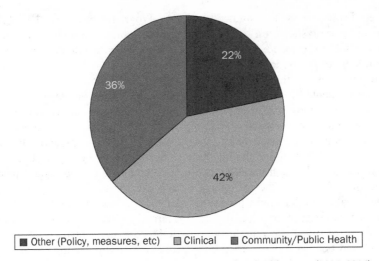

■ Other (Policy, measures, etc)　▨ Clinical　■ Community/Public Health

FIGURE 21.2 Funded NIH dissemination and implementation research in health grants (2006–2016).

grant portfolio (Figure 21.2). Topics being addressed in these grants include tobacco control, alcohol and substance abuse, nutrition and physical activity, obesity, cancer screening, diabetes, HIV/STIs, mental health, flu vaccinations, palliative care, bone health, autism, and chronic back pain.

The CDC has also increased dissemination and implementation research funding. Since 2006 they have funded approximately 66 grants with a primary focus on what they labeled as translational research. The majority of these translational research projects (45) focused on community and public health settings (Figure 21.3). Topics addressed in the CDC grants include asthma, diabetes, HIV, mental health, obesity, nutrition, cardiovascular disease, physical activity, substance abuse, tobacco control, emergency preparedness, motor vehicle safety, vaccinations, and cancer prevention.

Theories and Conceptual Frameworks in D&I Research

Previous chapters have described the different theories and approaches used in D&I research. It has been noted that there is no single underlying theory base or conceptual framework driving the field. Rather, D&I research draws on a range of theories and practices depending on the project underway. For example, in a recent rapid scoping review of dissemination and implementation theories, models, and frameworks applied in practice with respect to evidence-based programs and policies for the prevention and management of cancer and other chronic diseases,[57] 109 D&I

theories, models, and frameworks were identified from the 285 studies published between 2000 and 2016 that met the rapid scoping review inclusion criteria. With respect to the targeted level of change, all but three theories/models/frameworks were used for individual-level change (98%, 106/ 109). Conversely, 50% (54/109) were used for organization-level, 42% (46/109) for community-level, and 27% (29/109) for system-level change. A recent review of the use of the Consolidated Framework for Implementation Research (CFIR) (see chapter 5) in implementation research indicated several that were conducted in public health and primary care settings.[58]

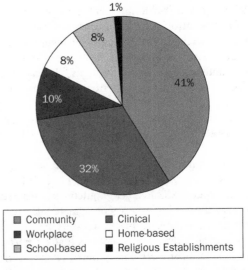

■ Community　■ Clinical
■ Workplace　□ Home-based
▨ School-based　■ Religious Establishments

FIGURE 21.3 Funded CDC dissemination and implementation research grants (2006–2014).

TABLE 21.1 NIH FUNDED DISSEMINATION AND IMPLEMENTATION GRANTS BY SETTING (2006–2016)

	RE-AIM	Diffusion of Innovation	CFIR	EPIS	PRISM	Interactive System Framework	Other
Clinical	7	4	1	1			6
Community	4	4	2		1		3
School-based	2			1		1	
Workplace	2	2					
Home-based	2						
TOTAL	17	10	3	2	1	1	9

With respect to NIH-funded D&I research grants, researchers applying for D&I research grant funding frequently continue to combine multiple theories and models or create a hybrid theory/model to meet specific project needs. The NIH's D&I Research in Health grants have encouraged grantees to focus on conceptual frameworks when designing their research studies, and it is interesting to examine the theories that have been used in the various research programs and how D&I research in public or community health research differs from those in primary care or specialty care. Previously, community and public health researchers utilized Rogers' Diffusion of Innovations Theory[59] most frequently.[57] However, a 2017 analysis of these awards indicated that clinical, community, and public health researchers are now utilizing the RE-AIM[60] model most frequently. The CFIR,[61] Exploration, Preparation, Implementation, and Sustainment (EPIS),[62] Practical Robust Implementation and Sustainability Model (PRISM),[63] and the Interactive Systems Framework (ISF)[64] were also present in the clinical and community research projects. Researchers in all areas continue to create and test new models despite the plethora of models that currently exist in this field.[65] (Table 21.1)

As noted previously, the CDC has also been funding grants to improve the translation of research into practice. Between 2006 and 2016 they funded 194 grants related to dissemination and implementation research. In an analysis limited to the abstracts and the specific aims, the majority did not identify a specific framework, theory, or model. Eighteen of those that mentioned theories or models in their abstracts incorporated the RE-AIM model in their research

design, five cited *Diffusion of Innovations,* and one cited the ISF.

D&I research being conducted in community and public health settings by and large do not appear to be initiated by community partners. Organizations that received funding for NIH D&I Research in Health grants focused on community and public health were all academic and/or research organizations. While they all had partners in the community, the funding was awarded through well-established research entities with histories of successfully applying for federal research grants. In the limited abstract analysis of the CDC-funded translation grants, 8 of the 166 awarded grants went to local government agencies (city or county) and one went to a community organization, while the rest were awarded to academic and/or research organizations. With the majority of D&I research largely based in academia, this continues to raise the question of how likely the findings from this research will be incorporated into community and public health practice settings if they are rarely the lead on the project.

GOVERNMENT/ACADAMIC CASE STUDY: PREVENTION RESEARCH CENTERS

Background

In 1984, the US Congress enacted Public Law 98-551, which established a program for Centers for Research and Demonstration of Health Promotion and Disease Prevention, currently known as the Prevention Research Center (PRC) program of the CDC. The program has evolved since its inception, expanding into 37 academic centers that maintain research-practice linkages with community members, practice, and policy settings in their respective communities.[44,66] In 1997 the IOM commissioned a report that reviewed the program's progress and discussed a vision for the future that explicitly placed dissemination research as one of its goals.[67] Dissemination research activities were included in the CDC's evaluation of the PRC program,[68] though as noted in the evaluation report, tracking indicators in dissemination and implementation has been difficult and highlights one area where further investment in D&I research activities can help sustain the program.

Context

The Cancer Prevention and Control Research Network (CPCRN) is one of five thematic research networks in the PRCs and is supported collaboratively by the Division of Cancer Prevention and Control at the CDC and the Division of Cancer Control and Population Science at the NCI. The CPCRN began in 2002 with a goal of accelerating the adoption of evidence-based cancer prevention and control in communities. The network provides the infrastructure to allow the funded research institutions to collaborate on community-based participatory D&I cancer research that spans academic and geographic boundaries (Figure 21.4). Composition of the network has changed over the years and there are currently eight research centers and one coordinating center.

Lessons Learned

The CPCRN has collaborated on research grant applications and has been able to partner on many D&I research projects. During the first funding cycle (2004–2009) the network produced 28 collaborative publications, partnered on 47 grant applications that received grant funding in excess of $26M, and had 125 collaborative research activities.[69] One example of a successful research project is the partnership with national 2-1-1 hotlines. 2-1-1 is a nationally designated 3-digit telephone number (like 9-1-1 for emergencies) that provides callers with access to information on social and health services in their community. A pilot project was initially developed in 2007 by the Washington University Network Center with the Missouri 2-1-1 hotline. The results of this pilot found that callers to the hotline were receptive to receiving health information and had greater cancer risk factors than the average person (higher smoking rates, lower screening rates, and lower rates of health insurance coverage).[70,71]

In 2008, after a successful initial pilot in Missouri, additional CPCRN centers from Harvard, University of North Carolina, University of Texas and University of Washington began working with 2-1-1 Centers in their states. The

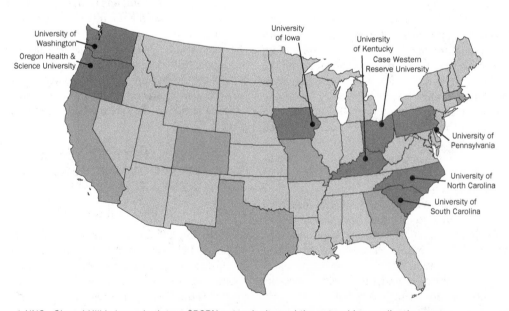

* UNC - Chapel Hill is home both to a CPCRN network site and the network's coordinating center.

FIGURE 21.4 Cancer Prevention and Control Research Network (CPCRN) map.

expanded pilot included giving callers a cancer control needs assessment and providing referrals for free or low-cost services as appropriate. In 2009, the University of Texas Network Center received funding to examine the use of phone navigators to provide counseling and navigation services to increase cancer screening and HPV vaccination rates by 25%.[72]

In 2014, CPCRN's D&I activities were retrospectively evaluated using the ISF.[64] The ISF is composed of three systems:

1. The Prevention Synthesis and Translation system summarizes existing evidence and customizes evidence-based products to be more easily accessible and usable by end users.
2. The Prevention Support system provides general and intervention-specific capacity building using the four components of the Evidence-based System for Innovation Support or EBSIS (tools, training, technical assistance, and quality assurance/quality improvement training) to build practitioner and organizational capacity to implement evidence-based interventions.
3. The Prevention Delivery system implements and delivers the evidence-based interventions.

The framework was designed to be used by different types of stakeholders (such as practitioners, funders, and researchers) to help them understand the respective needs of all stakeholders and systems.[73]

The CPCRN's D&I activities were mapped onto the three ISF systems to identify the roles of key stakeholders (researchers, practitioners, community partners) and thus "better conceptualize key systems, functions, and relationships affecting" the translation of evidence-based interventions into practice.[64] This study of the CCRN provides a real-world example of the application of ISF systems to show how the collaborative activities supported by the CPCRN "accelerated the synthesis and translation of evidence, built both general and innovation-specific capacity, and worked with delivery systems to advance cancer control research and practice." For example, CPCRN activities addressing all ISF systems included: (a) building the capacity of cancer control planners and public health professionals to locate, select, adopt, adapt, implement, and

evaluate evidence-based cancer prevention programs, policies, and practices through face-to-face training and technical assistance; (b) developing a training curriculum on using cancer evidence with slides, interactive exercises, and resources for cancer planners, which was delivered at national conferences and to local community partners; and (c) researching capacity-building models and evaluating training or technical assistance initiatives to translate evidence-based approaches into communities. Overall, the authors found "the ISF systems relevant and useful" and that their experience "confirms that developing research–practitioner–funder–consumer partnerships leads to an acceleration of knowledge creation around the Prevention Support system."

Directions for Future Research

The variability in structure, resources, and function of public health systems creates challenges as well as opportunities for D&I research. For example, while uniformity can facilitate the transfer of research-tested interventions across settings, variability creates "laboratories" for testing interventions under different conditions. A review of community based D&I research in cancer prevention,[74] which extended the work of a previous review by the AHRQ,[75] provides these recommendations for future research and practice that apply broadly to D&I research in community and public health settings:

- Standardize the terminology for D&I research.
- Evaluate the D&I of effective interventions targeting diverse populations and various community settings.
- Develop and use reliable and valid measures of D&I constructs.
- Use a combination of quantitative and qualitative data from multiple sources.
- Measure the real-world impact of D&I studies using standardized measures of stages of the D&I process, moderators, mediators, and outcomes.
- Apply appropriate study designs; RCT is not always the most appropriate or feasible.
- Active and multimodal D&I strategies are more likely to be effective than passive, single modal strategies.
- Add something on de-implementation/mis-implementation.

Other fields of research also hold promise in the future development of D&I research in community and public health settings. Community-based participatory research (CBPR) has been defined as "a collaborative approach to research that equitably involves all partners in the research process and recognizes the unique strength that each brings."[76] The strong focus on social and economic justice places it as a key concept in the development, implementation, and evaluation of interventions that address social determinants of health inequities.[77] Placed in the context of participatory research, core elements have been described as building mutual trust and respect, capacity, empowerment and ownership, accountability, and sustainability.[78] Given the heterogeneous settings for community health, applying CBPR methods by involving the community in early stages of study design should enhance success of the later stages of D&I.

The nascent but growing field of public health services and systems research (PHSSR) attempts to capitalize on the variability inherent in public health systems by investigating factors such as organizational, workforce, financial resources, and other characteristics of components of the public health system in relation to performance and outcomes.[79,80] A central focus of enhancing growth in the field has been the development of data resources,[81,82] including the PHSSR subset of the National Library of Medicine's health services research database.[83]

SUMMARY

Both the review in this chapter of what we know and the case examples of what is being done to close the gap between research discovery and program and policy delivery, suggest that a very small portion of the overall investment in research, practice, and policy work is being used to link the lessons learned from science with the lessons learned from policy and practice. From the research funding agency perspective, the NIH and CDC have supported dissemination and implementation research for the past several years. From the practice/policy funding perspective, the NIH and CDC have also provided support for such linkages as well as providing forums and IT tools to disseminate evidence-based intervention approaches and best practices both domestically and internationally. However, as has been noted previously,[35] these relatively small steps at their current level of support, and in and of themselves, are unlikely to accelerate closing the discovery–delivery gap.

To make significant change, each and every sector involved in public health will need to examine their funding priorities and decide what proportion of the investments will be focused on what they can do on their own versus what they should do in partnership with other sectors. For example, even as academic organizations recognize the potential for peer-reviewed funding and publications in this nascent field in public health, will they be willing to also provide academic credit and career advancement for faculty who choose to invest their time and energy in building coalitions and collaborating with public health practice and policy partners outside academia?

Similarly, government research and practice funding agencies face a similar choice: continue to expend most of their resources on their own initiatives, within their mission frameworks and comfort zones, versus make a significant investment in collaborative funding initiatives and sharing the credit and the responsibility for working together across departments, ministries, and jurisdictions. While it is much easier to coordinate within an agency, impact is greater with cooperation and collaborate across agencies, sectors, and regions.[84]

Absent a significant effort at redesigning and increasing investments in D&I research and knowledge translation on the part of science and service funding agencies, and a similar change in the academic rewards for research, practice, and policy partnerships, integrating the lessons learned from research with those learned from practice and policy, the ideal of research influencing practice and policy and vice versa will remain a side show to our seemingly unquenchable thirst for discovery.

SELECTED READINGS

Brownson RC, Fielding JE, Maylahn CM. Evidence-based public health: a fundamental concept for public health practice. *Annu Rev Public Health.* 2009;30:175–201.
Reviews the evolution of the concept of evidence-based public health and provides a typology of scientific evidence for public health practice. Also discusses organizational, political and structural barriers to implementing evidence-based practice in public health settings, and strategies for enhancing workforce competencies.

Dobbins M, Hanna SE, Ciliska D, et al. A randomized controlled trial evaluating the impact of knowledge translation and exchange strategies. *Implement Sci.* 2009; 4:61.

A randomized trial to evaluate the effectiveness of three different implementation strategies for improving knowledge translation and exchange in health departments.

Leeman J, Calancie L, Hartman MA, Escoffery CT, Herrmann AK, et al. What strategies are used to build practitioners' capacity to implement community-based interventions and are they effective?: a systematic review. *Implement Sci.* 2015;10: 80.

A systematic review of capacity-building interventions that builds on the Evidence-based System of Innovation Support EBSIS.

Pettman TL, Armstrong R, Jones K, Waters E, Doyle J. Cochrane update: building capacity in evidence-informed decision-making to improve public health. *J Public Health (Oxf).* 2013;35:624–627

Narrative description of methods and evaluation of trainings delivered by the Cochrane Public Health Group that support evidence-informed decision-making by public health practitioners and policymakers.

Rabin BA, Glasgow RE, Kerner JF, Klump MP, Brownson RC. Dissemination and implementation research on community-based cancer prevention: a systematic review. *Am J Prev Med.* 2010;38(4):443–456.

A systematic review of recent dissemination and implementation research of evidence-based interventions in smoking, healthy, diet, physical activity, and sun protection.

Contandriopoulos D, Lemire M, Denis JL, Tremblay E. Knowledge exchange processes in organizations and policy arenas: a narrative systematic review of the literature. *Milbank Q.* 2010;88(4):444–483.

A narrative literature review that provides a framework for analyzing context with respect to developing knowledge exchange strategies in organizations and policy arenas. It emphasizes the importance of contextual factors in three domains and the limitations of context-independent evidence resulting from randomized trials, providing direction to address some of the limitations discussed in Dobbins et al. 2009.[50]

Smith K. *Beyond evidence-based policy in public health: The interplay of ideas.* New York: Palgrave MacMillan; 2013.

This book explores the concept of evidence-based policymaking. It utilizes case studies on tobacco control and health inequalities in the United Kingdom to demonstrate the complex interplay between research and practice.

Selected Websites and Tools

Guide to Community Preventive Services. http://www.thecommunityguide.org/index.html

Federally sponsored website that provides guidance on selecting community-based programs and policies to improve health and prevent disease that are based on systematic reviews of the evidence.

National Registry of Evidence-based Programs and Practices. http://www.nrepp.samhsa.gov/

On-line registry of tested interventions that support mental health promotion, substance abuse prevention, and mental health and substance abuse treatment.

Cancer Control P.L.A.N.E.T. (Plan, Link, Act, Network with Evidence-based Tools). http://cancercontrolplanet.cancer.gov/

Web portal designed to provide cancer control practitioners with step-wise access to data and evidence-based resources to assist in planning and implementing evidence-based plans and programs.

Research to Reality. https://researchtoreality.cancer.gov/

Online community of practice designed to bring together cancer control practitioners and researchers to discuss moving evidence-based programs into practice.

Research-tested Interventions Programs (RTIPs) website. http://rtips.cancer.gov/rtips/index.do

Searchable database of cancer control interventions and program materials, designed to provide program planners and public health practitioners easy and immediate access to research-tested materials.

High Impact HIV/AIDS Prevention Project (HIP) website. http://www.effectiveinterventions.org/en/home.aspx

Website designed to bring science-based, community, group and individual-level HIV prevention interventions to community-based service providers and state and local health departments.

Center of Excellence for Training and Research Translation (UNC). http://www.center-trt.org/

Website focused on enhancing the impact of the WISEWOMAN program and the Nutrition and Physical Activity Program to Prevent Obesity and Other Chronic Diseases.

REFERENCES

1. Institute of Medicine. *The future of public health.* Washington, DC: Author; 1988.
2. Aday L. *Reinventing public health.* San Francisco: Jossey-Boss; 2005.
3. Scriven A. *Public health: Social context and action.* Berkshire, England: One University Press; 2007.
4. Institute of Medicine. The Future of the Public's Health in the 21st Century. 2003.
5. Turnock B. *Public health: What it is and how it works.* 5th ed. Burlington, MA: Jones & Bartlett Learning; 2012.
6. Rosenbaum. The patient protection and affordable care act: implications for public health policy and practice. *Public Health Rep.* 2011;126(1):130–135.

7. US Department of Health and Human Services (HRSA). Health Center Data & Reporting. https://bphc.hrsa.gov/datareporting/. Accessed August 9, 2017.

8. US Department of Health and Human Services. HRSA Health Center Program: Impact and Growth. https://bphc.hrsa.gov/about/healthcenter-program/index.html. Accessed February 13, 2017.

9. National Association of County and City Health Officials. 2016 National Profile of Local Health Departments. 2017.

10. Guide to Community Preventive Services. https://www.thecommunityguide.org/. Accessed February 13, 2017.

11. Brownson RC, Ballew P, Brown KL, et al. The effect of disseminating evidence-based interventions that promote physical activity to health departments. *Am J Public Health*. 2007;97(10):1900–1907.

12. Truman BI, Smith-Akin CK, Hinman AR, et al. Developing the Guide to Community Preventive Services--overview and rationale. The Task Force on Community Preventive Services. *Am J Prev Med*. 2000;18(1 Suppl):18–26.

13. Mullen PD, Ramirez G. The promise and pitfalls of systematic reviews. *Annu Rev Public Health*. 2006(27):81–102.

14. Zaza S, Briss PA, Harris KW, eds. *The guide to community preventive services: What works to promote health?* New York: Oxford University Press; 2005.

15. Mercer SL, Banks SM, Verma P, Fisher JS, Corso LC, Carlson V. Guiding the way to public health improvement: exploring the connections between The Community Guide's evidence-based interventions and health department accreditation standards. *J Public Health Manag Prac*. 2014;20(1):104–110.

16. National Registry of Evidence-based Programs and Practices. https://www.samhsa.gov/nrepp. Accessed February 13, 2017.

17. Cancer Control P.L.A.N.E.T. Links to comprehensive cancer control resources for public health professionals. https://cancercontrolplanet.cancer.gov/about.html. Accessed February 13, 2017.

18. Research-tested Intervention Programs. https://rtips.cancer.gov/rtips/index.do. Accessed February 13, 2017.

19. Centers for Disease Control and Prevention (CDC). Compendium of Evidence-based Interventions and Best Practices for HIV Prevention. https://www.cdc.gov/hiv/research/interventionresearch/compendium/index.html. Accessed February 13, 2017.

20. Effective Interventions: HIV Prevention That Works. High Impact HIV/AIDS Prevention Project (HIP). https://effectiveinterventions.cdc.gov/en/HighImpactPrevention/Interventions.aspx. Accessed February 13, 2017.

21. Center for Excellence for Training and Research Translation. http://www.centertrt.org/?p=about_who. Accessed February 13, 2017.

22. Center for Excellence for Training and Research Translation. Intervention Review Process. http://www.centertrt.org/?p=about_how_interventions_review. Accessed February 13, 2017.

23. Brownson RC, Fielding JE, Maylahn CM. Evidence-based public health: a fundamental concept for public health practice. *Annu Rev Public Health*. 2009;30(1):175–201.

24. Colditz GA, Emmons KM, Vishwanath K, Kerner JF. Translating science to practice: community and academic perspectives. *J Public Health Manag Pract*. 2008;14(2):144–149.

25. Yancey AK, Fielding JE, Flores GR, Sallis JF, McCarthy WJ, Breslow L. Creating a robust public health infrastructure for physical activity promotion. *Am J Prev Med*. 2007;32(1):68–78.

26. Dearing JW. Evolution of diffusion and dissemination theory. *J Public Health Manag Pract*. 2008;14(2):99–108.

27. Green LW, Ottoson JM, Garcia C, Hiatt RA. Diffusion theory and knowledge dissemination, utilization, and integration in public health. *Annu Rev Public Health*. 2009; 30:151–174.

28. Baker EA, Brownson RC, Dreisinger M, McIntosh LD, Karamehic-Muratovic A. Examining the role of training in evidence-based public health: a qualitative study. *Health Promot Pract*. 2009;10(3):342–348.

29. Dobbins M, Cockerill R, Barnsley J, Ciliska D. Factors of the innovation, organization, environment, and individual that predict the influence five systematic reviews had on public health decisions. *Int J Technol Assess Health Care*. 2001;17(4):467–478.

30. Dreisinger M, Leet TL, Baker EA, Gillespie KN, Haas B, Brownson RC. Improving the public health workforce: evaluation of a training course to enhance evidence-based decision making. *J Public Health Manag Pract*. 2008;14(2):138–143.

31. Jacobs JA, Dodson EA, Baker EA, Deshpande AD, Brownson RC. Barriers to evidence-based decision making in public health: a national survey of chronic disease practitioners. *Public Health Rep*. 2010;125(5):736–742.

32. Maylahn C, Bohn C, Hammer M, Waltz EC. Strengthening epidemiologic competencies among local health professionals in New York: teaching evidence-based public health. *Public Health Rep*. 2008;123(Suppl 1):35–43.

33. Brownson RC, Ballew P, Dieffenderfer B, et al. Evidence-based interventions to promote

physical activity: what contributes to dissemination by state health departments. *Am J Prev Med.* 2007;33(1 Suppl):S66–S73; quiz S74–68.

34. Glasgow RE, Marcus AC, Bull SS, Wilson KM. Disseminating effective cancer screening interventions. *Cancer.* 2004;101(5 Suppl):1239–1250.

35. Kerner JF. Integrating science with service in cancer control: closing the gap between discovery and delivery. In: Elwood M SS, ed. *Cancer control.* Oxford: Oxford University Press; 2010.

36. US Department of Health and Human Services. Community-based interventions for smokers: the COMMIT field experience. *NCI Monograph No.* 1995;6.

37. Campbell MK, Hudson MA, Resnicow K, Blakeney N, Paxton A, Baskin M. Church-based health promotion interventions: evidence and lessons learned. *Annu Rev Public Health.* 2007; 28:213–214.

38. Kerner JF HK. Research dissemination and diffusion: translation within science and society. *Res Social Work Pract.* 2009;19(5):519–530.

39. Kerner JF, Rimer BK, Emmons KM. Dissemination research and research dissemination: how can we close the gap? *Health Psychol.* 2005;24(5):443–446.

40. National Comprehensive Cancer Control Program (NCCCP). Increasing the Implementation of Evidence-based Cancer Survivorship Interventions to Increase Quality and Duration of Life Among Cancer Patients. https://www.cdc.gov/cancer/ncccp/dp15-1501.htm. Accessed February 10, 2017.

41. Kerner JF. Knowledge translation versus knowledge integration: a "funder's" perspective. *J Contin Educ Health Prof.* 2006;26(1):72–80.

42. Kerner JF. Integrating research, practice, and policy: what we see depends on where we stand. 2008;14(2):193–198.

43. Dopson S F. The active role of context. In: Dopson S FL, ed. *Knowledge to action? Evidence-based health care in context.* Oxford: Oxford University Press; 2005:79–103.

44. Green LW. The prevention research centers as models of practice-based evidence two decades on. *Am J Prev Med.* 2007;33(1 Suppl): S6–S8.

45. Ferlie E DS. Study complex organizations in health care. In: Dopson S FL, ed. *Knowledge to action? Evidence-based health care in context.* Oxford: Oxford University Press; 2005:8–26.

46. Jetha N, Robinson K, Wilkerson T, Dubois N, Turgeon V, DesMeules M. Supporting knowledge into action: The Canadian Best Practices Initiative for Health Promotion and Chronic Disease Prevention. *Can J Public Health.* 2008;99(5):1–8.

47. Public Health Accreditation Board. http://www.phaboard.org/. Accessed February 13, 2017.

48. Beitsch LM, Riley W, Bender K. Embedding quality improvement into accreditation: evolving from theory to practice. *J Public Health Manag Pract.* 2014;20(1):57–60.

49. Kronstadt J, Beitsch LM, Bender K. Marshaling the evidence: the prioritized public health accreditation research agenda. *Am J Public Health.* 2015;105(S2): S153–S158.

50. Dobbins M, Hanna SE, Ciliska D, et al. A randomized controlled trial evaluating the impact of knowledge translation and exchange strategies. *Implement Sci.* 2009;4:61.

51. Sorensen G, Thompson B, Basen-Engquist K, et al. Durability, dissemination, and institutionalization of worksite tobacco control programs: results from the Working Well trial. *Int J Behav Med.* 1998;5(4):335–351.

52. Glanz K, Steffen A, Elliott T, O'Riordan D. Diffusion of an effective skin cancer prevention program: design, theoretical foundations, and first-year implementation. *Health Psychol.* 2005;24(5):477–487.

53. Lewis E, Mayer JA, Slymen D, et al. Disseminating a sun safety program to zoological parks: the effects of tailoring. *Health Psychol.* 2005;24(5):456–462.

54. Rabin BA, Nehl E, Elliott T, Deshpande AD, Brownson RC, Glanz K. Individual and setting level predictors of the implementation of a skin cancer prevention program: a multilevel analysis. *Implement Sci.* 2010; 5:40.

55. Sood R, Ho PS, Tornow C, Frey W. Cancer Control P.L.A.N.E.T. Evaluation Final Report. 2007.

56. Breslau ES, Rochester PW, Saslow D, Crocoll CE, Johnson LE, Vinson CA. Developing partnerships to reduce disparities in cancer screening. *Prev Chronic Dis.* 2010;7(3):A62.

57. Stamatakis KA, Vinson CA, Kerner JF. Community and public health settings. In: Brownson R, Colditz G, Proctor E, eds. *Dissemination and implementation research in health: Translating science to practice.* New York: Oxford University Press; 2012:359–383.

58. Kirk MA, Kelley C, Yankey N, Birken SA, Abadie B, and Damschroder L. A systematic review of the use of the Consolidated Framework for Implementation Research. *Implement Sci.* 2016;11:72.

59. Rogers EM. *Diffusion of innovations.* 5th ed. New York: Free Press; 2003.

60. Dzewaltowski DA, Glasgow RE, Klesges LM, Estabrooks PA, Brock E. RE-AIM: Evidence-based standards and a web resource to improve translation of research into practice. *Annf Behav Med.* 2004;28(2):75–80.

61. Damschroder L, Aron D, Keith R, Kirsh S, Alexander J, Lowery J. Fostering implementation

of health services research findings into practice: a consolidated framework for advancing implementation science. *Implement Sci.* 2009; 4:50.

62. Aarons, G. A., Hurlburt, M., & Horwitz, S. M. Advancing a conceptual model of evidence-based practice implementation in public service sectors. *Adm Policy Ment Health Ment Health Serv Res.* 2011;38(1):4–23.

63. Feldstein AC GR. A practical, robust implementation and sustainability model (PRISM). *Jt Comm J Qual Patient Safety.* 2008;34(4):228–243.

64. Fernández ME, Melvin CL, Leeman J, Ribisl KM, Allen JD, Kegler MC, Bastani R, Ory MG, Risendal BC, Hannon PA. The cancer prevention and control research network: an interactive systems approach to advancing cancer control implementation research and practice. *Cancer Epidemiol Biomarkers Preven.* 2014;23(11):2512–2521.

65. Tabak RG, Khoong EC, Chambers DA, Brownson RC. Bridging research and practice: models for dissemination and implementation research. *Am J Prev Med.* 2012;43(3):337–350.

66. National Center for Chronic Disease Prevention and Health Promotion. Prevention research centers: building the scientific research base with community partners. 2010.

67. Stoto M, Green L, Bailey L, eds. *Linking research and public health practice: A review of CDC's program of Centers for Research and Demonstration of Health Promotion and Disease Prevention.*Washington, DC: National Academies Press; 1997.

68. Centers for Disease Control and Prevention. Prevention Research Centers Program. Evaluation Results: Program Indicators.2010.

69. Williams R. Cancer Prevention and Control Research Network Summary Progress Report: 9-30-04 to 9-29-09.

70. Cancer Prevention and Control Research Network. www.cpcrn.org. Accessed February 12, 2017.

71. Fernandez M, Ball-Ricks K, Vernon S, Savas L. Advancing dissemination and implementation research and practice: a collaboration between the CPCRN and 2-1-1. 2012.

72. Mullen PD, Savas LS, Bundy LT, Haardoefer R, Hovell M, Fernandez ME, Monroy JA, Williams RS, Kreuter MW, Jobe D, Kegler MC. Minimal intervention delivered by 2-1-1 information and referral specialists promotes smoke-free homes among 2-1-1 callers: a Texas generalized trial. *Tobacco Control.* 2016; Suppl 1(October):i10–i18.

73. Wandersman A, Duffy J, Flaspohler P, et al. Bridging the gap between prevention research and practice: the interactive systems framework for dissemination and implementation. *Am J Community Psychol.* 2008;41(3-4):171.

74. Rabin BA, Glasgow RE, Kerner JF, Klump MP, Brownson RC. Dissemination and implementation research on community-based cancer prevention: a systematic review. *Am J Prev Med.* 2010;38(4):443–456.

75. Agency for Healthcare Research and Quality. Diffusion and dissemination of evidence-based cancer control interventions. 2003.

76. Minkler M WN. *Community based participatory research for health.* San Francisco: Jossey-Bass; 2003.

77. Brennan Ramirez L, Baker E, Metzler M. Promoting health equity: a resource to help communities address social determinants of health. 2008.

78. Cargo M MS. The value and challenges of participatory research: strengthening its practice. *Annu Rev Public Health.* 2008;29:325–350.

79. Mays GP, Halverson PK, Scutchfield FD. Behind the curve? What we know and need to learn from public health systems research. *J Public Health Manag Pract.* 2003;9(3):179–182.

80. Mays GP, Smith SA, Ingram RC, Racster LJ, Lamberth CD, Lovely ES. Public health delivery systems: evidence, uncertainty, and emerging research needs. *Am J Prev Med.* 2009;36(3):256–260.

81. Scutchfield FD, Bhandari MW, Lawhorn NA, Lamberth CD, Ingram RC. Public health performance. *Am J Prev Med.* 2009;36(3):256–265.

82. Scutchfield FD, Lawhorn N, Ingram R, Perez DJ, Brewer R, Bhandari M. Public health systems and services research: dataset development, dissemination, and use. *Public Health Rep.* 2009;124(3):372–377.

83. National Information Center on Health Services Research and Health Care Technology (NICHSR). http://wwwcf.nlm.nih.gov/hsrr_search/index.cfm. Accessed February 12, 2017.

84. Himmelman AT. On coalitions and the transformation of power relations: collaborative betterment and collaborative empowerment. *Am J Commun Psychol.* 2001;29(2):277–284.

22

Dissemination and Implementation in Social Service Settings

J. CURTIS MCMILLEN AND DANIELLE R. ADAMS

INTRODUCTION

Social service sectors of care are uniquely positioned to disseminate and implement health prevention and intervention protocols to reach vulnerable populations. Social service agencies often are tasked with implementing complex protocols in complicated systems of care. Dissemination and implementation (D&I) work in this area provides important lessons learned for D&I work and research in other sectors. Before addressing these larger points, the authors propose some boundaries around the social services.

The term "social services" confuses many, even those who work within them. This is because the term is commonly used to represent a number of different sectors of nonmedical services designed to increase social well-being. Generally, the social services are thought to encompass:

- Child maltreatment investigations and remediation efforts, including foster care, residential services, and adoption
- Juvenile justice services (delinquency prevention, services to offending children, juvenile detention, residential services)
- Some adult justice services, such as probation, parole, and decarceration
- Income transfer programs for the poor, such as (in the United States), Temporary Aid for Needy Families and the Supplemental Nutritional Assistance Program
- Some housing programs for the impoverished
- Community long-term care services for older adults, generally designed to keep older adults living in the community and out of long-term care facilities
- Services for victims of interpersonal violence

For many people, the term also involves community-based mental health programming for those with serious and persistent mental health challenges. It generally excludes private practice psychiatric and counseling services.

These social services may be provided through large public agencies or through private (nongovernmental) social service entities. Often, the public agencies contract with the private social service agencies to provide the needed service.

THE POTENTIAL OF DISSEMINATION AND IMPLEMENTATION EFFORTS IN THE SOCIAL SERVICES

Developing structures and strategies to disseminate and implement health-focused prevention and intervention protocols in the social services is justified for three main reasons. First, there is often a primacy of relationships between social service workers and their clients. Second, social service clients often possess high need for improved health. Third, it is often of self-interest to social service systems of care to improve the health of their clients.

Another Primary Care

For many children, youth, and families deeply involved in social service sectors of care, the professional most primary to them—chief in importance, most frequently seen, and first seen in a sequence of help seeking behaviors—is a social service employee. In some sectors of care the social services case manager explicitly serves as the gatekeeper of other services, including medical care.[1] In these sectors, the social services case manager can be thought of as the primary care provider, a term usually reserved for a patient's first-line physician.

In contrast to other sectors of care, the combination of the frequency of contact and the degree of impairment of the client gives the social services case manager a role with high influence. These workers know what is going on with their clients, and the clients may not be capable of accessing care without the social service worker's assistance.

High Need

The second reason to consider a role for the social services in the D&I of health prevention and treatments is the level of need among social service clients. While we are all at risk of some diseases no matter our neighborhood, social class or ethnic group, two common denominators of health problems are emerging from a vast and complex literature—low income and early life adversity. People who grew up in families with low income and high levels of adversity such as maltreatment, parental substance abuse, and incarceration are at a higher risk of both social service involvement and health problems. This convergence points to the social services as a natural entry point for health interventions.

In many countries, including the United States, income and health are negatively and consistently related.[2-4] Studies like the Adverse Childhood Experiences Study provide convincing evidence that early adversity is predictive of a wide range of later health problems.[5,6] Increasingly, a life course perspective is taken to understand inequalities in health,[7,8] showing how low income and early adversity unfold over the life course to leave adults vulnerable to poor health. Some social services, like income transfer programs, are designed to lessen the impact of hardship. Others, like foster care and juvenile justice systems, strive to provide turning points that alter life courses in positive ways. In this sense, the social services are situated to see large numbers of people with health problems in a helping context.

The literature on the health needs of social service clients is underdeveloped, segmented by service sector, and largely hidden from traditional literature searches in government reports. But foster care services for older youth, the population focus of the first author of this chapter, can be exemplary. Estimates are that 35% of these young people are obese;[9] cigarette smoking is twice as common as among other teens;[10,11] and rates of past year major depression for foster youth[12] are three times as high as that of other youth.[13]

Self-Interest

Health is not the raison d'être of these social service sectors and thus rarely the primary focus of social service systems. Still, the D&I of evidence-supported health interventions might assist social service agencies in fulfilling their main functions. Income assistance programs are motivated to help their clients budget their meager means to last through the month. Therefore, they may want to help their clients stop smoking, in order for the financial assistance they provide to go further. They also want to help move their clients from the welfare rolls to employment. Therefore, they may want to help some clients lose weight, as high body weight may be a barrier in gaining employment.[14] The intersection between health concerns and service system mission will be different for each sector of care. An agency that provides in-home services to older adults may not be interested in smoking cessation, for example, but may be interested in depression-focused interventions, as preventing or treating depression may help keep older adults in their homes.

Sector self-interest may also drive funding battles for the implementation of evidence-supported health protocols, with service sectors preferring to cost-shift when possible. Medicaid, an entitled benefit, often becomes the preferred funder to avoid local or state battles over who should pay for a service that benefits social service consumers. Much of child welfare services, for example, are billed to Medicaid.[15] This is less of an option in juvenile justice, however, where a federal inmate exclusion clause does not allow Medicaid dollars to go to services for incarcerated youth.[16]

WHAT COULD AND SHOULD BE DISSEMINATED AND IMPLEMENTED IN THE SOCIAL SERVICES?

The justification for D&I work in the social services cited earlier suggests that there should be broad interest within social service sectors for evidence-supported health prevention and intervention protocols with the highest potential for affecting multiple disease processes. These protocols would target increased physical activity levels, healthy eating, the cessation or prevention of tobacco use, and chronic disease management. In some sectors of care, HIV prevention would be an important clinical target. The evidence-based protocols that appear on lists developed for social service sectors seem to prioritize behavioral health. It may be these sectors of care believe that better behavioral health will help them improve their primary outcomes of interest, such as recidivism, safety, and permanence in housing.

There are protocols for each of these health targets developed for other sectors of care that are available for adaptation in social service settings. Real-world uptake for them appears to be minimal, but implementation scientists have begun to study and document these adaptation processes.[17]

To date, the D&I action in the social services has been mostly focused on implementing complex protocols for multifaceted, difficult to treat conditions. Substance abuse, conduct disorder, depression, and posttraumatic stress disorder are common targets. The juvenile justice sector exemplifies this theme. In this sector, the most promoted programs are designed to decrease and prevent youth conduct problems. Many of these programs are proprietary, and the most promoted are complex clinical programs that possess evidence of their efficacy generated through multiple randomized clinical trials. The exception to this trend is in the sector of community services for older adults, where programs promoted for dissemination include those for physical activity and healthy eating.

Interestingly, some of the high-intensity, behaviorally oriented complex interventions being implemented in the social services to reduce social ills like criminality may have unexpected positive consequences on health outcomes, which complicates issues of who will pay for what services. For example, Multisystemic Treatment (MST) has been shown to reduce hospital admissions and costs for youth with type I diabetes[18] and Multidimensional Treatment Foster Care (MTFC) has reduced pregnancies among criminally involved girls.[19]

WHAT GROUPS HAVE COMPILED, DISSEMINATED, AND ENDORSED PROGRAMS FOR DISSEMINATION IN THE SOCIAL SERVICES?

Some of the social service sectors have established websites and organizations designed to increase awareness of information about known, evidence-supported interventions that are available for implementation within the sector. One model organization is the California Evidence-Based Clearinghouse for Child Welfare (CEBC; http://www.cebc4cw.org). It is unique in several ways.

First, it is state funded, through the California Department of Social Services. Second, it uses scientific experts to rate the quality and type of published, peer-reviewed research associated with a program. Third, it rates the relevance of the program for child welfare populations. Fourth, it also conducts reviews of programs in areas that are important to child welfare practice, but for which there are not yet evidence-supported interventions. This is done to inform administrators and consumers about programs that may market themselves as evidence-based, when they are not. As of December 27, 2016, the Clearinghouse listed 358 programs in 44 topic areas. Thirty of the programs received the Clearinghouse's best scientific rating of "well-supported by research." Activity levels, healthy eating, and smoking cessation are not among the topic areas covered to date.

The National Council on Aging lists 50 programs on its website (https://www.ncoa.org/resources/ebpchart/) that meet the standard of evidence required under the Older Americans Act and that can be implemented in community settings for old adults. The Council, however, has ceased adding new programs to their list. Most of these are directly health related, and include programs related to fall prevention, physical activity, and chronic disease management. The Council website provides ample implementation advice.

Multiple organizations have compiled and disseminated evidence-supported programs in the juvenile justice sector. The *Blueprints for Healthy Youth Development* program (http://www.colorado.edu/cspv/blueprints), affiliated with the University of Colorado at Boulder, aims to identify and promote a small number of programs with a very high scientific standard of effectiveness that are intended to reduce antisocial behavior and promote a healthy course of youth development. According to its website (as of December 27, 2016), it had assessed over 1,400 programs and certified 15 as model programs, meaning they have been shown to work for 12 months or longer in at least two studies. Two of these programs are certified as model plus, meaning that they have had at least one independent replication. They are *Life Skills Training*, a drug abuse prevention program for middle schoolers, and MST (described later in a case study). Forty-five additional programs are rated as promising. Among these are weight management and smoking cessation programs. The Blueprints program uses staff reviews followed by scientific reviews from an advisory board.

The U.S. Office of Juvenile Justice and Delinquency Prevention, on the other hand, lists 279 model programs in nine domains that it promotes for dissemination in juvenile justice settings (as of December 27, 2016; https://www.ojjdp.gov/mpg/). It rates 60 of these programs as "effective," its highest rating. Despite the number of available programs for dissemination, experts believe few juvenile offenders have the opportunity to benefit from programs with demonstrated efficacy or effectiveness.[20]

In mental health, the Substance Abuse and Mental Health Services Administration (SAMHSA) maintains a National Registry of Evidence-based Programs and Practices for the prevention and treatment of mental health and substance abuse problems (http://nrepp.samhsa.gov/01_landing.aspx). As of December 27, 2016, its registry included 405 programs, including 37 rated as possessing effective outcomes and another 87 with promising outcomes. SAMHSA used to rate the implementability of these programs, but no longer does.

To date, efforts to disseminate health prevention and intervention protocols through the social services have been focused on the juvenile justice, child welfare, mental health, and community long-term care services for older adults sectors of care. Professionals working in other social service sectors of care may need to rely on compilations of evidence-supported protocols that are health-topic specific. There are a number of these. Some are reviewed in chapters 21 and 23–26 of this book.

DISSEMINATION AND IMPLEMENTATION MODELS IN THE SOCIAL SERVICES

No one model of D&I has taken hold in the social services. In many cases, it has been the treatment developer that has been responsible for setting up organizations and strategies for both dissemination and implementation.

The Purveyor Organization

Several intervention developers working in social service sectors use separate training and technical assistance (TA) organizations to aid with D&I. An existing organization may agree to take on this task or a new, separate organization (i.e., a purveyor organization) may be developed. Care for Elders, a Houston-based TA agency for *Healthy Ideas* is an example of the former. Examples of purveyor organizations created explicitly for D&I work include Behavioral Tech, LLC, to

disseminate *Dialectical Behavior Therapy*, TFC, Inc. to disseminate MTFC, and MST Services to disseminate MST (see Case Study 1). Some of these are nonprofit and others are incorporated for-profit organizations.

The interventions these organizations disseminate tend to be complex enough to require substantial start-up assistance. In all known cases, the demand for training far outweighed the ability of the clinical innovator to provide it. These separate organizations are in charge of the D&I activities associated with the clinical innovation and thus allow the original treatment developers to create new innovations and run clinical trials. This chapter delineates two different models operating within these purveyor organizations, though there are undoubtedly other variations in operation.

Train + Implementation Technical Assistance

Some purveyor organizations provide substantially more implementation guidance than others. These developers have created implementation standards and guidance that they distribute to organizations that are adopting their intervention. Care for Elders, the disseminator of *Healthy Ideas*, offers a free initial consultation and readiness assessment tools for organizations interested in adopting their intervention. Once an adoption decision has been made, Care for Elders, for a one-time fee, will visit the organization, provide monthly telephone consultation on implementation designed to ensure that ongoing training, quality assurance, and fidelity measurement have been instituted, and provide program and implementation manuals, training videos, a variety of other tools, and unlimited email technical assistance.

Train + Consultation + Certification

Some of the purveyor organizations have more of a focus on consultation for clinical services. As an example, TFC Inc. trains clinical teams in their treatment foster care model during a week-long training program in Oregon, provides consultation on start-up and recruiting foster parents, then provides weekly supervision to the team by phone from their offices in Oregon for the first year of clinical services. During this year, clinical team and foster parent team meetings are audio-recorded and reviewed by the TFC, Inc. consultant, who provides guidance on adhering to the model. Some of the purveyor organizations offer a certification or accreditation process that designates an organization as an official provider of the intervention. After a year of ongoing consultation with TFC, Inc. and a site visit by the TFC, Inc. consultant, an MTFC team can be certified to provide these services for a specified period of time without TFC, Inc. consultation or additional site visits.

Such designations may prove useful in efforts to get funders to pay for the clinical service. For example, a state Medicaid office may agree to pay a lump sum for providing a complicated, multicomponent evidence-supported protocol, such as MTFC, rather than having the provider bill piecemeal for each service offered within it. But this lump sum reimbursement plan may only be made available to provider organizations certified by the purveyor. This keeps other certified organizations, theoretically those providing lesser services at lower costs, from being able to bill under the lump sum payment code.

The focus in this section to this point on purveyor organizations may suggest that there are purveyor organizations out there ready to assist social service agencies to adopt, adapt, and implement the evidence-supported protocols of their choice. This is not the case. Most evidence-based protocols exist more in theory and in manuals not accessible to agency providers. They often don't come in packages with trainers at-the-ready and someone eager to problem solve a site's unique implementation challenges. Some of the organizations that maintain lists of evidence-supported protocols, such as the CEBC, also provide information on what implementation supports are available. Often, there are none. Agencies are then left on their own to develop their own implementation strategies. Named, blended, implementation models may be particularly salient in these conditions, especially when these blended models fully define their implementation strategies. Some of these have been examined in research trials in the social services. Two are ARC and the Community Development Team Model.

ARC

Glisson's ARC model (Availability, Responsiveness, Continuity)[21] is a complex implementation model that blends interventions at three levels—community, administration, and clinical teams—and guides organizations through twelve components in three stages of work lasting 1 to 3 years. ARC components are (1) building organizational leadership, (2) building personal relationships, (3) accessing and facilitating organizational networks, (4) building teamwork in frontline clinical teams, (5) providing information and training related to a clinical innovation, (6) team decision-making and technical support, (7) establishing a data feedback mechanism, (8) implementing participatory decision making in frontline teams, (9) resolving staff conflicts, (10) goal setting and continuous quality improvement, (11) redesigning jobs, and (12) ensuring self-regulation and stabilization. Theoretically, ARC is designed to affect implementation through improved agency culture and climate, partnered with the introduction of new systems to monitor progress and confront problems as they are experienced. In a Tennessee-based randomized clinical trial ARC was tested in conjunction with implementation of MST in a large public agency, with counties randomized to ARC or implementation as usual. Youth who received MST in ARC counties experienced significantly greater decreases in problem behavior than youth in implementation as usual counties.[22]

The California Institute of Mental Health Community Development Team Model

The manual for the Community Development Team Model[23] describes a process that involves (a) outreach to agency directors to drum up interest in evidence-supported interventions, (b) partnerships with treatment developers to deliver clinical training, (c) agency-developed implementation plans, (d) individualized, technical assistance from centralized staff to agencies on issues of implementation, and (e) the development of peer-to-peer networks of agency staff who are implementing evidence-supported interventions to jointly problem solve implementation barriers and to share successful strategies. This model was used in a large clinical trial of MTFC in California and Ohio counties, with the counties randomized to receive implementation as usual or implementation using the Community Development Team Model. The Community Development Team counties were able to mount more successful treatment foster care teams and serve twice as many children as the usual implementation counties.[24]

DESIGNING DISSEMINATION AND IMPLEMENTATION INTERVENTIONS FOR THE SOCIAL SERVICES

The consolidated framework for implementation science proposed by Damschroder and colleagues[25] offers a useful tool for discussing the special considerations needed to disseminate and implement health interventions in social service settings. They propose five domains of influences on D&I: intervention characteristics, the outer setting, the inner setting, characteristics of individuals and process. We will discuss the first four of these domains.

Intervention Characteristics

Rogers's diffusion of innovation theory[26] proposed that innovations that have greater *relative advantage, compatibility, trialability*, and *observability*, along with less *complexity*, generally will be adopted over innovations that do not. There is no doubt that the complexity of the evidence-supported interventions now being implemented in the social services may challenge the most robust implementation strategies. MTFC, for example, is a 24-hour per day, 7 days per week, 365 days per year intervention delivered in teams of six program staff (a supervisor, therapist, family therapist, skills coach, foster parent recruiter, daily caller), plus foster parents, serving 10 clients at a time. Many of these interventions require intense training and substantial consultation through the learning phase. The *trialability* of this kind of intervention is exceptionally low. While not listed among Rogers' characteristics, the *fit* of a protocol with social service agency settings may be just as important in the adoption decision.[27]

The expense of these interventions is compounded by the complexity of the implementation strategies needed to make them work in the long term. Retraining, booster training, and ongoing monitoring of intervention processes for quality assurance are typical implementation requirements for complex interventions. For organizations that successfully implement these interventions, mounting less complex protocols, like smoking cessation programs, might be easier than for other organizations. On the other hand, organizations that attempt to launch these complex programs and fail might be hesitant to try to implement a less complex protocol.

Complex, expensive interventions with low trialability require high competitive advantage and high observability in order for adoption to take place. At this juncture, with low dissemination of evidence-supported programs, agencies may receive substantial competitive advantage just by advertising their adoption of an evidence-based program. Over time, however, documented improved outcomes will likely be required to sustain these programs.

Outer Setting Considerations— Social Service Consumers

Think about two kinds of social service consumers—chronic and temporary. Many people use a social service for a short time. Rank and Hirschl,[28] for example, found that half of Americans use food stamps at some point in their lifetime. Far fewer need food stamps for years at a stretch. Temporary users of social services can be thought of as resourceful, capable, often resilient people who experience a tough patch along the life course and turn to the social services for help. The social services may not be the most likely access point for delivering evidence-supported health interventions for the temporary social service client. They can be reached through other means (e.g., through their primary care physician).

It is the longer term user of a social service who may consider the social service case manager their "primary carer," and for whom the influence of this case manager to move clients toward evidence-supported health interventions is greatest. Chronic users of social services may need these evidence-supported health interventions for a variety reasons. For example, they may have fewer resources, come from difficult circumstances, and have more comorbid health problems. These complicating factors make implementing programs of any type more difficult. Will a weight loss program work for a client on psychotropic medications known to lead to weight gain? Will a smoking cessation program work for a person with poor emotion regulation? Will a chronic disease management program work for a client who lives on the streets for weeks at a time?

Some social service consumers may also have less competence in daily living and organizational skills than health service providers are accustomed or that some health protocols require. Chronic social service consumers may also enter health intervention activities with long service histories. While some are sensitized to respond to professional intervention through prior service successes, others may have a history of service failures that may need to be addressed in any new intervention effort.

These complexities introduced by the nature of social service consumers may require substantial program adaptation. These adaptations might include adding assessments for readiness, adding motivational interviewing to intervention protocols, using materials that require less literacy, parsing the intervention into less complicated processes, and scheduling changes. Some of these adaptation strategies may be uncovered by active attempts to gather consumer and service provider inputs into implementation planning.[17]

Other Outer Setting Considerations

Moving evidence-supported health protocols into the social services faces one challenge that overshadows all others. Who will pay for it? Other pressures can be leveraged to advocate for increased access to evidence-supported health interventions—from advocacy groups, consumer groups, and the press—but without means to pay for these interventions, they will likely not be adopted and sustained by social service agencies. Health interventions moved into social service settings will either need to pay for themselves—with a business case laid out before adoption—or they need to have payment worked out in advance.

Complex interventions, like those often implemented in social service sectors, bring complex payment options. Medicaid is the most common payer for many of the health interventions discussed in this chapter. Complex protocols can sometimes be broken down into billable parts using existing billing codes. MTFC, for example, can bill some of its services as psychotherapy. On other occasions, agencies can arrange for reimbursement for the entire package of a multicomponent intervention, through paying per case or per day;[29] often this occurs when the Medicaid agency is eager to support evidence-based approaches and the agency provider possesses good advocacy skills. Even more rare are instances where Medicaid provides a reimbursement sufficient to cover both the intervention and the necessary implementation strategies (e.g., trainings, consultation calls) needed to adopt and sustain it.

Inner Setting Considerations

Local context is a valid consideration in every implementation effort. Social service agencies vary, however, on every possible dimension. Some dimensions that may have the most relevance for D &I work include agency size, financial resources, accessibility to information, presence of a professionalized performance management workforce, a culture that emphasizes continuous improvement, history of successful implementation efforts, electronic case records, and leadership commitment. Public agencies often have difficulty freeing money from compartmentalized funding streams to innovate. Private agencies often operate with small margins on their service contracts and operate with limited reserves that can be tapped to move new initiatives forward.

Provider Considerations

The level of staff motivation needs to be assessed as part of any implementation effort in the social services. Social service employees are often stereotyped as underpaid and overworked. Social service caseworkers who are overworked are not good candidates for new innovations. They may only participate if the new intervention reduces their workload. Evidence suggests, however, that training in evidence-based protocols, when combined with a supportive coaching and monitoring program, may be protective in reducing staff turnover.[30]

Skill and educational levels vary in the social services. Juvenile justice and child welfare services are often delivered by frontline staff with bachelor's degrees. Intervention activities have to be commensurate with staff skill and allow sufficient time in training.

For all of these considerations, the D&I of evidence-supported health intervention and prevention programs into the social services will require careful collaboration. Community academic partnership models of research have poignant relevance in the social services.[31,32] Social services consumers and providers will be skeptical that researchers without practical experiences in their worlds will understand the social realities embedded in these sectors of care and will welcome efforts to establish partnerships of equals that promote colearning, address health from both positive and ecological perspectives, and disseminate findings and knowledge to all partners.

Two case studies from different perspectives are provided here. The first describes the buildout of a network of services to disseminate and implement a packaged intervention into social service sectors of care. The second describes an effort from a sector of care to bring an evidence-supported intervention into its system.

CASE STUDY ONE: DISSEMINATING MULTISYSTEMIC THERAPY

Like other interventions being implemented in the social services, MST is a complicated clinical intervention most often implemented in a sector of care not known for high quality services—juvenile justice. Also typical of work in the social services, MST is disseminated through a purveyor organization. MST is atypical in at least three ways. Its intervention model is more intense than most. MST has been the focus of substantial implementation science. And, its dissemination story is described in the literature.[21]

What Is Being Disseminated

MST is a manualized, complex, clinical intervention designed for youth with conduct problems and a history of juvenile offenses.[33] It is short term (3–5 months), intense, and includes 24/7 therapist availability. There is daily contact between MST therapists and families and am MST therapist sees only three to six families at a time. MST is focused on changing sequences of behavior between and among systems that maintain problem behaviors. It is strength based, action focused, and targets well-specified problems. It uses behavioral, cognitive, and systems concepts in its intervention protocol.

The Vehicles of Dissemination

MST has two primary vehicles for dissemination, MST Services and MST Network Partners. Like many other efforts, the dissemination of MST began ad hoc, with its treatment developers providing training on a moonlighting basis, supplementing their academic jobs. This led to a training agreement with the state of South Carolina (using the state's federal family preservation block grant dollars) to disseminate MST across the state. Out-of-state training continued ad hoc, until the demand became too great and the treatment developers sought a new solution. The result was a university-licensed, for profit organization, MST Services, launched in 1996 in the name of technology transfer and now seen as an exemplar of the purveyor dissemination organization. Through MST Services, agencies purchase initial and ongoing training, consultation, and quality assurance services, including a robust feedback system from their proprietary data system, and MST Services licenses teams at agencies to use their program. The MST Services website in 2016 listed 17 MST expert consultants on its staff.

By 2000, some agencies expressed a desire to train their own MST teams using a train-the-trainer model and expand their own programs. A new dissemination system, MST Network Partners, was developed to allow established MST organizations to carry out the entire MST dissemination and implementation process.[21] In some cases, MST Services helps organizations, states, and countries start a MST program and then MST Services transfers oversight to a nearby MST network partner. MST Services, however, also offers network partners a set of supports and monitoring from its own office and maintains a staff of professionals for this purpose. In 2016, MST Services listed 24 network partners on its website. Most network partners are private social service agencies, but there are three university units and one US state agency among its partners. Network partners are based in Australia, Denmark, Norway, Sweden, the United Kingdom, and the United States. An advisory council of network partners provides guidance to MST Services on better ways to build and maintain the MST intervention.

Dissemination and Penetration Process

MST Services works with agencies and state governments to develop the appropriate framework and context for MST service delivery. This includes assessment of agency finances, beliefs, other services, and community support for MST. The assessment procedures are used to build support for MST implementation and to identify unique barriers to be overcome and strengths to use in the implementation effort.[34] Novel foci include developing agency human resources policies that support a 24/7 service delivery model and developing a financial plan that puts into place reimbursement mechanisms that will allow MST to function.[21] This up-front work on financial arrangements is one thing that sets MST's dissemination efforts apart from others and likely contributes to longer term sustainment.

The MST implementation model likely fits in the training + consultation + certification category described earlier, but with some additional components. Training in MST includes an initial 5-day on-site training, quarterly booster trainings, weekly on-site supervision by a member of MST Services, as well as weekly phone consultations with an MST expert. What may truly set MST's implementation model apart from others, however, is its heavy accent on quality monitoring. In addition to therapist adherence to MST predicting consumer outcomes e.g.,[35,36] MST studies have shown that fidelity of the supervisor[37] and MST consultant[38] also contribute to consumer outcomes. Therefore, MST Services and their network partners accent adherence to MST protocols more than almost any other known implementation effort. Clinicians are monitored with consumer measures of adherence; supervisors are monitored with clinician measures of adherence; and consultants are monitored with measures completed by clinicians and supervisors and these rating are routinely fed back to MST teams from the MST data system.

Reach and Penetration

100 MST teams were established in the first five years, with 425 teams trained by 2008.[21] In 2016, the MST Services website noted 500 + active teams in 34 US states and 15 countries, treating more than 23,000 youth per year. Schoenwald,[21] however, suggests that even with these teams, a very small percentage of juvenile offenders receive MST.

CASE STUDY 2: IMPLEMENTING TRAUMA-FOCUSED COGNITIVE BEHAVIORAL THERAPY IN RESIDENTIAL TREATMENT FACILITIES IN PHILADELPHIA

Residential treatment facilities (RTFs) provide 24/7 residential or restrictive care and clinical interventions for youth with emotional and behavioral problems involved in child welfare, juvenile justice, and mental health service systems. Despite high rates of trauma and posttraumatic stress disorder among youth in RTFs, these youth rarely have access to evidence-based trauma-informed treatment.[39,40] This case study describes the implementation of an evidence-based trauma treatment for youth in mental health RTF settings in Philadelphia, highlighting barriers and facilitators to implementation and adaptations made to the intervention protocol to fit the context.

What Is Being Implemented

Trauma-Focused Cognitive Behavioral Therapy[41] (TF-CBT) is a structured psychotherapy for children and adolescents (and their caregivers) who have experienced trauma. A trained clinician moves a child and caregiver through a series of nine treatment components, pacing the progression of the treatment with client readiness. Multiple clinical trials have demonstrated its efficacy for improving posttraumatic symptoms for children and youth with the kinds of diverse trauma histories seen in RTFs.[42] Further, TF-CBT had been implemented in other RTFs.[43] More recently, TF-CBT has been the focus of some implementation science.[44–46]

Context of Philadelphia and the History of the Trauma Initiative

The TF-CBT D&I effort for RTFs in Philadelphia was nested within other change efforts. A 2012 grant from the Substance Abuse and Mental Health Services Administration formed the Philadelphia Alliance for Child Trauma Services (PACTS)[47] to increase the number of children who receive evidence-based trauma treatments in Philadelphia. The grantee, Philadelphia's Department of Behavioral Health and Intellectual disAbility Services, had initiated in 2005 a system transformation that prioritized creating a recovery and resiliency oriented system for people with behavioral health needs.[48,49] The 2012 award was preceded in 2011 with the city's "Trauma Initiative," which contracted with treatment developers to provide training for behavioral health agencies in trauma-specific evidence-based practices.[47] The Trauma Initiative's first D&I effort was aimed at adults. TF-CBT was chosen as the second intervention for the Trauma Initiative system transformation's focus on children and adolescents.

Implementation of TF-CBT in Residential Treatment Facilities

PACTS was designed to include all the agencies previously engaged in the larger Trauma Initiative; two ran RTFs as part of their service configuration. An additional agency that provided some RTF services (but is not a full RTF) was partnered with in 2015 for RTF focused trainings; in 2016, one of the RTFs closed.

As described elsewhere,[47] clinicians in the two RTFs and other participating agencies received the standard, developer-recommended package of TF-CBT training: a web-based learning course (http://tfcbt.musc.edu), a 2-day, in-person didactic training with a TF-CBT master trainer, and subsequent consultation phone calls as clinicians began delivering the intervention. In this implementation, consultation calls were biweekly over 9 months, 1 hour in duration, with up to 10 participants. Further, each agency designated a supervisor (also trained in TF-CBT) who provided weekly internal supervision to therapists. Finally, annual booster sessions were provided to keep therapists engaged in TF-CBT implementation.

Four alterations to the standard training package were made for RTFs:

1. RTF therapists were placed into the same consultation call group, to increase contextual relevance.
2. The *TF-CBT* master trainer also provided consultation calls for each participating agency, to provide feedback specific to context.
3. Despite these additions, RTF therapists requested and were provided even more training that increased contextual relevance. These trainings covered: engaging caregivers and family members in TF-CBT, complex trauma, vicarious trauma, and TF-CBT milieu staff training. According to the PACTS project director, a highlight of the additional training was participation from a parent advocate who shared with the trainees her struggles and lessons learned raising a child who was placed at an RTF. She encouraged therapists not to forget parents living apart from their children, to honor the voices of caregivers, and meet caregivers where they are (Arturo Zinny, email communication, October 21, 2016).
4. Additional consultation calls were scheduled with each RTF to address even more adaptation issues that arose: integrating caregivers in TF-CBT when the child is placed far from the caregiver; youth "stuck" on mother not believing their history of sexual abuse; how to prepare youth to be discharged to a "nonsupportive" parent; how to utilize milieu staff the child trusts to prevent aggressive behaviors; how to implement TF-CBT with fidelity while also providing other interventions delivered at the RTF (Arturo Zinny, email communication, October 21, 2016).

Barriers and Facilitators to Implementing TF-CBT in RTF Settings

Cohen and colleagues[39] identified factors where an RTF context may facilitate TF-CBT implementation. One, the 24/7 nature of RTFs, proved beneficial in the PACTS implementation. In the words of the PACTS director, Arturo Zinny, (phone communication, October 21, 2016):

In outpatient settings the therapist sees the child once a week if they're lucky. The therapist hopes the child will practice the skills, do their homework, etc., but isn't sure to what extent the child is doing this or having this reinforced at home. But when a child is in an RTF setting, you can monitor that they're practicing, doing their homework, and have the opportunity to strategize with other staff on how to have them engage in the treatment throughout their day.

The Project Director also noted a major and yet expected barrier to the implementation of TF-CBT in RTFs. Caregivers often lived far from the RTF, or may have had a conflicted relationship with the child. The Project Director estimated that around 20% of caregivers participated in TF-CBT treatment with their children (Arturo Zinny, phone communication, October 21, 2016). This led to additional conversations with the treatment developers, who coached therapists on how to proceed with TF-CBT without a caregiver if continued efforts at caregiver engagement were not effective. Sometimes, direct care RTF staff members were invited into the treatment.

Reach and Penetration

In total, 1,510 children and adolescents, as of January 26, 2017, had received TF-CBT through PACTS and over 715 have completed treatment; the Project Director estimated that approximately 10% of youth who received TF-CBT did so at one of the RTFs (Arturo Zinny, email communication, January 6, 2017). Throughout the PACTS initiative, 50 RTF therapists were trained in TF-CBT; eight of those are still employed by their RTF, for a retention rate of 16% (Arturo Zinny, email communication, January 6, 2017). This retention rate is likely due in large part to the closing of two of the RTF agencies in Philadelphia.

To us, these two case studies illustrate themes emphasized elsewhere in this book. Complex interventions require a complex set of D&I supports, especially related to ongoing consultation, problem solving, and monitoring. Sometimes, new organizations need to be created to offer these kinds of supports. To date, the D&I field has not figured out the best way to mount and configure these supporting organizations.

DIRECTIONS FOR FUTURE RESEARCH

Everything that can be written about the need for further D&I research in other settings can be written about D&I research in the social services. There is a need for better specification of implementation strategies and outcome measurement, a need for studying implementation over time, a need for comparative effectiveness studies of implementation strategies, a need to test theoretical models of implementation, and so on. Also, almost every research question important to the field of D&I in health could be addressed in research that is conducted in social service settings. Other questions can be generated from this brief review of D&I work in the social services. We'll mention five.

Are social service sectors of care interested in health intervention and prevention protocols? Given the competing demands inherent in doing health work in the social services, what is the acceptability of this work in social service settings to the different social service stakeholders? How are health concerns prioritized among other demands, including behavioral health, in these sectors? Given similar efforts to disseminate, are adoption and uptake rates of these interventions similar to those found in other sectors of care? What factors motivate social service agencies to seek out health intervention and prevention protocols for implementation?

Are intervention and prevention protocols designed for other sectors of care effective when implemented through social service sectors of care? Is it feasible to implement health prevention and intervention programs in social service settings? (This question underscores the need for research studies with hybrid designs that examine implementation along with effectiveness). What are the common adaptations needed to bring health prevention and intervention protocols into social service settings? Can successful implementation of health intervention and prevention protocols in the social services change the outcomes of most interest to social service administrators?

Are implementation protocols developed for complex social service systems of care effective in implementing intervention and prevention protocols in other sectors of care? Can the lessons learned, say, about fidelity in juvenile justice settings by the MST research teams, be transported to medical settings of care?

What are the active ingredients of complex, blended implementation efforts? Given some of the difficulties of bringing complex intervention protocols into less than ideal settings, the implementation strategies in use in the social service sectors have tended to be multi-faceted, multi-phased efforts. It is important to know what components of these interventions are the most important to successful implementation.

How are social service agencies funding the delivery and implementation of evidence-supported health interventions? What funding streams are being used? Are they negotiating for new billing codes from Medicaid? Are they sustaining grant funded efforts after the initial funding period? How are social service agencies funding the planning, training and implementation supports needed to mount and sustain these complex interventions?

SUMMARY

Social service settings offer numerous complexities in their staffing, consumers, and payer mix that require careful consideration in designing dissemination and implementation efforts. However, social services' unique access to vulnerable populations with health problems may prove vital in efforts to improve the health status of many of our citizens and reduce health disparities. While a number of well-developed, blended D&I models are being used in social service settings, they all require additional documentation, research, and field experience. Nonetheless, the lessons learned in the social services may help organizations in other sectors better implement health interventions with complex consumers in complex settings.

ACKNOWLEDGEMENTS

We would like to thank Arturo Zinny, Rinad S. Beidas, Kamilah Jackson, and Steve Berkowitz for their assistance and feedback with the TF-CBT case study.

SUGGESTED READINGS AND WEBSITES

Readings

Powell BJ, Beidas RS, Special issue editors. Special Issue: System level implementation of evidence-based practice. *Adm Policy Ment Health Ment Health Serv Res*, 2016:43(6).
This special issue provides some insight into the type of implementation science being applied in the social services today.

Damschroder LJ, Aron DC, Keith RE, Kirsh SR, Alesander JA Lowery JC. Fostering implementation of health services research findings into practice: a consolidated framework for advancing implementation science. *Implement Sci.* 2009;4:50–65.

This influential integrative article provides practitioners and researchers a useful framework to think through some of the issues that they might confront when taking on a D&I project in the social services.

Selected Websites and Tools

The website for *Blueprints for Healthy Youth Development* http://www.colorado.edu/cspv/blueprints

A project of the Center for the Study and Prevention of Violence at the University of Colorado, it serves as a resource for governments, foundations, businesses, and other organizations trying to make informed judgments about their investments in violence and drug prevention programs. The project has reviewed the research for programs designed to reduce youth antisocial behavior and promote a positive developmental pathway. It promotes the use of specific model programs with detailed program descriptions, introductory videos and contact information.

The California Evidence-Based Clearinghouse for Child Welfare http://www.cebc4cw.org

The Clearinghouse provides professionals access to information about the research evidence for programs being used or marketed. It rates programs on the strength of their evidence and their relevancy to child welfare populations and categorizes programs by content area. It has become a force in the dissemination world that a new positive rating or an improved rating based on updated research drives requests for training from purveyor organizations.

The Coalition for Evidence Based Policy www.top-tierevidence.org

The Coalition site seeks to identify social interventions for all sectors of care that are shown to produce sustained benefits to participants and/or society using a very high standard of evidence. It identifies 10 "top tier programs," including two that are directly health related, Carrerra Adolescent Pregnancy Prevention Program, and Staying Free, a smoking cessation program for hospitalized smokers. It categorizes another 10 as near top-tier, two that are health focused: Healthy Living Partnerships to Prevent Diabetes (HELP PD and Child Immunization Campaign with Incentives).

The *Community Tool Box* http://ctb.ku.edu

Created by the Work Group for Community Health and Development at the University of Kansas, it is a well-organized website that offers numerous tools for community development activities, including participatory community assessment and evaluation.

The *National Implementation Research Network* website http://nirn.fpg.unc.edu

This website is designed to contribute to the best practices of and science of implementation. It provides a primer on implementation, topical reviews, and guidance on a range of implementation topics.

The U.S. Office of Juvenile Justice and Delinquency Prevention maintains a Model Programs Guide at https://www.ojjdp.gov/mpg.

It is designed as a resource for practitioners and communities about what works, what is promising, and what does not work in juvenile justice, delinquency prevention, and child protection and safety.

The U.S. Substance Abuse and Mental Health Services Administration's National Registry of Evidence-based Programs and Practices http://nrepp.sam-hsa.gov/01_landing.aspx

This is a searchable online registry of substance abuse and mental health interventions. It also contains links to a number of resources of interest to programs wanting to learn about how to effectively implement programs.

REFERENCES

1. Stiffman AR, Psecosolido B, Cabassa L. Building a model to understand youth service access: The Gateway Provider Model. *Ment Health Serv Res.* 2004;6 (4):189–198.

2. Wilkinson RG. Putting the picture together: Prosperity, redistribution, health and welfare. In Marmot M, Wilkinson RG, eds. *The social determinants of health.* 2nd ed. Oxford: Oxford University Press; 2006: 256–273.

3. Williams RB. Lower socioeconomic status and increased mortality: early childhood roots and the potential for successful interventions. *JAMA.* 1998;279:1745–1746.

4. Ahnquist J, Wamala SP, Lindstrom M. Social determinants of health—a question of social or economic capital? Interaction effects of socioeconomic factors on health outcomes. *Soc Sci Med.* 2012;74:930–939.

5. Anda RF, Felitti VJ, Bremner JD, et al., The enduring effects of abuse and related adverse experiences in childhood: a convergence of evidence from neurobiology and epidemiology. *Eur Arch Psychiatry Clin Neurosci.* 2006;256:174–186.

6. Dube SR, Felitti VJ, Dong M, Giles WH, Anda RF. The impact of adverse childhood experiences on health problems: evidence from four birth cohorts dating back to 1900. *Prevent Med.* 2003;37:268–277.

7. Blane D. The life course, the social gradient, and health. In: Marmot M, Wilkinson RG, eds. *The social determinants of health*, 2nd ed. Oxford: Oxford University Press; 2006: 54–77.

8. Kuh D, Ben-Shlomo Y. *A life course approach to chronic disease epidemiology: Tracing the origins of ill health from early to adult life.* 2nd ed. Oxford: Oxford University Press; 2004.

9. Steele JS, Buchi KF. Medical and mental health of children entering the Utah foster care system. *Pediatrics.* 2008;1122,e703–e709.

10. Monitoring the Future. http://monitoringthefuture.org/data/09data.html#2009data-cigs. (Accessed August 16, 2010).

11. Vaughn M, Ollie M, McMillen JC, Scott LD, Munson, MR. Substance use and abuse among older youth in foster care. *Addictive Behaviors.* 2007;32:1929–1935.

12. McMillen JC, Zima BT, Scott LD, et al. The prevalence of psychiatric disorders among older youths in the foster care system. *J Am Acad Child Adolesc Psychiatry.* 2005;44:88–95.

13. Reinherz HZ, Giacona RM, Lefkowitz ES, Pakiz B, Frost AK. Prevalence of psychiatric disorders in a community sample of older adolescents. *J Am Acad Child Adolesc Psychiatry.* 1993;32:369–377.

14. Cawley J, Danziger S. *Obesity as a barrier to the transition from welfare to work.* National Bureau of Economic Research Working paper # W10508; 2004.

15. Raghavan, R, Inkelas, M, Franke, T 7 Halfon, N. Administrative barriers to the adoption of high-quality mental health services for children in foster care: a national study. *Adm Policy Ment Health Ment Health Serv Res,* 2007;34,191–201.

16. Acoca, L, Stephens, J, van Vleet, A. *Health coverage and care for youth in the juvenile justice system: The role of Medicaid and CHIP.* The Kaiser Commission on Medicaid and the Uninsured. Issue brief, 2014.

17. Hasche, LK, Lenze, S, Brown, T, Lawrence, L, Nickel, M, Morrow-Howell, Proctor, EK. Adapting collaborative depression care for public community long-term care: using research-practice partnerships. *Adm Policy Ment Health Ment Health Serv Res,* 2014;14:687–696.

18. Ellis D, Naar-King S, Templin R, Frey M, Cunningham P, Sheidow A, Cakan N, Idalski A. Mutisystemic therapy for adolescents with poorly controlled type 1 diabetes. *Diabetes Care,* 2008;31:1746–1747.

19. Kerr, DCR, Level, LD, Camberlain, P. Pregnancy rates among juvenile justice girls in two RCTs of Mulditidmensional Treatment Foster Care. *J Consult Clin Psychol,* 2009;77:588–593.

20. Greenwood P. Prevention and intervention programs for juvenile offenders: the benefits of evidence-based practice. *Future Child.* 2008;18:11–36.

21. Glisson C, Schoenwald SK. The ARC organizational and community intervention strategy for implementing evidence-based children's mental health treatments. *Ment Health Serv Res.* 2005;7(4):243–259.

22. Glisson C, Schoenwald SK, Hemmelgarn A, et al. Randomized trial of MST and ARC in a two-level evidence-based treatment implementation strategy. *J Consult Clin Psychol.* 2010;78: 537–550.

23. Sosna T, Marsenich L. *Community development team model: Supporting the model adherent implementation of programs and practices.* California Institute for Mental Health; Sacramento, CA. 2006.

24. Brown CH, Chamberlain P, Saldana L, Padgett, C, Wang W and Cruden, C. Evaluation of two implementation strategies in 51 child county public service systems in two states: results of a cluster randomized head-to-head implementation trial. *Implement Sci,* 9;134:2014.

25. Damschroder LJ, Aron DC, Keith RE, Kirsh SR, Alesander JA Lowery JC. Fostering implementation of health services research findings into practice: a consolidated framework for advancing implementation science. *Implement Sci.* 2009;4:50–65.

26. Rogers E. *Diffusion of innovation.* 4th ed. New York: Free Press; 1995.

27. Beidas, RS, Stewart, RE, Adams, DR et al. A multilevel examination of stakeholder perspectives of implementation of evidence-based practices in a large urban publicly funded mental health system. *Adm Policy Ment Health Ment Health Serv Res.* 2016;43:893–908.

28. Rank MR, Hirschl T. Likilihood of using food stamps during the adulthood years. *J Nutr Educ Behav.* 2005;37:137–146.

29. Schoenwald SK. From policy pinball to purposeful partnership: The policy contexts of Multisystemic Therapy transport. In Weisz JR, Kazdin AE, eds. *Evidence-based psychotherapies for children and adolescents.* 2nd ed. New York: Guilford Press; 2010: 538–553.

30. Aarons, GA, Domerfield, DHZ, HEch, DB, Silovsky, JF, Chaffin, MJ. The impact of evidence-based practice implementation and fidelity monitoring on staff turnover: evidence for a protective effect. *J Consult Clin Psychol,* 2009;77:270–280.

31. Drahota A, Meza RD, Brikho B, Naaf M., Estabillo JA, Gomez ED, Vejnoska Dufek S, Stahmer AC, Aarons GA. Community-academic partnerships: a systematic review of the state of the literature and recommendations for future research. Millbank Q, 2016;94:163–214.

32. Israel BA, Schulz AJ, Parker EA, Becker AB. Review of community-based research: assessing partnership approaches to improve public health. *Annu Rev Public Health.* 1998;19:173–202.

33. Henggeler SW, Schoenwald SK, Borduin CM, Rowland MD, Cunningham PB. *Multisystemic treatment of antisocial behavior in children and adolescents.* 2nd. ed. New York: Guilford Press; 2009.

34. Edwards DL, Schoenwald SK, Henggeler SW, & Strother KB. (2001). A multi-level perspective on the implementation of multisystemic therapy (*MST*): Attempting dissemination with fidelity. In Bernfield GA, Farrington DP, Leschied AW. eds. *Offender rehabilitation in practice: Implementing and evaluating effective programs.* London: Wiley; 2001: 97–120.

35. Henggeler SW, Pickrel SG, Brondino MJ. Multisystemic treatment of substance abusing and dependent delinquents: outcomes, treatment fidelity, and transportability. *Ment Health Serv Res.* 1999;1:171–184.

36. Schoenwald SK, Carter RE, Chapman JE, Sheidow AJ. Therapist adherence and organizational effects on change in youth behavior problems one year after multisystemic therapy. *Adm Policy Ment Health Ment Health Serv Res.* 2008;35:84–97.

37. Schoenwald SK, Sheidow AJ, Chapman JE. Clinical supervision in treatment transport: effects on adherence and outcomes. *J Consult Clin Psychol.* 2009;77:410–421.

38. Schoenwald, SK, Sheidow AJ, Letourneau, EJ Toward effective quality assurance in evidence-based practice: links between expert consultation, therapist fidelity, and child outcomes. *J Clin Child Adolesc Psychol.* 2004;33:94–104.

39. Cohen, JA, Mannarino AP, Jankowski K, Rosenberg S, Kodya S, Wolford GL. A randomized implementation study of trauma-focused cognitive-behavioral therapy for adjudicated teenagers in residential treatment facilities. *J Am Acad Child Adolesc Psychiatry.* 2016;55:S279–S280.

40. Hodgdon HB, Kinniburgh K, Gabowitz D, Blaustein ME, Spinazzola J. Development and implementation of trauma-informed programming in youth residential treatment centers using the ARC framework. *J Fam Violence,* 2013;28:679–692.

41. Cohen, JA, Mannarino, AP, Deblinger, E. *Treating trauma and traumatic grief in children and adolescents.* New York: Guilford Press; 2006.

42. Cary C, McMillen JC. The data behind the dissemination: a systematic review of trauma-focused cognitive behavioral therapy for use with children and youth. *Child Youth Serv Rev.* 2012;34:748–757.

43. Cohen JA, Mannarino AP, Navarro D. Residential treatment. In Cohen JA, Mannarino AP, & Deblinger E, eds. *Trauma-focused CBT for children and adolescents: Treatment applications.* New York: Guilford Press, 2012: 73–104.

44. Sigel, BA, Benton, AH, Lynch, CE, Kramer, TL. Characteristics of 17 statewide initiatives to disseminate trauma-focused cognitive-behavioral therapy (TF-CBT). *Psychol Trauma Theory Res Pract Policy.* 2013;5(4):323.

45. Cohen, J, Mannarino, AP. Disseminating and implementing trauma-focused CBT in community settings. *Trauma Violence Abuse.* 2008;9:214–226.

46. McMillen, JC, Hawley, KH, Proctor, EK. Mental health clinicians' participation in web-based training for an evidence supported intervention: signs of encouragement and trouble ahead. *Adm Policy Ment Health Ment Health Serv Res.* 2016;43:592–603.

47. Beidas, RS, Adams, DR, Kratz, HE, Jackson, K, Berkowitz, S, et al. Lessons learned while building a trauma-informed public behavioral health system in the City of Philadelphia. *Eval Progr Plan.* 2016;59:21–32

48. Achara-Abrahams I, Evans AC, King JK. (2010). Recovery-focused behavioral health system transformation: A framework for change and lessons learned from Philadelphia. In Kelly JF, White WL (Eds.), *Addiction recovery management.* Totowa, NJ: Humana Press; 2010: 187–208.

49. Powell BJ, Beidas RS, Rubin RM, Stewart RE, Wolk CB, Matlin SL, Weaver S, Hurford MO, Evans AC, Hadley TR, Mandell DS. Applying the policy ecology framework to Philadephia's behavioral health transformation efforts. *Adm Policy Ment Health Serv Res.* 2016;43:909–926.

23

Implementation Science in Health Care

ALISON B. HAMILTON AND BRIAN S. MITTMAN

INTRODUCTION

Among the many domains and sectors studied by implementation researchers during the past 30 to 40 years, the diversity of settings and volume of implementation science activity in health care are arguably among the richest. Health care implementation science has contributed valuable theory and empirical evidence, and has advanced efforts to identify and address important conceptual and methodological challenges. Implementation research in health care has also stimulated policy and practice interest and has facilitated the field's continuing transformation into a coherent, integrated body of research encompassing multiple disciplines and domains. Yet implementation science in health care continues to confront the full range of challenges facing the field more broadly, including an overabundance of terms and labels; shortcomings in the application of relevant theory; debates over appropriate research approaches, designs and methods; and gaps in research attention to important phenomena. This chapter briefly reviews key stages in the evolution and development of implementation science in health care, describes the range of settings and effective practices of interest to implementation researchers—and the implementation strategies and programs developed to facilitate improvements in health care processes and outcomes—and examines key challenges and future directions in the field. A case study describing an integrated program of implementation research illustrates many of the ideas discussed in the chapter.

EVIDENCE BASE AND THEORY

The field of implementation science in health care comprises a rich body of literature, much of which developed through separate streams of activity before its relatively recent coalescence into a more unified whole. Early implementation research within the field of clinical and health services research during the 1970s, 1980s, and continuing into the 1990s studied strategies for "changing physician behavior"[1,2] and was conducted primarily by physician researchers and a smaller group of social and behavioral scientists. Driven largely by concerns over excessive resource utilization and costs (e.g., duplicative or nonindicated diagnostic testing), this research assumed that individual physician decisions were the primary driver of most clinical practices and health care resource utilization, and that effective strategies for influencing individual physician practices were key to improving adherence to recommended practices, and thus for improving quality and outcomes.

Much of the early research in this period examined the effectiveness of passive information dissemination and conventional educational strategies such as continuing medical education,[3] based on the implicit assumption that physicians' clinical practices are driven primarily by information, knowledge, and education.[4] Other strategies studied during this period included financial incentives and chart-based reminder systems[5,6] intended to incentivize and prompt physicians to follow recommended practices and apply the knowledge they obtained via education and passive information dissemination. Accumulating evidence showing the lack of effectiveness of these methods helped stimulate a series of articles (beginning in the late 1980s and 1990s) discussing the limitations of passive information dissemination and education and examining the role of professional norms and related factors in influencing physician practices,[7,8] particularly in light of the high levels of uncertainty inherent in clinical decision-making.[9] These insights led to the development and testing of strategies such as opinion leader methods,[10] academic detailing,[11] and related approaches based on principles of social influence rather than models of rational, analytical decision-making.[12] Positive results from many of these studies, in contrast to the largely negative findings of studies evaluating educational strategies, prompted increased interest and continued research on social influence approaches.[13–17]

In addition to concerns over cost and resource utilization, research evaluating strategies for changing physician practices was also driven by evidence of significant geographic variations in health care practices and outcomes, and emerging research conceptualizing and measuring the quality of health care. Early research documenting variations in care across health care delivery settings and geographic regions[18] led to further studies showing that variations often reflected inappropriate use of specific medical procedures and services.[19] Research to define and measure "quality of care" began in the 1960s and accelerated in the 1970s and 1980s,[20,21] producing specific measures of quality, such as hospital mortality rates,[22] and the accumulation of additional evidence demonstrating gaps and deficiencies in health care quality and outcomes, including widely cited reports from the Institute of Medicine and other groups in the United States and abroad.[23–27]

Interest in the development of strategies for addressing quality problems was also strengthened by the introduction of appropriateness criteria,[28] clinical practice guidelines,[29,30] "practice parameters,"[31] and other tools and approaches associated with the emerging field of evidence-based medicine.[32] These tools combine research evidence with expert consensus to specify recommended "evidence-based" clinical practices and offer a focus for clinical decision aids, quality improvement and implementation efforts, as well as benchmarks for measuring health care quality and progress towards improvement. A significant share of implementation research in health care continues to focus on guideline implementation,[33–36] targeting guidelines listed in repositories such as the National Guidelines Clearinghouse and the Guidelines International Network's International Guidelines Database. Additional implementation and quality improvement efforts in health care target evidence-based practices identified through systematic reviews, including those produced by entities such as Cochrane Collaboration review groups, Agency for Healthcare Research and Quality (AHRQ) Evidence-based Practice Centers, and the University of York Center for Reviews and Dissemination. Interest in comparative effectiveness research (CER) and the establishment of the Patient-Centered Outcomes Research Institute in the United States in 2010 have produced additional clinical evidence and evidence-based guidance for health care practice, prompting additional interest in implementation research to guide CER implementation efforts.[37,38]

Concurrent with the growth of interest in health care quality and evidence-based medicine, the prevailing emphasis on individual clinician practices during the early decades of implementation science in health care was replaced by a focus on the role of organizational structures and policies ("systems") in the 1980s and 1990s, with an accompanying transition away from efforts to change individual physician behavior and toward strategies such as "continuous quality improvement" and "total quality management" employed in the manufacturing and service sectors.[39,40] This trend led to replacement of the label "changing physician practices" with the term "quality improvement research" to describe activity now labeled implementation research. This period also witnessed a significant increase in the volume of policy, practice, and research activity in health care quality improvement and significant growth in quality improvement research funding (e.g., following establishment of the Agency for Health Care Policy and Research in 1989, later renamed the Agency for Healthcare Research and Quality). Several new journals emerged in this period as well, including the *American Journal of Medical Quality*, 1986; *International Journal for Quality in Health Care*, 1989; and *Quality in Health Care*, 2000, subsequently retitled *Quality and Safety in Health Care* and later *BMJ Quality and Safety*.

The development and application of theories and conceptual frameworks guiding implementation strategies, and research evaluating specific techniques for changing behavior, evolved together with changes in emphasis from individual clinicians to organizations. Theories of individual decision-making and behavior change have been augmented by theories drawn from management research and by conceptual frameworks linked to the dominant quality improvement techniques such as continuous quality improvement and total quality management. Although key theories from the fields of management research and organization theory have been harnessed to design and study implementation strategies and processes,[41–46] the volume of activity to catalogue and explore the role and application of organizational theories in implementation lags that devoted to psychological theories.[47-49] Rogers' diffusion of innovations theory[50] and expansions of this theory,[51] as well as broader planning and evaluation frameworks such as RE-AIM,[52] have featured prominently in implementation studies throughout the history of the field, but development of newer theoretical frameworks has accelerated.[53-56] Among the most frequently used are the PARIHS framework,[57,58] Theoretical Domains Framework,[59,60] and Consolidated Framework for Implementation Research,[61-63] while newer approaches (e.g., Normalization Process Theory) continue to emerge and contribute to innovative implementation studies (also see chapter 5).[64-66]

The streams of research activity discussed represent only a portion of the overall body of activity comprising implementation science in health care. Developing largely in parallel with the health care quality improvement-oriented work, rich portfolios of implementation research activity in health have developed within related fields such as nursing research, health psychology and health promotion, research on substance use disorders, patient safety, health equity and disparities, and others. This research proceeds under labels such as "research utilization" (common in nursing research),[67,68] "technology transfer" (common in substance use disorders research),[69] and "operations research"[70] (common in research in global health and improvement of health systems). Overlapping bodies of research captured by the labels "dissemination and implementation research in health" in the United States, "knowledge translation" (largely in Canada) and related labels in Europe and elsewhere embody theories, research approaches, and empirical studies closely related to work labeled "quality improvement research in health" and, more recently, "improvement science." In the United States, the labels "quality improvement research," "patient safety research," and "improvement science" tend to be more common in studies funded by the AHRQ and by several foundations (e.g., Robert Wood Johnson Foundation, Commonwealth Fund), whereas "dissemination and implementation research" is more commonly seen in studies supported by the US National Institutes of Health and the US Department of Veterans Affairs. The latter body of studies generally differ from improvement science in their focus on implementation of evidence-based practices to overcome "translational roadblocks" or implementation gaps. These roadblocks—examined in depth by the Institute

of Medicine Clinical Research Roundtable[71,72] and constituting a key motivation for the development of the NIH Roadmap Initiative,[73,74] the NIH Clinical and Translational Science Award program, and related initiatives—are similar to the "quality chasm" and quality gaps examined by the Institute of Medicine's Quality Chasm report series. Thus, despite differences in their underlying policy and practice motivations and goals (i.e., an emphasis on increasing adoption of research-developed, evidence-based practices and innovations vs. an emphasis on improving quality and reducing quality gaps), improvement science and implementation science in health share many common theories, research approaches, and methods and pursue similar aims, questions, and hypotheses.[75-78]

DESIGNING DISSEMINATION AND IMPLEMENTATION PROGRAMS AND STRATEGIES IN HEALTH SETTINGS: THEORY, DIAGNOSIS, CONTEXT, AND ADAPTATION

Robust activity in implementation science in health has produced rich guidance for selecting and designing implementation strategies in health care. The Cochrane Collaboration Effective Practice and Organisation of Care (EPOC) review group[79] has published approximately 110 systematic reviews (as of August 2017) of implementation strategies in health care, including strategies incorporating financial incentives, educational programs, organizational policy and structure changes, and others. The EPOC collection includes systematic reviews focused on specific single-component implementation strategies and reviews examining strategies studied in reference to a specific type of implementation program or care setting. In the United States, the AHRQ Evidence-based Practice Centers program[80] has published several systematic reviews of implementation strategies under the topic "Quality Improvement and Patient Safety," including a multivolume series entitled "Closing the Quality Gap: A Critical Analysis of Quality Improvement Strategies." Additional compilations have been produced by individual research teams.[81-83]

The range of potential implementation strategies and multi-component (multi-strategy) implementation programs is limitless. Early work in the field typically employed single-component, narrowly focused, physician behavior change or quality improvement strategies found to be effective in changing clinical practices in previous studies. This approach was based on an implicit assumption that specific behavior change strategies could be identified that were inherently and broadly effective across diverse implementation problems and contexts. This generic approach, and the underlying assumption that robust implementation strategies exist, was eventually replaced by recognition that implementation strategies must be selected on the basis of identified, diagnosed causes of quality and implementation gaps[84] and an assessment of barriers and facilitators to practice change.[85] There is also growing recognition that implementation strategies must be guided by appropriate behavior change theory and conceptual models,[86–89] and sensitive to contextual factors beyond barriers and facilitators to change.[90,91] Furthermore, because most implementation or quality gaps have multiple causes and involve multiple barriers to change, implementation programs must generally include multiple components delivered at multiple levels.[92,93] New approaches for diagnosing implementation gaps to identify specific root causes and barriers and facilitators to change, to select and apply relevant theories, and to select and adapt a combination of implementation strategies to local needs and contextual factors continue to emerge. These include guidance by Powell and colleagues, who suggest four methods for matching implementation strategies to identified barriers and facilitators in particular practice settings: concept mapping, group model building, conjoint analysis, and intervention mapping.[94]

Work to better understand and guide adaptation to respond to the extreme heterogeneity of implementation problems and settings is particularly promising.[95–98] Maintaining the core purpose, or function, of an implementation strategy while adapting its format, or form, to local circumstances is a promising strategy for maintaining fidelity to the core functions of a multicomponent strategy while adapting features and details of its operationalization to conform to local circumstances.[99,100]

IMPLEMENTATION BARRIERS

Recognition of the importance of identifying and overcoming barriers to implementation in health care is well established: many of the key frameworks for planning and conducting implementation research in health care include specific research phases and activities in which barriers are explicitly assessed.[101] Numerous empirical studies in recent decades have documented and classified barriers to implementation,[102,103] including recent work examining patient perspectives on implementation barriers.[104] Although specific barriers vary across the range of health care delivery settings (e.g., small physician practices, hospitals), most result from a common set of fundamental characteristics of health care, including (1) high levels of uncertainty in diagnostic and treatment decision-making and in identifying causal links between treatment activities and outcomes, (2) the resulting dominance of professionals and professional norms and culture in health care delivery, and (3) the diverse range of constraints and influences on health care practices.

Uncertainty

The importance of professional autonomy and individual judgment in professionals' clinical decision-making and practices is driven largely by high levels of uncertainty in health care delivery and in cause-effect relationships.[105] High levels of variability in treatment outcomes, combined with the effects of psychological processes such as belief perseverance,[106] contribute to clinical inertia,[107,108] and considerable stability and resistance to change in clinicians' beliefs regarding clinical practices. Conservatism and resistance to change are reinforced by the prevalence of contradictory findings from clinical research:[109,110] clinicians trained prior to the era of meta-analyses and systematic reviews implicitly yet appropriately downgrade the weight of individual studies and thus published guidance, and approach clinical practice guidelines and other forms of published guidance with the same inherent skepticism.

Professionals and Professional Norms

The central role of professionals in health care delivery and the implications of professionalism for practice change were recognized at an early point in the development of the field. For implementation efforts targeting individual, autonomous clinicians (e.g., physicians in solo and small practices and working in community hospitals under traditional fee-for-service reimbursement), effective implementation requires changes in professional norms in addition to changes in individual clinicians' knowledge and beliefs, economic incentives, and other factors. Professional norms are typically highly stable and not easily influenced by outsiders. Physician resistance to improvement efforts led by insurers and other outside stakeholders is high: clinical practice guidelines developed by physicians' peers and professional communities (e.g., medical societies) are seen as more credible than those developed by government bodies or insurance companies.[111,112] Traditional norms of professionalism favor individual professional judgment and patient-by-patient decisions over standardized, codified policies and procedures, leading physicians to rely more heavily on their own individual judgment rather than clinical practice guidelines and related forms of evidence documented in systematic reviews. This led to early organized resistance to clinical practice guidelines by the American Medical Association, which employed the label "practice parameters" rather than "clinical practice guidelines" to convey the belief that guidelines should offer a voluntary, advisory set of parameters for use in clinical decisions rather than a more explicit form of guidance. Although more accepted now than during the 1990s, guidelines and other tools of evidence-based medicine continue to face strong resistance among many physicians and other health care professionals.

Professionalism and professional autonomy represent significant barriers to implementation in large organized delivery systems as well as individual settings. Conventional approaches to management employed in traditional complex organizations, in which authority increases in relation to higher positions in a traditional pyramid-shaped organization, are not applicable in health care delivery organizations (and other "professional bureaucracies")[113] in which front-line workers at the bottom of traditional organizational pyramids are highly educated, professional clinicians whose decisions and practices are more heavily influenced by outside professional communities and peers rather than organizational rules and policies. Although quality improvement strategies such as continuous quality improvement have been adapted successfully to accommodate the unique hierarchical features of health care organizations, the dominance of external professional norms over internal organizational policies remains a significant barrier to implementation efforts within organizations.

Multilevel Influences

Another significant source of challenges to implementation in health care is the multilevel nature of influences and constraints on health care practices. Several authors[114-116] have noted that health care practices are influenced by a broad range of factors operating at the level of the individual patient and patient–clinician dyad, at the level of clinical microsystems, clinics and larger organizations, within professional communities and regions, and at the national policy level. Individual implementation efforts typically involve behavior change strategies aimed at one or two levels (e.g., patients and clinicians); implementation researchers, clinical leaders, and others attempting to change clinical practices lack sufficient leverage and authority to influence the full range of factors constraining and influencing the target practices. The need for multilevel, coordinated approaches to implementation is increasingly recognized and has led to innovative programs such as the Robert Wood Johnson Foundation "Aligning Forces for Quality" initiative,[117] as well as calls for and examples of multilevel implementation approaches.[118-120]

IMPLEMENTATION RESEARCH CASE STUDY

Frameworks guiding the design and conduct of implementation studies, and portfolios of implementation research and texts offering broad overviews of implementation science in health,[121,122] describe a series of desirable research activities and study features important for achieving success in identifying, diagnosing, and closing quality and implementation gaps. Table 23.1 summarizes much of this guidance by listing key research activities and selected features of these activities.

Many of the recommended features of implementation research in health care are illustrated by a rich program of implementation studies targeting quality and implementation gaps for schizophrenia. Conducted by Young and colleagues based at the VA Greater Los Angeles Healthcare System and UCLA, this research encompasses a series of studies documenting and diagnosing gaps in quality and outcomes, and evaluating specific strategies for closing these gaps through implementation of evidence-based practices and other innovations in care delivery.

The fundamental motivation for this research program comprises studies documenting significant gaps in the quality of health care received by patients with schizophrenia.[123-125] This evidence, including more recent updated data on quality, implementation, and equity gaps[126,127] has stimulated a program of research to develop

TABLE 23.1 KEY FEATURES OF A COMPREHENSIVE IMPLEMENTATION RESEARCH PORTFOLIO AND FEATURES OF INDIVIDUAL STUDIES

Research activity	Desirable features and comments
Pre-implementation studies	
Clinical effectiveness research to develop evidence-based, innovative practices	Research design, methods, sampling and other features should maximize external validity and policy/practice relevance to increase acceptability to target clinicians and leaders.[160,161]
Development of evidence-based clinical practice guidelines	Guideline development processes should follow published recommendations for appropriate use of evidence, involvement of key stakeholder groups, sponsorship, etc.[111,112]
Development of other innovations	Innovation characteristics should facilitate adoption, incorporating features identified by research on the diffusion of innovations.[50]
Development of methods and measures for implementation studies	Important research tools include validated, casemix-adjusted measures of implementation outcomes (adherence, adoption) and appropriate data sources; study designs for quantitative impact evaluation with adequate external validity; and research approaches and methods for process evaluation.
Documentation of current practices and their determinants	Observational studies to understand current clinical practices and their influences incorporating quantitative and qualitative methods.
Measurement and diagnosis of quality or implementation gaps	Observational studies to compare current practices to desired practices and to identify determinants or "root causes" of quality and implementation gaps.
Observational implementation studies	
Studies of naturally occurring (policy- and practice-led) implementation processes	Observational studies maximize external validity, avoid artificial elements of researcher-led implementation trials, and offer opportunities to develop insights into barriers, facilitators, and key influences on routine implementation processes and success. Strong research designs are needed to achieve adequate internal validity.
Interventional implementation studies	
Phase 1 pilot studies of implementation programs	Pilot studies offer opportunities to develop initial evidence regarding the feasibility, acceptability and potential effectiveness of implementation strategies and to begin to identify key contextual influences and other factors influencing effectiveness. Emphasis on formative evaluation to modify the implementation program based on frequent measurement of impact and operation.
Phase 2 efficacy-oriented small-scale trials of implementation programs	Trials of implementation programs under idealized (efficacy-oriented) conditions, such as active research team facilitation and support for participating sites and grant funding for added costs, permit assessment of implementation program effectiveness under best-case conditions. Phase 2 studies feature initial formative evaluation to refine implementation program followed by emphasis on fidelity (with site-level adaptation guided by a predeveloped adaptation protocol).

(continued)

TABLE 23.1 CONTINUED

Research activity	Desirable features and comments
Phase 3 effectiveness-oriented large trials of implementation programs	Larger trials of implementation programs under routine conditions (e.g., limited or no research team technical assistance or grant support to participating sites) permit assessment of implementation program effectiveness when deployed under real-world conditions. Phase 3 studies feature site-level adaptation guided by a predeveloped adaptation protocol, and measurement of sustainment, scale-up/spread potential, costs and cost effectiveness, and a broad range of outcomes (implementation outcomes and, where feasible, system-level as well as clinical and patient outcomes [clinical, functional, quality of life, etc.]).
Phase 4 "postmarketing" study of implementation program	Research-led monitoring and evaluation of policy/practice-led scale-up and spread of an effective implementation program. Phase 4 studies generate feedback to policy/practice leaders to guide their management of an implementation and spread effort.

and evaluate specific implementation strategies to improve care, guided by a careful assessment of the key research needs and challenges and a roadmap specifying the research activities to be conducted.[128]

Consistent with frameworks for pre-implementation and implementation studies, Young et al. supplemented initial research to identify and quantify quality gaps with studies examining the determinants, and thus potential causes, of these gaps[125] and research to assess key stakeholders' views and recommendations regarding potential approaches for closing these gaps.[129,130] Additional pre-implementation and methods-development research included studies developing and assessing the validity of key measures of implementation program impacts such as quality of care,[131] clinician competencies,[132] and additional tools, methods, and measures required for implementation studies.[133]

A series of interventional implementation studies launched by Young and colleagues illustrates many of the desirable features of such studies, including extensive formative and process evaluation to examine implementation barriers, facilitators, and processes and thus to supplement and explain analyses of implementation program effectiveness. The research portfolio has included studies examining individual elements of a multicomponent approach to implementation, such as a computerized decision support system,[134] a consumer-led strategy targeting clinicians,[135] a family-targeted intervention,[136] and a weight management intervention.[137]

Additional studies (EQUIP-1, EQUIP-2) evaluated multicomponent, multilevel implementation programs building on the prior studies of individual components.[138–141] More recent work by this team has advanced patient-facing interventions for patients with serious mental illness, incorporating technology and consumer support to both strengthen patient-centered approaches to accessing care and to decrease burden on providers.[142] Collectively, this rich sequence of studies illustrates the progression from small-scale to larger implementation trials, as well as the value and use of extensive formative and process evaluation and other key features of implementation studies and phased research programs.

RESEARCH GAPS AND DIRECTIONS FOR FUTURE RESEARCH

Continued growth in research interest, activity and funding in health care implementation science offers considerable promise for continued progress in addressing the field's key challenges. Expanded activity and contributions from researchers trained in diverse disciplines and employing a broader range of research approaches and methods will continue to enrich the methodological toolkit, the range of theoretical perspectives, and the breadth of research epistemologies applied to the field's key questions, while simultaneously expanding the volume of empirical evidence and insights and the range of implementation problems and settings studied.

Future activity in the field is likely to help address several identified gaps, advance a number of key debates regarding the future of the field, and apply implementation science frameworks and insights to emerging areas of clinical research and innovation, such as precision medicine.[143,144] Important gaps include (1) the limited amount of research attention to challenges in achieving sustainment and routine scale-up and spread of effective practices following their initial adoption; (2) the need for increased research examining naturally occurring implementation processes (vs. investigator-led implementation); and (3) greater attention to implementation processes and mechanisms via approaches such as process evaluation and theory-based evaluation, to complement and help understand and interpret the results of impact-oriented research. Key challenges to progress in addressing these research gaps include ongoing debates regarding the need for research to inventory, classify, and guide the selection and effective use of theory; debates regarding research approaches and the nature of evidence required to better understand and guide implementation processes and evaluate the effectiveness of alternative implementation strategies and programs; and the need for improved methods for observational research on implementation.

Sustainment, Scale-up, and Spread

Interest in sustainment, scale-up, and spread has increased recently, based on recognition that successful implementation of effective practices through short-term research-led efforts (typically targeting a limited number of research sites) does not naturally lead to sustained adoption in the participating sites nor broader adoption in additional sites. Interventional implementation studies comparing an intensive, investigator-led multifaceted implementation strategy deployed in a sample of health care organizations against a low-intensity "usual care" implementation approach in a matched sample of settings can produce significant increases in rates of adoption of the target health care practice. Yet much of this increase might be due to temporary factors such as high levels of researcher attention, technical assistance and support for participating sites, grant funding for additional staff and resources (e.g., IT support for implementation), and others. Studies measuring long-term sustainment of resulting practice changes after withdrawal of these resources are rare, despite considerable evidence from management theory and related fields suggesting that professional and organizational changes may be temporary. Theory and research on phenomena such as organizational learning[145,146] and institutionalization[147] offer considerable value in explaining and predicting long-term patterns of behavior change, and should be explored as part of a broader program of theory development and empirical research to better understand sustainment phenomena and to guide efforts to design improved implementation strategies to increase the likelihood that short-term successes in changing health care practices will be sustained.[148]

A similar need exists for increased attention to scale-up and spread processes and strategies. A range of factors limit the external validity and transferability of the findings from interventional implementation studies assessing effectiveness of an investigator-led implementation program in a small number of sites. Factors limiting sustainment, such as temporary researcher attention and technical assistance and grant-provided funds for staff and IT, serve to limit spread of effective practices beyond sites participating in time-limited implementation research projects as well: responsibility for deploying effective implementation strategies on a large scale, including provision of technical assistance and other forms of facilitation and support provided by research teams in grant-funded implementation studies, is often unclear. Other factors contribute to limited spread, including non-representativeness of sites participating in research studies: these sites are often high-resource organizations whose ability to successfully adopt effective practices is likely to be high even in the absence of carefully designed practice change strategies. Research to understand barriers and facilitators to routine scale-up and spread and to develop effective scale-up strategies will help identify and characterize these and other limitations of current approaches to implementation research and will help develop new guidance for successful scale-up and spread.[149]

Observational Studies

Increased research attention to sustainment and scale-up and spread processes will help stimulate growth in observational research examining naturally occurring spread as well as phased implementation research programs[150] involving progression from small-scale efficacy-oriented implementation trials (involving high levels of researcher technical assistance and support for participating sites) to larger scale effectiveness-oriented trials and observational studies in which researchers have little or no role in facilitating implementation but serve mainly to evaluate the implementation process. Researcher-led implementation efforts are often highly artificial, addressing quality and implementation gaps viewed as important by researchers but not necessarily by participating sites, and involving a range of practice change strategies led by an external research team rather than internal staff. Insights into barriers and facilitators to practice change from research-led implementation efforts have limited external validity. Better insights are needed from appropriately-designed[151,152] observational studies of large-scale implementation efforts conducted by policy and practice entities, such as CDC, HRSA, and Medicare Quality Improvement Organizations in the United States, as well as practice-driven implementation efforts conducted by integrated health care delivery systems such as the VA, Kaiser Permanente, and national health systems outside the United States.

Impact versus Process and Mechanism Focus

Much of the research examining implementation in health care has pursued questions of implementation strategy effectiveness and has employed well-established experimental and quasi-experimental research approaches for assessing the effectiveness of various implementation strategies. Researchers are increasingly recognizing that effectiveness of implementation strategies is often highly dependent on contextual factors and features of the manner in which the implementation strategies are delivered and managed.[153] As a result, the main effect of an implementation strategy is often weak and dominated by multiple contextual and delivery factors, limiting the ability of standard evaluation approaches to estimate effectiveness of the core implementation program. Recent interest and efforts to define, conceptualize, and measure contextual factors[154,155] and to develop better analytical methods for examining their effects[156] is addressing the challenge of weak main effects, but the sample size requirements and other barriers to estimating implementation strategy effectiveness when main effects are small and the number of significant contextual factors is large will continue to challenge the field. In extreme (although arguably common) situations in which outcomes of implementation efforts are driven almost entirely by contextual factors and the manner in which implementation strategies are delivered, with essentially no detectable main effect of the implementation strategy, implementation research efforts must focus on developing insights into the processes and mechanisms of action, pursuing questions such as how, when, where, and why an implementation strategy is effective, rather than whether it is effective.[157-159] Research efforts to develop appropriate methods and approaches for these questions, including theory-based evaluation and realistic evaluation, and debates over the role and value of these approaches in quality improvement and implementation research, will help broaden the portfolio of such research and increase the likelihood that valid, useful insights and guidance will emerge and better contribute to ongoing efforts to reduce quality and implementation gaps and enhance the performance and beneficial impacts of health care delivery and health services.

SUMMARY

Implementation science in health care comprises over 30 years of rich and varied activity that has developed, refined, and applied implementation science concepts, theories, and research approaches. This body of activity has produced valuable empirical findings and has contributed to the continued development of the broader field of implementation science. This chapter describes key stages in the development and evolution of implementation science in health care. It discusses key settings, evidence-based practices, and implementation strategies studied by health care implementation researchers and examines key challenges and future directions in the field.

Continued growth in health care implementation science will require expanded attention to sustainment, scale-up, and spread of effective health care practices and attention to the study of routine, naturally-occurring implementation processes in addition to experimental evaluation of investigator-led implementation. Progress will also require increased attention to implementation processes and mechanisms of action, supplementing current interest in measuring the impacts and outcomes of implementation strategies. Implementation strategies are complex interventions characterized by high levels of heterogeneity and complexity, often showing weak main effects and strong contextual influences. Research approaches suitable for studying such complexity are needed to generate valuable guidance for decision-makers interested in effective implementation in their unique settings, requiring careful selection and adaptation of implementation strategies and active management of implementation settings and processes.

SUGGESTED READINGS AND WEBSITES

Readings

Eccles MP, Armstrong D, Baker R, Cleary K, Davies H, Davies S, Glasziou P, Ilott I, Kinmonth AL, Leng G, Logan S, Marteau T, Michie S, Rogers H, Rycroft-Malone J, Sibbald B. An implementation research agenda. *Implement Sci.* 2009;4:18.
Documents results of an expert panel convened to develop an agenda for research in implementation science in the UK.

Estabrooks CA, Derksen L, Winther C, Lavis JN, Scott SD, Wallin L, Profetto-McGrath J. The intellectual structure and substance of the knowledge utilization field: a longitudinal author co-citation analysis, 1945 to 2004. *Implement Sci.* 2008;3:49.
Describes the content and evolution of several subfields closely related to, and overlapping with, the field of implementation science. Provides a useful introduction and overview of these fields.

Glasgow RE, Vinson C, Chambers D, Khoury MJ, Kaplan RM, Hunter C. National Institutes of Health approaches to dissemination and implementation science: current and future directions. *Am J Public Health.* 2012;102(7):1274–1281.
Reviews research progress and successful examples of implementation science, discusses key issues, and offers recommendations for future progress.

Lobb R, Colditz GA. Implementation science and its application to population health. *Annu Rev Public Health.* 2013;34:235–251.
Discusses the history of implementation science and its progress, and discusses opportunities and strategies for continued research.

Remme JH, Adam T, Becerra-Posada F, D'Arcangues C, Devlin M, Gardner C, Ghaffar A, Hombach J, Kengeya JF, Mbewu A, Mbizvo MT, Mirza Z, Pang T, Ridley RG, Zicker F, Terry RF. Defining research to improve health systems. *PLoS Med.* 2010;7(11):e1001000.
Offers an overview and description of implementation research and related fields of research intended to improve health systems, health care, and public health from a global perspective.

Selected Websites and Tools
https://societyforimplementationresearchcollaboration.org/

The Society for Implementation Research Collaboration is a professional society supporting enhanced collaboration among researchers, policy and practice leaders to strengthen implementation research and its successful application. Key activities include a biennial conference, the SIRC Instrument Review Project, and activities to facilitate networking and mentorship.

https://cancercontrol.cancer.gov/IS/
The National Cancer Institute implementation science website offers an array of resources for implementation researchers, including links to funding opportunities, webinars, training programs, conferences, and others.

https://academyhealth.confex.com/academyhealth/2016di/meetingapp.cgi/ModuleSessionsByDay/0
The Annual NIH Conference on the Science of Dissemination and Implementation represents the largest annual gathering of dissemination and implementation researchers and research activity in the United States and internationally. The website for each year's conference offers copies of the agenda, participant list, presentations, and selected session summaries and videos.

https://www.queri.research.va.gov/default.cfm
The US Department of Veterans Affairs' Quality Enhancement Research Initiative (QUERI) website provides links to QUERI program activity and output, including implementation tools, QUERI webinars, and the QUERI Implementation Guide.

http://www.kusp.ualberta.ca/en/KnowledgeUtilizationColloquia.aspx
The Knowledge Utilization Colloquia Archive provides materials from the annual Knowledge Utilization Colloquium and periodic Knowledge Translation Forum. The Colloquium is a relatively small but intensive conference encompassing implementation research and practice in the fields of nursing research and broader domains of health and health care.

REFERENCES

1. Eisenberg JM. *Doctors' decisions and the cost of medical care: The reasons for doctors' practice patterns and ways to change them.* Ann Arbor, MI: Health Administration Press; 1986.
2. Smith WR. Evidence for the effectiveness of techniques to change physician behavior. Chest. 2000;118(2 Suppl):8S–17S.
3. Davis DA, Thomson MA, Oxman AD, Haynes RB. Evidence for the effectiveness of CME. A review of 50 randomized controlled trials. *JAMA.* 1992;268(9):1111–1117.
4. Davis DA, Thomson MA, Oxman AD, Haynes RB. Changing physician performance. A systematic review of the effect of continuing medical education strategies. *JAMA.* 1995;274(9):700–705.

5. McDonald CJ, Wilson GA, McCabe GP Jr. Physician response to computer reminders. *JAMA.* 1980;244(14):1579–1581.

6. Burack RC, Gimotty PA, George J, McBride S, Moncrease A, Simon MS, Dews P, Coombs J. How reminders given to patients and physicians affected pap smear use in a health maintenance organization: results of a randomized controlled trial. *Cancer.* 1998;82(12):2391–400.

7. Greer AL. The state of the art versus the state of the science. The diffusion of new medical technologies into practice. *Int J Technol Assess Health Care.* 1988;4(1):5–26.

8. Kanouse DE, Jacoby I. When does information change practitioners' behavior? *Int J Technol Assess Health Care.* 1988;4(1):27–33.

9. Eddy DM. Variations in physician practice: the role of uncertainty. *Health Aff (Millwood).* 1984;3(2):74–89.

10. Lomas J, Enkin M, Anderson GM, Hannah WJ, Vayda E, Singer J. Opinion leaders vs audit and feedback to implement practice guidelines. Delivery after previous cesarean section. *JAMA.* 1991;265(17):2202–2207.

11. Soumerai SB, Avorn J. Principles of educational outreach ("academic detailing") to improve clinical decision making. *JAMA.* 1990;263(4):549–556.

12. Mittman BS, Tonesk X, Jacobson PD. Implementing clinical practice guidelines: social influence strategies and practitioner behavior change. *QRB Qual Rev Bull.* 1992;18(12):413–422.

13. McIntosh KA, Maxwell DJ, Pulver LK, Horn F, Robertson MB, Kaye KI, Peterson GM, Dollman WB, Wai A, Tett SE. A quality improvement initiative to improve adherence to national guidelines for empiric management of community-acquired pneumonia in emergency departments. *Int J Qual Health Care.* 2011;23(2):142–150.

14. Ornstein S, Nemeth LS, Jenkins RG, Nietert PJ. Colorectal cancer screening in primary care: translating research into practice. *Med Care.* 2010t;48(10):900–906.

15. Huis A, Schoonhoven L, Grol R, Donders R, Hulscher M, van Achterberg T. Impact of a team and leaders-directed strategy to improve nurses' adherence to hand hygiene guidelines: a cluster randomised trial. *Int J Nurs Studies.* 2013;50(4):464–474.

16. Johnson MJ, May CR. Promoting professional behaviour change in healthcare: what interventions work, and why? A theory-led overview of systematic reviews. *BMJ Open.* 2015;5(9):e008592.

17. Mostofian F, Ruban C, Simunovic N, Bhandari M. Changing physician behavior: what works?. *Am J Manag Care.* 2015;21(1):75–84.

18. Wennberg J, Gittelsohn. Small area variations in health care delivery. *Science.* 1973;182(117):1102–1108.

19. Chassin MR, Kosecoff J, Park RE, Winslow CM, Kahn KL, Merrick NJ, Keesey J, Fink A, Solomon DH, Brook RH. Does inappropriate use explain geographic variations in the use of health care services? A study of three procedures. *JAMA.* 1987;258(18):2533–2537.

20. Donabedian A. Twenty years of research on the quality of medical care: 1964-1984. *Eval Health Prof.* 1985;8(3):243–265.

21. Donabedian A. The quality of care. How can it be assessed? *JAMA.* 1988;260(12):1743–1748. Review.

22. Dubois RW, Brook RH, Rogers WH. Adjusted hospital death rates: a potential screen for quality of medical care. *Am J Public Health.* 1987;77(9):1162–1166.

23. Schuster MA, McGlynn EA, Brook RH. How good is the quality of health care in the United States? *Milbank Q.* 1998;76(4):517–563, 509.

24. Institute of Medicine. *Crossing the quality chasm: A new health system for the 21st century.* Washington DC: National Academy Press; 2001.

25. McGlynn EA, Asch SM, Adams J, Keesey J, Hicks J, DeCristofaro A, Kerr EA. The quality of health care delivered to adults in the United States. *N Engl J Med.* 2003;348(26):2635–2645.

26. Hussey PS, Anderson GF, Osborn R, Feek C, McLaughlin V, Millar J, Epstein A. How does the quality of care compare in five countries? *Health Aff (Millwood).* 2004;23(3):89–99.

27. Levine DM, Linder JA, Landon BE. The quality of outpatient care delivered to adults in the United States, 2002 to 2013. *JAMA Intern Med.* 2016;176(12):1778–1790.

28. Brook RH, Chassin MR, Fink A, Solomon DH, Kosecoff J, Park RE. A method for the detailed assessment of the appropriateness of medical technologies. *Int J Technol Assess Health Care.* 1986;2(1):53–63.

29. Woolf SH. Practice guidelines: a new reality in medicine. I. Recent developments. *Arch Intern Med.* 1990;150(9):1811–1818.

30. Field MJ, Lohr KN. *Clinical practice guidelines: Directions for a new program.* Washington DC: National Academies Press; 1990.

31. Kelly JT, Swartwout JE. Development of practice parameters by physician organizations. *QRB Qual Rev Bull.* 1990;16(2):54–57.

32. Sackett DL, Rosenberg WM, Gray JA, Haynes RB, Richardson WS. Evidence based medicine: what it is and what it isn't. *BMJ.* 1996;312(7023):71–72.

33. Lomas J. Words without action? The production, dissemination, and impact of consensus recommendations. *Annu Rev Public Health.* 1991;12:41–65.

34. Grimshaw JM, Thomas RE, MacLennan G, Fraser C, Ramsay CR, Vale L, Whitty P, Eccles MP, Matowe L, Shirran L, Wensing M, Dijkstra R, Donaldson

C. Effectiveness and efficiency of guideline dissemination and implementation strategies. *Health Technol Assess.* 2004;8(6):iii-iv, 1–72.

35. Lineker SC, Husted JA. Educational interventions for implementation of arthritis clinical practice guidelines in primary care: effects on health professional behavior. *J Rheumatol.* 2010;37(8):1562–1569.

36. Gagliardi AR, Alhabib S. Trends in guideline implementation: a scoping systematic review. *Implement Sci.* 2015;10(1):54.

37. Naik AD, Petersen LA. The neglected purpose of comparative-effectiveness research. *N Engl J Med.* 2009;360(19):1929–1931.

38. Bonham AC, Solomon MZ. Moving comparative effectiveness research into practice: implementation science and the role of academic medicine. *Health Aff (Millwood).* 2010t;29(10):1901–1905.

39. Berwick DM. Continuous improvement as an ideal in health care. *N Engl J Med.* 1989;320(1):53–56.

40. Kritchevsky SB, Simmons BP. Continuous quality improvement. Concepts and applications for physician care. *JAMA.* 1991;266(13):1817–1823.

41. Ash J. Organizational factors that influence information technology diffusion in academic health sciences centers. *J Am Med Inform Assoc.* 1997;4(2):102–111.

42. Rosenheck R. Stages in the implementation of innovative clinical programs in complex organizations. *J Nerv Ment Dis.* 2001;189(12):812–821

43. Sheaff R, Pilgrim D. Can learning organizations survive in the newer NHS? *Implement Sci.* 2006;1:27.

44. Weiner BJ. A theory of organizational readiness for change. *Implement Sci.* 2009;4:67.

45. Simpson DD, Flynn PM. Moving innovations into treatment: a stage-based approach to program change. *J Subst Abuse Treat.* 2007;33(2):111–120.

46. Lukas CV, Holmes SK, Cohen AB, Restuccia J, Cramer IE, Shwartz M, Charns MP. Transformational change in health care systems: an organizational model. *Health Care Manage Rev.* 2007;32(4):309–320.

47. Michie S, Johnston M, Abraham C, Lawton R, Parker D, Walker A; "Psychological Theory" Group. Making psychological theory useful for implementing evidence based practice: a consensus approach. *Qual Saf Health Care.* 2005;14(1):26–33.

48. Godin G, Belanger-Gravel A, Eccles M, Grimshaw J. Healthcare professionals' intentions and behaviours: a systematic review of studies based on social cognitive theories. *Implement Sci.* 2008;3:36

49. Gardner B, Whittington C, McAteer J, Eccles MP, Michie S. Using theory to synthesise evidence from behaviour change interventions: the example of audit and feedback. *Soc Sci Med.* 2010;70(10):1618–1625.

50. Rogers EM. *Diffusion of innovations.* 5th ed. 2003. New York: Free Press.

51. Greenhalgh T, Robert G, Macfarlane F, Bate P, Kyriakidou O. Diffusion of innovations in service organizations: systematic review and recommendations. *Milbank Q.* 2004;82(4):581–629.

52. Glasgow RE, Vogt TM, Boles SM. Evaluating the public health impact of health promotion interventions: the RE-AIM framework. *Am J Public Health.* 199989(9):1322–1327.

53. Tabak RG, Khoong EC, Chambers DA, Brownson RC. Bridging research and practice: models for dissemination and implementation research. *Am J Prev Med.* 2012;43(3):337–350.

54. Nilsen P. Making sense of implementation theories, models and frameworks. *Implement Sci.* 2015;10:53.

55. Moullin JC, Sabater-Hernández D, Fernandez-Llimos F, Benrimoj SI. A systematic review of implementation frameworks of innovations in healthcare and resulting generic implementation framework. *Health Res Policy Syst.* 2015;13:16.

56. Milat AJ, Li B. Narrative review of frameworks for translating research evidence into policy and practice. *Public Health Res Pract.* 2017;27(1):pii: 2711704.

57. Harvey G, Kitson A. PARIHS revisited: from heuristic to integrated framework for the successful implementation of knowledge into practice. *Implement Sci.* 2016;11:33.

58. Stetler CB, Damschroder LJ, Helfrich CD, Hagedorn HJ. A guide for applying a revised version of the PARIHS framework for implementation. *Implement Sci.* 2011;6:99.

59. Michie S, Johnston M, Abraham C, Lawton R, Parker D, Walker A. Making psychological theory useful for implementing evidence based practice: a consensus approach. *Qual Safe Health Care.* 2005;14(1):26–33.

60. Mosavianpour M, Sarmast HH, Kissoon N, Collet JP. Theoretical domains framework to assess barriers to change for planning health care quality interventions: a systematic literature review. *J Multidiscip Healthc.* 2016;9:303.

61. Damschroder LJ, Aron DC, Keith RE, Kirsh SR, Alexander JA, Lowery JC. Fostering implementation of health services research findings into practice: a consolidated framework for advancing implementation science. *Implement Sci.* 2009;4(1):50.

62. Kirk MA, Kelley C, Yankey N, Birken SA, Abadie B, Damschroder L. A systematic review of the use of

the Consolidated Framework for Implementation Research. *Implement Sci.* 2016;11:72.

63. Birken SA, Powell BJ, Presseau J, Kirk MA, Lorencatto F, Gould NJ, Shea CM,Weiner BJ, Francis JJ, Yu Y, Haines E, Damschroder LJ. Combined use of the Consolidated Framework for Implementation Research (CFIR) and the Theoretical Domains Framework (TDF): a systematic review. *Implement Sci.* 201712(1):2.

64. May CR, Mair F, Finch T, MacFarlane A, Dowrick C, Treweek S, Rapley T, Ballini L, Ong BN, Rogers A, Murray E. Development of a theory of implementation and integration: Normalization Process Theory. *Implement Sci.* 2009;4(1):29.

65. McEvoy R, Ballini L, Maltoni S, O'Donnell CA, Mair FS, MacFarlane A. A qualitative systematic review of studies using the normalization process theory to research implementation processes. *Implement Sci.* 2014;9(1):2.

66. May C. Towards a general theory of implementation. *Implement Sci.* 2013;8(1):18.

67. Stetler CB. Research utilization: defining the concept. *Image J Nurs Sch.* 1985;17(2):40–44.

68. Champion VL, Leach A. Variables related to research utilization in nursing: an empirical investigation. *J Adv Nurs.* 1989;14(9):705–710.

69. Brown BS. Reducing impediments to technology transfer in drug abuse programming. *NIDA Res Monogr.* 1995;155:169–185.

70. Remme JH, Adam T, Becerra-Posada F, D'Arcangues C, Devlin M, Gardner C, Ghaffar A, Hombach J, Kengeya JF, Mbewu A, Mbizvo MT, Mirza Z, Pang T, Ridley RG, Zicker F, Terry RF. Defining research to improve health systems. *PLoS Med.* 2010;7(11):e1001000.

71. Sung NS, Crowley WF Jr, Genel M, Salber P, Sandy L, Sherwood LM, Johnson SB, Catanese V, Tilson H, Getz K, Larson EL, Scheinberg D, Reece EA, Slavkin H, Dobs A, Grebb J, Martinez RA, Korn A, Rimoin D. Central challenges facing the national clinical research enterprise. *JAMA.* 2003;289(10):1278–1287

72. Crowley WF Jr, Sherwood L, Salber P, Scheinberg D, Slavkin H, Tilson H, Reece EA, Catanese V, Johnson SB, Dobs A, Genel M, Korn A, Reame N, Bonow R, Grebb J, Rimoin D. Clinical research in the United States at a crossroads: proposal for a novel public-private partnership to establish a national clinical research enterprise. *JAMA.* 2004;291(9):1120–1126.

73. Zerhouni E. Medicine. The NIH Roadmap. *Science.* 2003;302(5642):63–72.

74. Zerhouni EA. Translational and clinical science—time for a new vision. *N Engl J Med.* 2005;353(15):1621–1623.

75. Djulbegovic B. A framework to bridge the gaps between evidence-based medicine, health outcomes, and improvement and implementation science. *J Oncol Pract.* 2014;10(3):200–202.

76. Brunner JW, Sankaré IC, Kahn KL. Interdisciplinary priorities for dissemination, implementation, and improvement science: frameworks, mechanics, and measures. Clin Transl Sci. 2015;8(6):820–823.

77. Yu J, Colditz GA. Defining issues in the study of process or quality improvement versus implementation science. *Ann Thorac Surg.* 2016;102(6):1774–1775.

78. Granger BB, Pokorney SD, Taft C. Blending quality improvement and research methods for implementation science, Part III: Analysis of the effectiveness of implementation. *AACN Adv Crit Care.* 2016;27(1):103–110.

79. Cochrane Effective Practice and Organisation of Care Group. http://epoc.cochrane.org. Updated December 21, 2010.

80. Evidence-based Practice Centers. Agency for Healthcare Research and Quality. http://www.ahrq.gov/clinic/epc. Updated October 2010.

81. Powell BJ, Waltz TJ, Chinman MJ, Damschroder LJ, Smith JL, Matthieu MM, Proctor EK, Kirchner JE. A refined compilation of implementation strategies: results from the Expert Recommendations for Implementing Change (ERIC) project. *Implement Sci.* 2015;10(1):21.

82. Powell BJ, Beidas RS, Lewis CC, Aarons GA, McMillen JC, Proctor EK, Mandell DS. Methods to improve the selection and tailoring of implementation strategies. J Behav Health Serv Res. 2015;21:1–8.

83. Chan WV, Pearson TA, Bennett GC, Cushman WC, Gaziano TA, Gorman PN, Handler J, Krumholz HM, Kushner RF, MacKenzie TD, Sacco RL. ACC/AHA Special Report: Clinical Practice Guideline Implementation Strategies: A Summary of Systematic Reviews by the NHLBI Implementation Science Work Group: A Report of the American College of Cardiology/American Heart Association Task Force on Clinical Practice Guidelines. *J Am Coll Cardiol.* 2017;69(8):1076–1092.

84. Cavanaugh JJ, Jones CD, Embree G, Tsai K, Miller T, Shilliday BB, McGuirt B, Roche R, Pignone M, DeWalt DA, Ratner S. Implementation science workshop: primary care-based multidisciplinary readmission prevention program. *J Gen Intern Med.* 2014;29(5):798.

85. Powell BJ, Beidas RS, Lewis CC, Aarons GA, McMillen JC, Proctor EK, Mandell DS. Methods to improve the selection and tailoring of implementation strategies. *J Behav Health Serv Res.* 2015;21:1–8.

86. Sales A, Smith J, Curran G, Kochevar L. Models, strategies, and tools. Theory in implementing evidence-based findings into health care practice. *J Gen Intern Med*. 2006;21 Suppl 2:S43–S49.

87. Grol RP, Bosch MC, Hulscher ME, Eccles MP, Wensing M. Planning and studying improvement in patient care: the use of theoretical perspectives. *Milbank Q*. 2007;85(1):93–138.

88. Improved Clinical Effectiveness through Behavioural Research Group (ICEBeRG). Designing theoretically-informed implementation interventions. *Implement Sci*. 2006;1:4.

89. Proctor EK, Powell BJ, McMillen JC. Implementation strategies: recommendations for specifying and reporting. *Implement Sci*. 2013;8(1):139.

90. Harvey G, Kitson A. Translating evidence into healthcare policy and practice: Single versus multi-faceted implementation strategies—is there a simple answer to a complex question? *Int J Health Policy Manag*. 2015;4(3):123–126.

91. Leeman J, Calancie L, Kegler MC, Escoffery CT, Herrmann AK, Thatcher E, Hartman MA, Fernandez ME. Developing theory to guide building practitioners' capacity to implement evidence-based interventions. *J Health Educ Behav*. 2017;44(1):59–69.

92. Mechanic D. Improving the quality of health care in the United States of America: the need for a multi-level approach. J Health Serv Res Policy. 2002;7(1_suppl):35–39.

93. Chaudoir SR, Dugan AG, Barr CH. Measuring factors affecting implementation of health innovations: a systematic review of structural, organizational, provider, patient, and innovation level measures. *Implement Sci*. 2013;8(1):22.

94. Powell BJ, Beidas RS, Lewis CC, Aarons GA, McMillen JC, Proctor EK, Mandell DS. Methods to improve the selection and tailoring of implementation strategies. *J Behav Health Serv Res*. 2015;21:1–8.

95. Stevens BJ, Yamada J, Promislow S, Stinson J, Harrison D, Victor JC. Implementation of multidimensional knowledge translation strategies to improve procedural pain in hospitalized children. *Implement Sci*. 2014;9(1):120.

96. Wensing M, Huntink E, van Lieshout J, Godycki-Cwirko M, Kowalczyk A, Jäger C, Steinhäuser J, Aakhus E, Flottorp S, Eccles M, Baker R. Tailored implementation of evidence-based practice for patients with chronic diseases. *PLoS One*. 2014;9(7):e101981.

97. Aarons GA, Green AE, Palinkas LA, Self-Brown S, Whitaker DJ, Lutzker JR, Silovsky JF, Hecht DB, Chaffin MJ. Dynamic adaptation process to implement an evidence-based child maltreatment intervention. *Implement Sci*. 2012;7(1):32.

98. Chambers DA, Norton WE. The adaptome: advancing the science of intervention adaptation. *Am J Prev Med*. 2016;51(4):S124–S131.

99. Hawe P, Shiell A, Riley T. Complex interventions: how" out of control" can a randomised controlled trial be?. *BMJ*. 2004;328(7455):1561.

100. Hawe P. Lessons from complex interventions to improve health. *Annu Rev Public Health*. 2015;36:307–323.

101. Craig LE, Churilov L, Olenko L, Cadilhac DA, Grimley R, Dale S, Martinez-Garduno C, McInnes E, Considine J, Grimshaw JM, Middleton S. Testing a systematic approach to identify and prioritise barriers to successful implementation of a complex healthcare intervention. *BMC Med Res Methodol*. 2017;17(1):24.

102. Cabana MD, Rand CS, Powe NR, Wu AW, Wilson MH, Abboud PA, Rubin HR. Why don't physicians follow clinical practice guidelines? A framework for improvement. *JAMA*. 1999;282(15):1458–1465.

103. Clarity C, Gourley G, Lyles C, Ackerman S, Handley MA, Schillinger D, Sarkar U, Conigliaro J. Implementation Science Workshop: Barriers and facilitators to increasing mammography screening rates in California's public hospitals. *J Gen Intern Med*. 2017;32(6):697–705.

104. Lingner H, Burger B, Kardos P, Criée CP, Worth H, Hummers-Pradier E. What patients really think about asthma guidelines: barriers to guideline implementation from the patients' perspective. *BMC Pulm Med*. 2017;17(1):13.

105. Pickles K, Carter SM, Rychetnik L, McCaffery K, Entwistle VA. General practitioners' experiences of, and responses to, uncertainty in prostate cancer screening: insights from a qualitative study. *PLoS One*. 2016;11(4):e0153299.

106. Ross L. The intuitive psychologist and his shortcomings: distortions in the attribution process. *Adv Exp Soc Psychol*. 1977;10:173–220.

107. Reach G. Clinical inertia, uncertainty and individualized guidelines. *Diabetes Metab*. 2014;40(4):241–245.

108. Phillips LS, Branch WT, Cook CB, Doyle JP, El-Kebbi IM, Gallina DL, Miller CD, Ziemer DC, Barnes CS. Clinical inertia. *Ann Intern Med*. 2001;135(9):825–834.

109. Altman DG. The scandal of poor medical research. *BMJ*. 1994;308(6924):283–284.

110. Ioannidis JP. Why most published research findings are false. *PLoS Med*. 2005;2(8):e124.

111. Tunis SR, Hayward RS, Wilson MC, Rubin HR, Bass EB, Johnston M, Steinberg EP. Internists' attitudes about clinical practice guidelines. *Ann Intern Med*. 1994;120(11):956–963.

112. Hayward RS, Guyatt GH, Moore KA, McKibbon KA, Carter AO. Canadian physicians' attitudes about and preferences regarding clinical practice guidelines. *CMAJ.* 1997;156(12):1715–923.

113. Mintzberg H. Organizational design, fashion or fit? *Harv Bus Rev.* 1981;59(1), 103–116.

114. Ferlie, E.B., Shortell, S.M. Improving the quality of health care in the United Kingdom and the United States: a framework for change. *Milbank Q.* 2001;79(2):281–315

115. Mechanic D. Improving the quality of health care in the United States of America: the need for a multi-level approach. *J Health Serv Res Policy.* 2002;7 Suppl 1:S35–S39.

116. Berwick DM. A user's manual for the IOM's "Quality Chasm" report. *Health Aff (Millwood).* 2002;21(3):80–90.

117. Aligning Forces for Quality. Robert Wood Johnson Foundation. Available at: www.forces4quality.org.

118. Williams NJ. Multilevel mechanisms of implementation strategies in mental health: integrating theory, research, and practice. *Adm Policy Ment Health.* 2016;43(5):783–798.

119. Rabin BA, Nehl E, Elliott T, Deshpande AD, Brownson RC, Glanz K. Individual and setting level predictors of the implementation of a skin cancer prevention program: a multilevel analysis. *Implement Sci.* 2010;5:40.

120. Oishi SM, Marshall N, Hamilton AB, Yano EM, Lerner B, Scheuner MT. Assessing multilevel determinants of adoption and implementation of genomic medicine: an organizational mixed-methods approach. *Genet Med.* 2015;17(11):919–926.

121. Grol R, Wensing M, Eccles M, Davis D. *Improving patient care: the implementation of change in health care.* 2nd ed. Oxford, UK: Wiley; 2013.

122. Straus SE, Tetroe J, Graham ID. *Knowledge translation in health care: moving from evidence to practice.* 2nd ed. Oxford, UK: Wiley-Blackwell, 2013.

123. Young AS, Sullivan G, Burnam MA, Brook RH. Measuring the quality of outpatient treatment for schizophrenia. *Arch Gen Psychiatry.* 1998;55(7):611–617.

124. Lehman AF. Quality of care in mental health: the case of schizophrenia. *Health Aff.* 1999;18:52–65.

125. Young AS, Sullivan G, Duan N. Patient, provider, and treatment factors associated with poor-quality care for schizophrenia. *Ment Health Serv Res.* 1999;1(4):201–211.

126. Young AS, Niv N, Cohen AN, Kessler C, McNagny K. The appropriateness of routine medication treatment for schizophrenia. *Schizophr Bull.* 2010;36(4):732–739.

127. Rost K, Hsieh YP, Xu S, Menachemi N, Young AS. Potential disparities in the management of schizophrenia in the United States. *Psychiatr Serv.* 2011;62(6):613–618.

128. Young AS. Evaluating and improving the appropriateness of treatment for schizophrenia. *Harv Rev Psychiatry.* 1999;7(2):114–118.

129. Henderson C, Jackson C, Slade M, Young AS, Strauss JL. How should we implement psychiatric advance directives? Views of consumers, caregivers, mental health providers and researchers. *Adm Policy Ment Health.* 2010;37(6):447–458.

130. Young AS, Niv N, Chinman M, Dixon L, Eisen SV, Fischer EP, Smith J, Valenstein M, Marder SR, Owen RR. Routine outcomes monitoring to support improving care for schizophrenia: report from the VA Mental Health QUERI. *Community Ment Health J.* 2011;47(2):123–135.

131. Cradock J, Young AS, Sullivan G. The accuracy of medical record documentation in schizophrenia. *J Behav Health Serv Res.* 2001;28(4):456–465.

132. Chinman M, Young AS, Rowe M, Forquer S, Knight E, Miller A. An instrument to assess competencies of providers treating severe mental illness. *Ment Health Serv Res.* 2003;5(2):97–108.

133. Chinman M, Hassell J, Magnabosco J, Nowlin-Finch N, Marusak S, Young AS. The feasibility of computerized patient self-assessment at mental health clinics. *Adm Policy Ment Health.* 2007;34(4):401–409.

134. Young AS, Mintz J, Cohen AN, Chinman MJ. A network-based system to improve care for schizophrenia: the Medical Informatics Network Tool (MINT). *J Am Med Inform Assoc.* 2004;11(5):358–367.

135. Young AS, Chinman M, Forquer SL, Knight EL, Vogel H, Miller A, Rowe M, Mintz J. Use of a consumer-led intervention to improve provider competencies. *Psychiatr Serv.* 2005;56(8):967–975.

136. Cohen AN, Glynn SM, Hamilton AB, Young AS. Implementation of a family intervention for individuals with schizophrenia. *J Gen Intern Med.* 2010;25 Suppl 1:32–37.

137. Niv N, Cohen AN, Hamilton A, Reist C, Young AS. Effectiveness of a psychosocial weight management program for individuals with schizophrenia. *J Behav Health Serv Res.* 2014;41(3):370–380.

138. Brown AH, Cohen AN, Chinman MJ, Kessler C, Young AS. EQUIP: implementing chronic care principles and applying formative evaluation methods to improve care for schizophrenia: QUERI Series. *Implement Sci.* 2008;3:9.

139. Hamilton AB, Cohen AN, Young AS. Organizational readiness in specialty mental health care. *J Gen Intern Med.* 2010;25 Suppl 1:27–31.

140. Hamilton AB, Cohen AN, Glover DL, Whelan F, Chemerinski E, McNagny KP, Mullins D, Reist C, Schubert M, Young AS. Implementation of evidence-based employment services in specialty mental health. *Health Serv Res.* 2013;48(6 Pt 2):2224–2244.

141. Cohen AN, Chinman MJ, Hamilton AB, Whelan F, Young AS. Using patient-facing kiosks to support quality improvement at mental health clinics. *Med Care.* 2013;51(3 Suppl 1):S13–S20.

142. Young AS, Cohen AN, Goldberg R, Hellemann G, Kreyenbuhl J, Niv N, Nowlin-Finch N, Oberman R, Whelan F. Improving weight in people with serious mental illness: the effectiveness of computerized services with peer coaches. *J Gen Intern Med.* 2017;32(Suppl 1):48–55.

143. Roberts MC, Kennedy AE, Chambers DA, Khoury MJ. The current state of implementation science in genomic medicine: opportunities for improvement. *Genet Med.* 2017 Jan 12. [Epub ahead of print]

144. Eccles MP, Armstrong D, Baker R, Cleary K, Davies H, Davies S, Glasziou P, Ilott I, Kinmonth AL, Leng G, Logan S, Marteau T, Michie S, Rogers H, Rycroft-Malone J, Sibbald B. An implementation research agenda. *Implement Sci.* 2009;4:18.

145. Argote L, Epple D. Learning curves in manufacturing. *Science.* 1990;247(4945):920–924.

146. Huber G. Organizational learning. *Organ Sci.* 1991;2(1):88–115.

147. May CR, Mair F, Finch T, MacFarlane A, Dowrick C, Treweek S, Rapley T, Ballini L, Ong BN, Rogers A, Murray E. Development of a theory of implementation and integration: Normalization Process Theory. *Implement Sci.* 2009;4(1):29.

148. Wiltsey Stirman S, Kimberly J, Cook N, Calloway A, Castro F, Charns M. The sustainability of new programs and innovations: a review of the empirical literature and recommendations for future research. *Implement Sci.* 2012;7:17.

149. Norton WE, McCannon CJ, Schall MW, Mittman BS. A stakeholder-driven agenda for advancing the science and practice of scale-up and spread in health. *Implement Sci.* 2012;7:118.

150. Campbell NC, Murray E, Darbyshire J, Emery J, Farmer A, Griffiths F, Guthrie B, Lester H, Wilson P, Kinmonth AL. Designing and evaluating complex interventions to improve health care. *BMJ.* 2007;334(7591):455–459.

151. Eccles M, Grimshaw J, Campbell M, Ramsay C. Research designs for studies evaluating the effectiveness of change and improvement strategies. *Qual Saf Health Care.* 2003;12(1):47–52.

152. Speroff T, O'Connor GT. Study designs for PDSA quality improvement research. *Qual Manag Health Care.* 2004;13(1):17–32.

153. Ovretveit JC, Shekelle PG, Dy SM, McDonald KM, Hempel S, Pronovost P, Rubenstein L, Taylor SL, Foy R, Wachter RM. How does context affect interventions to improve patient safety? An assessment of evidence from studies of five patient safety practices and proposals for research. *BMJ Qual Saf.* 2011;20(7):604–610.

154. Kaplan HC, Brady PW, Dritz MC, Hooper DK, Linam WM, Froehle CM, Margolis P. The influence of context on quality improvement success in health care: a systematic review of the literature. *Milbank Q.* 2010;88(4):500–559.

155. Taylor SL, Dy S, Foy R, Hempel S, McDonald KM, Ovretveit J, Pronovost PJ, Rubenstein LV, Wachter RM, Shekelle PG. What context features might be important determinants of the effectiveness of patient safety practice interventions? *BMJ Qual Saf.* 2011;20(7):611–617.

156. Shekelle PG, Pronovost PJ, Wachter RM, Taylor SL, Dy SM, Foy R, Hempel S, McDonald KM, Ovretveit J, Rubenstein LV, Adams AS, Angood PB, Bates DW, Bickman L, Carayon P, Donaldson L, Duan N, Farley DO, Greenhalgh T, Haughom J, Lake ET, Lilford R, Lohr KN, Meyer GS, Miller MR, Neuhauser DV, Ryan G, Saint S, Shojania KG, Shortell SM, Stevens DP, Walshe K. Advancing the science of patient safety. *Ann Intern Med.* 2011;154(10):693–696.

157. Walshe K, Freeman T. Effectiveness of quality improvement: learning from evaluations. *Qual Saf Health Care.* 2002;11(1):85–87.

158. Walshe K. Understanding what works--and why--in quality improvement: the need for theory-driven evaluation. *Int J Qual Health Care.* 2007;19(2):57–59.

159. Berwick DM. The stories beneath. *Med Care.* 2007;45(12):1123–1125.

160. Glasgow RE, Lichtenstein E, Marcus AC. Why don't we see more translation of health promotion research to practice? Rethinking the efficacy-to-effectiveness transition. *Am J Public Health.* 2003;93(8):1261–1267.

161. Green LW, Glasgow RE. Evaluating the relevance, generalization, and applicability of research: issues in external validation and translation methodology. *Eval Health Prof.* 2006;29(1):126–153.

24

Health Dissemination and Implementation Within Schools

REBEKKA M. LEE AND STEVEN L. GORTMAKER

INTRODUCTION

Schools hold great promise for the promotion of health. In much of the world, individuals spend the majority of their formative years within school settings. Thus, schools are ideal places to initiate healthy behaviors early on to promote lifelong health. A healthy school environment can promote norms about foods and beverages children consume, physical activity participation, and appropriate social behavior. These healthy environments can be created by local school practices or mandated by top-down policies. In addition to providing healthy environmental defaults and cues, schools are optimal settings for disseminating health education messages discouraging risk-taking behaviors (e.g. smoking, drinking, drug use, or unprotected sex) and can be an important place for delivering basic preventive services (e.g., vaccines, vision screening, mental health assessments). Elementary, middle, and high schools as well as preschools and afterschool programs are fundamental settings for establishing healthy habits early on for optimal prevention of childhood health risks as well as chronic disease later in life. With sound implementation, schools have the potential for tremendous reach and impact. Careful implementation and dissemination research is necessary to ensure that the full promise of schools for health promotion is achieved, considering the important public health objectives of improving population health and simultaneously narrowing health disparities.

Education, in and of itself, has been targeted as a key factor for future health and poverty reduction across the globe. In fact, the United Nations named universal primary education as one of their eight Millennium Development Goals, achieving an increase in enrolment from 83% in 2000 to 91% in 2015.[1] Furthermore, they recently adopted the 2030 Agenda for Sustainable Development, which includes "inclusive and equitable quality education and lifelong learning opportunities for all."[2] The World Health Organization has identified the school setting as particularly important for promoting intersectoral action to address child and adolescent health.[3] Their Health Promoting Schools Framework—a holistic approach that includes health education curriculum, school environments that promotes health, and school engagement with communities and families—has been taken up by countries throughout the world over the past three decades. These efforts have demonstrated modest effects, with the potential for wide population reach in improving health outcomes such as physical activity, smoking, bullying, and body mass index.[4]

In the United States, education has been considered a public good since it became mandatory by all states at the close of World War I. On the other hand, while deliberate health promotion by the state has been encouraged since the 1800s, countries today vary dramatically in their role as provider of health services and preventive programs to their citizens.[5,6] By weaving health promotion, above and beyond the delivery of health services, into the public school agenda, there is the opportunity to reach the whole population, including underserved groups (e.g., rural, low-income, people of color), with health messages and services that other settings may miss. Moreover, the amount of time that children spend in school is incomparable to other settings such as primary care. Consider, for instance, the difference between the 30 minutes a doctor might spend with a child at an annual well visit exam compared with the roughly 75,600 minutes (7 hours/day over 180 days) children spend within school walls each year. Thus, promoting health within schools has the potential to reinforce the messages of health professionals in a sustained manner, changing norms and everyday behaviors with accumulating effects across the early years of life (Table 24.1). However, there is a flip side to this potential. Roughly half of funding for schools in the United States comes from local sources.[7] This translates into differences in public school resources and quality. Without careful planning and attention to issues of implementation and dissemination, situating health promotion efforts in schools could actually exacerbate health disparities because communities with fewer resources may not be able to afford to implement health interventions. In this vein, increased attention should be paid toward selecting low-cost solutions for schools and families that will be most acceptable and feasible for dissemination across schools with varying resources.

There is still much to be learned about what interventions (e.g., policies, practices, services, and curricula) are best to implement and disseminate within schools, as well as by whom, when, and how. This chapter seeks to review the school-based dissemination and implementation evidence base and discuss the specific challenges that schools face in their quest to promote health.

EVIDENCE BASE AND THEORY

Current State of School-Based Health Intervention Evidence

Identifying evidence-based interventions is a crucial first step for accelerating implementation and dissemination of programs most likely to impact population health. The Centers for Disease Control and Prevention (CDC) has set forth guidance for how schools can best create healthy school environments and integrate health promotion services, education and programs for

TABLE 24.1 TYPOLOGY OF HEALTH INTERVENTION IMPLEMENTED AND DISSEMINATED WITHIN SCHOOLS

Type	Definition	Examples
Health promoting policies	Regulations implemented at the national, state, district, or school level intended to promote children's health within schools	• District wellness policies • State law mandating physical activity time • Healthy Hunger Free Kids Act: National mandate for improved school meals, access to free potable drinking water, and Smart Snacks nutrition standards for competitive foods [8]
Environmental change strategies	School practices that are intended to create healthy environments for children	• Active recess • Enhanced physical education • Classroom-based social skills development (e.g., Responsive Classroom) • Safe Routes to School
Health education messages	Health lessons and messages designed to lay the foundation for lifelong health	• Physical education • Sexual health education • Classroom-based nutrition and physical activity curricula (e.g., Planet Health) • Substance use prevention lessons • Violence prevention programs • Healthy messaging directed toward students, staff and parents on posters, newsletters etc.
Health programs & services	Delivery of prevention and clinical care within the school setting	• School food service • Afterschool sports • Immunization • Vision, healthy, body mass index, and scoliosis screening • Mental health assessment & counseling • Contraceptive and pregnancy care

children.[9] It also hosts the Guide to Community Preventive Services online resource, which publishes systematic reviews and recommendations for public use along with supporting materials and considerations for implementation.[10] The National Institutes of Health has funded web initiatives such as the Research-Tested Intervention Programs (RTIPs) that scores the evidence base and ease of implementation of cancer prevention programs with tailored searches for school-based programs.[11] For identifying evidence-based programs that target mental health, substance use, sexual health, and violence, the Blueprints for Healthy Youth Development web resource allows users to search for ratings of school-based program, and reviews the benefits and costs of implementation.[12]

Review of these resources and the peer-reviewed literature points to evidence for a wide range of school-based health interventions. These include programs designed to address mental and emotional health, substance use, healthy eating and nutrition, and sexual health.[13–25] Environmental intervention in schools such as Safe Routes to School[26] and cafeteria-based behavioral economics approaches[27] have shown some effectiveness in promoting physical activity and nutrition among children. School-based health policies have also shown evidence for effectiveness.[28–32] Finally, schools are an important setting for delivering prevention and clinical services such as vaccines,[33,34] asthma care management,[35,36] mental health counseling,[37,38] and contraceptive and pregnancy care.[39,40] While there is much research on the efficacy of specific school-based health interventions and numerous web-based resources for identifying evidence-based intervention, too few interventions have been replicated or taken to scale.

Implementation and Dissemination Quality Gap

A large gap remains between the programs, policies, curricula, and services that are suggested as best practices and those that are currently being implemented within schools. In 2006, the School Health Programs and Policies Study (SHPPS) estimated the following: only 61% of schools required health education in at least one specific grade; 78% of schools required students to take some physical education, but less than 10% required daily physical education across the school year; 86% of schools had a school nurse, yet only 14% of schools provided immunizations

and less than 5% of high schools made condoms available to students.[41–43] Recent data indicate that "junk foods" and beverages are still available in many schools.[44]

The broad adoption of programs like DARE (Drug Abuse Resistance Education) over more effective prevention programs is an illustration of how the dissemination and implementation gap can work in reverse. Although this program showed little to no efficacy for preventing substance use behavior, it was the only curriculum endorsed in the 1986 Drug-Free Schools and Communities Act and has been disseminated to over half of US school districts, costing at least $1 billion each year.[45,46] Further underscoring this issue, a 2016 national survey on obesity prevention and wellness found that less than 3% schools were implementing evidence-based programs, and schools were conducting initiatives like weight loss competitions and calorie counting that may unintentionally exacerbate student weight stigma in their place (personal correspondence, Kenny 2016). Research also shows that formal sexual health education in the United States has declined in recent years.[47] While one step toward creating schools that promote health is to continue to build the evidence base for efficacy of new interventions, addressing the dissemination gap and identifying strategies for de-implementation of ineffective and potentially harmful health initiatives are essential for future public health research.

Organizations Accelerating Implementation & Dissemination in Schools

National and regional organizations throughout the world, such as the CDC and Schools for Health in Europe provide leadership in promoting evidence-based health programming within schools as well as resources to support delivery. The CDC and the Association for Supervision and Curriculum Development recommend the Whole School, Whole Community, Whole Child approach as a means for systematically achieving better health for students,[48] consisting of 10 components: health education, physical education and physical activity, health services, nutrition environment and services, counseling and psychological services, social and emotional climate, physical environment, employee wellness, family engagement, and community involvement.[48] The CDC also helps schools implement and disseminate effective, low-cost programming with their school guidance documents for topics such as chronic disease management for asthma and diabetes, tobacco and prevention, and healthy eating and physical activity as well as self-assessment tools (e.g., School Health Index and Physical Education Curriculum Analysis Tool).[49]

Similar school-based health guidance, implementation tools, and assessments are promoted by the Schools for Health in Europe (SHE) network.[50,51] SHE's Health Promoting schools takes a similar whole school approach to the United States, encompassing school policy, school physical environment, school social environment, individual health skills and actions, and community links and health services in their five-step guide to take action for optimal child health. The network focuses on healthy eating, physical activity, mental health, substance use, sexual health, and physical safety themes and provides a rapid assessment tool schools can used to identify current strengths and areas need improvement.[51]

Theory Base

With school-based public health implementation and dissemination research still in its development, much literature to date lacks an explicit theoretical framework. That being said, three key frameworks—the RE-AIM framework, the Diffusion of Innovations theory, and the Consolidated Framework for Implementation Research—have been successfully applied to dissemination and implementation research within schools. Additionally, social ecological models are useful for thinking through the appropriate level at which to intervene within schools, and cost considerations are a critical aspect of interventions, their implementation, feasibility, and evaluation.[52,53]

The RE-AIM framework has been effectively used as a guide for evaluating implementation within the school context (see chapter 19).[54–57] RE-AIM identifies five elements that are key for measuring the success of interventions in real-world settings—reach, efficacy, adoption, implementation, and maintenance.[54] In the context of school-based health promotion, reach would refer to the number of children who are served water or fruits and vegetables every day in the school cafeteria or how many children participate in physical education class. Efficacy would refer to changes in children's behavior (beverage or fruit and vegetable consumption or physical activity level) that can be attributable to a given

school-based intervention. Adoption would refer to the number of schools that order water coolers to promote water consumption, change their lunch menus, or schedule more hours of physical education. Implementation, although closely linked to adoption, refers specifically to whether planned changes in practice or policy are translated into action. For example, implementation studies would assess if foods and beverages served match those on menus, or if scheduled physical activity blocks run successfully. Finally, maintenance refers to the degree to which initiatives like more nutritious offerings at lunch and improved physical education continue over time.[55]

Everett Rogers' *Diffusion of Innovations* aims to describe how ideas or practices perceived as new (e.g., policies, practices, curricula, or services) are communicated through a variety of channels over time among members of a social system (see chapter 3).[58] For example, school-based researchers following diffusion of innovation would measure the initial adoption of a new physical education curricula (e.g., ordering new materials or equipment), the planned effort to introduce the new curricula within a given number of school, the maintenance of the practices across multiple school years, the sustainability of the curriculum after initial funding is used up, and its institutionalization within all physical education classes in a given school district. Diffusion of innovations describes the multitude of factors that can influence the likelihood of implementation and dissemination of health interventions within schools as it has been successfully applied within education and health fields for decades.[58] Diffusion of innovations also implicitly points to the role of cost in the implementation and dissemination of new interventions. Applying diffusion of innovations to school settings encourages research on the factors that inhibit or facilitate schools to implement and disseminate health promoting initiatives, an important domain of study for the investigation of health disparities.[57,59]

In recent years, the Consolidated Framework for Implementation Research (CFIR) has been applied to the school setting.[60] The CFIR brings together a variety of theories and frameworks to comprehensively consider the contextual influences on implementation. These domains of influence include the "outer" setting, characteristics of the individual(s) implementing the intervention, characteristics of the intervention, the "inner" setting (in this case, factors related to the school such as the climate and leadership), and processes of implementation such as approaches to planning and engagement of teachers, parents, and students.[60] The framework has been used to understand barriers and facilitators to creating an expanded medical home by connecting primary care with school-based health centers [61] as well as to school-based parental support intervention for nutrition and physical activity.[62]

Ecological theories of change are unique in their consideration of many levels of influence on human behavior. They share the common assumption that the best public health solutions include behavior-specific intervention on **both** the individual and the environment.[63] Stokols articulated these concepts in his social ecological model, which points to interpersonal, intrapersonal, organizational, community, and policy as different levels at which behavior change can occur.[64] This theoretical orientation is important for deciding the appropriate level or levels of intervention for implementation and dissemination research within schools.

DISSEMINATION AND IMPLEMENTATION CHALLENGES SPECIFIC TO SCHOOL SETTINGS

Adapting Interventions to Diverse School Settings and Student Populations

As researchers choose their targets for implementation and dissemination research within schools, it is essential that they are designed with enough flexibility so they can adapt to have local relevance and account for the norms and culture within schools. Examples of adaptations to diverse communities include: considering regional differences in the availability of fruits and vegetables, inaccessibility to drinking fountains due to lead in water pipes in low- income communities,[65] or differences in weather and facilities that would impact physical education curricula or policy changes. Interventions that explicitly seek to identify and change local norms about children's food preferences, the safety of drinking water, or the importance of physical activity will also have a greater chance to be implemented and sustained as they will be more relevant to teachers, children, parents, and members of the community. This focus on diversity should also be considered within a given school setting: for instance, using sexual health education curricula and contraceptive services that are inclusive of gay and transgender youth, or tailoring school-based environmental and policy interventions to consider contextual factors identified by communities, such as the availability of healthy foods to ensure equity for low-income students and students of color.[66] While school priorities and cultures will vary across space and time, one key factor to keep in mind as researchers develop school-based interventions is the importance of aligning with the primary mission of learning. Thus, all policies, environmental change strategies, health education, programs, and services should be designed to fit easily into current school practices and, if possible, aim to promote academic as well as health objectives.

Considering Economic Cost & Impacts Beyond Health

School-based health promotion research has seldom explicitly applied economic concepts to investigate issues of dissemination and implementation. Cost is a major factor that influences implementation (see chapter 6), especially within public schools where budgets are tight and resources have to be allocated carefully. Although Levin started to apply cost-effectiveness within education in the 1970s and 1980s, few studies have applied the strategy to compare the relative costs and effects of interventions in schools.[52,67,68] Within the health field, Weinstein was among the first to develop cost-effectiveness guidelines to inform resource distribution decisions.[69,70] Recent cost-effectiveness research has begun to be applied to health promotion within the school setting. The CHOICES project has identified aspects of the Healthy Hunger Free Kids Act of 2010—including Smart Snacks—as particularly cost-effective dietary policy interventions,[71] and a recent cost-effectiveness assessment of physical activity interventions identified some of the most cost-effective approaches to increasing child physical activity in schools.[72] This cost-effectiveness approach costs out all resources used in providing an intervention, including personnel (e.g., wages and additional time for teachers, administrators, and volunteers), equipment (e.g. curriculum, water coolers, parent newsletters), and travel. These costs are partitioned out in terms of costs to the health sector, costs to government sectors (in this case, education), and costs incurred by children, families, and staff.[72] Finding cost-effective strategies is particularly important for making health promotion appealing to education leaders, teachers, policymakers, and tax payers.

A report designed to direct available resources in Australia ranked 160 health interventions and found that policies that have a broad reach and make use of existing personnel and infrastructure can be particularly cost-effective and may even by cost-saving in the long run. Providing evidence for cost-effectiveness and benefits beyond health can be important for achieving buy-in and continuing support since academics are the number one priority for schools. Policies and practices that do not require extra staff and limited training and equipment are appealing to administrators as they keep costs down and can be more easily maintained once a research project is complete. Planet Health, for instance, was able to keep costs low by incorporating the curriculum into existing class time, requiring just one book per teacher, and calling for minimal extra materials in lessons (see Planet Health case study for more details).[20] In the realm of school health services, while all interventions may seem beneficial on the surface, they could vary greatly in their cost-effectiveness. For example, there is evidence supporting the cost-effectiveness of providing Hepatitis B vaccinations in schools versus through HMO's; however, vision and hearing screenings in schools may largely duplicate efforts and end up being cost inefficient.[73] A nutrition curriculum that includes grade- and subject-specific academic lessons, a physical activity programs that provides 10-minute classroom activity breaks, or a water campaign that combines messages about environmental responsibility are a few examples of innovative approaches that consider the multitude of priorities within the school setting.

Targeting Multiple Levels of Change

Careful consideration of the level of change is also important in the design of interventions that are to be successfully implemented within the school setting.[64] School-based health promotion interventions could be implemented at a national, state, or district policy level; as a change in school practice; or via one-on-one services delivered by teachers, counselors, nurses, etc. Each of these strategies has different implications for the reach, dose, and cost of implementation. For instance, a district wellness policy may be able to be disseminated broadly across a large school system. This change could likely cost very little and reach a large number of children with a small change for each child. School food services changing to provide more fruits and vegetables during lunches across a district would have similar reach with perhaps a higher cost to implement but a larger gain to each individual child. As interventions rely more on teachers and counselors, training and implementation time and costs decrease, and reach is likely to increase but the potential benefit to an individual may be larger. This is all to say that weighing the level of intervention with the costs linked to that strategy is essential for designing policies, programs, and curricula that can be easily implemented and disseminated within schools.

Overcoming Challenges: Strategies for Designing School-Based Health Interventions

Developing partnerships with teachers and administrators via community-based participatory research (CBPR) strategies is essential for developing initial buy-in for interventions, institutionalizing new school policies, sustaining curricula usage, or maintaining healthy school environments.[74-76] Employing CBPR means including key stakeholders in all stages of the research process—the development of research questions, the choice of intervention strategies and measurement decisions, as well as the review of findings in a manner that can be useful for future planning and intervention. By engaging classroom teachers, superintendents, physical education teachers, counselors, and school food service personnel; school-based health interventions are likely to be implemented with greater attention to the real-world barriers to change within schools and be better sustained once any formal study of the intervention is complete.

Beyond designing interventions that can be implemented and sustained, researchers should ensure that they can be disseminated with ease once efficacy is established. In the end, what's the good of creating a health-promoting policy, environmental change, curriculum, or service that can never be replicated? Again, formative research with teachers and administrators is key; understanding the ways that education policies are made within a district or teacher's preferred strategies for adopting new curricula can make or break the ultimate success of school-based interventions. Costs also play a major role here, as initial implementation of a service is one way schools may have a marginal financial impact, but hiring new personnel to carry it out across a city or state could be expensive. Conversely, implementing policies via school board mandates or programs via low-cost training programs will likely bode well for large-scale dissemination. Finally, dissemination cannot be undertaken by a researcher alone. Collaboration with school or health organizations, publishers, and community groups can help to promote successful interventions more broadly.

Choosing the appropriate study design is essential for researchers to conduct sound dissemination and implementation research (see chapter 13). As diffusion of innovations and the RE-AIM framework emphasize, it is important to conduct a thorough process evaluation concurrent with a traditional outcome evaluation in order to look beyond what changes can be attributable to the intervention and understand *how* interventions work in real-world settings. While randomized controlled trials are the most rigorous study designs to investigate the efficacy and effectiveness of interventions within schools, natural and quasi-experimental designs can also produce valuable and valid results.[77]

Care should be taken to develop reliable and valid measures of implementation processes and health outcomes, regardless of study design (see chapter 14).[24,77] There are benefits and drawbacks to the variety of measurement strategies that are currently utilized in school-based implementation research. Whenever possible, it is beneficial to collect data on the implementation process prospectively to avoid collecting retrospective data that could be influenced by the experience of the participation in the intervention. Most school implementation studies to date rely on self-reports of implementation barriers and facilitators via questionnaire to determine the factors that influence successful change. These self-reports can provide insight into the perceptions of those who are responsible for implementing the interventions, but could be subject to bias; recent research, for example, indicates little problem with water access when reported by school officials, but half of schools were found to have access problems when measured objectively.[78] Researchers should consider who they are collecting reports from when they develop questionnaires to ensure they understand the realities of implementation within the school. For instance, classroom teachers and principals may have differing perspectives of the barriers they face in implementation of a nutrition curriculum—teachers may emphasize resistance from students while administrators focus more on budget costs. Observations and in-depth

interviews may lend important information to measurement in implementation for future studies.[79] The stages or levels of implementation are also generally self-reported, although they could also come from more objective sources such as purchasing reports for curricula, attendance at trainings, online reporting systems, or purchases made through school food service. Finally, the measurement of costs has great potential for prioritizing school-based health solutions; however, more research is needed to assess the validity and reliability of these measurement strategies.

CONTEXTUAL INFLUENCES ON IMPLEMENTATION AND DISSEMINATION OF HEALTH INTERVENTIONS IN SCHOOL SETTINGS

A range of policies, environmental change strategies, curricula, and services within schools have been shown to be effective for creating health change,[13-24,27-30,80] and a number of these interventions provide evidence for cost-effectiveness and, as such, can provide additional information when considering implementation and dissemination.[71-73,81-84] However, the gap between determining efficacy within the research setting and effectiveness in the real world is substantial, and much research is still needed to investigate how interventions can be effectively implemented and sustained within schools. Here we turn to the research to date, organized according to the CFIR, on specific factors that influence the success of interventions within school settings.

Characteristics of individuals implementing interventions in schools such as age, years of experience, education, personality, expectations and attitudes about a given intervention, role responsibility, coping style, self-efficacy, motivation to implement, and leadership experience are common factors hypothesized to influence effective implementation of interventions within schools.[85-90] Also linked to the influence of providers is the impact of teacher and staff turnover on implementation success. Interventions at the interpersonal level would likely be more influenced by individual differences among teachers or counselors, whereas policy and practices changes would rely more on initial strong leadership and a system for accountability thereafter.

Characteristics of the interventions themselves have also been investigated as they relate to real-world effectiveness in schools. These attributes include standardization of a particular curriculum or service, the degree of integration within the school day, and the cost and time associated with the intervention.[87] The adaptability of interventions, cultural tailoring, and the perceived usefulness and acceptability to parents, teachers, school nurses, and students have emerged as themes important for successful implementation and dissemination.[62,91,92] The quality and quantity of training associated with intervention implementation has also been investigated, but little attention has been paid to the time and cost associated with these trainings that may make sustainability over time difficult.[87,88] Using existing staff to deliver school health interventions may be one way to balance these cost and training concerns.

Finally, the school inner setting (e.g., organizational capacity, size, support from principals and superintendents; competing demands, resources such as space and equipment), and outer setting (e.g., community poverty, high patient need) have also been studied in their relation to implementation success.[61,85–87,90,93,94] These factors could be specific to the intervention, such as having access to an on-site school kitchen to serve healthy beverages afterschool[90] or more general measures of capacity.[95]

Considering these different factors in conjunction is an important step for understanding the most important drivers of successful implementation. For instance, Payne et. al. determined that structural influences predict quality implementation more than factors related to personnel or school and community climate.[87] Additionally, investigation of contextual influences in an afterschool group randomized trial found that characteristics of the individuals (site director's years of experience), the outer setting (perceived support from the school), and the inner setting (a kitchen available on site), all influenced changes in children's water consumption.[90]

RESEARCH GAPS AND DIRECTIONS FOR THE FUTURE

There is much need for more research in the field of school-based implementation and dissemination. While there is solid evidence for the efficacy of interventions and policies that are designed to promote health in schools, many have not been translated from "best practice" to "common practice." More research is needed to identify effective strategies for implementing and disseminating evidence-based interventions in schools and understanding how to de-implement current practices that are ineffective or even harmful to child health. Investigating the factors that influence the implementation and dissemination of efficacious interventions into real-world settings should be a top research priority. While a handful of studies have attempted to tease out the different influences of personnel, setting, and intervention features on intervention effectiveness; this research is limited in scope. Similar to the inconsistent measurement of implementation and dissemination processes, these moderating factors that make or break the success of an intervention within schools are infrequently measured.[24] When assessed, they vary considerably in how they are operationalized within studies. One major step toward addressing this research gap is for investigators to broaden the traditional intervention effectiveness study that narrowly focuses on short-term behavioral and attitudinal outcomes to include more rigorous study of the intervention implementation process and the factors that positively and negatively affect uptake at each stage. These studies should be rooted in comprehensive theories or frameworks, such as Diffusion of Innovations, Consolidated Framework for Implementation Research, and RE-AIM, and employ strong study designs. Finally, in order to take advantage of the potential schools have as settings for narrowing health disparities, research should focus on developing strong school and community partnerships and emphasize the importance of cost-effective strategies for health promotion.

SUMMARY

In sum, this chapter began by emphasizing the enormous potential schools hold for impacting population health. Considering the constant presence of school in children's lives for over 12 years, it is important to conduct research and plan programs that can work together across the life course to promote health and seek to understand how schools can help to link children to services beyond the school walls.[96] A large gap between the evidence for effectiveness of school-based health interventions and the types of programs, policies, and services that currently influence the lives of children must be addressed. In this effort, the excitement of translating public health research findings into practice should be balanced by the realities of the educational system and the implementation barriers and facilitators specific to schools. Future school-based dissemination and implementation research cannot overestimate the importance of developing strategies that are compatible with the primary aims of schools: promoting learning through reading, writing, math, etc. Equally important is considering policy and environmental change strategies at the national, state, and district level to promote health within schools. Policies that make use of existing personnel and infrastructure can be particularly cost effective.[97] Research within schools should investigate the factors that influence quality of implementation and assess the impact of interventions that have been adapted to local contexts and to accommodate real-world barriers.

PLANET HEALTH CASE STUDY

Background

The prevalence of childhood obesity in the United States has increased rapidly to historically high levels over recent decades, and has only begun to begun to plateau among children aged 2 to 5 and in some communities and states.[98] Moreover, higher rates of obesity persist among minority and economically disadvantaged youth.[98] Obesity is associated with significant health problems in early life, including high cholesterol and hypertension, and is a significant risk factor for adult morbidity and mortality.[99]

Context

Planet Health, conducted in the mid-1990s, was the first field trial of a middle school-based obesity prevention program.[20] It aimed to move beyond the evidence for efficacy of obesity prevention interventions to show effectiveness within a real-world context. Moreover, process evaluations of Planet Health helped to investigate how the program was implemented and disseminated within schools.[76,100]

The intervention had a group randomized design with 10 middle schools matched on area characteristics (e.g., school system) and then randomized to receive the intervention.[20] The communities in the sample had a mean income similar to the US average and the intervention followed boys and girls in grades 6 to 8 over 2 school years. The primary endpoint for the intervention was obesity prevalence. Secondary endpoints included moderate and vigorous physical activity; TV viewing; dietary intake of fat, fruits, and vegetables; and total energy intake.

The interdisciplinary curriculum took a population approach to disease prevention and was guided by behavioral choice and social cognitive theories. Intervention components included staff trainings, classroom lesson plans, and materials for physical education teachers, staff wellness sessions, and small funds to put toward fitness improvements.

Findings and Lessons Learned
Intervention Effectiveness

The 2-year Planet Health intervention was effective across a range of outcomes. It reduced TV watching among boys and girl as well as decreased obesity prevalence, decreased daily calories consumed, and increased fruit and vegetable intake among girls.[20] Girls in the intervention were also less likely to report weight control behavior disorders.[101]

Evidence for Successful Dissemination and Implementation

After the program was shown to be effective, the Boston Public Schools expressed interest in disseminating Planet Health. In a process evaluation of this dissemination effort, teachers delivered the program at intended levels, indicating that Planet Health can be implemented at the intended dose over 3 school years.[76] Despite reported challenges of planning time and conflicts with school meals programs, vending machines, and home environments, over 75% of teachers planned to continue teaching Planet Health the next year and self-reported feasibility and acceptability was high.[76] Collecting theory-based process measures of feasibility, acceptability, and sustainability in the dissemination phase of Planet Health helped to show the promise of how similar interventions can be implemented and sustained within a school system.[76] Following this successful dissemination effort, as of 2010, more than 10,000 copies of Planet Health have been purchased in all 50 states and more than 20 countries. Moreover, the program has been shown to be cost effective for reducing obesity in middle-school age youth and has been recommended by Cancer Control P.L.A.N.E.T. and the Guide to Community Preventive Services as an effective intervention for reducing screen time and improving weight-related outcomes.[83] Most recently, when Planet Health was part of a multicomponent community-based intervention in 45 middle schools, there was evidence for increases in fruit and vegetable consumption as well as physical activity, decreases in television viewing, as well as decreases in the proportion of overweight and obese children over 3 years.[102]

Lesson #1: School Context Is Challenging for Study Design and Measurement

The Planet Health intervention faced numerous research challenges due to the unique context of the school setting. First, like many school-based interventions, measurement of health behaviors was limited to self-report.[20] This strategy is often more feasible for a field trial, but has limited reliability and validity, especially among children. Evaluation of school-based programs is also complicated due to the difficulty of tracking changes over time. Planet Health investigators were careful to select a sample of students that would be relatively stable over time and chose implementation measures that would withstand any school or personnel changes over a 2-year time period. Although the study did face these design challenges, the benefits of evaluating the intervention for effectiveness in a real-world setting outweigh these limitations.

Lesson #2: Benefits of Adapting Interventions to Diverse School Settings

Considering the various competing demands within school was important to ensure that the curriculum appealed to teachers and administrators and was implemented as intended. Accordingly, lesson evaluations and focus groups were conducted with teachers during the development of the units.[20] One finding from this formative research was that teachers preferred text books to web-based materials. Producing a curriculum that teachers are likely to perceive as advantageous and easy to utilize may seem like an obvious step; however, most research does not build in time to discover these implementation preferences and could miss similar factors and end up developing a program that would not be readily adopted by schools and teachers.

Researchers also spent years building authentic school and community partnerships that help to explain the effectiveness of the intervention in a middle-school setting and the positive process evaluation finding. The importance of developing partnerships and working within a community based participatory research framework also stands out as crucial for moving Planet Health beyond a field trial to dissemination throughout the state and across the country.[76]

Lesson #3: Benefits of Considering Economic Cost and Impacts Beyond Health

Researchers took an interdisciplinary approach that incorporates subject and grade-specific learning objectives in the development of Planet Health. The design of the intervention also considered the limited resources available to schools for health promotion. Its low-cost, population approach weaves nutrition and physical activity messaging into math, English, science, and social studies material with existing classroom teachers.[20,100] Each lesson is designed to promote literacy, and the curriculum aligns with the Massachusetts Department of Education Curriculum Frameworks, which is consistent with learning standards in many other states.[103] A recent research study in two communities also found that training approaches can considerably impact the cost of Planet Health intervention; training costs were considerably lower when a small number of health teachers were trained to implement the curriculum throughout the school rather than all middle school classroom teachers.[104] In addition to the curriculum, the intervention provided small Fitness Funds to purchase items that would help to sustain changes beyond the study period.[20] By designing a curriculum that was inexpensive and supported the school's primary objective, researchers made the curriculum more appealing to teachers and administrators and likely aided initial implementation, maintenance, and dissemination.[105]

Conclusion

The findings from Planet Health hold several key implications for teachers, policymakers, and researchers. First, the importance of building partnerships with schools cannot be overstated. If researchers want to develop programs that will outlive their evaluation, they must collaborate with the people who will be responsible for delivery down the road from the onset. Specific factors that are likely to carry over to other school-based programs are those that are low-cost and easy to integrate into existing classroom practices. These principles have also been adopted in the development of the Harvard T.H. Chan School of Public Health Prevention Research Center Food & Fun Afterschool curriculum. Developed in collaboration with the largest provider of afterschool programming, the YMCA of the USA, these nutrition and physical activity lessons are designed to be easily integrated into a variety of out-of-school time programs and are available free-of-charge at www.foodandfun.org and www.osnap.org.

SUGGESTED READINGS AND WEBSITES

Readings

Estabrooks P, Dzewaltowski DA, Glasgow RE, Klesges LM. Reporting of validity from school health promotion studies published in 12 leading journals, 1996-2000. *J Sch Health.* 2003;73(1):21–28.

The authors of this study used the RE-AIM framework to evaluate school-based studies emphasizing good nutrition, physical activity, and smoking prevention published over a four-year period. The article recommends more frequent reporting of representativeness criteria in order to increase applicability outside of the research setting.

Gortmaker SL, Wang YC, Long MW, Giles CM, Ward ZJ, Barrett JL, Kenney EL, Sonneville KR, Afzal AS, Resch SC, Cradock AL. Three interventions that reduce childhood obesity are projected to save more than they cost to implement. *Health Aff (Millwood).* 2015;34(11):1932–1939.

This paper describes the CHOICES modeling approach used to assess the cost-effectiveness of dietary intervention, including policy changes within school settings due to the Healthy Hunger Free Kids Act. It examines impact on both cost effectiveness metrics, total costs, and population health outcomes.

Klimes-Dougan B, August GJ, Lee C-YS, Realmuto GM, Bloomquist ML, Horowitz JL, Eisenberg TL. Practitioner and site characteristics that relate to fidelity of implementation: the early risers prevention program in a going-to-scale intervention trial. *Prof Psychol Res Pract.* 2009;40(5):467–475.

Authors of this study examine the influence of practitioner characteristics (e.g. experience, personality, beliefs, coping) and perceived school climate/culture on implementation fidelity among 27 elementary schools taking a prevention program to scale. The study demonstrates how researchers can operationalize and systematically investigate the influence of a variety of contextual factors on intervention success in the real world.

Payne AA, Eckert R. The relative importance of provider, program, school, and community predictors of the implementation quality of school-based prevention programs. *Prev Sci.* 2010;11(2):126–141.

This study examines implementation factors such as program structure, school climate, and community structure in school-based prevention programs. Using national data from over 500 schools, the authors concluded that program structure characteristics (e.g., supervision, use of standardized materials, high quality training) had the greatest impact on program quality.

Rabin BA, Glasgow RE, Kerner JF, Klump MP, Brownson RC. Dissemination and implementation research on community-based cancer prevention: a systematic review. *Am J Prev Med.* 2010;38(4):443–456.

A systematic review of dissemination and implementation research of evidence-based interventions in smoking, healthy diet, physical activity and sun protection. This review highlights, among other recommendations, the need for studies that cover a broader range of populations and settings, more consistent terminology use, more practice-based evidence, and measures with higher validity and reliability.

Stokols D. Translating social ecological theory into guidelines for community health promotion. *Am J Health Promot.* 1996;10(4):282–298.

This article describes how the core principles of social ecological theory can be translated into practical guidelines for research conducted in real-world settings. The author describes how researchers can intervene within organizations to achieve optimal implementation, emphasizes the importance of creating change at multiple levels of influence, and highlights the need for more assessment of intervention sustainability over time.

Selected Websites and Tools

Centers for Disease Control and Prevention: Healthy Schools. https://www.cdc.gov/healthyschools/.
The CDC Healthy Schools page provides links to data and statistics, training opportunities, state programs, and tools for promoting health within the school setting. There are specific areas devoted to nutrition, physical activity, obesity prevention, chronic health conditions, and wellness policies.

Schools for Health in Europe. http://www.schoolsforhealth.eu/
Schools for Health in Europe aims to support organizations and professionals to further develop and sustain school health promotion by providing the European platform for school health promotion. The network is coordinated by the Netherlands Institute for Health Promotion, as a WHO Collaborating Centre for School Health Promotion.

Harvard T.H. Chan School of Public Health Prevention Research Center. http://www.hsph.harvard.edu/research/prc/
The Harvard School of Public Health Prevention Research Center website includes links to sample lessons from Planet Health and Eat Well and Keep Moving (a similar curriculum designed for elementary grades). The HPRC Food and Fun Afterschool materials also include planning tools designed to improve implementation of nutrition and physical activity changes in resource-tight settings.

Change Lab Solutions: Healthier Schools. http://www.changelabsolutions.org/childhood-obesity/schools

ChangeLab Solutions provides community-based solutions for America's most common and preventable diseases. Their Healthier Schools page provides practical tools that can support school-based implementation such as a strategy guide for wellness policy enforcement and a Safe Routes to School roadmap.

Research-tested Intervention Programs (RTIPs). https://rtips.cancer.gov/rtips/

RTIPs is a database of evidence-based interventions and program materials designed for cancer prevention. School-based practitioners can search by setting to identify program materials, ratings provided by external experts, and assessments of implementation metrics according to the RE-AIM framework.

Blueprints for Healthy Youth Development. http://www.blueprintsprograms.com

The Blueprints website provides a database of evidence-based programs for positive youth development. Practitioners interested in school-based interventions can narrow their search using the program selector by setting. The site provides ratings of evidence as well as information about costs and funding strategies.

REFERENCES

1. United Nations. Millenium Goals. http://www.un.org/millenniumgoals/education.shtml. Accessed December 23, 2016.
2. United Nations. Transforming our world: the 2030 Agenda for Sustainable Development In: Assembly G, ed. *70/12015.*
3. WHO. *European strategy for child and adolescent health and development.* Copenhagen: WHO Regional Office for Europe; 2008.
4. Langford R, Bonell C, Jones H, et al. The World Health Organization's Health Promoting Schools framework: a Cochrane systematic review and meta-analysis. *BMC Public Health.* 2015;15(1):130.
5. Young I. Health promotion in schools--a historical perspective. *Promot Educ.* 2005;12(3-4):112-117, 184-190, 205-111.
6. Chadwick E. *Report of the sanitary conditions of the labouring population of Great Britain.* London: Poor Law Commission;1842.
7. U.S. Department of Education National Center for Education Statistics. Common Core of Data (CCD), "National Public Education Financial Survey," 2002–03 through 2012–13. https://nces.ed.gov/programs/coe/pdf/coe_cma.pdf. Accessed January 3, 2017.
8. Healthy, Hunger-Free Kids Act of 2010, Public Law No 111-296.
9. Schools for Health in Europe. http://www.schoolsforhealth.eu/. Accessed March 9, 2017.
10. Guide to Community Preventive Services. 2016. https://www.thecommunityguide.org/about/about-community-guide. Accessed December 26, 2016.
11. National Cancer Institute and Substance Abuse and Mental Health Services Administration. Research-tested Interventions Programs website. http://rtips.cancer.gov/rtips/. Accessed March 5, 2017.
12. Center for the Study and Prevention of Violence. Blueprints for Youth Development website http://www.blueprintsprograms.com. Accessed March 5, 2017.
13. Wilson SJ, Lipsey MW, Derzon JH. The effects of school-based intervention programs on aggressive behavior: a meta-analysis. *J Consult Clin Psychol.* 2003;71(1):136–149.
14. Neil AL, Christensen H. Efficacy and effectiveness of school-based prevention and early intervention programs for anxiety. *Clin Psychol Rev.* 2009;29(3):208–215.
15. Botvin GJ, Baker E, Dusenbury L, Botvin EM, Diaz T. Long-term follow-up results of a randomized drug abuse prevention trial in a white middle-class population. *JAMA.* 1995;273(14):1106–1112.
16. Thomas RE. PR. School-based programmes for preventing smoking (Review). *The Cochrane Library.* 2008(4).
17. Faggiano F. V-TF, Versino E., Zambon A., Borraccino A., Lemma P. School-based prevention for illicit drugs' use (Review). *The Cochrane Library.* 2008(3).
18. Mytton JA. DiGuiseppi C, Gough D., Taylor RS., Logan S. School-based secondary prevention programmes for preventing violence (Review). *The Cochrane Library.* 2009(4).
19. Luepker RV, Perry CL, McKinlay SM, et al. Outcomes of a field trial to improve children's dietary patterns and physical activity. The Child and Adolescent Trial for Cardiovascular Health. CATCH collaborative group. *JAMA.* 1996;275(10):768–776.
20. Gortmaker SL, Peterson K, Wiecha J, et al. Reducing obesity via a school-based interdisciplinary intervention among youth: Planet Health. *Arch Pediatr Adolesc Med.* 1999;153(4):409–418.
21. Dobbins M. De Corby K, Robeson P, Husson H, Tirilis D. School-based physical activity programs for promoting physical activity and fitness in children and adolescents aged 6-18 (Review). *The Cochrane Library.* 2009(3).
22. Oringanje C, Meremikwu MM, Eko H, Esu E, Meremikwu A, EhirI JE. Interventions for preventing unintended pregnancies among adolescents (Review). *The Cochrane Library.* 2010(1).
23. Institute of Medicine. *Bridging the evidence gap in obesity prevention: A framework to inform decision*

making. Washington DC: The National Academies Press; 2010.

24. Rabin BA, Glasgow RE, Kerner JF, Klump MP, Brownson RC. Dissemination and implementation research on community-based cancer prevention: a systematic review. *Am J Prev Med.* 2010;38(4):443–456.

25. Kibbe DL, Hackett J, Hurley M, et al. Ten years of TAKE 10!(R): integrating physical activity with academic concepts in elementary school classrooms. *Prev Med.* 2011;52:S43–S50.

26. Boarnet MG, Anderson CL, Day K, McMillan T, Alfonzo M. Evaluation of the California Safe Routes to School legislation—Urban form changes and children's active transportation to school. *Am J Prev Med.* 2005;28(2):134–140.

27. Hanks AS, Just DR, Wansink B. Smarter lunchrooms can address new school lunchroom guidelines and childhood obesity. *J. Pediatr.* 2013;162(4):867–869.

28. Evans-Whipp T, Beyers JM, Lloyd S, et al. A review of school drug policies and their impact on youth substance use. *Health Promot Int.* 2004;19(2):227–234.

29. Jaime PC, Lock K. Do school based food and nutrition policies improve diet and reduce obesity? *Prev Med.* 2009;48(1):45–53.

30. Kahn EB, Ramsey LT, Brownson RC, et al. The effectiveness of interventions to increase physical activity: a systematic review. *Am J Prev Med.* 2002;22(4, Supplement 1):73–107.

31. Cradock AL, McHugh A, Mont-Ferguson H, et al. Effect of school district policy change on consumption of sugar-sweetened beverages among high school students, Boston, Massachusetts, 2004-2006. *Prev Chronic Dis.* 2011;8(4):A74.

32. Mozaffarian RS, Gortmaker SL, Kenney EL, et al. Assessment of a districtwide policy on availability of competitive beverages in Boston Public Schools, Massachusetts, 2013. *Prev Chronic Dis.* 2016;13:9.

33. Paul P, Fabio A. Literature review of HPV vaccine delivery strategies: Considerations for school- and non-school based immunization program. *Vaccine.* 2014;32(3):320–326.

34. Kwong JC, Ge H, Rosella LC, et al. School-based influenza vaccine delivery, vaccination rates, and healthcare use in the context of a universal influenza immunization program: an ecological study. *Vaccine.* 2010;28(15):2722–2729.

35. Coffman JM, Cabana MD, Yelin EH. Do School-based asthma education programs improve self-management and health outcomes? *Pediatrics.* 2009;124(2):729–742.

36. Bruzzese JM, Sheares BJ, Vincent EJ, et al. Effects of a school-based intervention for urban adolescents with asthma a controlled trial. *Am J Respir Crit Care Med.* 2011;183(8):998–1006.

37. Bains RM, Diallo AF. Mental health services in school-based health centers: systematic review. *J School Nurs.* 2016;32(1):8–19.

38. Cappella E, Frazier SL, Atkins MS, Schoenwald SK, Glisson C. Enhancing schools' capacity to support children in poverty: an ecological model of school-based mental health services. *Adm Policy Ment Health Ment Health Serv Res.* 2008;35(5):395–409.

39. Daley AM. Rethinking school-based health centers as complex adaptive systems maximizing opportunities for the prevention of teen pregnancy and sexually transmitted infections. *Adv Nurs Sci.* 2012;35(2):E37–E46.

40. Ethier KA, Dittus PJ, DeRosa CJ, Chung EQ, Martinez E, Kerndt PR. School-based health center access, reproductive health care, and contraceptive use among sexually experienced high school students. *J Adolesc Health.* 2011;48(6):562–565.

41. Kann L, TellJohann, Wooley SF. Health education: results from the School Health Policies and Programs Study 2006. *J Sch Health.* 2007;77(8):408–434.

42. Brener ND, Weist M, Adelman H, Taylor L, Vernon-Smiley M. Mental health and social services: results from the School Health Policies and Programs Study 2006. *J Sch Health.* 2007;77(8):486–499.

43. Lee SM, Burgeson CR, Fulton JE, Spain CG. Physical education and physical activity: results from the School Health Policies and Programs Study 2006. *J Sch Health.* 2007;77(8):435–463.

44. Chriqui JF, Turner L, Taber DR, Chaloupka FJ. Association between district and state policies and US public elementary school competitive food and beverage environments. *JAMA Pediatr.* 2013;167(8):714–722.

45. Ennett ST, Tobler NS, Ringwalt CL, Flewelling RL. How effective is drug abuse resistance education? A meta-analysis of Project DARE outcome evaluations. *Am J Public Health.* 1994;84(9):1394–1401.

46. Shepard EM. *The economic costs of D.A.R.E.* Syracuse, NY: Institute of Industrial Relations; 2001.

47. Lindberg LD, Maddow-Zimet I, Boonstra H. Changes in adolescents' receipt of sex education, 2006-2013. *J Adolesc Health.* 2016; 58(6):621–627.

48. Lewallen TC, Hunt H, Potts-Datema W, Zaza S, Giles W. The Whole School, Whole Community, Whole Child Model: a new approach for improving educational attainment and healthy development for students. *J Sch Health.* 2015;85(11):729–739.

49. Centers for Disease Control and Prevention. Healthy Schools—Tools and Resources. 2015;

https://www.cdc.gov/healthyschools/resources.htm. Accessed December 23, 2016.

50. Burgher MS, Rasmussen VB, Rivett D. *The European Network of Health Promoting Schools: The alliance of education and health.* WHO Regional Office for Europe: Copenhagen Denmark. 1999.

51. Schools for Health in Europe. http://www.schools-for-health.eu/she-network. Accessed December 23, 2016.

52. Levin HM. Waiting for godot: Cost-effectiveness analysis in education. *New Direct Eval.* 2001;90:55–68.

53. Carter R, Moodie M, Markwick A, et al. Assessing cost-effectiveness in obesity (ACE-obesity): an overview of the ACE approach, economic methods and cost results. *BMC Public Health.* 2009;9(1):419.

54. Glasgow RE, Vogt TM, Boles SM. Evaluating the public health impact of health promotion interventions: The RE-AIM framework. *Am J Public Health.* 1999;89(9):1322–1327.

55. Dunton GF, Lagloire R, Robertson T. Using the RE-AIM framework to evaluate the statewide dissemination of a school-based physical activity and nutrition curriculum: "Exercise Your Options." *Am J Health Promo.* 2009;23(4):229–232.

56. Estabrooks P, Dzewaltowski DA, Glasgow RE, Klesges LM. Reporting of validity from school health promotion studies published in 12 leading journals, 1996-2000. *J Sch Health.* 2003;73(1):21–28.

57. McGoey T, Root Z, Bruner MW, Law B. Evaluation of physical activity interventions in youth via the Reach, Efficacy/Effectiveness, Adoption, Implementation, and Maintenance (RE-AIM) framework: a systematic review of randomised and non-randomised trials. *Prev Med.* 2015;76:58-67.

58. Rogers EM. *Diffusion of innovations.* 5th ed. New York: Free Press; 2003.

59. Downs SM, Farmer A, Quintanilha M, et al. From paper to practice: barriers to adopting nutrition guidelines in schools. *J Nutr Educ Behav.* 2012;44(2):114–122.

60. Damschroder LJ, Aron DC, Keith RE, Kirsh SR, Alexander JA, Lowery JC. Fostering implementation of health services research findings into practice: a consolidated framework for advancing implementation science. *Implement. Sci.* 2009;4:50.

61. Riley M, Laurie AR, Plegue MA, Richarson CR. The adolescent "expanded medical home": school-based health centers partner with a primary care clinic to improve population health and mitigate social determinants of health. *J Am Board Fam Med.* 2016;29(3):339–347.

62. Norman A, Nyberg G, Elinder LS, Berlin A. One size does not fit all-qualitative process evaluation of the Healthy School Start parental support programme to prevent overweight and obesity among children in disadvantaged areas in Sweden. *BMCc Public Health.* 2016;16:11.

63. Sallis JF, Owen N, Fisher EB. Ecological models of health behavior. In: Glanz K, Rimer BK, Viswanath K, eds. *Health behavior and health education: Theory, research, and practice.* 4th ed. San Francisco: Jossey-Bass; 2008:465–482.

64. Stokols D. Translating social ecological theory into guidelines for community health promotion. *Am J Health Promot.* 1996;10(4):282–298.

65. Cradock AL, Wilking CL, Olliges SA, Gortmaker SL. Getting back on tap the policy context and cost of ensuring access to low-cost drinking water in Massachusetts schools. *Am J Prev Med.* 2012;43(3):S95–S101.

66. Kumanyika SK, Swank M, Stachecki J, Whitt-Glover MC, Brennan LK. Examining the evidence for policy and environmental strategies to prevent childhood obesity in black communities: new directions and next steps. *Obes Rev.* 2014;15:177–203.

67. Levin HM, Glass GV, Meister GR. Cost-effectiveness of computer-assisted instruction. *Eval Rev,* 1987;11: 50–72.

68. Hummel-Rossi B, Ashdown J. The state of cost-benefit and cost-effectiveness analyses in education. *Rev Educ Res.* 2002;72(1):1–30.

69. Weinstein MC, Siegel JE, Gold MR, Kamlet MS, Russell LB. Recommendations of the Panel on Cost-effectiveness in Health and Medicine. *JAMA.* 1996;276(15):1253–1258.

70. Mandelblatt JS, Fryback DG, Weinstein MC, Russell LB, Gold MR. Assessing the effectiveness of health interventions for cost-effectiveness analysis. Panel on Cost-Effectiveness in Health and Medicine. *J Gen Intern Med.* 1997;12(9):551–558.

71. Gortmaker SL, Wang YC, Long MW, et al. Three interventions that reduce childhood obesity are projected to save more than they cost to implement. *Health Aff (Millwood).* 2015;34(11):1932–1939.

72. Cradock AL, Barrett JL, Kenney EL, et al. Using cost-effectiveness analysis to prioritize policy and programmatic approaches to physical activity promotion and obesity prevention in childhood. *Prev Med.* 2017;05 Suppl:S17–S27.

73. Deuson RR, Hoekstra EJ, Sedjo R, et al. The Denver school-based adolescent hepatitis B vaccination program: a cost analysis with risk simulation. *Am J Public Health.* 1999;89(11):1722–1727.

74. Israel BA, Schulz AJ, Parker EA, Becker AB. Review of community-based research: assessing partnership approaches to improve public health. *Annu Rev Public Health.* 1998;19:173–202.

75. Leung MW, Yen IH, Minkler M. Community based participatory research: a promising approach for increasing epidemiology's relevance in the 21st century. *Int J Epidemiol.* 2004;33(3):499–506.

76. Wiecha JL, El Ayadi AM, Fuemmeler BF, et al. Diffusion of an integrated health education program in an urban school system: planet health. *J Pediatr Psychol.* 2004;29(6):467–474.

77. Shadish WR, Cook TD, Campbell DT. *Experimental and quasi-experimental designs for generalized causal inference.* Belmont, CA: Wadsworth Cengage Learning; 2002.

78. Kenney EL, Gortmaker SL, Cohen JF, Rimm EB, Cradock AL. Limited school drinking water access for youth. *J Aolesc Health.* 2016;59(1):24–29.

79. Resnicow K, Davis M, Smith M, et al. How best to measure implementation of school health curricula: a comparison of three measures. *Health Educ Res.* 1998;13(2):239–250.

80. Lonsdale C, Rosenkranz RR, Peralta LR, Bennie A, Fahey P, Lubans DR. A systematic review and meta-analysis of interventions designed to increase moderate-to-vigorous physical activity in school physical education lessons. *Prev Med.* 2013;56(2):152–161.

81. Wang LY, Crossett LS, Lowry R, Sussman S, Dent CW. Cost-effectiveness of a school-based tobacco-use prevention program. *Arch Pediatr Adolesc Med.* 2001;155(9):1043–1050.

82. Wang LY, Davis M, Robin L, Collins J, Coyle K, Baumler E. Economic evaluation of Safer Choices: a school-based human immunodeficiency virus, other sexually transmitted diseases, and pregnancy prevention program. *Arch Pediatr Adolesc Med.* 2000;154(10):1017–1024.

83. Wang LY, Yang Q, Lowry R, Wechsler H. Economic analysis of a school-based obesity prevention program. *Obes Res.* 2003;11(11):1313–1324.

84. Gortmaker SL, Long MW, Resch SC, et al. Cost effectiveness of childhood obesity interventions evidence and methods for CHOICES. *Am J Prev Med.* 2015;49(1):102–111.

85. Klimes-Dougan B, August GJ, Lee C-YS, Realmuto GM, Bloomquist ML, Horowitz JL, Eisenberg TL. Practitioner and site characteristics that relate to fidelity of implementation: the early risers prevention program in a going-to-scale intervention trial. *Prof Psychol Res Pract.* 2009;40(5):467–475.

86. Ransford C, Greenberg MT, Domitrovich CE, Small M, Jacobson L. The role of teachers' psychological experiences and perceptions of curriculum supports on the implementation of a social and emotional learning curriculum. *School Psychol Rev.* 2009;38(4):510–532.

87. Payne AA, Eckert R. The relative importance of provider, program, school, and community predictors of the implementation quality of school-based prevention programs. *Prev Sci.* 2010;11(2):126–141.

88. Rohrbach LA, D'Onofrio CN, Backer TE, Montgomery SB. Diffusion of school-based substance abuse prevention programs. *Am Behav Sci.* 1996;39:919–934.

89. Harris BR, Shaw BA, Sherman BR, Lawson HA. Screening, brief intervention, and referral to treatment for adolescents: attitudes, perceptions, and practice of New York school-based health center providers. *Subst Abus.* 2016;37(1):161–167.

90. Lee RM, Okechukwu C, Emmons KM, Gortmaker SL. Impact of implementation factors on children's water consumption in the Out-of-School Nutrition and Physical Activity group-randomized trial. *New Direct Youth Dev.* 2014;2014(143):79–101.

91. Robbins SCC, Ward K, Skinner SR. School-based vaccination: a systematic review of process evaluations. *Vaccine.* 2011;29(52):9588–9599.

92. Alhassan S, Greever C, Nwaokelemeh O, Mendoza A, Barr-Anderson DJ. Facilitators, barriers, and components of a culturally tailored afterschool physical activity program in preadolescent African American girls and their mothers. *Ethnicity Disease.* 2014;24(1):8–13.

93. Hoyle TB, Bartee RT, Allensworth DD. Applying the process of health promotion in schools: a commentary. *J School Health.* 2010;80(4):163–166.

94. Hastmann TJ, Bopp M, Fallon EA, Rosenkranz RR, Dzewaltowski DA. Factors influencing the implementation of organized physical activity and fruit and vegetable snacks in the HOP'N After-School Obesity Prevention Program. *J Nutr Educ Behav.* 2013;45(1):60–68.

95. Halgunseth L, Carmack C, Childs S, Caldwell L, Craig A, Smith E. Using the interactive systems framework in understanding the relation between general program capacity and implementation in afterschool settings. *Am J Community Psychol.* 2012;50(3-4):311–320.

96. Greenberg MT. Current and future challenges in school-based prevention: the researcher perspective. *Prev Sci.* 2004;5(1):5–13.

97. Vos T, Carter R, Barendregt J, et al. *Assessing cost-effectiveness in prevention (ACE–Prevention): Final report.* University of Queensland, Brisbane and Deakin University, Melbourne; 2010.

98. Ogden CL, Carroll MD, Lawman HG, et al. Trends in obesity prevalence among children and adolescents in the United States, 1988-1994 through 2013-2014. *JAMA.* 2016;315(21):2292–2299.

99. Freedman DS, Dietz WH, Srinivasan SR, Berenson GS. The relation of overweight to cardiovascular

risk factors among children and adolescents: the Bogalusa Heart Study. *Pediatrics.* 1999;103(6 Pt 1):1175–1182.

100. Franks A, Kelder SH, Dino GA, et al. School-based programs: lessons learned from CATCH, Planet Health, and Not-On-Tobacco. *Prev Chronic Dis.* 2007;4(2).

101. Austin SB, Field AE, Wiecha J, Peterson KE, Gortmaker SL. The impact of a school-based obesity prevention trial on disordered weight-control behaviors in early adolescent girls. *Arch Pediatr Adolesc Med.* 2005;159(3):225–230.

102. Peterson KE, Spadano-Gasbarro JL, Greaney ML, et al. Three-year improvements in weight status and weight-related behaviors in middle school students: The Healthy Choices Study. *PLoS One.* 2015;10(8):12.

103. Carter J, Wiecha JL, Peterson KE, Nobrega S, Gortmaker SL. *Planet Health: An interdisciplinary curriculum for teaching middle school nutrition and physical activity.* 2nd ed. Champaign, IL: Human Kinetics; 2007.

104. Blaine RE, Franckle RL, Ganter C, et al. Using school staff members to implement a childhood obesity prevention intervention in low-income school districts: the Massachusetts Childhood Obesity Research Demonstration (MA-CORD Project), 2012-2014. *Prev Chronic Dis.* 2017;14:E03.

105. Kenney EL, Wintner S, Lee RM, Austin SB. Low dissemination of evidence-based obesity prevention interventions in U.S. public schools, 2016: are schools filling the gap with programs that promote weight stigma? *Prevent Chronic Dis.* In press.

25

Dissemination and Implementation Research in Worksites

PEGGY A. HANNON AND JEFFREY R. HARRIS

INTRODUCTION

The workplace is a powerful socioecological environment for adult health promotion. This chapter uses the term "health promotion" broadly, to encompass primary prevention through lifestyle behaviors (such as healthy eating and engaging in physical activity) and vaccinations, early detection of disease through screening, and treatment and management of chronic illness. The socioecological model states that health behavior is influenced by intrapersonal, interpersonal, institutional, community, and public policy-level factors.[1] The majority of US adults are employed,[2] and their workplaces can function at multiple levels of the socioecological model. As an institution, the workplace shapes the daily environment in which health-related choices are made and interpersonal interactions occur.[3] Workplace policies, formal and informal, affect access to healthy foods, time and facilities to be physically active, and places to use tobacco. In the United States, most adults under the age of 65 obtain health insurance through an employer (their own or a family member's), so the workplace also impacts access to health care. Employers, especially those providing and paying for health insurance, have an incentive to address health behavior across levels of the socioecological model in order to increase the health and productivity of their workforce and potentially contain health insurance costs. Table 25.1 shows examples of how the workplace can impact health behavior across different levels of the socioecological model, using both clinical and lifestyle behaviors as examples.

Workplaces are not all created equal in their willingness, capacity, and resources to implement health promotion programs. Thus, in spite of the range of opportunities available to worksites to support the health of their employees, we see tremendous variation in the amount and effectiveness of health promotion programs that workplaces implement. These differences are often driven in part by the resources available to the workplace, such that workplaces in industries with low profit margins offer fewer health promotion opportunities to their employees. As these employees are more likely to be in low-wage jobs, these differences in health promotion opportunities at and through the workplace have the potential to exacerbate health disparities.

The term "workplace health promotion (WHP) programs" is used broadly here, to refer to a variety of benefit, communication, policy, and program approaches. To aid readers, it is useful to define and distinguish among employers, workplaces, and worksites. *Employers* are organizations, public or private, with employees. A *workplace* includes not only the physical location of work, but also the social, cultural, and policy environment created by an employer. More broadly defined workplaces, often with multiple locations, are deliberately differentiated from more narrowly defined physical *worksites*, the locations where employees actually work.

This chapter first addresses the current state of WHP practice and research. It describes how current WHP programs are structured, which employers are most likely to offer such programs, whether the programs are evidence-based, and who the key players are. This sets the stage for describing dissemination and implementation challenges specific to evidence-based WHP programs. It then provides an overview of dissemination and implementation research in workplace health promotion. The chapter closes with two case studies, one focused on a large employer's approach to WHP and the other focused on disseminating evidence-based interventions (EBIs) to small workplaces. Occupational health and safety research is beyond the scope of this chapter;

TABLE 25.1 WORKPLACE HEALTH BEHAVIOR INTERVENTION EXAMPLES ACROSS SOCIOECOLOGICAL MODEL LEVELS

Socioecological Model Level	Definition	Clinical Example: Influenza Vaccination	Lifestyle Example: Physical Activity
Intrapersonal	Characteristics of the individual such as knowledge, attitudes, skills, etc.	Small media promoting flu shots	Workplace provides information about physical activity guidelines
Interpersonal	Formal and informal social network and social support systems, including family, work group, and friends	Managers communicate vaccination opportunities to their direct reports	Workplace sponsors team physical activity program or challenge
Institutional	Social institutions with organizational characteristics, and formal and informal rules and regulations for operation	On-site flu shot clinics, to maximize convenience of vaccination for employees	Workplace offers on-site physical activity facilities and/or subsidized gym memberships
Community	Relationships among organizations, institutions, and informal networks	Workplace partners with local pharmacies and visiting nurse services to maximize opportunities for vaccination	Workplace promotes and holds events at nearby community parks, YMCAs, or other locations that support physical activity
Public Policy	Local, state, and national laws and policies	Employer-sponsored health insurance covers flu shots with no co-pays, under the Affordable Care Act	Incentives to be physically active/discounts on health insurance premiums allowed under the Affordable Care Act

however, it briefly addresses Total Worker Health, which aims to integrate occupational health and safety with WHP.[4,5]

CURRENT STATE OF WORKPLACE HEALTH PROMOTION

The state of WHP was well described in 2012 in a RAND Corporation review commissioned by the U.S. Departments of Labor and Health and Human Services as part of planning for implementation of the Affordable Care Act.[6] This section summarizes and builds on the RAND findings to answer six questions related to the current state of WHP programs: How are WHP programs structured? Which employers have the programs? Who administers the programs? Are the programs evidence-based? Do the programs save money? What role do

industry organizations, governmental agencies, and regulators play?

The RAND review included a systematic literature review, a national survey of employers, employer case studies, and an analysis of claims data.[6] Because the RAND review is several years old, the authors use more recent employer-survey results where available. At least four entities survey employers annually about their health insurance and health promotion offerings: the Kaiser Family Foundation and Health Research & Educational Trust (KFF/HRET),[7,8] the National Business Group on Health and Willis Towers Watson,[9] Mercer,[10] and PriceWaterhouseCoopers.[11] Greatest use was made of the KFF/HRET survey because it is recent, has a large sample size (1,687 responders in 2016), has broad employer-size coverage (three or more workers), and provides detailed description of its methods.

How are WHP Programs Structured?

There is no consensus on a classification system for the components of WHP programs,[6] but the Workplace Health Model from the CDC (Figure 25.1) offers a comprehensive, systematic, and stepwise framework with four intuitive components: *assessment, planning and management, implementation, and evaluation.*[12] The *assessment* component measures the current state at three levels: individual (e.g., demographics, health risks, and use of preventive care), organization (e.g., workplace infrastructure, current practices, and environment), and community (e.g., transportation, parks and recreation). Aggregate, national information on employers' assessment at the individual level comes from the 2016 KFF/HRET survey, which found that 33% of employers offer a health risk assessment to measure employee behaviors, and that 22% offer biometric screening through blood collection or measurement of physical attributes like body mass index.[8] Little or no aggregate information was found on how many employers assess at the organization or community levels, though there are comprehensive organization-assessment tools available for free: e.g., the CDC Worksite Health ScoreCard,[13] the Health Enhancement Research Organization Scorecard,[14] and the National Business Group on Health Wellness Impact Scorecard.[15]

The *planning and management* component assures readiness for implementation by addressing five infrastructural needs: leadership support, management capacity, dedicated resources, communications capacity, and a plan for workplace health improvement. As with organization-level assessment, we found little information on the extent of use of this component, though the organization-level assessment tools discussed[13–16] provide some or all of this information to users. In the communications area, the 2014 KFF/HRET survey found that 39% of employers (with three or more employees and health insurance benefits) offered web-based resources for healthy living, and 34% had a wellness newsletter;[7] the KFF/HRET survey no longer collects this information.

The *implementation* component includes health-promoting processes in four areas: programs (e.g., group walks), benefits (e.g., coverage or provision of influenza vaccination), environmental support (e.g., on-site exercise facilities), and policies (e.g., prohibition of tobacco use in the workplace). The 2014 KFF/HRET survey found that 74% of employers had offerings in at least one of these areas.[7] Programs offered included lifestyle or behavioral coaching (23% of employers), nutrition classes (20%), smoking

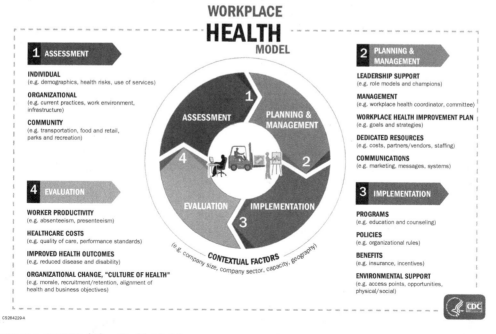

FIGURE 25.1 CDC Workplace Health Model.

cessation (27%), and weight loss (19%). In the benefits area, 53% offered influenza vaccinations. In the environmental-support area, 28% offered gym membership discounts or on-site exercise facilities. The KFF/HRET survey does not report on policies. The authors' 2012 national survey of mid-sized employers (100–4,999 employees) in low-wage industries found that 48% had a written policy about tobacco use in the workplace.[17]

The *evaluation* component measures outcomes in four areas: worker productivity, health care costs, improved health, and organizational culture. The RAND review concluded that formal program *evaluation* is rare.[6]

Which Employers Have WHP Programs?

The offerings and comprehensiveness of WHP programs increase with employer size. In 2016, the KFF/HRET survey[8] found that, among employers offering health-insurance benefits, large employers (200 or more workers) were significantly more likely than small employers (3–199 workers) to offer each of the program components covered by the survey: health risk assessments (59% vs. 32%, large vs. small), biometric screening (53% vs 20%), smoking cessation programs (74% vs 37%), weight-loss programs (68% vs 33%), and lifestyle/behavioral coaching (73% vs 36%). Offerings also increased stepwise with employer size, for example, 34% of employers with 3 to 49 workers offered smoking cessation programs, as did 58% of those with 50 to 199 workers, 72% of those with 200 to 999 workers, 82% of those with 1,000 to 4,999 workers, and 89% of those with 5,000 or more workers. The U.S. Department of Health and Human Services also periodically surveys employers about their offerings and measures program comprehensiveness[18] by asking about five elements: health education, supportive social and physical environment, integration, linkage to related programs, and worksite screening. Here again, there are significant differences by size; in 2004, 4.6% of employers with 50 to 99 workers offered programs with all five elements, while 24.1% of employers with 750 or more workers did.

The 2016 KFF/HRET survey[8] also found significant differences in offerings by industry. For example, 20% of employers in finance, retail, and wholesale offer weight-loss programs, compared with 52% of employers in health care and state and local government. In between, 34% of employers in the service industry offer weight-loss programs, as do 40% in agriculture,

communications, construction, manufacturing, mining, transportation, and utilities.

Who Administers the Programs?

It is difficult to find comprehensive information on who administers WHP programs. The KFF/HRET survey last asked this question in 2014, found that employers rely heavily on their health plans, and found that reliance on health plans is inversely related to employer size.[7] Among employers offering both health insurance and a wellness program, 74% of those with 3 to 24 workers said that most wellness benefits are provided by their health plan, as did 77% of those with 25 to 199 workers, 56% of those with 200 to 999 workers, 47% of those with 1,000 to 4,999 workers, and 46% of those with 5,000 or more workers.

The other administrators of WHP programs are the employers themselves and vendors.[6] A growing wellness industry[6] includes vendors ranging from those offering a full range of services to those that are highly specialized, for example, those conducting health risk assessments only, or those offering HRAs along with web-based lifestyle-management tools. The vendors serving large employers are relatively few in number and often serve a national market.[6] The vendors serving small and midsized employers not surprisingly serve more local markets. For example, in 2015, the authors identified 13 vendors serving small and midsized employers in Washington State; nine of these were based in the state.[19] Three recent trends were revealed from a national survey of large health plans and vendors offering WHP.[20] First, the workplace-wellness industry is becoming more diverse and competitive. Second, there is an increased focus on affecting employee health by modifying workplace culture. Third, employers are increasingly interested in assessing broad measures of program value beyond reduction of health care costs; these measures include employee retention, job satisfaction, and productivity.

Employers usually purchase WHP and other insurance services via intermediaries.[21] The intermediaries used most commonly by large employers are consulting firms[21] such as Mercer and the others listed earlier as conducting annual surveys. The intermediaries used most commonly by small and mid-sized employers are insurance brokers.[21] These brokers are served by a national organization, the National Association of Health Underwriters, and operate under state regulation that varies dramatically from state to state; we know very little about how they sell WHP services (www.nahu.org). Small and mid-sized employers also commonly purchase health insurance in groups via aggregators such as chambers of commerce and trade associations.[22] A Washington State study indicated that these groups are receptive to purchasing work health promotion services but perceive little demand from their employer members.[22]

Are the Programs Evidence Based?

The RAND review of the evidence concluded that WHP programs can sustainably reduce unhealthy behaviors such as smoking, and increase healthy behaviors such as physical activity and weight control.[6] The RAND review did not find evidence that these programs aid cholesterol control.

Another way to look at the evidence base for WHP programs is to look at systematic reviews of WHP interventions, as well as interventions tested elsewhere and applicable to workplace settings. The CDC's *Guide to Community Preventive Services* has conducted systematic reviews and recommends the following five interventions specifically for the workplace:[23] health assessments with feedback and health education; on-site, reduced-cost, actively promoted influenza vaccinations; tobacco-cessation incentives and competitions combined with additional interventions; tobacco-free policies; and weight control programs. The Community Guide found insufficient evidence to support three interventions: health assessments alone; off-site, actively promoted influenza vaccinations; and tobacco-cessation incentives and competitions alone. Other Community Guide recommendations, such as those for promoting cancer screening and group physical activity programs, are also applicable in the workplace.[24,25] A recent systematic review of Total Worker Health interventions combining both health protection and health promotion identified 16 studies with significantly improved health promotion outcomes, including smoking, weight, cholesterol, and physical activity.[26]

In the international context, the Cochrane Collaboration lists eight systematic reviews of interventions for primary or secondary prevention in the workplace (http://www.cochranelibrary.com/cochrane-database-of-systematic-reviews/index.html). Interventions with at least low-quality evidence of effectiveness include: increased worker control of work

scheduling to improve health outcomes, including sleep; workplace provision of smoking cessation medications and counseling; workplace-based deposit-refund incentive programs to promote smoking cessation; sit-stand desks to reduce sitting; and workplace HIV voluntary counseling and testing programs to increase testing and decrease risky sexual behaviors and sexually transmitted infections. Interventions with insufficient evidence of effectiveness include: workplace pedometer interventions for physical activity, support of breastfeeding for employed women, and workplace programs aimed at increasing commuting by walking or cycling.

Although the RAND review concluded that the evidence supports the effectiveness of WHP programs, neither it nor any source we found identified the proportion of current WHP interventions that are evidence-based.

Do Employees Participate in the Programs?

For WHP programs to be maximally effective, employees must participate in them, and the RAND review found that participation is often low.[6] Even though health assessments do not change behaviors on their own, many employers use them as gateways to participation. The 2016 KFF/HRET survey found that 41% of employees in large companies (≥200 employees) complete the offered health assessments (small companies were not asked this question).[8] The 2012 RAND survey of employers looked at participation in other program components and found lower levels: 21% for fitness, 16% for disease management, 11% for weight management, and 7% for smoking cessation (among smokers only).[6]

Many employers are providing employees incentives to increase these low participation levels. The 2016 KFF/HRET survey found that, among large companies, 54% offer an incentive for health-assessment completion, 59% for biometric screening, and 42% for participation in wellness programs.[8] Common incentive offerings include lowered premium contributions, reduced cost sharing, cash, gift cards, merchandise, and contributions to health savings accounts and health retirement accounts.[8] The RAND review concluded that incentives, particularly above $50, are effective in promoting health assessments and biometric screening.[6] On the other hand, it concluded that evidence supporting use of incentives for participation in wellness programs is weak.

Factors Influencing Program Effectiveness

The RAND review ended with five key factors associated with program effectiveness: (1) use of existing resources and relationships, (2) leadership engagement at all levels,(3) effective communication strategies, (4) opportunity for employees to engage, and (5) continuous evaluation.[6] These five factors somewhat echo the seven factors identified by Goetzel et al. in their 2008 review of the literature on WHP programs of large employers: (a) integrating WHP programs into the organization's central operations; (b) addressing individual, environmental, policy, and cultural factors affecting health and productivity; (c) targeting several health issues simultaneously; (d) tailoring programs to address specific needs of the population; (e) attaining high participation rates; (f) rigorously evaluating outcomes; and (g) effectively communicating these outcomes to key stakeholders.[27] Both point toward the importance of taking advantage of the workplace as a socioecological environment that can operate at both interpersonal and institutional levels to effect employee behavior change.

Do the Programs Save Money?

Reviews of cost evaluations of WHP programs have largely concluded that these programs, if well implemented, can provide a positive return on investment (ROI), both in lowered health care costs and increased worker productivity. A recent meta-analysis of 22 published studies by Baicker et al. found a 3.27 ROI in reduced health care costs and a 2.73 ROI in reduced absenteeism.[28] The RAND review included an analysis of claims data and found a small, statistically insignificant downward trend in health care costs in program participants.[6] The RAND review pointed out that very few programs are evaluated for effectiveness, or effects on health care cost or employer productivity, and cautioned about generalizing from limited findings.

Since the RAND review, the cost-effectiveness of WHP programs has been the subject of heated debate,[29,30] much of it driven by concerns over the potentially coercive nature and large size of the program-participation incentives authorized by the Affordable Care Act.[6,31] A careful look at the findings from Baicker's meta-analysis suggests that employers looking for savings in health care costs from WHP programs need to be realistic about the size of the potential savings. Baicker found that employers spent $144 per employee per year on WHP. Multiplying this expenditure by a 3.27 ROI yields $471 in annual savings in health care costs, substantial but small compared with the $18,142 in annual premiums for family coverage for employer-sponsored health insurance.[8] In addition to these savings in health care costs, employers can expect a similar, additional return from productivity gains.[28]

What Role Do Industry Organizations, Governmental Agencies, and Regulators Play?

The US workplace wellness industry is often estimated to generate $6 billion in annual revenue,[32] but it is loosely organized and largely unregulated. There is no national trade association of vendors, though there is a small professional association, the International Association for Worksite Health Promotion. There are two prominent annual conferences serving the industry in the United States. One is the Art and Science of Health Promotion Conference (www.health-promotionconference.com), and the other is organized by the Health Enhancement Research Organization (hero-health.org). Largely in response to the Affordable Care Act, the CDC has developed the Workplace Health Model (see Figure 25.1),[12] an organization-level assessment tool,[13] and a research network, but this work has recently been curtailed because of loss of Congressional funding support. Another federal agency, the National Institute for Occupational Safety and Health, part of the CDC, has developed its Total Worker Health approach, which supplements its traditional focus on health protection in the workplace with a new emphasis on health promotion,[5] though it is evolving.[4] The industry regulator is the National Committee for Quality Assurance, a private nonprofit organization that has developed its Wellness & Health Promotion Accreditation (www.ncqa.org/Portals/0/Programs/Recognition/wellness-web.pdf). To receive accreditation, health insurers and vendors are assessed on 12 infrastructure standards, such as the ability to maintain privacy and confidentiality, and 10 process-oriented performance measures, such as employee participation. To be accredited, insurers and vendors must pay a fee, so the number of accredited organizations is small and largely limited to those serving national employers.

DISSEMINATION AND IMPLEMENTATION CHALLENGES SPECIFIC TO WORKPLACE SETTINGS

"Workplace" describes a diverse array of settings, resources, job activities, and workforce characteristics. At one end of the spectrum, there are large employers with multiple locations and employees in the thousands. At the other end of the spectrum, there are small independent businesses that may only have a single location and less than five employees. The nature of job activities can vary both within and across workplaces, and may impact the health interests of employers and employees. For example, employers with a sedentary workforce may be interested in physical activity and/or weight management; in contrast, employers with employees in physically active and demanding jobs often display little interest in increasing their employees' physical activity. Employers who retain employees for the long term and have an aging workforce are likely to prioritize chronic disease prevention and management. Employers with a young and/or high-turnover workforce may lack interest in chronic diseases and be more willing to address health issues that affect their short-term costs, such as influenza vaccination and tobacco use.[33] Many employers face substantial logistical challenges to adopting and implementing WHP. These include employees spread across multiple worksites, employees without access to computers at work, and employees with limited English proficiency.[34,35] Smaller employers may find these challenges more difficult to address, given their limited capacity for WHP.[34]

OVERVIEW OF DISSEMINATION AND IMPLEMENTATION RESEARCH IN WORKPLACE SETTINGS

There are far fewer studies specific to disseminating and implementing evidence-based WHP programs than studies investigating the effectiveness of new programs. Drawing from key constructs in the dissemination and implementation literature, several factors are covered next that may influence dissemination and implementation of effective WHP programs. These factors include employers' and employees' needs and motivations to adopt health promotion programs; workplace readiness and capacity to adopt programs; the extent to which effective programs are actively disseminated, offer implementation support, and can be adapted to fit workplace needs; and the extent to which effective programs are sustained.

Employer and Employee Motivations to Adopt WHP Programs

Employers and employees may have different motivations and interests in WHP programs. One of employers' primary motivations to adopt these programs is containing health care costs.[29] Much of the controversy cited hinges on health care cost ROI as *the* metric of WHP success. The authors find additional motivations for WHP in their work with employers, including recruitment and retention of employees, improving employee productivity, improving morale, and reducing employee turnover. Some also cite altruistic motives, wishing to implement WHP programs to help improve employees' health, or generally believing it's the right thing to do.[34,36] One of these studies was replicated with employers in Kansas, and found similar motives—reducing health care costs, improving employee health, and improving productivity.[37] As noted, employee participation in programs is often low. A common approach is to deliver incentives for participation, but a first step is to discover whether employees see programs as relevant to their needs. The topics most wellness programs address are aligned with behaviors that employees need to change, want to change, and are actively trying to change. These behaviors include healthy eating, physical activity, weight management/loss, and to a lesser extent, smoking cessation and stress management.[35,38,39] Another important topic is the strategy the programs employ to address these behaviors. We find that employees in low-wage jobs often place strong emphasis on the need for convenience and on-site resources (for example, the importance of offering flu shots on-site rather than using pharmacy vouchers, even if both are free),[33,35] which is consistent with the Community Guide review on effective workplace interventions.[23]

Readiness and Capacity to Implement Effective WHP Programs

Readiness at the organizational level is characterized in Weiner's theory of organizational readiness to change.[40] The theory identifies two facets of readiness for change: change commitment (a shared resolve among organizational members to implement a change) and change efficacy (a shared belief among organizational members that they have a collective capability to implement a change). Change commitment and change efficacy are influenced by change valence (how much organizational members value the proposed change) and informational assessment (organizational members' perceptions of the tasks and resources needed to implement the change). Change valence and informational assessment are predicted by contextual factors, such as the organizational culture, resources, and past experiences with change. Change commitment and change efficacy predict change-related effort, which in turn predicts implementation success.

Small and medium-sized worksites exhibit less readiness and capacity for WHP than larger worksites; we also see differences by industry.[17,41] These differences in readiness and capacity may explain differences in implementation between smaller and larger worksites described earlier. However, there are limited tools to measure readiness and capacity for worksite health promotion. A simple three-item index measuring the presence or absence of (1) a wellness budget, (2) a paid staff position (part-time or full-time) for wellness, and (3) a wellness committee is strongly associated with current WHP implementation in small and medium-sized workplaces in low-wage industries.[17,41] The authors developed a readiness and capacity measurement tool based on Weiner's theory[41] and are assessing whether it predicts implementation success. Developing readiness and capacity tools with predictive validity would be a key facilitator to successfully implementing effective programs, as it would allow researchers and practitioners to (a) identify the workplaces ready to implement programs and (b) offer guidance to less-ready workplaces interested in implementing programs.

Adapting WHP Programs to Fit Different Workplace Contexts

Effective WHP programs need to be adapted to fit various workplace populations and contexts, but often there is little guidance on how to make adaptations without compromising the core elements that make the program effective. Many programs are tested via rigorous randomized controlled trials that have strict participation criteria; workplaces willing to participate in such trials are often not representative of workplaces in general.[42] One study examined "beta testing" as a critical step in disseminating a program for firefighters.[43] The PHLAME program showed positive impact on healthy eating, well-being, and reduced weight gain.[44] Elliot and colleagues beta-tested the PHLAME program with six sites following the successful trial. They define beta testing as selecting new adopters to try the program, reporting their experience, and using these findings to adapt the program. The original program was designed to take place over 12 months. However, in the course of working with six sites (each of which had multiple units, fire stations), the researchers found that few could maintain enthusiasm over 12 months and few completed all sessions. Thus, the researchers made a major adaptation—they shortened the intervention to 3 months. The beta test phase uncovered additional insights about the most effective change agents for the PHLAME program and effective strategies for enrolling new sites. This study makes a compelling case for using beta testing as a strategy to learn how to market and adapt an intervention for dissemination to an audience that will likely be different than the original testing audience.

Sustainability of WHP Programs

Maintenance is a key aspect of successful implementation. NIH is placing increasing emphasis on studying sustainability as part of dissemination and implementation research,[45] yet few articles were found studying whether WHP programs were sustained long-term. One study examined whether tobacco control activities were sustained for 2 years following the intervention period. In general, tobacco control activities were not sustained 2 years later.[46] In contrast, the Seattle 5 a Day study showed small positive effects on fruit and vegetable intake after 2 years with no intervention contact.[47] The first case study is an example of a WHP program that a large employer has sustained and grown over the course of decades. We need more research that helps us understand which programs are sustainable, and which conditions promote sustainability of WHP programs.

RESEARCH GAPS AND DIRECTIONS FOR THE FUTURE

There are many WHP interventions and programs that have a significant, positive impact on workplace culture of health and employees' health behavior. Yet, as noted earlier, the majority of workplaces do not have a comprehensive WHP program in place. There are almost six million employers in the United States; 89% have fewer than 20 employees[48] and have limited capacity to adopt and implement evidence-based health promotion programs. A common strategy is to work through intermediaries, especially to reach smaller employers. Research on how to best collaborate with employers and intermediaries is limited. Several intermediaries and vendors in the authors' region were not interested in working with smaller employers on health promotion.[22] A separate study found a disconnect between small employers' and intermediaries' perceptions of who small employers are connected with and what would motivate them to participate in a program about preventing workplace violence.[49] As noted, employers rely on their insurers for much of their WHP programs and resources, especially small employers.[7] The authors partnered with two insurers to help recruit small employers to our studies,[24] and referrals from insurers were more successful than cold calls.[50] We need more research on effective partnerships to reach small and mid-sized employers with evidence-based health promotion.

Across all sizes and types of workplaces, there are several phases of adopting and implementing WHP. First, employers must be motivated to adopt WHP (this is often assumed, but often employers are not motivated to adopt WHP). Second, employers have to be able to choose sound, evidence-based programs that fit the health needs of their workforce. Ideally, these choices are informed by assessments of their employees, their organizational resources, and the resources in the community, as in CDC's Workplace Health Model.[12] Many employers lack access to data about their employees' health and health behaviors, and lack capacity to assess organizational and community resources. This lack of capacity may limit their awareness of available programs and their ability to evaluate available programs. Thus, they often rely on their insurers, brokers, and consultants to tell them what's best. Third, they have to successfully implement the programs. Fourth, employees have to be aware of the programs, resources, or policies and actually take advantage of them. Fifth, employers have to sustain these efforts for the long term, and their motivation to do so often wanes if they see only a few employees participating, do not evaluate program success, or do not see the changes they want. There are relatively few studies looking at all of these steps, except for case studies that usually focus on very large employers.

CASE STUDY 1: IMPLEMENTING AND EVALUATING WHP AT JOHNSON & JOHNSON

Background

The first case study is the workplace health program at Johnson & Johnson, a large, publicly owned, multinational manufacturer of medical devices and consumer and pharmaceutical products, with 125,000 employees in 60 countries.[51] The Johnson & Johnson program is profiled because it is one of the best known and longest running in the United States.[52] The program has been the site of substantial implementation research on program effectiveness and cost-effectiveness.[52-54] It is also often cited by those trying to disseminate effective implementation practices to others.[27,28]

Johnson & Johnson has a long history of corporate social responsibility embodied in "The Credo" developed by one of its three founding brothers, Robert Wood Johnson, who also founded his namesake foundation, the largest philanthropic organization dedicated to health and health care in the United States.[55] "The Credo" included a strong commitment to employee health and safety.[51] That commitment persists and today is embodied in Johnson & Johnson's "Culture of Health,"[56] a strong part of the company's overall organizational culture.

History

In 1979, Johnson & Johnson's chief executive officer, James Burke, created the "Live for Life" program to make Johnson & Johnson's employees "the healthiest in the world."[53] The program had two goals: (1) to provide employees with information about, and programs to control, their behavioral health risks, and (2) to provide employees with health care as efficiently as possible.[52] The program was voluntary and enrolled a minority of employees. Evaluations in the 1980s compared participants and nonparticipants and thus risked selection bias.[52] Nevertheless, they concluded that the program "was associated with improved employee health, reduced inpatient health care spending, decreased employee absenteeism, and better employee attitudes."[53]

In 1995, Johnson & Johnson dramatically increased employee participation to approximately 90% by offering a $500 credit toward health insurance premiums to those employers who participated in the health assessment and followed up with targeted health improvement programs.[52] In 2002, an external evaluation compared health care utilization of nearly 9,000 participating employees 4 years before and 5 years after program enrollment[54] and found lowered inpatient use, fewer mental health visits, and fewer outpatient visits, resulting in health care savings of $225 per employee per year. Employee participation in programs continued at a high level, in the range of 80% to 85%,[52] and there was evidence of long-term change in risk factors. Between the periods 1995–1999 and 2007–2010, sedentariness decreased from 39% to 20.8%, tobacco use from 12% to 3.8%, hypertension prevalence from 14% to 6.1%, and high cholesterol from 19% to 5.7%.[52]

The most recent external evaluation for the period 2002–2008 attempted to remove selection bias by comparing the health care costs of Johnson & Johnson employees to propensity-matched employees at 16 other large, self-insured manufacturing companies.[53] The annual growth rate in health care spending was 3.7% lower at Johnson & Johnson compared with the other companies, and the prevalence of health risks was lower for hypertension, poor nutrition, obesity, physical inactivity, and tobacco use, but not for mental health issues including alcohol use, depression, and stress.

The Johnson & Johnson program has become increasingly comprehensive and integrated with other health-related services. In 2013, the program included: offerings related to improving physical activity (such as on-site fitness centers, reimbursement for exercise expenditures, a pedometer program, and seasonal fitness challenges), guidance on nutrition (offering healthy cafeteria choices and online weight-management tools, and subsidizing Weight Watcher's membership), lifestyle management, computerized coaching programs (health coaching for blood pressure management, tobacco cessation, and blood lipid control), and chronic disease management.[52] Today, there are 12 "Culture of Health" program components: "tobacco free, HIV policy, health profile, employee assistance, physical activity, healthy eating, medical surveillance, health promotion, stress and energy management, cancer awareness, return-to-work, and travel health."[56]

Implications

Because it is a single company, the nearly four-decade experience at Johnson & Johnson provides more insights on implementation than dissemination. Although the published research on even the Johnson & Johnson program provides fewer implementation details than one might want, the program seems to have addressed all five factors that the RAND review found contribute to program effectiveness.[6] First, the program is integrated into operations and represents a remarkable investment—up to $300 per employee annually, totaling tens of millions of dollars since 1979.[53] Second, there has been leadership engagement throughout the organization, with a strong emphasis on a culture of wellness. Third, there has been substantial communication. Fourth, employee engagement has been high, though there have been ups and downs. Employee participation was very high in the 1990s. In 2010, however, only 30% of employees completed a health assessment and "knew their numbers"; in 2015, that proportion had risen to 92%.[56] Fifth, there has been frequent evaluation and reformulation. This attention to implementation has resulted in substantial payoff--all evaluations have shown behavior change, with health care savings, and positive return on investment.

CASE STUDY 2: DISSEMINATING EVIDENCE-BASED PROGRAMS TO SMALL WORKSITES VIA HEALTHLINKS

Background

Employers that are most likely to offer worksite health promotion programs are those with 1,000 or more employees,[18,57,58] yet most employers are smaller.[59] Small worksites face two major barriers in adopting and implementing evidence-based programs for their employees: (1) lack of information needed to find, choose, and adapt programs for their worksites; and (2) lack of resources required to implement programs. Small employers need help in selecting programs, and they need programs that are low cost or free and take little time to implement.

Despite the challenges described, many evidence-based programs spanning several health behaviors are feasible for small worksites. The Community Guide lists evidence-based strategies for cancer screening, healthy eating, physical activity, and tobacco cessation that worksites can adopt and implement.[60-64] Many of these are policy and environmental changes. The evidence is mixed on whether policy and environmental changes at the worksite are sufficient to change employees' health behaviors, but does suggest that these changes combined with other programs are effective.[65] All 50 states provide breast and cervical cancer screening and treatment free-of-charge for low-income and uninsured women, as well as telephone quitlines for tobacco cessation for smokers. These programs are underused, serving only a small proportion of those eligible to receive these services.[66,67] Very few worksites promote these services.[68,69]

HealthLinks Intervention and Research to-Date

The American Cancer Society and the Health Promotion Research Center (HPRC) at the University of Washington collaborated to develop and test *HealthLinks* as a means to disseminate evidence-based programs to small employers and provide implementation assistance. The HPRC Dissemination and Implementation Framework[70] guides our partnership and dissemination research activities. Worksites participating in *HealthLinks* complete activities with the assistance of a trained interventionist. In the Assessment phase, the interventionist measures current worksite implementation of cancer screening, nutrition, physical activity, and tobacco cessation programs. In the Recommendations phase, the interventionist creates a tailored *Recommendations Report* and delivers the report in a face-to-face meeting with the employer. At the *Recommendations Report* meeting, the interventionist provides *Implementation Toolkits* for each of the recommended programs. During the *Implementation Phase*, the employer begins adopting the recommended programs and promoting them to employees. The interventionist contacts worksites at least once per month by email or telephone during this phase to offer implementation assistance.

ACS and the HPRC have collaborated on three *HealthLinks* studies, and the intervention period ranges from 6 to 15 months across these studies.[24,71,72] The primary outcome is worksite-level adoption and implementation of evidence-based programs. We measure programs by asking several questions about each one, and then using a scoring algorithm to calculate a score ranging from 0% to 100% implementation for each program. A total implementation score is also created, also on a 0% to 100% scale. In each *HealthLinks* study, total worksite implementation increased at least 20% (absolute) from baseline to follow-up.[71,72]

Lessons Learned

One of the core elements of *HealthLinks* is in-person (and telephone and email) assistance

from a trained interventionist. *HealthLinks* is offered as a free service, and this in-person component makes scale-up challenging. The authors are pilot-testing a training model in which local health department staff members (for example, health educators and public health nurses) are distance-trained to deliver *HealthLinks* to worksites in their communities. Staff from several local health departments in Washington State were trained and they have been successfully recruiting worksites in their communities and helping them adopt and implement EBIs through *HealthLinks*. The authors are now exploring paths are now being explored for national scale-up of this model.

Recruiting worksites is a consistent challenge. There are three reasons many small worksites hesitate to engage with *HealthLinks*. First, there are often contextual issues at play in the worksite: its mission may not include health and well-being, its workforce may be perceived as young and healthy, and its employee turnover may be so great that the business case for preventing future chronic diseases may seem weak. Second, for many small employers, capacity for wellness is so low that even taking the time to participate in a free wellness program may seem impossible. Third, there is always a research component that requires, at minimum, a follow-up assessment of whether *HealthLinks* EBIs were adopted. Several WHP programs have recognition programs that reward employers for higher levels of EBI implementation.[16] The authors pilot-tested a recognition program with two of the local health departments with which they did *HealthLinks*, and it motivated many employers to complete evaluation and aim to "level-up" to the next recognition tier on future assessments.

Implications for Practitioners, Policymakers, and Researchers

HealthLinks disseminates a simple three-step process of implementing EBIs and provides free in-person assistance from a trained interventionist. One of the most frequent questions we receive is why not just make the whole program available online as a self-directed website. First, as noted, many such self-directed tools are already available. Second, employers who participate in *HealthLinks* say that the in-person assistance was the critical factor that helped them make changes. One of the key challenges for practice and research is to match the level of assistance given with the level needed for employers to be successful in implementing programs. The authors' partnership with the American Cancer Society and use of a specific dissemination and implementation framework helped build a program of research around small worksites that includes formative research with small employers and their employees, efficacy testing of *HealthLinks*, building out and testing additional implementation strategies such as wellness committees, and new partnerships to attempt scale-up.

SUMMARY

The workplace gives us an opportunity to reach more than 60% of adults in the United States with evidence-based health promotion. There is a lot of research on the effectiveness of specific WHP programs, but comparatively little research on disseminating and implementing effective WHP programs. There are many intriguing tensions in the world of WHP dissemination and implementation research. For example, there is a thriving for-profit workplace wellness industry offering health promotion interventions at a much quicker pace than that generally achieved by academic researchers. Many of these interventions are creative and appealing; fewer have evaluation results that are clearly vetted by outside experts. Most of the for-profit vendors are focused on working with large employers, and with good reason—they can reach large numbers of people more efficiently. Unfortunately, this focus on large employers leaves almost half of the workforce out, and that half is disproportionately at risk for health disparities. There are unique opportunities in WHP dissemination and implementation research for partnerships between academic researchers, employers, and both for-profit and not-for-profit vendors to identify (and create) effective WHP programs, tailor them to meet the needs and capacities of employers across size and industry categories, market them effectively, provide appropriate levels of implementation assistance, and evaluate impact and use the results to improve the programs and increase their reach.[70,73]

ACKNOWLEDGEMENTS

Development of this chapter was supported by cooperative agreement no. U48DP005013 from the Centers for Disease Control and Prevention. Additional support was provided by the James W. Mifflin University Professorship at the University of Washington.

SUGGESTED READINGS AND WEBSITES

Suggested Readings

Goetzel RZ, Henke RM, Tabrizi M, et al. Do workplace health promotion (wellness) programs work? *J Occup Environ Med.* 2014;56:927–964.

The authors summarize research evaluating the effectiveness of workplace health promotion programs, as well as the recent controversy over whether these programs are effective. They make several recommendations for employers considering adopting workplace health promotion programs.

Harris JR, Hannon PA, Beresford S, McClellan D, Linnan L. Health promotion in smaller workplaces in the United States. *Ann Rev Pub Health.* 2014;35:327–342.

This review paper summarizes research on small and medium-sized workplaces in the United States. The authors summarize the challenges smaller employers in identifying and implementing evidence-based wellness programs, and identify research and policy priorities for this large population of employers.

Mattke S, Liu H, Caloyeras JP, et al. *Workplace wellness programs study, final report.* Santa Monica, CA: RAND Corporation; 2013.

This federally commissioned state-of-the-art review of WHP programs includes a systematic literature review, a national survey of employers, employer case studies, and an analysis of claims data. It summarizes evidence of the effectiveness and cost-effectiveness of WHP programs and also focuses on the effectiveness of incentives for increasing employee participation.

Fonarow GC, Calitz C, Arena R, et al. Workplace wellness recognition for optimizing workplace health: a presidential advisory from the American Heart Association. *Circulation.* 2015;131(20):e480–e497.

This position statement by the American Heart Association compares and contrasts the tools that the Centers for Disease Control and Prevention, the Health Enhancement Research Organization, and the National Business Group on Health offer to assess organization-level implementation of WHP. It then surveys employer-recognition systems based on these and other assessments and announces the Association's new approach to assessment and recognition.

Sorensen G, Landsbergis P, Hammer L, et al. Preventing chronic disease at the workplace: a workshop report and recommendations. *Am J Public Health.* 2011;101:S196–S207.

This paper summarizes a workshop sponsored by CDC and NIH to identify research priorities to effectively reduce chronic disease risk. Workshop participants developed a conceptual framework and research agenda to integrate health promotion and disease protection in the workplace, as a means to preventing chronic disease.

Selected Websites and Tools

Centers for Disease Control and Prevention. Workplace Health Promotion. http://www.cdc. gov/workplacehealthpromotion/

This website provides information on CDC's workplace health promotion activities and tools. It includes their Workplace Health Model and Workplace Health Scorecard, both cited in this review, as well as links to evidence-based policies, programs, and communications; data and surveillance; and other tools and resources to support workplace health promotion practitioners and researchers.

Cochrane Database of Systematic Reviews. http:// www.cochranelibrary.com/cochrane-database-of- systematic-reviews/index.html

This searchable database of systematic reviews uses literature from global sources, including both high- income and lower-and-middle-income countries. At the time of writing of this chapter, there were eight reviews on primary and secondary prevention in workplace settings.

The Community Guide, Worksite Health. https://www. thecommunityguide.org/topic/worksite-health

This website summarizes the recommendations and systematic reviews related to workplace health promotion from CDC's Community Guide. Links are provided to stories from the field and other resources. It is worth exploring other topics on the Community Guide's website, as evidence-based strategies in other topic areas are often relevant to workplace health promotion. For example, several strategies for cancer screening (distributing small media or home test kits) can be implemented in the workplace.

Kaiser Family Foundation/Health Research and Education Trust. Employer Health Benefits Survey. http://kff.org/health-costs/report/ 2016-employer-health-benefits-survey/

This website summarizes the 2016 KFF/HRET survey. Links are provided to the full report, published articles, and interactive graphics that allow users to explore changes over time. Survey reports and resources from prior KFF/HRET surveys (1998–2015) are also available.

REFERENCES

1. McLeroy KR, Bibeau D, Steckler A, Glanz K. An ecological perspective on health promotion programs. *Health Educ Q.* 1988;15(4):351–377.

2. Labor force statistics from the Current Population Survey. 2016; http://data.bls.gov/timeseries/ LNS12300000. Accessed Oct 8, 2016.

3. Tabak RG, Hipp JA, Marx CM, Brownson RC. Workplace social and organizational environments and healthy-weight behaviors. *PLoS One.* 2015;10(4):e0125424.

4. Howard J, Chosewood LC, Hudson HL. The perils of integrating wellness and safety and health and the possibility of a worker-oriented alternative. *New Solut.* 2016;26:345–348.

5. Sorensen G, Landsbergis P, Hammer L, et al. Preventing chronic disease at the workplace: a workshop report and recommendations. *Am J Public Health.* 2011;101:S196–S207.

6. Mattke S, Liu H, Caloyeras JP, et al. *Workplace wellness programs study, final report.* Santa Monica, CA: RAND Corporation; 2013.

7. Kaiser Family Foundation and Health Research & Educational Trust. *Employer health benefits. 2014 annual survey.* Menlo Park, CA: Author; 2014.

8. Kaiser Family Foundation and Health Research & Educational Trust. *Employer health benefits. 2016 annual survey.* Menlo Park, CA: Author; 2016.

9. National Business Group on Health and Willis Towers Watson. *High-performance insights—best practices in health care.* Washington DC: National Business Group on Health; 2015.

10. Mercer. Living with Health Reform, 2016 employer survey. 2016; www.mercer.com/our-thinking/ health-care-reform-survey.html. Accessed Nov 10, 2016.

11. PriceWaterhouseCoopers. *Health and well-being touchstone survey results.* London: PriceWaterhouseCoopers; 2016.

12. Centers for Disease Control and Prevention. Workplace health model. www.cdc.gov/work-placehealthpromotion/pdf/workplacehealth-model-update.pdf. Accessed Nov 18, 2016.

13. Centers for Disease Control and Prevention. The CDC Worksite Health ScoreCard: an assessment tool for employers to prevent heart disease, stroke, and related health conditions. 2014; www.cdc. gov/dhdsp/pubs/docs/hsc_manual.pdf. Accessed Nov 21, 2016.

14. Health Enhancement Research Organization. HERO Scorecard. hero-health.org/scorecard. Accessed Nov 21, 2016.

15. National Business Group on Health. WISCORE, the wellness impact scorecard. https://www. businessgrouphealth.org/pub/?id=f316447f- 2354-d714-515f-e943301f22f0. Accessed Nov 21, 2016.

16. Fonarow GC, Calitz C, Arena R, et al. Workplace wellness recognition for optimizing workplace health: a presidential advisory from the American Heart Association. *Circulation.* 2015;131(20):e480–e497.

17. Hannon PA, Garson G, Harris JR, Hammerback K, Sopher CJ, Clegg-Thorp C. Workplace health promotion implementation, readiness, and capacity among midsize employers in low-wage

industries: a national survey. *J Occup Environ Med.* 2012;54(11):1337–1343.

18. Linnan L, Bowling M, Childress J, et al. Results of the 2004 National Worksite Health Promotion Survey. *Am J Public Health.* 2008;98(8):1503–1509.

19. Rooke, L. E. (2015). *An analysis of services offered by comprehensive wellness vendors in washington state* (Order No. 1600459). Available from Dissertations & Theses @ University of Washington WCLP; ProQuest Dissertations & Theses Global. (1732168264). Retrieved from https://search.pro-quest.com/docview/1732168264?accountid=14784.

20. Abraham J, White KM. Tracking The changing landscape of corporate wellness companies. *Health Aff (Millwood).* 2017;36(2):222–228.

21. Marquis MS, Long SH. Who helps employers design their health insurance benefits? *Health Aff (Millwood).* 2000;19(1):133–138.

22. Harris JR, Hammerback KR, Hannon PA, et al. Group purchasing of workplace health promotion services for small employers. *J Occup Environ Med.* 2014;56(7):765–770.

23. Task Force on Community Preventive Services. Guide to Community Preventive Services. www.thecommunityguide.org. Accessed Feb 9, 2017.

24. Hannon PA, Hammerback K, Allen CL, et al. HealthLinks randomized controlled trial: design and baseline results. *Contemp Clin Trials.* 2016;48:1–11.

25. Hannon PA, Harris JR. Interventions to improve cancer screening: opportunities in the workplace. *Am J Prev Med.* 2008;35(1 Suppl):S10–S13.

26. Anger KW, Elliot DL, Bodner T, et al. Effectiveness of Total Worker Health interventions. *J Occup Health Psychol.* 2015;20:226–247.

27. Goetzel RZ, Ozminkowski RJ. The health and cost benefits of work site health-promotion programs. *Annu Rev Public Health.* 2008;29:303–323.

28. Baicker K, Cutler D, Song Z. Workplace wellness programs can generate savings. *Health Aff (Millwood).* 2010;29(2):304–311.

29. Goetzel RZ, Henke RM, Tabrizi M, et al. Do workplace health promotion (wellness) programs work? *J Occup Environ Med.* 2014;56(9):927–934.

30. Lewis A, Khanna V, Montrose S. Workplace wellness produces no savings. 2014; healthaffairs.org/blog/2014/11/25/workplace-wellness-produces-no-savings/.

31. Consensus Statement of the Health Enhancement Research Organization, American College of Occupational and Environmental Medicine, American Cancer Society and American Cancer Society Cancer Action Network, American Diabetes Association, Americam Heart Association. Guidance for a reasonably designed, employer-sponsored wellness program using outcomes-based incentives. *J Occup Environ Med.* 2012;54(7):889–896.

32. RAND Corporation. Do workplace wellness programs save employers money? www.rand.org/content/dam/rand/pubs/research_briefs/RB9700/RB9744/RAND_RB9744.pdf. Accessed Nov 23, 2016.

33. Allen CL, Hammerback K, Harris JR, Hannon PA, Parrish AT. Feasibility of workplace health promotion for restaurant workers, Seattle, 2012. *Prev Chronic Dis.* 2015;12:E172.

34. Hannon PA, Hammerback K, Garson G, Harris JR, Sopher CJ. Stakeholder perspectives on workplace health promotion: a qualitative study of midsized employers in low-wage industries. *Am J Health Promot.* 2012;27(2):103–110.

35. Parrish A, Hammerback K, Hannon PA, Mason C, Wilkie MN, Harris JR. *Supporting the health of low socioeconomic status employees: qualitative perspectives from employees and large companies* (submitted manuscript, 2016). University of Washington.

36. Hughes MC, Patrick DL, Hannon PA, Harris JR, Ghosh DL. Understanding the decision-making process for health promotion programming at small to midsized businesses. *Health Promot Pract.* 2011;12(4):512–521.

37. Witt LB, Olsen D, Ablah E. Motivating factors for small and midsized businesses to implement worksite health promotion. *Health Promot Pract.* 2013;14(6):876–884.

38. Hammerback K, Hannon PA, Harris JR, Clegg-Thorp C, Kohn M, Parrish A. Perspectives on workplace health promotion among employees in low-wage industries. *Am J Health Promot.* 2015;29(6):384–392.

39. Kilpatrick M, Sanderson K, Blizzard L, et al. Workplace health promotion: what public-sector employees want, need, and are ready to change. *J Occup Environ Med.* 2014;56(6):645–651.

40. Weiner BJ. A theory of organizational readiness for change. *Implement Sci.* 2009;4:67.

41. Hannon PA, Helfrich CD, Chan KG, et al. Development and pilot test of the Workplace Readiness Questionnaire, a theory-based instrument to measure small workplaces' readiness to implement wellness programs. *Am J Health Promot.* 2017;31(1):67–75.

42. Glasgow RE, Klesges LM, Dzewaltowski DA, Bull SS, Estabrooks P. The future of health behavior change research: what is needed to improve translation of research into health promotion practice? *Ann Behav Med.* 2004;27(1):3–12.

43. Elliot DL, Kuehl KS, Goldberg L, DeFrancesco CA, Moe EL. Worksite health promotion in six varied US sites: beta testing as a needed

translational step. *J Environ Public Health.* 2011;2011:797646.

44. Elliot DL, Goldberg L, Kuehl KS, Moe EL, Breger RK, Pickering MA. The PHLAME (Promoting Healthy Lifestyles: Alternative Models' Effects) firefighter study: outcomes of two models of behavior change. *J Occup Environ Med.* 2007;49(2):204–213.

45. National Institutes of Health. Dissemination and Implementation. https://prevention.nih.gov/prevention-research/research-highlights/dissemination-and-implementation. Accessed Dec 1, 2016.

46. Sorensen G, Thompson B, Basen-Engquist K, et al. Durability, dissemination, and institutionalization of worksite tobacco control programs: results from the Working Well trial. *Int J Behav Med.* 1998;5(4):335–351.

47. Beresford SA, Thompson B, Bishop S, Macintyre J, McLerran D, Yasui Y. Long-term fruit and vegetable change in worksites: Seattle 5 a Day follow-up. *Am J Health Behav.* 2010;34(6):707–720.

48. United States Census Bureau. 2014 SUSB annual data tables by establishment industry. 2016; https://www.census.gov/data/tables/2014/econ/susb/2014-susb-annual.html. Accessed Dec 6, 2016.

49. Bruening RA, Strazza K, Nocera M, Peek-Asa C, Casteel C. How to engage small retail businesses in workplace violence prevention: perspectives from small businesses and influential organizations. *Am J Ind Med.* 2015;58(6):668–678.

50. Hammerback K, Hannon PA, Kohn MJ, Parrish A, Allen CL, Harris JR. *Comparing methods for recruiting small, low-wage worksites for community-based health promotion research.* (Unpublished manuscript. 2016). University of Washington.

51. About Johnson & Johnson. https://www.jnj.com/about-jnj. Accessed Dec 9, 2016.

52. Isaac F. A role for private industry: comments on the Johnson & Johnson's wellness program. *Am J Prev Med.* 2013;44(1 Suppl 1):S30–S33.

53. Henke RM, Goetzel RZ, McHugh J, Isaac F. Recent experience in health promotion at Johnson & Johnson: lower health spending, strong return on investment. *Health Affairs.* 2011;30(3):490–499.

54. Ozminkowski RJ, Ling D, Goetzel RZ, et al. Long-term impact of Johnson & Johnson's Health & Wellness Program on health care utilization and expenditures. *J Occup Environ Med.* 2002;44(1):21–29.

55. Robert Wood Johnson Foundation. www.rwjf.org. Accessed Dec 9, 2016.

56. Johnson & Johnson. Our strategic framework: culture of health. http://www.jnj.com/caring/citizenship-sustainability/strategic-framework/culture-of-health. Accessed Dec 9, 2016.

57. Bondi MA, Harris JR, Atkins D, French ME, Umland B. Employer coverage of clinical preventive services in the United States. *Am J Health Promot.* 2006;20(3):214–222.

58. Rosenthal MB, Landon BE, Normand SL, Frank RG, Ahmad TS, Epstein AM. Employers' use of value-based purchasing strategies. *JAMA.* 2007;298(19):2281–2288.

59. Harris JR, Lichiello PA, Hannon PA. Workplace health promotion in Washington State. *Prev Chronic Dis.* 2009;6(1):A29.

60. Hopkins DP, Razi S, Leeks KD, Priya Kalra G, Chattopadhyay SK, Soler RE. Smokefree policies to reduce tobacco use. A systematic review. *Am J Prev Med.* 2010;38(2 Suppl):S275–S289.

61. Sabatino SA, Lawrence B, Elder R, et al. Effectiveness of interventions to increase screening for breast, cervical, and colorectal cancers: nine updated systematic reviews for the guide to community preventive services. *Am J Prev Med.* 2012;43(1):97–118.

62. Soler RE, Leeks KD, Buchanan LR, Brownson RC, Heath GW, Hopkins DH. Point-of-decision prompts to increase stair use. A systematic review update. *Am J Prev Med.* 2010;38(2 Suppl):S292–S300.

63. Soler RE, Leeks KD, Razi S, et al. A systematic review of selected interventions for worksite health promotion. The assessment of health risks with feedback. *Am J Prev Med.* 2010;38(2 Suppl):S237–S262.

64. Anderson LM, Quinn TA, Glanz K, et al. The effectiveness of worksite nutrition and physical activity interventions for controlling employee overweight and obesity: a systematic review. *Am J Prev Med.* 2009;37(4):340–357.

65. Kahn-Marshall JL, Gallant MP. Making healthy behaviors the easy choice for employees: a review of the literature on environmental and policy changes in worksite health promotion. *Health Educ Behav.* 2012;39(6):752–776.

66. Finkelstein JB. Screening program serves fraction of those eligible. *J Natl Cancer Inst.* 2007;99(4):270–271.

67. Cummins SE, Bailey L, Campbell S, Koon-Kirby C, Zhu SH. Tobacco cessation quitlines in North America: a descriptive study. *Tob Control.* 2007;16 Suppl 1:i9–i15.

68. Boles M, Dowler D. *Washington State healthy worksite survey: Statewide results.* Salem, OR: Program Design and Evaluation Services, Oregon Dept of Human Services; 2007.

69. Hughes MC, Yette EM, Hannon PA, Harris JR, Tran NM, Reid TR. Promoting tobacco cessation

via the workplace: opportunities for improvement. *Tob Control.* 2011;20(4):305–308.

70. Harris JR, Cheadle A, Hannon PA, et al. A framework for disseminating evidence-based health promotion practices. *Prev Chronic Dis.* 2012;9:E22.

71. Hannon PA, Hammerback K, Teague S, et al. Employees' perceptions of evidence-based approaches to wellness in low-wage industries. Annual meeting of the American Public Health Association; November, 2014; New Orleans, LA

72. Laing SS, Hannon PA, Talburt A, Kimpe S, Williams B, Harris JR. Increasing evidence-based workplace health promotion best practices in small and low-wage companies, Mason County, Washington, 2009. *Prev Chronic Dis.* 2012;9:E83.

73. Kreuter MW, Bernhardt JM. Reframing the dissemination challenge: a marketing and distribution perspective. *Am J Public Health.* 2009;99(12):2123–2127.

26

Policy Dissemination Research

JONATHAN PURTLE, ELIZABETH A. DODSON,
AND ROSS C. BROWNSON

INTRODUCTION

Policies, in the form of laws and administrative regulations, have profound effects on population health. For example, a review of the 10 greatest public health achievements of the 20th century[1] shows that each was influenced by policy change, such as seat belt laws and regulations governing workplace exposures. In addition to physical health and safety, public policies have tremendous effects on population mental health by shaping the social determinants of mental health and the likelihood that a person has timely access to quality mental health services.[2] However, as noted in a 2016 National Academies report,[3] the development of public policy is extremely complex and the product of scientific, administrative, economic, social, and political forces and the inter-play of factors that influence policymakers' decisions are especially complicated.[4-7] Policy dissemination research seeks to understand these complexities and increase the likelihood that research evidence reaches policymakers and influences their decisions so that the population health benefits of scientific progress are maximized.

In this chapter, adapting the definition of dissemination research used in the 2016–2019 National Institutes of Health's dissemination and implementation (D&I) research program announcement, *we define policy dissemination research as the study of the targeted distribution of scientific evidence to policymakers to understand how to promote the adoption and sustainment of evidence-based policies.* This chapter focuses primarily on "Big P" policies (i.e., laws and administrative regulations) as opposed to "small p" policies (i.e., organizational policies and professional guidelines), although many of the same principles apply to either type of policy translation.[8,9] The term "policymaker" in this chapter refers to elected officials (e.g., legislators) and administrative officials (e.g., agency leaders in the executive branch of government) at federal, state, and local, but not organizational, levels.

This chapter is organized into several sections. First, it briefly discusses the state of policy dissemination research and defines two broad types of policy dissemination studies. Then, for context, it provides a high-level overview of evidence-based policymaking and challenges to integrating research evidence into policymaking processes. Then, it synthesizes information on theories, frameworks, methods, and measures that are used in policy dissemination research. Although an exhaustive review of policy dissemination research studies is beyond the scope of this chapter, it provides examples of such studies throughout each section. The chapter concludes by discussing future directions for policy dissemination research.

THE STATE OF POLICY DISSEMINATION RESEARCH

Policy dissemination research is relatively underdeveloped compared with other areas within the field of research in the United States. For example, a content analysis of all projects funded by the National Institutes of Health through D&I program announcements between 2007 and 2014 found that only 12 policy D&I projects had been funded, accounting for 8.2% of all projects.[14] Just four of these projects were focused on policy dissemination research. Although policy dissemination research can be considered an emerging area within the contemporary D&I enterprise in the United States, policy dissemination research is not a new field and is more developed in countries outside of the United States. Since at least the 1970s, social scientists (e.g., Carol Weiss, Nathan Caplan) have investigated the role research evidence plays in policymaking and how it can have a greater influence.[15-17] In countries such as Canada, Australia, and the United Kingdon, researchers in the field of knowledge transfer and exchange often focus on policymaker audiences. International journals such as *Evidence & Policy* and *Health Research Policy and Systems* are devoted to topics related to policy dissemination research, although the term is rarely, if ever, mentioned.

Policy dissemination studies can be classified according to two broad categories. First are *audience research studies*. These studies are formative, often cross-sectional, assessments of policymakers' knowledge and attitudes about research evidence, practices of using it, preferences for receiving it, and the sociopolitical context in which policy decisions are made. For example, an audience research study might survey policymakers about their attitudes toward specific evidence-based policies,[10] interview policymakers and their staff to understand how research evidence was used in a policymaking process,[11] or analyze news media to shed light on the sociopolitical context surrounding an evidence-based policy proposal (e.g., assess public opinion and arguments for and against a policy proposal).[12] The purpose of audience research studies is to inform the design of policymaker-focused dissemination strategies. Second are *intervention studies*. These studies test the effectiveness of different policymaker-focused dissemination strategies. For example, an intervention study might randomize policymakers to receive a data-focused or narrative-focused policy brief and then assess their support for the evidence-based policy that was discussed in the brief.[13]

DEFINING EVIDENCE-BASED POLICY

An evaluation of the existing evidence base for policy dissemination research reveals that while public policy has vast potential to influence population health, there is limited evidence on how precisely it may do so. In this way, public policy illustrates the "inverse evidence law," which states that the interventions most likely to influence whole populations (e.g., policy change) are least valued in an evidence matrix emphasizing randomized designs.[18,19] For example, knowledge is growing about the ways policy can be used to facilitate healthy decision-making and reduce risk of obesity.[20,21] There is still much more to learn about which policies work and which do not, how policies should be developed

and implemented, and the best ways to combine quantitative and qualitative methods for evaluation of so-called "upstream" risk factors.[22] These knowledge gaps are unlikely to be addressed by randomized designs and are more likely to be addressed through the use of quasi-experimental designs.[23]

Brennan and colleagues propose a four-level evidence typology that incorporates a range of evidence levels that can include the highest quality systematic reviews, research and evaluation reports, and new innovations.[24] The first level includes "Tier 1" effective strategies. Leading sources for such information include The Guide to Community Preventive Services[25] and the Cochrane Collaboration Reviews,[26] which consist of a range of interventions that have been evaluated by systematic review. The second level includes "Tier 2" effective strategies, which include published, peer-reviewed studies indicating considerable health impacts. The third level includes promising strategies, which may show important, probable health impacts in published or unpublished studies. The fourth level includes emerging strategies, which come from innovative, untested interventions with some face validity. A similar typology has also been developed by the University of Wisconsin Population Health Institute (http://whatworksforhealth.wisc.edu/evidence.php). Applying such typologies to existing policy interventions can help dissemination researchers appropriately identify those worthy of potential dissemination.

Another framework that may be useful for the dissemination of evidence-based policy is shown in Figure 26.1. Each phase of this framework has specific characteristics that are important for effective dissemination. Carefully assessing the phase of each target population can help tailor dissemination activities and inform the development of policy dissemination research questions. The framework starts with the definition of evidence-based policies, and then illustrates how both active and passive dissemination may take place. In the innovation development phase, members from the target audience provide critical feedback on policies and the rationale is built for evidence-based policies. The awareness stage defines the actions taken to make target audiences aware of the innovative policies across sites and settings.[27,28] Adoption can be defined as "a decision to make full use of an innovation as the best course of action available."[29] The adoption phase examines factors that influence the decision to

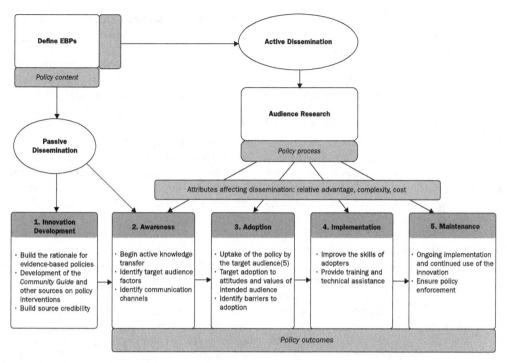

FIGURE 26.1 A framework for dissemination of evidence-based policies.

undertake the innovation by an individual or organization.[28] Implementation can be defined as the extent to which an innovation is carried out with completeness and fidelity. This phase involves improving the skills of adopters through training and technical assistance. Maintenance refers to the extent to which an innovation, such as a program, becomes embedded into the normal operation of an organization.[30] This phase also involves ensuring policy enforcement. This framework provides a helpful guide to studying various steps in the policy dissemination process.

CHALLENGES TO EVIDENCE-BASED POLICYMAKING

There are substantial challenges in developing, implementing, and evaluating evidence-based policies. Others have written about these in detail.[31-35] In part, these challenges reflect what has been learned from Diffusion Theory (Table 26.1).[29] While these attributes have been applied to multiple disciplines (e.g., agriculture, business)[36] and some public health programs,[37,38] their use in policy settings is limited. Building on these

TABLE 26.1 POLICY ATTRIBUTES THAT AFFECT DISSEMINATION

Characteristic	Description/rationale
Relative Advantage	More beneficial than available alternatives
Complexity	More easily communicated the better
Comparability	More consistent with the new environment or setting
Flexibility	Policy is robust to modification, or can be subdivided, and still be effective
Reversibility	For a policy that is not working, the old approach can be resumed.
Risk	The less the uncertainty about the results of the policy, the better.
Cost	Benefits of the policy outweigh the costs.

attributes, this section highlights several challenges most relevant to effectively disseminating research evidence in policy settings.

Clash of Cultures

Perhaps most importantly, the cultures and decision-making processes for researchers and policymakers are significantly different.[17] Researchers rely on experimental and observational studies to test specific hypotheses in a systematic way. Their influence is based on their specialized knowledge, and their timelines to action are long. On the other hand, policymaking is built on a history of related policies and demands from stakeholders.[39] Policymakers have to sell, argue, advocate, and get re-elected in light of the available political capital. Decisions are often the result of compromise. Their interests are often shorter term and keyed to an election cycle, leaving little room for interaction with the, slower, calculated pace of researchers.

Poor Timing

Scientific studies are not always conducted at the right time to influence policy decisions. Research tends to progress in a deliberate, although not always predictable pace. Frequently, research projects take 3 to 6 years to complete and as many as 8 to 10 years may pass from the time of the initial hypothesis or research question to publication and dissemination of findings. Contrast this with the policy process, which moves much more quickly, and where public officials are elected every 2 to 6 years and often are dealing with hundreds of policy issues in a single legislative cycle. By the time that research findings are sufficient to support policy changes, the political and social climates may not be receptive or the issues/problems may have subsided or disappeared from public concern.

Ambiguous Findings

Policymakers often become frustrated with the ambiguity of findings that researchers present (e.g., "confidence intervals" around their estimates). Policymakers prefer "point estimates" (e.g., a precise estimate) of the effect. The Congressional Budget Office, which is charged by the US Congress to project future changes in the budget, has for years documented the difficulty in projecting the future health costs of Medicare and explained that their projections are uncertain. Nevertheless, when Congress passed the Medicare Modernization Act, they passed the policy with a one-point estimate of the budget costs, not a range of budget estimates.

Balancing Objectivity and Advocacy

There has been considerable dialogue and disagreement among researchers regarding the degree to which scientists should be involved in the policymaking process. Largely, the differences focus on the role of scientists as advocates. Even the definition of advocacy is ambiguous,[40] ranging from raising awareness of an issue, to communicating research results to policymakers, to actively lobbying for a particular policy. Some argue that researchers who take a public stance on a given health policy issue may face real or perceived loss of objectivity that may adversely affect their research.[41] Objectivity implies that a researcher seeks to observe things as they are, without falsifying observations to match some preconceived view. Objectivity may be influenced by the research questions in which a researcher is personally interested.[42] Even if a D&I researcher is not involved in all stages along the advocacy continuum, they can still study the policy process and raise awareness of important health policy issues.

Information Overload

Multiple demands compete for the time of a policymaker, and the number of demands has grown at a steady pace over the years. A fundamental tenet of the communication process is that people are limited in how much information they can process. A policymaker in the United States is typically exposed to hundreds of messages from multiple sources on a daily basis. A study of 292 state policymakers supported the notion that much of the information provided to policymakers is not assimilated.[43] Among surveyed policymakers, 27% read the information they receive in detail, 53% skim the information for general content, and 35% "never get to" material. Some have suggested that many policymakers "read people" not written reports.[44] In addition, scientists may be ill-equipped to communicate complex information to policymakers in effective ways.[45]

Lack of Relevant Data

Data can be powerful in shaping policy decisions, yet the type of evidence needed often varies across research and policy audiences.[46,47] Epidemiologic data, whether from etiologic research or from surveillance systems, are often not in the form most useful for policymakers. Many datasets provide disease or risk factor data at the national, state, or county level. Surveillance data are often compiled in reports that can be hundreds of pages in length. In a study of directors of applied research organizations in Canada, 67% of organizations reported targeting policymakers with their research knowledge.[48] Among these groups, only 49% tailored materials to specific policy audiences. Policymakers often look for data that: (1) show public support for a particular issue; (2) demonstrate priority for an issue over many others; (3) show relevance at the local (voting district) level; and (4) personalize an issue by telling a compelling story of how peoples' lives are affected. In a political setting, a good anecdote or intuitive argument may carry more weight than a plethora of statistics or research results. Anecdotes are especially persuasive to the audiences policymakers speak with (their constituents), who often are not sophisticated consumers of statistical evidence.[49]

The Mismatch of Randomized Thinking with Nonrandom Situations

In biomedical research, the most rigorous design for hypothesis testing is the randomized controlled trial;[50] thus, systematic reviews (e.g., Cochrane Review) tend to favor such designs. As such, randomized controlled trials are often more likely to be funded and their results are more likely to be published. However, well-designed observational studies can also be powerful tools by which to estimate risk and understand disease.[51,52] Further, a randomized design is seldom useful in policy-related dissemination research because the scientist cannot randomly assign exposure (the policy) and problems are often qualitative—thus, alternative research designs are often superior in framing policy-relevant questions.

THEORIES AND FRAMEWORKS FOR POLICY DISSEMINATION RESEARCH

Few well-established theories or frameworks for policy dissemination research exist. In their 2012 review of theories and frameworks for D&I research, Tabak and colleagues identified 61 different models, but only eight gave consideration to the policy level and even fewer were focused on policy contexts.[53] While new policy-relevant D&I models have been created since the review was conducted, policy dissemination researchers often find themselves needing to adapt D&I frameworks to suit the context of their study and research questions. Highlighted here are two frameworks that are particularly useful for policy dissemination research.

Multiple Streams Framework

Developed by John Kingdom, multiple streams is a political science framework that is widely used in the social sciences.[54] A recent review found that the framework was used in 311 peer-reviewed studies published between 2000 and 2013.[55] Multiple streams is founded on the premise that countless issues are constantly competing for policymakers' attention and posits that three "streams" influence if and how issues are addressed by public policy: (1) a problem stream, consisting of issues that are perceived by policymakers and the public as needing to be addressed; (2) a policy stream, consisting of potential solutions to these problems; and (3) a political stream, consisting of public opinion and the broader sociopolitical context in which policymaking occurs. When these three streams converge around an issue, a "policy window" opens and "policy entrepreneurs" (e.g., advocates, researchers seeking to implement evidence-based policy) can advance their policy proposals. Multiple streams is generally regarded as a D&I framework,[53] but was not created with the intent of structuring D&I research and thus might require adaptation. Such adaptation is acceptable because the framework was rated by Tabak and colleagues as having high construct flexibility for D&I research.[53]

An example of such adaptation is provided by Purtle and colleagues, who modified the multiple streams framework for a policy dissemination audience research study focused on comprehensive state mental health parity legislation (C-SMHPL)—a policy intervention that requires health insurers to provide the same level of coverage for all mental and physical health benefits. In this study, the problem stream is focused on inadequate insurance coverage for mental health services, the policy stream is focused on C-SMHPL, and the political stream is focused on public opinion and interest group pressure related to C-SMHPL, mental illness, and evidence-based mental health treatments. For the purpose of the audience research study, a deficit of multiple streams was that it did not sufficiently account for the individual characteristics of state policymakers (i.e., the adopters of C-SMHPL). These characteristics were important because

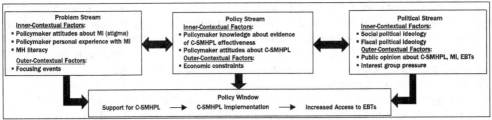

MH = mental health, MI = mental illness, EBTs = evidence-based mental health treatments, C-SMHPL = comprehensive state mental health parity legislation

FIGURE 26.2 A conceptual framework for an exploratory audience research to disseminate C-SMHPL evidence to state policymakers

they were conceived as mutable targets that could be altered by a future dissemination intervention. Thus, multiple streams was supplemented with the concepts of inner- and outer-contextual factors from Aarons' Model of Evidence-Based Implementation in Public Sectors.[56] Inner-contextual factors are individual attributes of the adopters of an intervention, whereas outer-contextual factors constitute features of the external environment that affect adoption. Figure 26.2 shows the adapted multiple streams framework for the audience research study.

The SPIRIT Action Framework

Developed in the field of knowledge transfer and exchange, the SPIRIT Action Framework[57] is the product of an extensive literature review,[58] interviews with policymakers,[59] and an interactive framework development process. The SPIRIT Action and multiple streams frameworks are similar in that they both emphasize the importance of considering sociopolitical context when disseminating research evidence to policymakers. Whereas multiple streams is a *descriptive framework* designed to characterize the policymaking process, the SPIRIT Action Framework is a *predictive framework* designed to identify factors that can be modified by interventions to promote evidence-informed policymaking. As Redman and colleagues describe, the SPIRIT Action Framework was developed with the explicit purpose "to guide the development and testing of strategies to increase to use of research in policy."

The SPIRIT Action Framework proposes a four step process through which research evidence influences policy and improves population health. First, the framework posits that a *catalyst* is needed to prompt policymaker engagement with research evidence. Potential catalysts include public demand or government requirements for research use or an emergent policy problem for

which new information is needed to develop a policy solution. Second, the framework hypothesizes that the response to the catalyst is mediated by the *capacity* of the policymaking agency to use research evidence (e.g., organizational climate supporting evidence-based policymaking, infrastructure supporting access to research information). Third, when capacity is sufficient, the framework proposes that policymakers are more likely to undertake one or more of four *research engagement actions*: access research evidence, evaluate research findings, conduct new research, and communicate with researchers. Fourth, after these engagement actions take place, *research use* occurs and increases the likelihood that research evidence informs policy development and that improvements in population health will be achieved.

OUTCOMES AND MEASURES FOR POLICY DISSEMINATION RESEARCH

Standardized outcomes and measures are less established for policy dissemination research than other areas in the field of D&I research. Nevertheless, validated instruments exist and comparable outcomes measures are often used across studies. Here, three main domains of outcomes and measures for policy dissemination research are synthesized: self-report policymaker research utilization, self-report policymaker support for evidence-based policies, and observed policymaker research utilization.

Self-Report Policymaker Research Utilization

Self-report measures of policymakers' research utilization practices and preferences are the most frequently studied outcomes in policy dissemination research. In formative audience research studies, these measures can inform the design of dissemination strategies that promote evidence-informed policymaking. For example, a study of US state legislators used Bogenschneider's measures of research utilization[60,61] to examine differences in research utilization between state legislators who prioritized behavioral health issues and those who did not.[62] A similar study compared research utilization activities between US state legislators who did and did not prioritize cancer control activities.[63] Both of these studies found significant differences between groups, suggesting that topic-specific dissemination strategies are warranted.

At the state-level outside of the United States, Zardo and Collie developed new self-report measures of research utilization and surveyed administrative public health policymakers in Victoria, Australia.[64,65] In one study, these measures were used to determine if academic research was used differently than other forms of information (e.g., internal data and reports) in policymaking.[64] In another study, these measures were used to identify individual- and organizational-level factors that predicted the utilization of academic research among policymakers.[65] Amara and colleagues surveyed administrative policymakers in the province of Quebec, Canada about their utilization of academic research evidence and classified responses according to instrumental, enlightenment, and symbolic uses.[66] Landry and colleagues used the same dataset to examine how research utilization varied across different stages of the policymaking process.[67] Finally, the Staff Assessment of enGagement with Evidence (SAGE) is a newly developed instrument that involves a 40-minute structured interview in which a policymaker describes how research was used in the development of a discrete policy document and includes a scoring instrument to quantify research utilization.[68,69]

Although most self-report utilization measures assess how policymakers have used research evidence in *past* policymaking activities, some measures assess policymakers' plans to use research evidence in *future* policymaking. For example, Boyko and colleagues used constructs from the Theory of Planned Behavior to develop a 15-item instrument that evaluates policymakers' intentions to use research when making policy deicisions.[70] In a study that tested the effects of disseminating narrative- versus data-focused policy briefs, Brownson and colleagues used Likert scale items to assess state policymakers' intention to use the policy brief or share it with a colleague.[71]

Self-Report Policymaker Support for Evidence-Based Policies

Policymakers' level of support for specific evidence-based policies can serve as an outcome measure in experiments that test the effectiveness of dissemination strategies. Support for an evidence-based policy, typically measured on a Likert scale, is frequently used as the main outcome in communication experiments with the general public that test the effects of different message frames. Examples include experiments that have measured public support for evidence-based policies that reduce sugar-sweetened beverage consumption,[72] increase access to naloxone,[73] prevent obesity,[74] and improve the social determinants of health.[75] In a communications experiment with state legislators, Niederdeppe and colleagues tested the effects of various combinations of narratives and statistical maps on state legislators' support for policies that improve access to healthy foods.[13]

Policymaker support for evidence-based policies can also be used in audience research studies to identify factors associated with support and inform the design of tailored dissemination strategies. For example, Welch and colleagues surveyed US state legislators and assessed policy support by asking them to indicate, on a three point scale, the likelihood that they would vote for 17 different evidence-based obesity reduction policies.[10]

Observed Policymaker Research Utilization

If policymaker-focused dissemination interventions are truly effective, one should observe policymakers taking actions that support the implementation of evidence-based policies. As with the self-report measures described above, direct observations of policymaker research utilization can serve as outcome variables when testing policy dissemination interventions and also have utility in audience research studies to inform the design of such interventions. The approach used by Gollust and colleagues in their study of childhood obesity policymaking in Minnesota provides an example of how research use in policymaking can be directly assessed.[76] First, key informant interviews were conducted and legislative databases were reviewed to identify relevant childhood obesity bills. Then, the state legislature's website and legislative library were used to collect all documents that were circulated at hearings on these bills (e.g., fact sheets, letters, reports, media articles) and audio/video recorded testimonies of the hearings. A coding instrument (available as an online appendix) was then developed and content analysis was conducted to describe if and how research evidence was used in each bill's policymaking processes. Yanovitzky and colleagues used a similar approach to examine the use of research in federal childhood obesity policymaking, with a focus on the knowledge brokers that supply research evidence.[77]

For legislative policies—such as those enacted by US Congress, state legislatures, or city councils—the voting behaviors of elected officials can serve as measures of support for evidence-based policies. Like the text of policy proposals, elected officials' roll call voting records are typically available on the Internet. While studies have identified policymaker characteristics that are associated with voting in favor of evidence-based public health policies,[78,79] no studies that we are aware of have used elected officials' voting behaviors as an outcome variable in a policy dissemination intervention study. Assessment of such "hard outcomes" is analogous to the use of prescribing behavior as an outcome variable in clinical D&I research and represents an important next phase of policy dissemination research.

Methodological Challenges and Opportunities in Policy Dissemination Research

There are unique methodological challenges, as well as some opportunities, to conducting policy dissemination research. One challenge is that the recruitment of policymakers, especially elected officials, can be difficult given their busy schedules and competing demands. Policy dissemination research conducted with elected officials in the United States, however, has shown that satisfactory response rates can be achieved with assertive recruitment and follow-up techniques. A response rate of 46% was achieved with US state legislators through exclusively telephone-based methods and each legislator being called up to 10 times.[62,63] An exclusively post-mail survey of US state legislators with three follow-up attempts achieved a response rate of 31%.[10] An experiment that compared post-mail and e-mail recruitment methods with US state legislators achieved response rates of 32% and 12%, respectively, and found that the characteristics of survey respondents were not significantly different according to the mode of survey completion.[80] Potential strategies to increase policymaker

response rates include obtaining endorsements from organizations that are respected by specific policymaker audiences (e.g., the Council of State Governments) and contacting policymakers' staff and administrative assistants. Although monetary incentives for survey completion often improve response rates, policymakers are generally not allowed to accept such incentives because of ethics laws.

One benefit to conducting policy dissemination research is that many artifacts of policymaking processes are publically available on the Internet and can serve as data sources to assess research use and the outcomes of policy dissemination interventions. For example, the text of policy proposals, legislative testimony, committee hearings and reports, and policymaker voting histories are usually available in searchable databases. The contact information for policymakers is also publically available and can be purchased in database format from trade organizations such as the National Conference of State Legislators and the National Conference of Mayors.

CASE STUDIES IN POLICY DISSEMINATION RESEARCH

Throughout, this chapter has highlighted specific features of policy dissemination research studies (e.g., recruitment strategies, measures and outcomes). Here, the methods of two policy dissemination research studies are described in greater detail.

Case Study 1: Audience Research Study

Purtle and colleagues conducted a mixed method, multilevel (policymaker, state) study that combined surveys of elected and administrative policymakers with semistructured interviews to inform the design of interventions to disseminate mental health evidence to US state policymakers. Specifically the study focused on comprehensive state mental health parity legislation (C-SMHPL)—an evidence-based policy, recommended by the US Community Preventive Services Taskforce, that requires health insurers to provide the same level of coverage for all mental and physical health benefits. The aims of the study were to: (1) characterize state policymakers' knowledge and attitudes about C-SMHPL and identify individual- and state-level attributes associated with support for C-SMHPL; and (2) integrate quantitative and qualitative data to develop a conceptual framework to disseminate information about C-SMHPL, evidence-based mental health treatments, and mental illness to state policymakers. The study was guided by John Kingdon's multiple streams framework (see Figure 26.2).

Study Population and Design

First, 10 legislators (n = 500) and two administrative policymakers (n = 100) from each state were recruited via post-mail, phone, and e-mail to complete a 15-minute survey. Legislators were randomly selected, and administrative policymakers in the position of state mental health program director and state insurance commissioner were purposively selected. Policymakers' survey responses were linked to state-level variables about the sociopolitical context for mental health policy in their state. After multilevel quantitative analyses were complete, semistructured interviews were conducted with a purposive sample of survey respondents (n ≈ 30) to explore survey findings in greater depth. Then, through a systematic process, quantitative and qualitative findings were integrated and a conceptual framework was developed.

Outcomes and Measures

The primary dependent variable was policymaker support for C-SMHPL (measured on a five point Likert scale) and secondary dependent variables were support for specific components of C-SMHPL (e.g., mental health benefits covered at parity, such as co-pays and visit limits; mental illnesses covered at parity, such as schizophrenia and depression). The primary independent variables were measures of knowledge and attitudes that were postulated to be associated with C-SMHPL support. These included knowledge of C-SMHPL effectiveness (e.g., that it increases appropriate utilization of mental services) and mental health literacy (e.g., knowledge about prevalence of mental illness in their state). Secondary independent variables were political ideology, personal experience with mental illness, research utilization practices, and dissemination preferences. State-level variables were selected on the basis of prior research about factors that potentially influence state policymakers' support for C-SMHPL. These included, but were not limited to, state government ideology, interest group pressure for C-SMHPL, and state per capita spending on mental health services.

Case Study 2: Intervention Trial

Lavis and colleagues used a sequential explanatory mixed method design that combined a randomized controlled trial with qualitative interviews to determine the effects of a "full-service" evidence intervention on administrative health policymakers' research utilization practices and intentions to use research evidence.[81] The intervention was structured upon Health Systems Evidence (www.healthsystemsevidence.org), a database of 1,400 research synthesis documents (i.e., systematic reviews, summaries of systematic reviews, and policy briefs) on topics relevant to health policy decisions (e.g., structure and financing of health systems, health care implementation strategies).

Study Population and Design

Administrative health policymakers in Ontario, Canada (n ≈ 170 potential study participants) were recruited to participate in the study. All participants completed a baseline survey and received "self-service" access to Health Systems Evidence for the first 2 months of the study. Then, participants who were randomized to the intervention group received "full-service" access to Health Systems Evidence for 6 months. "Full-service" access included two intervention components that "self-service" did not: (1) monthly e-mail alerts with information about new additions to Health Systems Evidence and hyperlinks to access these resources, and (2) access to the full text of all resources in Health Systems Evidence. Following this 6-month period, control group participants also received "full-service" access for 2 months. After quantitative analysis of the trial data, 15 semistructured interviews were conducted with participants from each arm of the study (n = 30). The interviews focused on topics such as participants' experiences using the evidence service, whether and how it influenced their policymaking activities, and recommendations for improving the service.

Outcomes and Measures

The primary dependent variable was utilization of the evidence service and was measured with data automatically collected by the web-based Health Systems Evidence platform. Each study participant was assigned a unique user ID to log into the database. These login credentials allowed for differences in utilization between the intervention and control groups to be tracked. Specific measures of research utilization included the mean number of visits to Health Systems Evidence, the mean number of minutes per month that participants were logged in, the number of times that specific sections of the database were accessed (e.g., user-friendly evidence summaries, full-text reports), and the number of times that monthly e-mails were forwarded. The secondary dependent variable was the change in participants' self-reported intention to use research evidence, measured by Boyko's 15-item theory of planned behavior instrument,[70] between baseline and the end of the intervention period.

DIRECTIONS FOR FUTURE RESEARCH

The field of policy dissemination research is an emerging area within the contemporary D&I enterprise and replete with opportunities for future research. Here are highlighted five areas that the authors perceive as priorities.

Understanding the Role of Social Media in Policymaking

Social media platforms, such as Facebook and Twitter, play an influential role in politics and policymaking, but have not yet been the focus of policy dissemination research studies. One relevant study, conducted in 2014, found that almost all US Congresspersons on federal health committees had Twitter accounts, and that some of these Congresspersons were very active on their accounts, using Twitter to both disseminate information and engage in dialogue with their constituents.[82] There are at least two main ways that social media can be used in policy dissemination research. First, social media can serve as a channel to disseminate research evidence to policymakers (although some researchers might be hesitant to engage in this activity themselves).[83,84] An intervention study could test the effect of Twitter versus e-mail evidence dissemination on policymakers' research utilization practices. Second, social media posts of policymakers and the general public can provide an indication of the sociopolitical environment surrounding a policy issue. An audience research study might analyze the content of tweets at policymakers about an issue and policymakers' responses to these tweets, to inform the design of a policy dissemination intervention. The fact that Twitter data are publically available support the feasibility of such approaches.

Understanding the Role of Public Opinion on Policymaker Research Utilization

It is well-established that public opinion influences public policy,[84,85] but little is known about how the general public can promote evidence-based policymaking. A growing body of research in the field of science communication is shedding light on how research evidence can be most effectively communicated to the general public and mobilize them to advocate for evidence-based policy change.[86] Policy dissemination research studies should investigate the impact of these policy advocacy activities on policymaker utilization of research evidence and support for evidence-based policies. As proposed in the SPIRIT Action Framework, a catalyst is often needed to spur research utilization in policymaking and public demand for evidence-based policies could potentially satisfy that need.

Understanding Factors that Influence the Production of Policy-Relevant Research Evidence

The rationale for policy dissemination research hinges upon the assumption that research evidence is relevant to the decisions that policymakers face. The overwhelming majority of policy dissemination research has focused on policymakers and factors that influence the "consumption" of research evidence in policy contexts, not researchers and the factors that influence the "production" of research evidence in academic contexts.[87] Future research should investigate how organizational- and individual-level factors influence the production and dissemination of timely, policy-relevant research evidence.

Understanding Who Should Disseminate Research Evidence to Policymakers, and Why

As described in chapter 1, dissemination represents a gap in the research-to-practice supply chain. This challenge is just as large in policy dissemination as it is in other areas. While some studies have begun to examine the questions of who is best positioned to disseminate research evidence to policymakers (e.g., advocacy organizations, academic researchers, constituents) and what incentive structures and institutional arrangements facilitate such activities,[87a] these remain important policy dissemination research questions that have yet to be sufficiently investigated.

Developing the Field of Policy Implementation Research

As with policy dissemination research, policy implementation research is a relatively understudied area in the contemporary field of D&I health research, but has a rich history in the fields of political science and public administration research.[88-92] Developing the field of policy implementation research, and identifying interrelationships between dissemination and implementation activities, represents an important area for future research. Two recent policy implementation studies in Canada[93] and Sweden[94] offer examples of methodological approaches in this area. Implementation science training programs—such as the Implementation Research Institute and the Mentored Training for Dissemination and Implementation Research in Cancer programs at Washington University in St. Louis—are available to help develop researchers who are interested in public policy-focused implementation research.

SUMMARY

In summary, there are myriad barriers to translating research findings into public policies that improve population health. Policy dissemination research is focused on understanding and addressing these barriers and can be defined as: the study of the targeted distribution of scientific evidence to policymakers to understand how to promote the adoption and sustainment of evidence-based policies. Policy dissemination research studies can be classified as audience research studies—which are formative assessments of policymakers' knowledge, attitudes, and uses of research evidence and policy contexts—and intervention studies, which test the effectiveness of different policymaker-focused dissemination strategies. Outcomes of policy dissemination research studies include self-report policymaker research utilization, self-report policymaker support for evidence-based policies, and observed policymaker research utilization. Challenges to conducting policy dissemination research include the recruitment of policymakers and a limited number of established theories and frameworks to guide data collection and analysis. Looking forward, future directions for policy dissemination research include understanding the role of social media in policymaking, the role of public opinion on policymaker research utilization, factors that influence the production of policy-relevant research evidence, and identifying who is best positioned and incentivized to disseminate evidence to policymakers. There is also a need to grow the field of policy implementation research and integrate theories, frameworks, and methods across the fields of public administration

research, political science, and implementation science.

Among the topics covered in this book, policy dissemination research is among the least developed. To maximize the population benefits of health research, evidence is needed about how to most effectively package and communicate research findings to various policymaker audiences in different contexts. Policy dissemination research and help address these knowledge gaps and inform the design of strategies to promote evidence-based policymaking.

SUGGESTED READINGS AND WEBSITES

Readings

Bogenschneider K, Corbett TJ. *Evidence-based policymaking: insights from policy-minded researchers and research-minded policymakers*. Abingdon, United Kingdom: Routledge; 2011.
Describes differences between the worlds of researchers and state policymakers and presents data and measures from a number of studies aimed at promoting evidence-based policy.

Brownson RC, Royer C, Ewing R, McBride TD. Researchers and policymakers: travelers in parallel universes. *Am J Prev Med*. 2006;30(2):164–172.
Examines reasons why public health research may not be effectively translated into policy. Compares and contrasts the complex worlds of research and policymaking.

Kingdon JW. *Agendas, alternatives, and public policies*. New York: Addison-Wesley Educational Publishers, Inc.; 2003.
Kingdon's seminal work on agenda setting and policy formation is informed by interviews with individuals working in and around the U.S. government.

Purtle J, Peters R, Brownson RC. A review of policy dissemination and implementation research funded by the National Institutes of Health, 2007–2014. *Implement Sci*, 2016;11(1):1.
Presents the results of study that used the NIH RePORTER tool to identify and describe all policy dissemination and implementation research projects funded by NIH between 2007 and 2014.

Selected Websites and Tools

The World Health Organization. The Evidence-Informed Policy Network (EVIPNet). http://www.who.int/evidence/en/
EVIPNet is a network established by the World Health Organization to promote the systematic use of research evidence in health policymaking.

The Sax Institute. https://www.saxinstitute.org.au/
The Sax Institute is an Australian-based organization that aims to bridge to gap between researchers and policymakers.

National Conference of State Legislatures. http://ncsl.org.
The NCSL is a bipartisan organization providing resources, technical assistance, and other services to the legislators and staffs of all 50 state governments. Their website offers extensive resources, such as information on myriad topics, webinars, networks, and access to policy specialists.

THOMAS. http://thomas.gov
A site detailing the daily activities of the United States Congress. THOMAS was launched under the leadership of the 104th Congress, when it instructed the Library of Congress to make federal legislative information publically available. THOMAS now includes information about bills and resolutions, Congressional activity, committees, and schedules.

The Canadian Partnership Against Cancer's Cancer View Canada Prevention Policies Directory. www.cancerview.ca/preventionpolicies
This searchable catalogue includes Canadian policies and legislation regarding primary modifiable risk factors for cancer and relevant chronic diseases. The database is based on environmental scans tracking policies and legislation from 1997 to the present.

REFERENCES

1. Centers for Disease Control and Prevention. Ten great public health achievements--United States, 1900-1999. *MMWR Morb Mortal Wkly Rep.* 1999;48(12):241-243.
2. Purtle J, Brownson RC, Proctor EK. Infusing science into politics and policy: the importance of legislators as an audience in mental health policy dissemination research. *Adm Policy Ment Health Ment Health Serv Res.* 2017;44(2):160-163.
3. National Academies of Sciences, Enginering, and Medicine; Division of Behavioral and Social Sciences and Education;. *Communicating science effectively: A research agenda.* Washington, DC: National Academies Press; 2017.
4. Spasoff RA. *Epidemiologic methods for health policy.* New York: Oxford University Press; 1999.
5. Jewell CJ, Bero LA. "Developing good taste in evidence": facilitators of and hindrances to evidence-informed health policymaking in state government. *Milbank Q.* 2008;86(2):177-208.
6. Liverani M, Hawkins B, Parkhurst JO. Political and institutional influences on the use of evidence in public health policy. A systematic review. *PLoS One.* 2013;8(10):e77404.
7. Council Nr. *Using science as evidence in public policy.* Washington, DC: National Academies Press; 2012.
8. Milio N. Glossary: healthy public policy. *J Epidemiol Commun Health.* 2001;55(9):622-623.
9. Schmid TL, Pratt M, Howze E. Policy as intervention: environmental and policy approaches to the prevention of cardiovascular disease. *Am J Public Health.* 1995;85(9):1207-1211.
10. Welch PJ, Dake JA, Price JH, Thompson AJ, Ubokudom SE. State legislators' support for evidence-based obesity reduction policies. *Prevent Med.* 2012;55(5):427-429.
11. Waddell C, Lavis JN, Abelson J, et al. Research use in children's mental health policy in Canada: maintaining vigilance amid ambiguity. *Soc Sci Med.* 2005;61(8):1649-1657.
12. Niederdeppe J, Gollust SE, Jarlenski MP, Nathanson AM, Barry CL. News coverage of sugar-sweetened beverage taxes: pro-and antitax arguments in public discourse. *Am J Public Health.* 2013;103(6):e92-e98.
13. Niederdeppe J, Roh S, Dreisbach C. How narrative focus and a statistical map shape health policy support among state legislators. *Health Commun.* 2016;31(2):242-255.
14. Purtle J, Peters R, Brownson RC. A review of policy dissemination and implementation research funded by the National Institutes of Health, 2007-2014. *Implement Sci.* 2016;11(1):1.
15. Weiss CH. The many meanings of research utilization. *Public Admin Rev.* 1979;39(5):426-431.
16. Weiss CH. Research for policy's sake: the enlightenment function of social research. *Policy Anal.* 1977:531-545.
17. Caplan N. The two-communities theory and knowledge utilization. *Am Behav Scientist.* 1979;22(3):459.
18. Nutbeam D. How does evidence influence public health policy? Tackling health inequalities in England. *Health Promot J Aust.* 2003;14:154-158.
19. Ogilvie D, Egan M, Hamilton V, Petticrew M. Systematic reviews of health effects of social interventions: 2. Best available evidence: how low should you go? *J Epidemiol Commun Health.* 2005;59(10):886-892.
20. Sallis JF, Cervero RB, Ascher W, Henderson KA, Kraft MK, Kerr J. An ecological approach to creating active living communities. *Annu Rev Public Health.* 2006;27:297-322.
21. Story M, Kaphingst KM, Robinson-O'Brien R, Glanz K. Creating healthy food and eating environments: policy and environmental approaches. *Annu Rev Public Health.* 2008;29:253-272.
22. McKinlay JB. Paradigmatic obstacles to improving the health of populations--implications for health policy. *Salud Publica Mex.* 1998;40(4):369-379.

23. Wholey J, Hatry H, Newcomer K, eds. *Handbook of practical program evaluation*. 2nd ed. San Francisco, CA: Jossey-Bass; 2004.

24. Brennan L, Castro S, Brownson RC, Claus J, Orleans CT. Accelerating evidence reviews and broadening evidence standards to identify effective, promising, and emerging policy and environmental strategies for prevention of childhood obesity. *Annu Rev Public Health*. 2011;32:199–223.

25. Zaza S, Briss PA, Harris KW, eds. *The guide to community preventive services: what works to promote health?* New York: Oxford University Press; 2005.

26. The Cochrane Collaboration. 2010; http://www.cochrane.org/. Accessed August 28, 2010.

27. Kar SB. Implications of diffusion research for planned change. *Int J Health Educ*. 1976;17:192–220.

28. McCormick LK, Steckler AB, McLeroy KR. Diffusion of innovations in schools: a study of adoption and implementation of school-based tobacco prevention curricula. *Am J Health Promot*. 1995;9(3):210–219.

29. Rogers EM. *Diffusion of innovations*. 5th ed. New York: Free Press; 2003.

30. Goodman RM, Tenney M, Smith DW, Steckler A. The adoption process for health curriculum innovations in schools: a case study. *J Health Educ*. 1992;23:215–220.

31. Brownson RC, Royer C, Ewing R, McBride TD. Researchers and policymakers: travelers in parallel universes. *Am J Prev Med*. 2006;30(2):164–172.

32. Feldman PH, Nadash P, Gursen M. Improving communication between researchers and policy makers in long-term care: or, researchers are from Mars; policy makers are from Venus. *Gerontologist*. 2001;41(3):312–321.

33. Lavis JN, Posada FB, Haines A, Osei E. Use of research to inform public policymaking. *Lancet*. 2004;364(9445):1615–1621.

34. Hennink M, Stephenson R. Using research to inform health policy: barriers and strategies in developing countries. *J Health Commun*. 2005;10(2):163–180.

35. Jewell CJ, Bero LA. "Developing good taste in evidence": facilitators of and hindrances to evidence-informed health policymaking in state government. *Milbank Q*. 2008;86(2):177–208.

36. Dearing J. Evolution of diffusion and dissemination theory. *J Public Health Manag Pract*. 2008;14(2):99–108.

37. King L, Hawe P, Wise M. Making dissemination a two-way process. *Health Promot Int*. 1998;13(3):237–244.

38. Dearing JW. Improving the state of health programming by using diffusion theory. *J Health Commun*. 2004;9 Suppl 1:21–36.

39. Choi BC, Pang T, Lin V, et al. Can scientists and policy makers work together? *J Epidemiol Commun Health*. 2005;59(8):632–637.

40. Stoto MA, Hermalin AI, Li R, Martin L, Wallace RB, Weed DL. Advocacy in epidemiology and demography. *Ann N Y Acad Sci*. 2001;954:76–87.

41. Poole C, Rothman KJ. Epidemiologic science and public health policy. *J Clin Epidemiol*. 1990;43(11):1270–1271.

42. Zalta E. *Stanford encyclopedia of philosophy*. Palo Alto CA: Stanford University; 2005.

43. Sorian R, Baugh T. Power of information: closing the gap between research and policy. When it comes to conveying complex information to busy policy-makers, a picture is truly worth a thousand words. *Health Aff (Millwood)*. 2002;21(2):264–273.

44. Weiss C. Congressional committees as users of analysis. *J Policy Anal Manag*. 1989;8:411–431.

45. Matanoski GM, Boice JD, Jr., Brown SL, Gilbert ES, Puskin JS, O'Toole T. Radiation exposure and cancer: case study. *Am J Epidemiol*. 2001;154(12 Suppl):S91–S98.

46. Green LW, Ottoson JM, Garcia C, Hiatt RA. Diffusion theory, and knowledge dissemination, utilization, and integration in public health. *Annu Rev Public Health*. 2009;30:159–174.

47. Kerner JF. Integrating research, practice, and policy: what we see depends on where we stand. *J Public Health Manag Pract*. 2008;14(2):193–198.

48. Lavis JN, Robertson D, Woodside JM, McLeod CB, Abelson J. How can research organizations more effectively transfer research knowledge to decision makers? *Milbank Q*. 2003;81(2):221–248, 171–222.

49. Peterson M. How health policy information is used in Congress. In: Mann T, Ornstein N, eds. *Intensive care*. Washington, DC: Brookings Institution; 1995.

50. Porta M, ed *A Dictionary of epidemiology*. 5th ed. New York: Oxford University Press; 2008.

51. Concato J, Shah N, Horwitz RI. Randomized, controlled trials, observational studies, and the hierachy of research designs. *N Engl J Med*. 2000;342:1887–1892.

52. Colditz GA, Taylor PR. Prevention trials: their place in how we understand the value of prevention strategies. *Annu Rev Public Health*.31:105–120.

53. Tabak RG, Khoong EC, Chambers DA, Brownson RC. Bridging research and practice: models for dissemination and implementation research. *Am J Prev Med*. 2012;43(3):337–350.

54. Kingdon JW. *Agendas, alternatives, and public policies*. New York: Addison-Wesley Educational Publishers, Inc.; 2003.

55. Jones MD, Peterson HL, Pierce JJ, et al. A river runs through it: a multiple streams meta-review. *Policy Stud J.* 2016;44(1):13–36.

56. Aarons GA, Hurlburt M, Horwitz SM. Advancing a conceptual model of evidence-based practice implementation in public service sectors. *Adm Policy Ment Health Ment Health Serv Res.* 2011;38(1):4–23.

57. Redman S, Turner T, Davies H, et al. The SPIRIT Action framework: a structured approach to selecting and testing strategies to increase the use of research in policy. *Soc Sci Med.* 2015;136:147–155.

58. Moore G, Redman S, Haines M, Todd A. What works to increase the use of research in population health policy and programmes: a review. *Evid Policy.* 2011;7(3):277–305.

59. Huckel Schneider C, Campbell D, Milat A, Haynes A, Quinn E. What are the key organisational capabilities that facilitate research use in public health policy? *Public Health Res Pract.* 2014;25(1):pii, e2511406.

60. Bogenschneider K, Corbett TJ. *Evidence-based policymaking: Insights from policy-minded researchers and research-minded policymakers.* Routledge; 2011.

61. Bogenschneider K, Little OM, Johnson K. Policymakers' Use of social science research: looking within and across policy actors. *J Marriage Fam.* 2013;75(2):263–275.

62. Purtle J, Dodson EA, Brownson RC. Uses of research evidence by State legislators who prioritize behavioral health issues. *Psychiatr Serv.* 2016;67(12):1355–1361.

63. Brownson RC, Dodson EA, Kerner JF, Moreland-Russell S. Framing research for state policymakers who place a priority on cancer. *Cancer Causes Control.* 2016;27(8):1035–1041.

64. Zardo P, Collie A. Type, frequency and purpose of information used to inform public health policy and program decision-making. *BMC Public Health.* 2015;15(1):1.

65. Zardo P, Collie A. Predicting research use in a public health policy environment: results of a logistic regression analysis. *Implement Sci.* 2014;9(1):1.

66. Amara N, Ouimet M, Landry R. New evidence on instrumental, conceptual, and symbolic utilization of university research in government agencies. *Sci Commun.* 2004;26(1):75–106.

67. Landry R, Lamari M, Amara N. Extent and determinants of utilization of university research in public administration. *Public Admin Rev.* 2003;63(2):191–204.

68. Makkar SR, Brennan S, Turner T, Williamson A, Redman S, Green S. The development of SAGE: a tool to evaluate how policymakers' engage with and use research in health policymaking. *Res Eval.* 2016;25(3):315–328.

69. Makkar SR, Williamson A, Turner T, Redman S, Louviere J. Using conjoint analysis to develop a system to score research engagement actions by health decision makers. *Health Res Policy Syst.* 2015;13(1):1.

70. Boyko JA, Lavis JN, Dobbins M, Souza NM. Reliability of a tool for measuring theory of planned behaviour constructs for use in evaluating research use in policymaking. *Health Res Policy Syst.* 2011;9(1):1.

71. Brownson RC, Dodson EA, Stamatakis KA, et al. Communicating evidence-based information on cancer prevention to state-level policy makers. *J Nat Cancer Inst.* 2011;103(4):306–316.

72. Gollust SE, Tang X, White JM, French SA, Runge CF, Rothman AJ. Young adults' responses to alternative messages describing a sugar-sweetened beverage price increase. *Public Health Nutr.* 2017;20(1):46–52.

73. Bachhuber MA, McGinty EE, Kennedy-Hendricks A, Niederdeppe J, Barry CL. Messaging to increase public support for naloxone distribution policies in the United States: results from a randomized survey experiment. *PloS One.* 2015;10(7):e0130050.

74. Barry CL, Brescoll VL, Brownell KD, Schlesinger M. Obesity metaphors: how beliefs about the causes of obesity affect support for public policy. *Milbank Q.* 2009;87(1):7–47.

75. Gollust SE, Lantz PM, Ubel PA. The polarizing effect of news media messages about the social determinants of health. *Am J Public Health.* 2009;99(12):2160–2167.

76. Gollust SE, Kite HA, Benning SJ, Callanan RA, Weisman SR, Nanney MS. Use of research evidence in state policymaking for childhood obesity prevention in Minnesota. *Am J Public Health.* 2014;104(10):1894–1900.

77. Chambers, D., Lisa S., Gila N., Ulrica von T. S., Antoinette Percy-Laurry, Gregory A. Aarons, Ross Brownson et al. Proceedings from the 9 th annual conference on the science of dissemination and implementation. *Implementation Science.* 2017;12(1):48.

78. Tung GJ, Vernick JS, Reiney EV, Gielen AC. Legislator voting and behavioral science theory: a systematic review. *Am J Health Behav.* 2012;36(6):823–833.

79. Purtle J, Goldstein ND, Edson E, Hand A. Who votes for public health? US senator characteristics associated with voting in concordance with public health policy recommendations (1998–2013). *SSM-Popul Health.* 2017;3:136–140.

80. Fisher SH, Herrick R. Old versus newL the comparative efficiency of mail and internet surveys of state legislators. *State Polit Policy Q.* 2013;13(2):147–163.

81. Lavis JN, Wilson MG, Grimshaw JM, et al. Effects of an evidence service on health-system policy makers' use of research evidence: a protocol for a randomised controlled trial. *Implement Sci.* 2011;6(1):1.

82. Kapp JM, Hensel B, Schnoring KT. Is Twitter a forum for disseminating research to health policy makers? *Ann Epidemiol.* 2015;25(12):883–887.

83. Grande D, Gollust SE, Pany M, et al. Translating research for health policy: researchers' perceptions and use of social media. *Health Affairs.* 2014;33(7):1278–1285.

84. Burstein P. The impact of public opinion on public policy: a review and an agenda. *Polit Res Q.* 2003;56(1):29–40.

85. Page BI, Shapiro RY. Effects of public opinion on policy. *Am Polit Sci Rev.* 1983;77(01):175–190.

86. Farrer L, Marinetti C, Cavaco YK, Costongs C. Advocacy for health equity: a synthesis review. *Milbank Q.* 2015;93(2):392–437.

87. Haynes AS, Derrick GE, Chapman S, et al. From "our world" to the "real world": exploring the views and behaviour of policy-influential Australian public health researchers. *Soc Sci Med.* 2011;72(7):1047–1055.

87a. Otten, J. J., Dodson, E. A., Fleischhacker, S., Siddiqi, S., & Quinn, E. L. (2015). Peer Reviewed: Getting Research to the Policy Table: A Qualitative Study With Public Health Researchers on Engaging With Policy Makers. *Preventing Chronic Disease*, 12.

88. Sabatier P, Mazmanian D. The implementation of public policy: a framework of analysis. *Policy Stud J.* 1980;8(4):538–560.

89. May PJ, Winter SC. Politicians, managers, and street-level bureaucrats: Influences on policy implementation. *J Public Adm Res Theor.* 2009;19(3):453–476.

90. Hill M, Hupe P. *Implementing public policy: An introduction to the study of operational governance.* Thousand Oaks, CA: Sage; 2008.

91. Tummers L, Steijn B, Bekkers V. Explaining the willingness of public professionals to implement public policies: content, context, and personality characteristics. *Public Admin.* 2012;90(3):716–736.

92. Tummers L, Bekkers V. Policy implementation, street-level bureaucracy, and the importance of discretion. *Public Manag Rev.* 2014;16(4):527–547.

93. Valaitis R, MacDonald M, Kothari A, et al. Moving towards a new vision: implementation of a public health policy intervention. *BMC Public Health.* 2016;16(1):1.

94. Strehlenert H, Richter-Sundberg L, Nyström M, Hasson H. Evidence-informed policy formulation and implementation: a comparative case study of two national policies for improving health and social care in Sweden. *Implement Sci.* 2015;10(1):1.

Dissemination and Implementation Research among Racial/Ethnic Minority and Other Vulnerable Populations

ANTRONETTE (TONI) YANCEY, BETH A. GLENN, CHANDRA L. FORD, AND LASHAWNTA BELL-LEWIS

INTRODUCTION

Public health efforts to prevent chronic disease do not address the needs of the whole population equally. While the health of the overall US population has improved substantially over the last 100 years as evidenced by a 30-year increase in average life expectancy[1], racial and ethnic minorities continue to lag behind the general population on many health metrics, including incidence, prevalence, morbidity and mortality rates of most chronic conditions; life expectancy; and, quality-of-life indicators.[2,3] As the WHO's Commission on the Social Determinants of Health explains, the root causes of the persistent disparities are avoidable societal inequalities that exacerbate the vulnerability of minority populations.[4] Historical injustices can influence present day disease patterns. For instance, discriminatory laws, which historically restricted African Americans' access to basic goods and services including medical care, arguably continue to impose a burden on the health of this population.[5,6] They also help explain how African Americans came to reside in underresourced neighborhoods and why distrust of providers remains a challenge in this population. Similarly, American Indian populations also lag behind on multiple health indices, and historically they were subjected to discrimination and genocide. Trauma due to these experiences may affect intervention D&I.[7] Immigration trends over the past century have also helped shape the health of some U.S. ethnic minority populations.[8] In the past, "selective migration" prevailed such that US emigres were healthier than their nonimmigrant counterparts; however, more recent immigrants have substantially poorer access to medical care, particularly preventive services, and they may reside in health-compromising neighborhoods.[9,10]

Furthermore, their risk for common diseases increases over time, with their presumed adoption of unhealthy American lifestyle with exposure to negative aspects of the social environment (e.g., racial discrimination).[11–14]

To identify effective interventions that promote uptake of preventive health strategies, studies must therefore involve members of the populations who will receive the interventions; however, much of this research has been conducted in settings (e.g., academic settings) where relatively few racial/ethnic minorities and socioeconomically disadvantaged persons are present.[15] Thus, findings from these studies may not be applicable to these populations. Even when research occurs in settings that serve diverse populations, the tendency to rely on randomized designs, which require strict protocols and narrow eligibility criteria, can diminish the generalizability of the findings.[15]

For example, an intervention to promote physical activity that is effective in a randomized trial setting conducted primarily among affluent, non-Latino whites may not yield the same results when implemented in a community setting or among members of a diverse population. Part of the challenge is that intervention strategies and messages developed for mainstream populations may be less appropriate and effective among racial/ethnic minority populations.

Though, as discussed in chapters 14 and 23, going beyond language translation to make cultural adaptations of existing interventions to facilitate their use in new settings and populations is important, but how to do so is poorly understood. In addition, interventions or emerging technologies may have the potential to be equally effective across diverse populations may nevertheless be disseminated unevenly. Inequitable and uneven dissemination can lead to low uptake among the most vulnerable members of a population.[15]

This chapter provides a focused, narrative review of dissemination and implementation (D&I) efforts among vulnerable populations in five key areas of prevention, and it proposes future directions to move the field forward. The chapter begins with a discussion of models that can be used to conceptualize and guide the D&I process in racially/ethnically diverse contexts such as the United States. It goes on to discuss challenges specific to D&I in underserved groups, then summarizes the literature in five prevention areas (physical activity/obesity/ nutrition, tobacco, cancer screening, HIV/STIs, childhood immunizations). Finally, it presents a successful case study of D&I in ethnic minority and underserved populations and provides a list of useful resources.

MODELS FOR CONCEPTUALIZING D&I IN DISADVANTAGED GROUPS

A small but growing number of models aim to explain the process of D&I within racially/ethnically diverse and other vulnerable populations. As described later, these heuristics aid researchers in understanding how the dissemination process occurs and they provide points of entry that help the interventions achieve reductions in health disparities. Typically, they are broad in scope and not designed to test the component parts of a particular study. The summaries below illustrate potential applications of these models to D&I research in special populations, but they do not attempt to evaluate the models based on empirical evidence. Few disparities-specific D&I models exist. Although this may be considered a limitation, it offers an opportunity to consider how widely used D&I models might be modified for application among specific racial/ethnic minorities and other vulnerable populations.

Established Models

Socioecologic frameworks, community-based participatory research (CBPR), and culturally targeted approaches derived from social cognitive theory (SCT) and social marketing have been used to guide intervention research in disease prevention among vulnerable populations, and they will continue to be valuable in conceptualizing the process of D&I in these groups. Socioecologic frameworks emphasize the importance of context

in shaping individuals' behaviors and outcomes. According to these frameworks, macrolevel factors help to drive individuals' behaviors by, for instance, constraining the behavior change options available to them. Models that address potential synergy between environmental-level and individual-level change are preferred over models that focus solely on individual level factors, because these models typically do not account for the powerful influence environment (i.e., policy, social, built, political) has on health.[17-20] Environmental influences may play an even more important role in D&I research than in traditional efficacy and effectiveness studies.

One of SCT's assertions is that individuals learn by observing and imitating others individuals perceived as worthy of emulation (i.e., role models).[25] A key premise of the theory is that certain sociodemographic similarities exist between individuals and their role model choices; for example, they may share ethnic, socioeconomic status (SES), and/or gender backgrounds. Thus, approaches based on SCT confirm the importance of engaging community representatives who can serve as "role models" or champions in strengthening D&I efforts.

Although numerous broad-based models have been developed to explain the complex process of implementation and dissemination (see chapter 5 for an in-depth discussion of D&I models), few have been adapted for health disparities research. One exception is the RE-AIM framework (a.k.a., Reach, Effectiveness, Adoption, Implementation, and Maintenance). Glasgow and colleagues[16a] illustrated how the RE-AIM framework can be used to conceptualize key issues in conducting D&I research aimed at reducing health disparities. The authors describe how the RE-AIM Framework guided the "Be Fit, Be Well" study, a randomized trial to promote weight loss and hypertension self-management in community health center patients.[16a] Examining the key constructs (e.g., Reach, Maintenance) within specific patient subgroups (e.g., racial/ethnic groups, income level, language preference) revealed some differences between vulnerable groups, which can inform both future research and dissemination efforts. Future research is needed to assess the value of the RE-AIM Framework compared with other D&I models for guiding health disparities research.

While building trust with the members of a community in order to carry-out a particular study can be difficult, implementing effective prevention strategies across an entire population can present even greater challenges. For example, community partners may be willing to "try out" a particular strategy in a limited number of settings for a trial period as part of a study, but due to a variety of concerns including uncertainty about the acceptability of the strategy to the broader community, limited resources, and competing priorities be reluctant to support dissemination of an intervention to the broader community for an indefinite time period.

The CBPR paradigm can be helpful in such situations. CBPR recalls the historical roots of public health, where problems are identified and addressed through collaboration with the "public" or community for the common good (covered in more detail in chapter 17).[21] Group members play an integral role in shaping the research process, the content of interventions, the scope of the evaluation, and the dissemination of the findings. By developing strong, respectful partnerships with communities, researchers can foster the trust and mutual respect necessary for true participation in the development and evaluation of interventions. A true partnership, which is characterized by shared decision-making, resources and recognition or "credit" with "cultural insider" key informants, marketing messengers, and investigators or research team members, creates a foundation for institutionalizing the organizational support necessary for intervention sustainability.[23] CBPR partnerships also cultivate leadership by training group members in research skills and assisting them in developing collaborations that reach beyond the initial research goals. A key component of CBPR is direct intervention by incorporating research findings into community change efforts. CBPR has been integral in guiding health disparities research across a variety of contexts and continues to be highly relevant for D&I research efforts.

Social marketing and other client-centered approaches that originated with commercial marketing are consistent with CBPR approaches and may be valuable for guiding D&I efforts.[24] These strategies account for both individual and organizational factors. For example, how best to frame an intervention to promote physical activity in a community setting may depend on the target community. Based on these social marketing approaches, some interventions may be more acceptable to certain communities when framed as fun, non-strenuous and enjoyable rather than as involving high levels of exertion.

Emerging Models

Inclusiveness, cultural appropriateness, equity, and diversity are common themes of the emerging models, which seek to clarify the processes by which population-level dissemination and implementation occur, though each model has a slightly different focus. This section explores three such models: the Meta-Volition Model, Health Impact Pyramid, and Public Health Critical Race Praxis (PHCRP). The Meta-Volition Model (MVM) illuminates the processes by which innovations may be taken to scale; the Health Impact Pyramid specifies a hierarchy in which interventions influencing socioeconomic determinants of health are most sustainable and scalable. The Public Health Critical Race praxis accounts for ways that racial oppression in society may affect the nature, effectiveness and sustainability of D&I processes and components.

Meta-Volition Model

The MVM dissects public health movements of the past few decades to discern the critical elements and the sequencing of efforts that drive their success. Meta-volition refers to leaders' and decision-makers' motivation to protect or enhance the interests of their own organizations. The MVM posits that population-wide behavior change will occur only by shifting the primary driver of change from individual motivation and self-efficacy (the focus of most health promotion models) to a collective and overarching volition and efficacy.

One critical element shared by successful public health initiatives—such as those limiting tobacco consumption, reducing alcohol consumption while driving, instituting and promoting the use of seat restraints in cars, and promoting breastfeeding—is that changes in the social environment and, in particular, in social norms help catalyze the changes to the physical environment that are necessary to promote and sustain population-wide behavior change. Another prominent feature is the presence of "push" strategies, which are behavioral economic levers that make the healthier options easier to choose and the unhealthy ones more difficult for to choose.[26] Organization-level approaches have several advantages. Building on an organization's existing infrastructure provides a ready means of delivering targeted messages within the organization's physical or socio-cultural "micro-environments" or communities. Organizational environments may be more malleable than they seem. As few as one influential leader within an organization can set the process of organizational change into motion. Compared to efforts targeting society at large, those occurring within organizations may produce widespread behavior change more directly and efficiently.

The MVM is dynamic rather than static, integrating biological influences with psychological factors, and socio-cultural influences with organizational and larger societal processes. It specifies a sequence of six levels or orders of dissemination: initiating (leader-leader); catalyzing (organizational-individual); viral marketing (individual-organization); accelerating (organization-organization); anchoring (organizational-community); and institutionalizing (community-individual). These levels can be used as points of entry for efforts to facilitate dissemination of interventions across a variety of health content areas. The model has been most completely explicated for physical activity, in proposing brief bouts of activity incorporated into organizational routine as the equivalent of smoking bans in spurring tobacco control; however, it also recognizes the weaknesses and gaps in these movements, for example, the persistent disparities in smoking prevalence among low-income and immigrant populations.

The MVM embeds an intrinsic cultural proficiency to align public health aims with those of a diversity of organizations, necessitating building interdisciplinary and inter-sectoral cultural competency to promote understanding of and ongoing attention to and working through differing motivators and risks. It is important to recognize at the outset of movement-building a community's cultural contexts and value systems. This encourages culturally grounded, assets-based intervention approaches that "bubble up" from within diverse communities and settings; it contrasts with approaches that impose externally developed interventions that were developed based on the needs of mainstream audiences. For example, in physical activity promotion, the content area for which the model is most fully developed, structured group activity breaks are promoted because they resonate culturally for the sedentary majority, for example, women, less affluent people, ethnic minority groups,[27] less fit, less agile, and overweight or obese individuals, though it has also been implemented among young children.[28] Basing interventions in a cultural context from the outset as proposed by MVM is critical

for maximizing reach, adoption, and sustainability of prevention programs over time.

Health Impact Pyramid
The Health Impact Pyramid is a five-tiered hierarchical schematic capturing the impact of different types of public health interventions.[29] Given the importance of social determinants of health in causing health disparities, interventions aimed at influencing socioeconomic factors appear at the base of the pyramid, reflecting the promise of these strategies to promote health equity. In ascending order, reflecting decreasing impact, are interventions that change the context to make individuals' default decisions healthy; clinical interventions that require limited contact but confer long-term protection; ongoing direct clinical care; and health education and counseling. Approaches concentrated at the lower levels of the pyramid tend to be more sustainable and have a greater impact because they reach broader segments of society, require less effort from individual participants, and may be more likely to reduce health disparities.

Public Health Critical Race Praxis
The PHCRP is an emerging approach that encourages researchers to remain attentive to issues of racial equity throughout the entire research process.[31] According to PHCRP, racism may influence both a community's need for an intervention as well as the processes and outcomes of D&I research. PHCRP enables researchers to assess and address systematically racism-related factors that may inadvertently influence how intervention research is carried out.[30] It may be used as a standalone framework guiding research or combined with other theories or methods.[30]

According to PHCRP, intervention sustainability is unlikely in minority communities unless researchers subject the D&I process and each of its elements to continual assessment of any racialized power differentials between, for instance, researchers at predominately white institutions who are conducting the research and the racial/ethnic minority communities within which the research is conducted. A growing body of research acknowledges racism's contribution to health disparities. PHCRP adds that racism may also inform efforts to understand and address them. Specifically, it may undergird the assumptions, methods, and theories on which researchers rely and thus effect the diffusion/dissemination/implementation continuum.

These issues are surmountable. Working together, researchers and communities can correct processes and elements of each D&I research endeavor to ensure the process itself is equitable. In light of the tendency to minimize racism's potential contributions to disparities, PHCRP outlines a process by which researchers and interventionists develop "racism consciousness" (also referred to as *race consciousness*) as they begin each project.[30,31] Racism consciousness enables interventionists to develop sensitivity to the ways that specific racial phenomena may be at work within a particular D&I endeavor.

The approach emphasizes the need to ground all efforts in the perspectives of the marginalized communities of interest. Community members play an important role in developing and implementing interventions that address the root causes of identified disparities. Interventions developed based on PHCRP may target either key community factors or the disciplinary conventions used to study the problem (e.g., the tendency to view minority populations from a deficits perspective).

As the evidence-base for D&I research in marginalized communities expands, existing models will continue to be refined and new models will emerge. D&I researchers should also seek to expand ways in which existing models not specifically developed to address disparities can better serve these purposes.

DISSEMINATION AND IMPLEMENTATION CHALLENGES IN WORKING IN ETHNIC MINORITY AND OTHER DISADVANTAGED COMMUNITIES

Ethnic minority, lower income, rural, aged, and other socioeconomically marginalized groups have sometimes been considered "hard to reach" by public health researchers because of their non-responsiveness to audiovisual and print health promotion materials and messages that target "general" (i.e., younger, white, urban, affluent) audiences.[15,32] in D&I research to date, as has been previously noted.[16,19] Some of the factors contributing to the underrepresentation of racial/ethnic minority communities in D&I research include:

- Investigators' failure to engage these populations. Recruitment, implementation, and evaluation success requires long-term relationship building activities. This

investment of time and energy is poorly rewarded among researchers working in academic institutions, and funding to support these activities can be difficult to obtain. In addition, dissemination and implementation research is complex and often involves the collection of large amounts of data from organizations, which may not be feasible in low-resource settings (e.g., safety net clinics, county health department units) where underserved minorities can be reached. As a consequence, many D&I studies are conducted in higher resource settings, but may yield findings that hold little relevance for the underserved populations. Furthermore, the composition of research teams often does not reflect the cultural diversity of targeted population, which may result in a lack of relevance (or perceived lack of relevance) of the interventions for the racial/ethnic minority communities.[15,33–36]

- Insufficient capacity or infrastructure to absorb opportunity or transactional costs among organizations that serve disadvantaged populations. An unsuitably trained workforce, inadequate space and staffing for the workload, unstable financing, outdated information technology, and a poorly maintained built environment are all examples of challenges organizations in low-resource communities frequently face. Because of these challenges, low-resource settings may be approached for participation in D&I research infrequently. Further, if asked to participate they may be less likely to do so if research is not a part of the organizational mission.[20]

- Use of research methods that are not culturally appropriate. Researchers may need to modify their methods in order to engage disadvantaged and ethnic minority communities effectively. This may include altering the survey administration method (e.g., interviewer administered vs. self-administered for low literacy populations), oversampling subgroups of interest, and modifying existing data collection instruments, beyond simple translation, to be more appropriate for special populations. Failure to consider the specific needs of the population of interest may lead to low quality data or alienation of the community under study.

- Conscious nonparticipation by group members. Disinterest in or suspicion about participating in research among people in underserved groups may stem from prior exploitation.[37,38] These attitudes are common even when the incidents engendering mistrust occurred in the distant past. Poor framing of disease prevention efforts may distort perceptions about costs associated with participating, the potential benefits, and perceived irrelevance of the effort for a particular population. Messages may also be insufficiently targeted to the values and contexts of the lives of their intended audiences and they compete poorly as compared to well-designed commercial communications.[39] Daily survival needs and obligations may overshadow future-oriented prevention concerns. In addition, incentives may be inadequate to offset the difficulties of participating in research. For example, transportation may be unreliable or participation may require people to take uncompensated time off from work.

THE IMPORTANCE OF TRUST AND COMMUNITY PARTNERSHIPS FOR DISSEMINATION AND IMPLEMENTATION EFFORTS IN ETHNIC MINORITY POPULATIONS

Although establishing trust is important when working with any community, it is particularly important to do so when working with under-served, racial/ethnic minority communities. Both the message and the messenger are important and can influence the process. Though underserved communities are routinely targeted for research, they may receive few lasting benefits of their participation in it, resulting in disinterest or distrust of research in these communities.[40,41] How long it takes to establish trust varies from project to project. In general, the greater the potential for an intervention to stigmatize communities (e.g., because they involve stigmatized diseases such as HIV/AIDS or populations such as sex workers) or the more invasive the approach, the more resistance can be expected. Ford et al.[42] reported

spending more than a year building rapport with the community for an HIV/STD prevention project and this duration of time was similar to that reported by other HIV prevention researchers.[42] Matching outreach workers by race or ethnicity can boost community members' levels of trust, but researchers will still have to address any intra-racial power dynamics (e.g., due to SES differences) that remain. Further, even racially matched investigators may require training to ensure their work is culturally relevant and responsive.

Partnering with communities in some of their other ongoing efforts can enhance trust and reach. Using innovative settings for health promotion (e.g., churches; YMCAs and YWCAs; Women, Infants, and Children (WIC) clinics; barbers and beauty shops) broadens the reach of interventions by connecting people, including those with higher levels of need who may be less likely to seek out services where they are. Other established institutions with credibility among priority populations include ethnic minority media, including newspapers, television, magazines and newsletters, radio, websites, and Listservs.[21]

OVERVIEW AND SYNTHESIS OF EMPIRICAL DISSEMINATION AND IMPLEMENTATION RESEARCH

A growing number of D&I studies have been conducted in low-resource settings that serve a substantial proportion of racial/ethnic minorities.[15,16,24,43–47] In this section, community-based D&I efforts are summarized in five prevention areas (physical activity/nutrition/obesity, tobacco, cancer screening, HIV/STIs, immunizations), with a specific focus on describing work within ethnic minority and marginalized communities. The goal is to provide a snapshot of documented efforts in this small but rapidly expanding literature rather than to critique individual studies.

Physical Activity, Nutrition, and Obesity Prevention and Control

Historically, the majority of intervention studies in the areas of physical activity, nutrition, and obesity prevention and control have evaluated the effects of individually focused strategies.[15,16,35] A large proportion of these studies were focused on non-Latino white and/or more affluent populations, which created challenges for dissemination to the broader population.[15,16,35] However, school-based interventions have been one exception. School-based efforts such as the Child and Adolescent Trial for Cardiovascular Health,[48,49] Take10,[50-54] and Action Schools! BC, are examples of school-based interventions, that have been effectively disseminated to diverse populations.[55,56] In addition, a growing number of studies have focused on preschool or childcare settings, often targeting settings that serve low-income and ethnic minority children.[57,58]

Another area of relative success has been efforts to evaluate the effectiveness of large-scale initiatives, such as *5 A Day for Better Health*, in underserved and low socioeconomic communities.[59] Churches have been utilized in targeting adults and families. *Body and Soul* is an example of one church-based intervention, which increased fruit and vegetable consumption among African Americans by 1.4 servings per day, which has been disseminated broadly.[60,61] Factors underlying the successful dissemination of *Body and Soul* likely included the early partnership between the academic investigators and the American Cancer Society, an entity with national reach and the positioning of the intervention in a culturally respected institution, African American churches. In addition, the intervention approach was consistent with SCT and elements of CBPR, engaging members of the church community in implementing the intervention and modeling healthy behaviors, which in turn likely facilitated subsequent dissemination. The church infrastructure likely fostered the maintenance and institutionalization of the intervention.

Over the past decade, obesity prevention and control efforts have shifted away from individually focused interventions toward policy and community-level efforts in order to reduce the disproportionate burden of obesity in racial/ethnic minority communities. This shift has been precipitated in part by the efforts of organizations such as the Centers for Disease Control and Prevention (CDC) to increase funding for these types of initiatives.[62,63] Examples of policy- and community-level obesity prevention and control efforts include increasing the number of community gardens, improving access to safe space for physical activity, increasing the availability of healthy foods in restaurants and grocery stores,[64,65] eliminating or reducing advertising of unhealthy food items,[39] and building supermarkets and organic and whole food stores.[64,66,67] The reach of these types of approaches has grown considerably in the past decade given numerous local, state, and federally funded initiatives,

a focus of several large foundations (e.g., Robert Wood Johnson Foundation) to fund these efforts, and development of relevant collaboratives such as the Healthy Eating Active Living initative.[22,23] Although promising, the contribution of these efforts on reducing disparities in obesity, physical activity, and nutrition is largely unknown at this point as they have not been rigorously evaluated.[23]

Tobacco Control

Relative to other disease prevention areas, a fair amount of D&I research has been conducted in the area of tobacco cessation though many studies have been descriptive in nature, and conducted in clinical settings. One of the most promising dissemination strategies outside of clinical settings is the promotion of tobacco cessation quitlines or telephone hotlines (Cancer Information Service, CIS). A number of dissemination studies aimed at referring study participants to quitlines specifically focused on ethnic minorities. Boyd and colleagues[68] evaluated the use of television and radio commercials as well as direct community outreach to increase the number of callers to the CIS in African American communities. Marin and colleagues evaluated the effect of media strategies to increase awareness and use of smoking cessation services among Latinos in San Francisco.[69-71] Although these studies provide evidence to inform future dissemination activities, few yield much data about quit rates among the population of users of these services or were unable to compare quit rates among users and nonusers. Cummins and colleagues, however, were able to enhance the accessibility and effectiveness of an existing quitline for use by Asian populations by translating the efficacious quitline's materials and resources for use by Chinese-, Korean-, and Vietnamese-speaking smokers. Such strategies hold promise for tobacco prevention in the populations experiencing disparities.

The evidence summarized in recent systematic reviews suggests many school-based programs are effective in preventing tobacco use among youth in the short term;[72] however, questions remain about their long-term effectiveness and sustainability.[73] Although most of these studies were not specifically focused on underserved populations, school-based interventions may be more inclusive of low-income and ethnic minorities than studies conducted within clinical settings are. These studies have compared the effects of different methods of training teachers and others involved in delivering the interventions and have examined factors related to program compliance, level of adoption, and changes in knowledge and attitudes.[74-78] Not-On-Tobacco, a program initially developed by West Virginia University, is one of the most widely used evidence-based tobacco use prevention programs for schools. Trainings for the program have been conducted in at least 47 states as well as in Europe and Canada, and the program has been delivered to over 100,000 adolescents to date. Factors that have attributed to its success include involvement of multiple stakeholders and integration of dissemination as a goal of the program since its outset, and partnership with the American Lung Association, an organization with national reach.[24a]

Based on the evidence regarding tobacco use prevention, disparities with respect to two other substances, e-cigarettes and marijuana, which has been legalized in a growing number of states, are likely to emerge in the near future. Some data suggests e-cigarettes may serve as a gateway to the use of conventional tobacco products among Latino youth.[79]

As additional states and municipalities around the country legalize marijuana use, interventionists and researchers should begin to chart ways in which D&I efforts to reduce marijuana consumption may parallel versus diverge from efforts to prevent the consumption of conventional tobacco products. One effective tobacco control strategy, which could easily be extended to encompass e-cigarette and marijuana use, has been the passage of clean indoor air laws.[80] This type of policy-level intervention holds the promise of reducing health disparities given its intention to provide benefit to the greater population and make the unhealthy choice (i.e., smoking) more difficult. However, there is evidence to suggest disadvantaged communities may have weaker or less restrictive ordinances, [81] which may reduce the benefits for these groups. Future research is needed to assess enforcement of clean air policies, which is likely not uniform across communities.

Cancer Screening

A substantial number of D&I studies conducted over the past 10 years has focused on cancer screening.[43,82,83] The evidence base from efficacy studies for the promotion of breast and cervical cancer screening, conducted in both clinical and community settings, is quite robust, based on a relatively large number of randomized trials conducted over several decades.[84,85] Data regarding the most effective methods of promoting colorectal cancer screening and informed decision-making regarding prostate cancer screening has emerged more recently.[85] Representation of ethnic minorities in efficacy studies has varied by group, with more studies including African American, Latinos, and Asians over time; fewer studies involve American Indian populations.[86] The CDC-funded *National Breast and Cervical Cancer Early Detection Program* (NBCCEDP) is one of the few federal dissemination initiatives to provide low-income, uninsured, and underserved women access to low-cost or free breast and cervical cancer screening.[87] The program has placed increasing emphasis on evaluating the best strategies to increase both effectiveness and reach of the program. The CDC recently expanded this initiative to include access to colorectal cancer screening in the 22 states and 4 tribal territories. To date, however, relatively few of the interventions have been evaluated.[87] The program has placed increasing emphasis on evaluating the best strategies to increase both effectiveness and reach of the program. The CDC recently expanded this initiative through the establishment of the Colorectal Cancer Control Program (CRCCP), which recently awarded funding to 24 states, 6 universities, and 4 tribal territories to promote colorectal cancer screening among men and women 50 years and older, with a particular focus on low-income, uninsured, underinsured, racial/ethnic minority groups disproportionately affect by colorectal cancer and individuals facing geographic barriers to screening.[88] A growing number of studies have evaluated the implementation and the impact of both the NBCCEDP and the CRCCP.[89-94] Results of these studies have revealed substantial variation with regard to the reach and impact of the NBCCEDP program and suggest that the program only reaches a modest proportion of eligible women. Given the recent establishment of the CRCCP, only a few studies have evaluated it. They focus primarily on assessing program implementation rather than the impact on screening rates, stage at diagnosis, or mortality.[89,91]

In addition to evaluations of these initiatives, numerous other D&I studies have examined cancer screening. Many of these studies have been conducted in low-resource settings, targeting racial/ethnic minority, low-income, and other vulnerable communities. A large number of studies have evaluated a variety of community-based strategies to disseminate effective cancer screening promotion interventions including church-based strategies.[95,96] Slater and colleagues (2005) described the process by which an effective multicomponent intervention, developed through a National Cancer Institute (NCI)-funded trial, was adapted by the American Cancer Society to increase mammography use among women living throughout the state of Minnesota.[96a] Bencivenga and colleagues[97] found that disseminating an evidence-based intervention through collaborations with food pantries and other community-based organizations in rural Appalachia was effective in increasing mammography rates. Kreuter and colleagues[98] tracked patterns of use and characteristics of users of computer kiosks, located in 40 different St. Louis community sites, generating individually tailored breast health education. Prior research found this method was effective in increasing mammography rates; however, factors associated with kiosk use had not yet been studied. The results suggested that the use of lay health workers,[99–102] and information kiosks in public places such as laundromats, libraries, and social services agencies[103] may be promising strategies for cancer screening promotion among urban, African American women.

A growing number of studies have investigated 2-1-1- hotlines in multiple states/counties/cities as a venue for promotion of cancer screening and other prevention strategies.[104–106] In addition, numerous studies have utilized a D&I framework to examine the best strategies for increasing cancer screening rates in clinical settings, with much of this work being conducted in safety net settings.[107–110]

A substantial portion of the research conducted in low-resource settings and targeted to ethnic minority and underserved populations has been led by investigators affiliated with the CDC/NCI-funded Cancer Prevention and Control Research Network (CPCRN). The CPCRN is a national network funded by the National Center for Chronic Disease Prevention and Health Promotion at the CDC and the Division of Cancer Control & Population Sciences of the NCI. The mission of CPCRN is to accelerate the use of evidence-based interventions in communities and to promote collaborative dissemination and implementation research among funded sites, particularly in low-resource settings and with underserved populations. Initially funded in 2002, this network has included more than 15 academic sites located throughout the country, each affiliated with a CDC-funded Prevention Research Center. Several published manuscripts[111,112] have summarized CPCRN accomplishments, including a recent paper that concluded the network was successful in promoting multisite collaborations in the form of peer-reviewed manuscripts and publications in several important areas of cancer prevention in underserved populations.[112a]

HIV/STIs

The CDC's Diffusion of Effective Behavioral Interventions (DEBI) initiative packages and distributes theory-based HIV interventions that are proven effective through randomized efficacy trials.[113] The packages are intended to be implemented with few or no changes, which ensures implementation occurs with fidelity to the proven models. Sometimes adaptations are necessary to improve the fit for specific communities. If intervention results are unexpected, however, it can be difficult to determine whether this reflects lack of fidelity to the proven intervention, poor fit to the new population or context, or failure of an appropriate and correctly implemented intervention to have an impact.[113,114] The CDC's Replicating Effective Programs framework helps to address these challenges by guiding the process by which researchers decide whether to keep an intervention exactly as designed or adapt it per local needs.[115] As of 2016, approximately 30 such interventions had been packaged and disseminated to more than 1,100 organizations for implementation.[116] Key challenges to dissemination and implementation of HIV-related interventions include the rapid pace at which the evidence on and treatments for HIV/AIDS are changing; policy-related issues, which may make it difficult to implement interventions in different regions or locales; and the persistence of HIV stigma and disparities.[116] Community-based organizations, including those that provide HIV services, are among the many types of stakeholders involved with HIV prevention and treatment; therefore, D&I efforts based on partnerships with them are recommended.[117]

D&I of HIV/STI interventions occur in three main types of settings. Street outreach is helpful for connecting with members of "hidden" populations (e.g., homeless persons, injection drug users).[42] Clinical settings provide efficient access to high-prevalence groups (e.g., STD patients) and those among whom HIV risk may be overlooked.[118] Organizational settings (e.g., community centers, churches) extend prevention efforts through existing support networks.[42,119]

Community-wide implementation and dissemination can improve intervention effectiveness and sustainability, and bolster community capacity to provide HIV/STI services, increase awareness of disparities, may improve rates of screening, and may reduce HIV/STI stigma. For example, the National HIV Testing Day promotes HIV testing without regard to actual or perceived risk and helps reduce HIV stigma. Whether community-wide implementation and dissemination affect condom use, incident infections, and numbers of sexual partners, however, remain unclear.

Many interventions targeting racial/ethnic minorities are gender specific. Those developed for women have been demonstrated to improve HIV knowledge, self-efficacy, and risk reduction behaviors (e.g., condom use) in sexual partnerships. Efforts for minority men primarily target those who self-identify as heterosexual but engage in sexual risk behaviors with other men.[120,121] The greatest challenge to HIV/STI prevention in this population is that the population remains hidden and stigmatized. Strategies for reaching these men include intercepting them online (e.g., in chat rooms where men go to meet other men for sex); using respondent-driven sampling to reach members of a social network; and, targeting places (e.g., parties) where they gather. While the number of D&I studies in this population is growing, the impact on preventive outcomes is still unclear, though studies have established that interventions and prevention messages developed for or disseminated via the white gay community are not necessarily effective for minority men.[122]

HIV prevention interventions rely on a wide range of psychosocial and behavioral theories. Most interventions aim to change individual-level psychosocial factors (e.g., HIV knowledge) or behaviors (e.g., unprotected sex). Others aim to diffuse effects through social/sexual networks or communities. These approaches draw on the resources available within social networks or communities, and the capacity of peers (e.g., lay health workers) or leaders (e.g., ministers) to influence members of their networks. Increasingly, interventions also target structural inequities and the social determinants of health. Some, such as SISTA, which is a culturally grounded, empowerment model initially developed for use among African American women, acknowledge the racial context in which the behaviors occur, even though they target individual-level behavior change.[123] By addressing the intersecting nature of racial and gender

oppression, SISTA aims to empower women to make decisions and take actions that reduce their risk of HIV transmission.[124]

Childhood Immunizations/ Vaccinations

Universal coverage programs for childhood vaccinations have been in place since the 1940s in the United States.[125] Coverage rates have increased over time and generally remain quite high (>90%) across most childhood vaccines with the exceptions of the flu vaccine.[126] The high level of vaccine coverage was achieved through a combination of activities, primarily at the policy level including coordinated efforts at the federal, state, and local level to promote vaccination, state-based immunization registries, recommendations from professional organizations regarding importance of vaccination, systematic collection of data to measure coverage, and prioritization of immunizations by governmental and professional bodies.[125,127,128] However, gaps in immunization rates between white and ethnic minority children were first identified in the 1970s and continue to persist today, although they have narrowed over time.[125,127–130] Disparities in childhood vaccination rates by poverty level also persist. Based on data from the 2014 National Immunization Survey, children living below the poverty level have significantly lower coverage rates for 8 of the 10 vaccines measured, although the magnitude of the differences was relatively modest (<5% point difference, on average).[126] Research has also documented significantly lower rates among foreign-born compared with US-born children.[131] Policy-level efforts specifically aimed at improving vaccination rates in underserved populations have included federal funding for low-cost or free vaccine through the Vaccines for Children Program, linkages between WIC and immunization activities, enhancement of payment for immunization services for children covered by Medicaid, and partnerships with minority health organizations.[128,130]

Within the larger context of vaccine promotion activities at the local, state, and national level, however, relatively few studies have rigorously evaluated vaccine promotion efforts intended for ethnic minority communities. Thus, the evidence base is somewhat limited, which may limit the effectiveness of future D&I research. Examples of interventions aimed at increasing vaccination coverage among underserved populations in nonclinical settings have included several randomized trials among families enrolled in WIC programs that found that linking food vouchers to immunization and escorting a child to a local vaccination clinic both led to significant increases in vaccination coverage.[132,133] The New York State Department of Health found that their efforts partnering with community-based organizations to reach underimmunized children successfully increased vaccination rates in New York City. The overall high rates of adherence to childhood vaccinations likely reflects widespread use of evidence-based strategies in clinical settings such as immunization information systems, client and provider reminders, provider assessment and feedback, and use of standing orders.[134] These system-level strategies likely contributed to recently documented declines in childhood vaccinations; however, they may not eliminate disparities.[135] Though promising, relatively few intervention efforts have been "taken to scale" or disseminated to the broader population. A recent review by Galea and colleagues [128] noted that without moving beyond trials to implementation and dissemination studies, sustainable increases in vaccination rates among underserved and ethnic minority populations will not occur.

Reduced access to health care may be one contributing factor, which will necessitate more upstream approaches to improve access to care. Community-focused approaches are another promising strategy for vaccine promotion among families that are not routinely accessing the health care system. For example, a substantial amount of prior research has examined the effectiveness of vaccine promotion interventions set in the WIC program.[134] In 2015, the Community Preventive Services Task Force recommended vaccination interventions in WIC settings based on strong evidence of their effectiveness. A recent study conducted in New York observed promising results for an educational intervention aimed at improving vaccination rates among children from low-income households that was delivered in partnership with the Salvation Army.[136] Although promising, these community-based efforts have not been "taken to scale" or disseminated to the broader population. A review by Galea and colleagues[128] noted that without moving beyond trials to implementation and dissemination studies, sustainable increases in vaccination rates among underserved and ethnic minority populations will not occur. Another recent international systematic review concluded that locally designed, multicomponent interventions were most effective for reducing inequalities in underserved, racial/ethnic minority communities.[137] Although potentially effective, locally designed and implemented efforts may pose challenges for widespread dissemination. It has been noted that a factor promoting the success of other evidence-based prevention interventions such as *Body and Soul* has been the ability to "open the box and get started" without substantial additional work on the part of the organization.[26] The higher the degree of local-level adaptation recommended, the more challenging implementation may be perceived by some organizations.

Although the majority of these efforts have focused on childhood vaccinations, initiatives for adolescents have grown with the recent HPV, tetanus/diphtheria/pertussis (Tdap) and meningococcal vaccines, and the "catch-up" hepatitis B vaccinations.[137-141] Efforts to increase uptake of the seasonal flu vaccine among adults, particularly the elderly, have also intensified, especially in clinical settings.[139,142-145] Racial/ethnic and socioeconomic disparities in vaccinations may be more pronounced in adults than in children.[139,143]

Emerging Issues

Though not elaborated on here, several emerging issues are important to mention, including mental health and homelessness among veterans; human trafficking; and health disparities affecting lesbian, gay, bisexual and transgender (LGBT) persons. D&I challenges in these populations include the poor understandings researchers have of the structure and nature of these social networks, which may make it difficult to evaluate the extent of dissemination across an entire population. Vulnerable, sometimes hard-to-reach populations, and racial/ethnic minorities are disproportionately affected by this consideration. Further, mistrust as well as psychosocial and legal barriers may exacerbate D&I efforts in these populations.[27] Each of these issues is also likely to become more important in the coming years. For instance, among veterans, especially those returning from war, rates of posttraumatic stress disorder, depression, homelessness, and suicide are elevated and have been increasing. Domestically and globally, human trafficking of children and adults for the purposes of sexual exploitation or labor is a rapidly expanding illegal enterprise that encompasses many public health issues. LGBT persons are an increasingly visible population whose prevention-related needs are poorly understood. In 2011, the Institute of Medicine called for research to understand and address health disparities affecting LGBT populations.[146] The available evidence suggests the LGBT population experiences extremely high rates of some disparities, including violence; however, very little D&I research has been conducted in this population as a whole. As the knowledge regarding LGBT health disparities grows, so too will the need to develop culturally targeted D&I strategies for the overall LGBT population and for specific subpopulations (e.g., transgender women).

CASE STUDY: ADOLESCENT VACCINATION

Background

As described earlier, adherence to recommendations for childhood vaccinations has been relatively high over the past several decades and racial/ethnic disparities in childhood vaccination rates appear to be narrowing.[150] However, achievement of the current coverage level and reduction of racial/ethnic disparities in coverage was a lengthy process, given that childhood vaccinations were first recommended in the 1940s. The "adolescent vaccine platform" was first introduced by the Advisory Committee on Immunization Practices in 1997, primarily as an opportunity for "catch-up" vaccination for childhood vaccines and as a "hook" for delivery of routine primary care to this age group.[151]

It was not until 2006 that the adolescent vaccine platform included the schedule of the three currently recommended vaccines: meningococcal, Tdap, and HPV. The introduction of the current adolescent vaccination schedule was perceived as an undertaking that could pose considerable challenges to the health care and public health system.[151] Potential barriers to adolescent vaccination identified at the time of its introduction included patient/parent barriers such as lack of interest and motivation to be vaccinated and infrequent visits to a health care provider, and provider and system-level factors including inadequate time and compensation for vaccine counseling and administration and prioritization of other preventive care needs. Historically, there have been numerous examples of uneven dissemination of preventive care recommendations across the population, with adherence to recommendations highest among more affluent and non-Latino white populations and substantial lags (of up to decades, in some cases) among underserved and ethnic/

minority populations. Examples of this phenomenon include childhood vaccination as well as screening for cervical, breast, and colorectal cancer, among others.

Despite these perceived challenges, vaccination coverage rates in 2015 reveal minimal racial/ethnic and socioeconomic disparities in the Tdap, meningococcal, and HPV vaccines.[141] Coverage with the Tdap vaccine was high and equivalent for non-Latino whites (86.6%), non-Latino blacks (86%), Latinos (85%), American Indians (87.6%), and Asians (86%). Furthermore, no differences in Tdap coverage rates were observed by poverty status. No differences were observed for coverage for the first dose of the meningococcal vaccine between non-Latino whites, African Americans, American Indian/Alaskan Native, and Asians, with rates hovering at around 80%, whereas Latino adolescents had a higher rate of coverage (85%) compared with non-Latino whites (80%). Rates of coverage for the first dose of the HPV vaccine were significantly higher among African American and Latino females and males compared with non-Latino whites. Rates among American Indians/Alaskan Natives and Asians were equivalent to the rates among non-Latino whites. In addition, rates of coverage for the first HPV vaccine dose were significantly higher among both females and males living below the poverty level compared with their more affluent counterparts. Rates of coverage for the meningococcal booster and the second and third doses of the HPV vaccine were considerably lower; however, no disparities were observed by race/ethnicity or poverty status.

The absence of disparities by race/ethnicity and poverty status for the three recommended adolescent vaccinations represents a success story in public health, providing a striking illustration of rapid and even dissemination of a new preventive care recommendation over a short time period (around a decade). A number of factors have likely contributed to this success. In promoting the adolescent vaccination schedule, the immunization community was able to take advantage of the strong existing infrastructure developed for childhood vaccinations, including state-based vaccine registries that assist in tracking and monitoring vaccination rates over time. A second important facilitator was the presence of the Vaccines for Children (VFC) program from the start. VFC was introduced in 1994, nearly half a century after the first childhood vaccinations were recommended.[152] School mandates for vaccination, which are considered to be a major contributor to the achievement of high coverage rates for many childhood vaccinations, likely only facilitated coverage rates for Tdap and, to a lesser degree, meningococcal vaccine coverage.[153] Tdap is required for secondary school entry in 46 states and the District of Columbia, whereas 27 states and the District of Columbia have a school mandate for the first dose of the meningococcal vaccine. Although there has been considerable interest in school mandates for the HPV vaccine, with proposed legislation in a large number of states, these efforts have been largely unsuccessful. with school mandates for the HPV vaccine being enacted in only three regions to date: Rhode Island, Virginia, and the District of Columbia (Immunize.org). The inclusion of adolescent vaccinations as a Healthcare Effectiveness Data and Information Set (HEDIS) measure may also have contributed to the successful dissemination of adolescent vaccinations.[154] More than 90% of health plans in the United States, including Medicare, Medicaid, and the Children's Health Insurance Program, report HEDIS measures, which are linked to accreditation and reimbursement.[155] In 2010, Tdap and meningococcal vaccines were first included as a HEDIS measure, with HPV vaccination coverage for females added in 2011. Recent changes have been made to the HEDIS adolescent vaccination measures to capture HPV vaccine coverage data for males and to better integrate HPV vaccine coverage data.

Findings and Lessons Learned

The case of diffusion of adolescent vaccinations is somewhat unique and thus poses challenges when trying to apply "lessons learned" to other priority health areas. However, as has been previously documented, widespread policy-level efforts to increase rates of vaccination among adolescents has been an integral part of reducing disparities in this area, which suggests one possible direction for increasing uptake of other preventive health services.

DIRECTIONS FOR FUTURE RESEARCH

Clearly, much remains to be studied in order to advance health equity at a population level. Future research should explore how to adapt effective interventions to improve the fit for communities without losing fidelity to the original models, which often are developed for use in mainstream, non-minority communities. It is also important to identify and evaluate promising practice-based interventions from within the communities experiencing the disparities. In addition to efforts targeting individuals, organizations, and communities, models are needed that target providers and more structural factors, such as health systems.[149] Finally, future research should clarify which processes, strategies, and sequences optimize D&I in specific underserved and vulnerable communities.

SUMMARY

The evidence base on intervention D&I for racial/ethnic minority communities is expanding rapidly. Although the strength of the evidence varies depending on the health outcome, some general trends are apparent. Key lessons include that cultural appropriateness enhances community "buy-in" of interventions. Increasingly, interventions are expected to be culturally appropriate. This requires that both the message and the messenger are well suited for the community. Targeting captive audiences can reduce the cost to the individual of participating. Interventions that reflect a community's cultural values and that are implemented in ubiquitous settings are also associated with success. CBPR approaches that share power and decision-making are gaining in prominence. They suggest that intervention sustainability is enhanced when community members are actively involved as equal partners in all phases of research, implementation, and dissemination. Efforts that account for place characteristics (e.g., neighborhood geography, intervention setting) can also improve the uptake of interventions. In contrast to the individually focused models of early prevention efforts, emerging approaches (e.g., see Rudolph et al.[147]) target social networks or whole communities and attempt to address macrolevel factors that may influence multiple health outcomes. Despite impressive advances in the dissemination of effective interventions, disparities persist. One reason may be that interventions primarily target proximal factors (e.g., knowledge, attitudes, and behaviors) only. As the WHO Commission on the Social Determinants of Health concluded, however, to eradicate health disparities necessitates interventions that target the structural causes of the disparities (e.g., policies). These factors fundamentally shape all individual-level risk factors.[148] Therefore, they should be incorporated into future D&I endeavors.

In contrast to tightly controlled randomized trials that evaluate intervention efficacy, maximizing external validity is an essential goal of D&I research. This work focuses on disseminating evidence-based protocols to broader audiences in order to further our understanding of the potential public health impact of interventions. Nevertheless, few D&I studies specifically focus on the implications for underserved and ethnic minority communities.[16]

In conclusion, the importance of inclusivity and equity in public health efforts to prevent and control disease is paramount. The participation of ethnic minority and other underserved populations in leadership and as targets of such research and service efforts must be central, rather than marginal, weak, and fragmented. The best way to achieve social justice *and* improve the health of the entire population is to ensure that the strategies most effective in preventing disease are disseminated within the populations at greatest risk.

ACKNOWLEDGMENT

During the period between production of the original version of this chapter and the second edition, we lost our close friend and colleague Dr. Toni Yancey. Toni was an outstanding individual, gone too soon, and we appreciate the tremendous work she did to promote community-driven strategies to eliminate health disparities.

SUGGESTED READINGS AND WEBSITES

Readings

Israel BA, Schulz AJ, Parker EA, Becker AB. Review of community-based research: assessing partnership approaches to improve public health. *Annu Rev Public Health.* 1998;19:173–202.
One of the most cited papers on community-based participatory research (CBPR) in the health field. This paper introduces CBPR, its core principles, as well as some of the challenges entailed in their implementation. In addition to providing a review of the literature, this work uses early lessons of the Detroit Community-Academic Research Center to explicate CBPR principles and their implementation.

Ford CL, Airhihenbuwa CO. The public health critical race methodology: praxis for antiracism research. *Soc Sci Med.* 2010;71(8):1390–1398.
Introduces the Public Health Critical Race praxis (PHCR), developed by the authors as an aid for studying modern day racial phenomena. This model provides potential tools for finding and eradicating race-based health disparities.

Thomas SB, Quinn SC, Butler J, Fryer CS, Garza MA. Toward a fourth generation of disparities research to achieve health equity. *Annu Rev Public Health.* 2011;32:399–416.
This paper outlines ways to apply the Public Health Critical Race Praxis (PHCRP) to efforts to address racial and ethnic health disparities.

Frieden T. A framework for public health action: the health impact pyramid. *Am J Public Health.* 2010;100(4):590–595.
Describes a framework that uses a 5-tier pyramid to prioritize public health interventions with regard to their potential impact on population health and health disparities. The author suggests that interventions at each level are needed to maximize sustainable population health benefits.

Welch V, Tugwell P, Petticrew M, et al. How effects on health equity are assessed in systematic reviews of interventions. *Cochrane Database Syst Rev.* 2010;12.
A systematic review of methods to assess effects of health equity within systematic reviews of effectiveness of health care interventions. The authors propose clarifying the definition of health equity in order to accurately report health equity effects in systematic reviews.

Yancey A. The meta-volition model: organizational leadership is the key ingredient in getting society moving, literally! *Prev Med.* 2009;49(4):342–351.
Introduces a dynamic population health behavior change conceptual model (MVM) derived from key drivers of successful social movements. The model specifies a cascade of changes from initiation to institutionalization that must be sparked by "healthy by default" organizational practices and policies such as smoking bans, in-patient postnatal breastfeeding support and elimination of formula distribution, and structural integration of brief physical activity bouts.

Allicock M, Campbell MK, Valle CG, Carr C, Resnicow K, Gizlice Z. Evaluating the dissemination of Body & Soul, an evidence-based fruit and vegetable intake intervention: challenges for dissemination and implementation research. *J Nutr Educ Behav.* 2012;44(6):530–538.
This paper reports the results of an effort to disseminate the Body & Soul intervention to a sample of churches located throughout the country using a real-world approach.

Bowen D, Sorensen G, Weiner B, Campbell M, Emmons K, Melvin C. Dissemination research in cancer control: where are we and where should we go? *Cancer Causes Control.* 2009;20(4):473–485.
This paper explores various definition and models of dissemination, common designs used in dissemination studies, and potential research questions in dissemination research in cancer prevention and control.

Selected Websites and Tools

1. Cancer Control P.L.A.N.E.T. (Plan, Link, Act, Network with Evidence-based Tools). http://cancercontrolplanet.cancer.gov/

This website is intended for use by planners, program staff, and researchers seeking data and other resources to guide the design, implementation, and evaluation of evidence-based cancer control programs.

2. Centers for Disease Control and Prevention (CDC). Compendium of Evidence-Based Interventions and Best Practices for HIV Prevention. https://www.cdc.gov/hiv/research/interventionresearch/compendium/index.html

This website provides information about and access to tested evidence-based interventions and best practices for HIV prevention identified through systematic reviews that were conducted as part of the CDC's Prevention Research Synthesis (PRS) Project.

3. Centers for Disease Control and Prevention (CDC). Diffusion of Effective Behavioral Interventions (DEBI). http://effectiveinterventions.org/en/home.aspx

This website provides evidence-based, user-friendly information and resources to promote high impact HIV/AIDS prevention in the communities and groups (e.g., men who have sex with men) most impacted by HIV/AIDS.

4. Guide to Community Preventive Services. http://www.thecommunityguide.org/index.html

This website provides access to content from the Guide to Community Preventive Services (The Community Guide), a collection of evidence-based findings from the Community Preventive Services Task Force (Task Force). The Guide was developed to serve as a resource to guide organizations in selecting interventions designed to improve health and prevent disease that can be implemented within diverse settings in the community.

5. National Breast and Cervical Cancer Early Detection Program (NBCCEDP). http://www.cdc.gov/cancer/nbccedp/

This website provides information about the CDC's NBCCEDP program. The website contains information on the history of the program, how to find local NBCCEDP providers, how to access resources for NBCCEDP providers, papers reporting the results of research on the program, and other topics.

6. Vaccines for Children Program (VFC). https://www.cdc.gov/vaccines/programs/vfc/index.html

This website provides information about the CDC's Vaccines for Children Program including a description of the program and links for parents and VFC providers to learn more about the program.

7. World Health Organization Commission on the Social Determinants of Health. http://www.who.int/social_determinants/thecommission/finalreport/en/

This website explains what the social determinants of health are. Further, it provides reports, summaries, and media information to encourage researchers and practitioners to move beyond studying disparities toward address their root causes.

REFERENCES

1. National Center for Health Statistics (U.S.). Health, United States, 2004. Atlanta: Centers for Disease Control and Prevention, 2004.

2. Harper S, Lynch J, Burris S, Davey Smith G. Trends in the black-white life expectancy gap in the United States, 1983-2003. *JAMA.* 2007;297(11):1224–1232.

3. National Center for Health Statistics (US). Health, United States, 2015: With Special Features on Racial and Ethnic Health Disparities. Hyattsville, MD: 2016 Contract No.: Report No.: 2016-1232.

4. World Health Organization Commision on Social Determinants of Health. *Achieving health equity: From root causes to fair outcomes.* Geneva: World Health Organization; 2007.

5. Byrd W, Clayton L. *An American health dilemma: Race, medicine, and health care in the United States.* New York: Routledge; 2002.

6. Ford CL, Harawa NT. A new conceptualization of ethnicity for social epidemiologic and health equity research. *Soc Sci Med.* 2010;71(2):251–258.

7. Jones D. The persistence of American Indian health disparities. *Am J Public Health.* 2006;96(12):2122–2134.

8. Heart MY, Chase J, Elkins J, Altschul DB. Historical trauma among Indigenous Peoples of the Americas: concepts, research, and clinical considerations. *J Psychoactive Drugs.* 2011;43(4):282–290.

9. Gee G, Ford C. Structural racism and health inequities: old issues, new directions. *Du Bois Rev: Soc Sci Res Race.* 2011;8(1):115–132.

10. Derose K, Escarce J, Lurie N. Immigrants and health care: sources of vulnerability. *Health Aff (Millwood).* 2007;26(5):1258–1268.

11. Osypuk T, Roux A, Hadley C, Kandula N. Are immigrant enclaves healthy places to live? The Multi-ethnic Study of Atherosclerosis. *Soc Sci Med.* 2009;69(1):110–20.

12. Koya D, Egede L. Association between length of residence and cardiovascular disease risk factors among an ethnically diverse group of United States immigrants. *J Gen Intern Med.* 2007;22(6):841–846. doi: 10.1007/s11606-007-0163-y.

13. Williams DR. The health of U.S. racial and ethnic populations. *J Gerontol B Psychol Sci Soc Sci.* 2005;60 Spec No 2:53-62. doi: 60/suppl_Special_Issue_2/S53 [pii].

14. Viruell-Fuentes EA. Beyond acculturation: immigration, discrimination, and health research among Mexicans in the United States. *Soc Sci Med.* 2007;65(7):1524–1535.

15. Yancey A, Ortega A, Kumanyika S. Effective recruitment and retention of minority research participants. *Annu Rev Public Health.* 2006;27:1–28.

16. Yancey A, Ory M, Davis S. Dissemination of physical activity promotion interventions in underserved populations. *Am J Prev Med.* 2006;31(4 Suppl):S82–S91.

16a. Glasgow RE, Askew S, Purcell P, Levine E, Warner ET, Stange KC, Colditz GA. Use of RE-AIM to address health inequities: Application in a low-income community health center-based weight loss and hypertension self-management program. *Transl Behav Med.* 2013;3(2):200–2010.

17. Matson-Koffman DM, Brownstein JN, Neiner JA, Greaney ML. A site-specific literature review of policy and environmental interventions that promote physical activity and nutrition for cardiovascular health: what works? *Am J Health Promot.* 2005;19(3):167–193.

18. Lobstein T, Baur L, Uauy R. Obesity in children and young people: a crisis in public health. *Obes Rev.* 2004;5 Suppl 1:4–104.

19. Kersh R, Morone J. The politics of obesity: seven steps to government action. *Health Aff (Millwood).* 2002;21(6):142–153.

20. Heintzman J, Gold R, Krist A, Crosson J, Likumahuwa S, DeVoe JE. Practice-based research networks (PBRNs) are promising laboratories for conducting dissemination and implementation research. *J Am Board Fam Med.* Nov-Dec 2014;27(6):759–762.

21. Israel BA, Schulz AJ, Parker EA, Becker AB. Review of community-based research: assessing partnership approaches to improve public health. *Annu Rev Public Health.* 1998;19:173–202.

22. Green L, Daniel M, Novick L. Partnerships and coalitions for community-based research. *Public Health Rep.* 2001;116 Suppl 1:20–31.

23. Yancey A, Miles O, Jordan A. Organizational characteristics facilitating initiation and institutionalization of physical activity programs in a multi-ethnic, urban community. *J Health Educ.* 1999;30(2):S44–S51.

24. Grier S, Bryant CA. Social marketing in public health. *Annu Rev Public Health.* 2005;26:319–339.

24a. Franks A, Kelder S, Dino GA, Horn KA, Gortmaker SL, Wiecha JL, Simoes EJ. School-based Programs: Lessons Learned from CATCH, Planet Health, and Not-on-Tobacco. In: Hassan N, ed. *School Nutrition and Activity: Impacts on Well-Being.* Oakville, ON, Canada: Apple Academic Press 2015.

25. Bandura A. *Social foundations of thought and action: a social cognitive theory.* Englewood Cliffs, NJ: Prentice-Hall; 1986.

26. Allicock M, Campbell MK, Valle CG, Carr C, Resnicow K, Gizlice Z. Evaluating the dissemination of Body & Soul, an evidence-based fruit and vegetable intake intervention: challenges for dissemination and implementation research. *J Nutr Educ Behav.* Nov-Dec 2012;44(6):530–538.

27. Crawford ND, Galea S, Ford CL, Latkin C, Link BG, Fuller C. The relationship between discrimination and high-risk social ties by race/ethnicity: examining social pathways of HIV risk. *J Urban Health.* Feb 2014;91(1):151–161.

28. Alhassan S, Nwaokelemeh O, Mendoza A, Shitole S, Whitt-Glover MC, Yancey AK. Design and baseline characteristics of the Short bouTs of Exercise for Preschoolers (STEP) study. *BMC Public Health.* 2012;12:582.

29. Frieden T. A framework for public health action: the health impact pyramid. *Am J Public Health.* 2010;100(4):590–595.

30. Ford C, Airhihenbuwa C. The public health critical race methodology: praxis for antiracism research. *Soc Sci Med.* 2010;71(8):1390–1398.

31. Ford CL, Airhihenbuwa CO. Critical Race Theory, race equity, and public health: toward antiracism praxis. *Am J Public Health.* 2010;100 Suppl 1:S30–S35

32. Freimuth VS, Mettger W. Is there a hard-to-reach audience? *Public Health Rep.* 1990;105(3):232–238. PubMed PMID: 2113680.

33. Ory M, Kinney Hoffman M, Hawkins M, Sanner B, Mockenhaupt R. Challenging aging stereotypes: strategies for creating a more active society. *Am J Prev Med.* 2003;25(3 Suppl 2):164–171.

34. Yancey AK. Building capacity to prevent and control chronic disease in underserved communities: expanding the wisdom of WISEWOMAN in intervening at the environmental level. *J Womens Health (Larchmt).* 2004;13(5):644–649.

35. Yancey A, Kumanyika S, Ponce N, McCarthy W, Fielding J, Leslie J, Akbar J. Population-based interventions engaging communities of color in healthy eating and active living: a review. *Prev Chronic Dis.* 2004;1(1):A09.

36. Herring P, Montgomery S, Yancey AK, Williams D, Fraser G. Understanding the challenges in recruiting blacks to a longitudinal cohort study: the Adventist health study. *Ethn Dis.* 2004;14(3):423–430.

37. Bell L, Butler T, Herring R, Yancey A, Fraser G. Recruiting blacks to the Adventist health study: do follow-up phone calls increase response rates? *Ann Epidemiol.* 2005;15(9):667–672.

38. Thomas S, Curran J. Tuskegee: from science to conspiracy to metaphor. *Am J Med Sci.* 1999;317(1):1–4.

39. Yancey A, Cole B, Brown R, Williams J, Hillier A, Kline R, Ashe M, Grier S, Backman D, McCarthy W. A cross-sectional prevalence study of ethnically targeted and general audience outdoor obesity-related advertising. *Milbank Q.* 2009;87(1):155–184.

40. Herek GM, Capitanio JP. Conspiracies, contagion, and compassion: trust and public reactions to AIDS. *AIDS Educ Prevent.* 1994;6(4):365–375.

41. Corbie-Smith G, Ford CL. Distrust and poor self-reported health. Canaries in the coal mine? *J Gen Intern Med.* 2006;21(4):395–397.

42. Ford CL, Miller WC, Smurzynski M, Leone PA. Key components of a theory-guided HIV prevention outreach model: pre-outreach preparation, community assessment, and a network of key informants. *AIDS Educ Prev.* 2007;19(2):173–186.

43. Rabin B, Glasgow R, Kerner J, Klump M, Brownson R. Dissemination and implementation research on community-based cancer prevention: a systematic review. *Am J Prev Med.* 2010;38(4):443–456.

44. Aisenberg E. Evidence-based practice in mental health care to ethnic minority communities: has its practice fallen short of its evidence? *Soc Work.* 2008;53(4):297–306.

45. Whitt-Glover M, Kumanyika S. Systematic review of interventions to increase physical activity and physical fitness in African-Americans. *Am J Health Promot.* 2009;23(6):S33–S56.

46. Yancey A, Tomiyama A. Physical activity as primary prevention to address cancer disparities. *Semin Oncol Nurs.* 2007;23(4):253–263.

47. Agency for Healthcare Research and Quality. Diffusion and *Dissemination of Evidence-based Cancer Control Interventions. 2003 Summary,* Evidence Report/Technology Assessment: Number 79.

48. Perry C, Sellers D, Johnson C, Pedersen S, Bachman K, Parcel G, Stone E, Luepker R, Wu M, Nader P, Cook K. The child and adolescent trial for cardiovascular health (CATCH): intervention, implementation, and feasibility for elementary schools in the United States. *Health Educ Behav.* 1997;24(6):716–735.

49. Perry C, Stone E, Parcel G, Ellison R, Nader P, Webber L, Luepker R. School-based cardiovascular health promotion: the child and adolescent trial for cardiovascular health (CATCH). *J Sch Health.* 1990;60(8):406–413.

50. Tsai P, Boonpleng W, McElmurry B, Park C, McCreary L. Lessons learned in using TAKE 10! with Hispanic children. *J Sch Nurs.* 2009;25(2):163–172.

51. Barry M, Mosca C, Dennison D, Kohl H, Hill J. TAKE 10! program and attraction to physical activity and classroom environment in elementary school students. *Med Sci Sport.* 2003;35:S134.

52. Kohl H, Moore B, Sutton A, Kibbe D, Schneider D. A curriculum-integrated classroom physical activity promotion tool for elementary schools: teacher evaluation of TAKE 10!. *Med Sci Sport.* 2001;33:S179.

53. Mahar M, Rowe D, Kenny R, Fesperman D. Evaluation of the TAKE 10! classroom based physical activity program. *Med Sci Sport.* 2003;35:S135.

54. Stewart J, Dennison D, Kohl H, Doyle J. Exercise level and energy expenditure in the TAKE 10! in-class physical activity program. *J Sch Health.* 2004;74(10):397–400.

55. Naylor P, Macdonald H, Reed K, McKay H. Action Schools! BC: a socioecological approach to modifying chronic disease risk factors in elementary school children. *Prev Chronic Dis.* 2006;3(2):A60.

56. Naylor P, Scott J, Drummond J, Bridgewater L, McKay H, Panagiotopoulos C. Implementing a whole school physical activity and healthy eating model in rural and remote first nations schools: a process evaluation of action schools! BC. *Rural Remote Health.* 2010;10(2):1296.

57. Fitzgibbon ML, Stolley MR, Schiffer L, Van Horn L, KauferChristoffel K, Dyer A. Hip-Hop to Health Jr. for Latino preschool children. *Obesity (Silver Spring).* 2006;14(9):1616–1625.

58. Fitzgibbon ML, Stolley MR, Schiffer LA, Braunschweig CL, Gomez SL, Van Horn L, Dyer AR. Hip-Hop to Health Jr. Obesity Prevention Effectiveness Trial: postintervention results. *Obesity (Silver Spring).* 2011;19(5):994–1003.

59. Stables G, Young E, Howerton M, Yaroch A, Kuester S, Solera M, Cobb K, Nebeling L. Small school-based effectiveness trials increase vegetable and fruit consumption among youth. *J Am Diet Assoc.* 2005;105(2):252–256.

60. Resnicow K, Campbell M, Carr C, McCarty F, Wang T, Periasamy S, Rahotep S, Doyle C, Williams A, Stables G. Body and soul. A dietary intervention conducted through African-American churches. *Am J Prev Med.* 2004;27(2):97–105.

61. Allicock M, Campbell MK, Valle CG, Carr C, Resnicow K, Gizlice Z. Evaluating the dissemination of Body & Soul, an evidence-based fruit and vegetable intake intervention: challenges for dissemination and implementation research. *J Nutr Educ Behav.* 2012;44(6):530–538.

62. Maxwell AE, Yancey AK, AuYoung M, Guinyard JJ, Glenn BA, Mistry R, McCarthy WJ, Fielding JE, Simon PA, Bastani R. A midpoint process

evaluation of the Los Angeles Basin Racial and Ethnic Approaches to Community Health across the US (REACH US) Disparities Center, 2007-2009. *Prev Chronic Dis.* 2011;8(5):A115.

63. Pollack KM, Schmid TL, Wilson AL, Schulman E. Advancing translation and dissemination research and practice through the physical activity policy research network plus. *Environ Behav.* 2016;48(1):266–272.

64. Galvez M, Morland K, Raines C, Kobil J, Siskind J, Godbold J, Brenner B. Race and food store availability in an inner-city neighbourhood. *Public Health Nutr.* 2008;11(6):624–631.

65. Grier S, Kumanyika S. Targeted marketing and public health. *Annu Rev Public Health.* 2010;31:349–369.

66. Powell L, Slater S, Mirtcheva D, Bao Y, Chaloupka F. Food store availability and neighborhood characteristics in the United States. *Prev Med.* 2007;44(3):189–195.

67. Ford P, Dzewaltowski D. Disparities in obesity prevalence due to variation in the retail food environment: three testable hypotheses. *Nutr Rev.* 2008;66(4):216–228.

68. Boyd N, Sutton C, Orleans C, McClatchey M, Bingler R, Fleisher L, Heller D, Baum S, Graves C, Ward J. Quit Today! A targeted communications campaign to increase use of the cancer information service by African American smokers. *Prev Med.* 1998;27(5 Pt 2):S50–S60.

69. Marín G, Marín B, Pérez-Stable E, Sabogal F, Otero-Sabogal R. Changes in information as a function of a culturally appropriate smoking cessation community intervention for Hispanics. *Am J Community Psychol.* 1990;18(6):847–864.

70. Marín G, Pérez-Stable E. Effectiveness of disseminating culturally appropriate smoking-cessation information: Programa Latino Para Dejar de Fumar. *J Natl Cancer Inst Monogr.* 1995;(18):155–163.

71. Pérez-Stable E, Marín B, Marín G. A comprehensive smoking cessation program for the San Francisco Bay Area Latino community: Programa Latino Para Dejar de Fumar. *Am J Health Promot.* 1993;7(6):430–442, 75.

72. Dobbins M, DeCorby K, Manske S, Goldblatt E. Effective practices for school-based tobacco use prevention. *Prev Med.* 2008;46(4):289–297.

73. Wiehe S, Garrison M, Christakis D, Ebel B, Rivara F. A systematic review of school-based smoking prevention trials with long-term follow-up. *J Adolesc Health.* 2005;36(3):162–169.

74. Basen-Engquist K, O'Hara-Tompkins N, Lovato C, Lewis M, Parcel G, Gingiss P. The effect of two types of teacher training on implementation of

Smart Choices: a tobacco prevention curriculum. *J Sch Health.* 1994;64(8):334–339.

75. Perry C, Murray D, Griffin G. Evaluating the statewide dissemination of smoking prevention curricula: factors in teacher compliance. *J Sch Health.* 1990;60(10):501–504.

76. Parcel G, Eriksen M, Lovato C, Gottlieb N, Brink S, Green L. The diffusion of school-based tobacco-use prevention programs: project description and baseline data. *Health Educ Res.* 1989;4:111–124.

77. Parcel G, O'Hara-Tompkins N, Harrist R, Basen-Engquist K, McCormick L, Gottlieb N, Eriksen M. Diffusion of an effective tobacco prevention program. Part II: Evaluation of the adoption phase. *Health Educ Res.* 1995;10(3):297–307.

78. Brink S, Basen-Engquist K, O'Hara-Tompkins N, Parcel G, Gottlieb N, Lovato C. Diffusion of an effective tobacco prevention program. Part I: Evaluation of the dissemination phase. *Health Educ Res.* 1995;10(3):283–295.

79. Lanza ST, Russell MA, Braymiller JL. Emergence of electronic cigarette use in US adolescents and the link to traditional cigarette use. *Addict Behav.* 2016;67:38–43.

80. Levy D, Chaloupka F, Gitchell J. The effects of tobacco control policies on smoking rates: a tobacco control scorecard. *J Public Health Manag Pract.* 2004;10(4):338–353.

81. Ferketich A, Liber A, Pennell M, Nealy D, Hammer J, Berman M. Clean indoor air ordinance coverage in the Appalachian region of the United States. *Am J Public Health.* 2010;100(7):1313–1318.

82. Bowen D, Sorensen G, Weiner B, Campbell M, Emmons K, Melvin C. Dissemination research in cancer control: where are we and where should we go? *Cancer Causes Control.* 2009;20(4):473–485.

83. Tinkle M, Kimball R, Haozous EA, Shuster G, Meize-Grochowski R. Dissemination and implementation research funded by the US National Institutes of Health, 2005-2012. *Nurs Res Pract.* 2013;2013:909606.

84. Baron R, Rimer B, Coates R, Kerner J, Kalra G, Melillo S, Habarta N, Wilson K, Chattopadhyay S, Leeks K, Services TFoCP. Client-directed interventions to increase community access to breast, cervical, and colorectal cancer screening a systematic review. *Am J Prev Med.* 2008;35(1 Suppl):S56–S66.

85. Centers for Disease Control and Prevention. Guide to community preventive services. Cancer prevention and control: client-oriented screening interventions. Atlanta, GA: 2009.

86. Kolahdooz F, Jang SL, Corriveau A, Gotay C, Johnston N, Sharma S. Knowledge, attitudes, and

behaviours towards cancer screening in indigenous populations: a systematic review. *Lancet Oncol.* 2014;15(11):e504–e516.

87. Centers for Disease Control and Prevention National Breast and Cervical Cancer Early Detection Program (NBCCEDP).

88. Centers for Disease Control and Prevention. Colorectal Cancer Control Program (CRCCP). 2016; Available from: https://www.cdc.gov/cancer/crccp/.

89. Escoffery C, Hannon P, Maxwell AE, Vu T, Leeman J, Dwyer A, Mason C, Sowles S, Rice K, Gressard L. Assessment of training and technical assistance needs of Colorectal Cancer Control Program Grantees in the U.S. *BMC Public Health.* 2015;15:49.

90. Escoffery CT, Kegler MC, Glanz K, Graham TD, Blake SC, Shapiro JA, Mullen PD, Fernandez ME. Recruitment for the National Breast and Cervical Cancer Early Detection Program. *Am J Prev Med.* 2012;42(3):235–241.

91. Hannon PA, Maxwell AE, Escoffery C, Vu T, Kohn M, Leeman J, Carvalho ML, Pfeiffer DJ, Dwyer A, Fernandez ME, Vernon SW, Liang L, DeGroff A. Colorectal Cancer Control Program grantees' use of evidence-based interventions. *Am J Prev Med.* 2013;45(5):644–648.

92. Subramanian S, Tangka FK, Ekwueme DU, Trogdon J, Crouse W, Royalty J. Explaining variation across grantees in breast and cervical cancer screening proportions in the NBCCEDP. *Cancer Causes Control.* 2015;26(5):689–695.

93. Tangka FK, Howard DH, Royalty J, Dalzell LP, Miller J, O'Hara BJ, Sabatino SA, Joseph K, Kenney K, Guy GP, Jr., Hall IJ. Cervical cancer screening of underserved women in the United States: results from the National Breast and Cervical Cancer Early Detection Program, 1997-2012. *Cancer Causes Control.* 2015;26(5):671–686.

94. Wu M, Austin H, Eheman CR, Myles Z, Miller J, Royalty J, Ryerson AB. A comparative analysis of breast cancer stage between women enrolled in the National Breast and Cervical Cancer Early Detection Program and women not participating in the program. *Cancer Causes Control.* 2015;26(5):751–758.

95. Allen JD, Torres MI, Tom LS, Leyva B, Galeas AV, Ospino H. Dissemination of evidence-based cancer control interventions among Catholic faith-based organizations: results from the CRUZA randomized trial. *Implement Sci.* 2016;11(1):74.

96. Holt CL, Tagai EK, Scheirer MA, Santos SL, Bowie J, Haider M, Slade JL, Wang MQ, Whitehead T. Translating evidence-based interventions for implementation: experiences from Project HEAL in African American churches. *Implement Sci.* 2014;9:66.

96a. Slater J, Finnegan JR, Madigan SD. Incorporation of a successful community-based mammography intervention: Dissemination beyond a community Trial. *Health Psychol.* 2005;24(5):463–469.

97. Bencivenga M, DeRubis S, Leach P, Lotito L, Shoemaker C, Lengerich E. Community partnerships, food pantries, and an evidence-based intervention to increase mammography among rural women. *J Rural Health.* 2008;24(1):91–95.

98. Kreuter M, Black W, Friend L, Booker A, Klump P, Bobra S, Holt C. Use of computer kiosks for breast cancer education in five community settings. *Health Educ Behav.* 2006;33(5):625–642.

99. Hou SI, Roberson K. A systematic review on US-based community health navigator (CHN) interventions for cancer screening promotion-- comparing community- versus clinic-based navigator models. *J Cancer Educ.* 2015;30(1):173–186.

100. Nguyen BH, Stewart SL, Nguyen TT, Bui-Tong N, McPhee SJ. Effectiveness of lay health worker outreach in reducing disparities in colorectal cancer screening in Vietnamese Americans. *Am J Public Health.* 2015;105(10):2083–2089.

101. Maxwell AE, Danao LL, Bastani R. Dissemination of colorectal cancer screening by Filipino American community health advisors: a feasibility study. *Health Promot Pract.* 2013;14(4):498–505.

102. Maxwell AE, Danao LL, Cayetano RT, Crespi CM, Bastani R. Adoption of an evidence-based colorectal cancer screening promotion program by community organizations serving Filipino Americans. *BMC Public Health.* 2014;14:246.

103. Joshi A, Trout K. The role of health information kiosks in diverse settings: a systematic review. *Health Info Libr J.* 2014;31(4):254–273.

104. Bennett GG. Connecting eHealth with 2-1-1 to reduce health disparities. *Am J Prev Med.* 2012;43(6 Suppl 5):S509–S511.

105. Hall KL, Stipelman BA, Eddens KS, Kreuter MW, Bame SI, Meissner HI, Yabroff KR, Purnell JQ, Ferrer R, Ribisl KM, Glasgow R, Linnan LA, Taplin S, Fernandez ME. Advancing collaborative research with 2-1-1 to reduce health disparities: challenges, opportunities, and recommendations. *Am J Prev Med.* 2012;43(6 Suppl 5):S518–S528.

106. Kreuter MW, Eddens KS, Alcaraz KI, Rath S, Lai C, Caito N, Greer R, Bridges N, Purnell JQ, Wells A, Fu Q, Walsh C, Eckstein E, Griffith J, Nelson A, Paine C, Aziz T, Roux AM. Use of cancer control referrals by 2-1-1 callers: a randomized trial. *Am J Prev Med.* 2012;43(6 Suppl 5):S425–S434.

107. Highfield L, Rajan SS, Valerio MA, Walton G, Fernandez ME, Bartholomew LK. A

non-randomized controlled stepped wedge trial to evaluate the effectiveness of a multi-level mammography intervention in improving appointment adherence in underserved women. *Implement Sci.* 2015;10:143.

108. James AS, Richardson V, Wang JS, Proctor EK, Colditz GA. Systems intervention to promote colon cancer screening in safety net settings: protocol for a community-based participatory randomized controlled trial. *Implement Sci.* 2013;8:58.

109. Larkey L, Szalacha L, Herman P, Gonzalez J, Menon U. Randomized controlled dissemination study of community-to-clinic navigation to promote CRC screening: study design and implications. *Contemp Clin Trials.* 2016.

110. Tu SP, Young VM, Coombs LJ, Williams RS, Kegler MC, Kimura AT, Risendal BC, Friedman DB, Glenn BA, Pfeiffer DJ, Fernandez ME. Practice adaptive reserve and colorectal cancer screening best practices at community health center clinics in 7 states. *Cancer.* 2015;121(8):1241–1248.

111. Fernandez ME, Melvin CL, Leeman J, Ribisl KM, Allen JD, Kegler MC, Bastani R, Ory MG, Risendal BC, Hannon PA, Kreuter MW, Hebert JR. The cancer prevention and control research network: an interactive systems approach to advancing cancer control implementation research and practice. *Cancer Epidemiol Biomarkers Prev.* 2014;23(11):2512–2521.

112. Harris JR, Brown PK, Coughlin S, Fernandez ME, Hebert JR, Kerner J, Prout M, Schwartz R, Simoes EJ, White C, Wilson K. The cancer prevention and control research network. *Prev Chronic Dis.* 2005;2(1):A21.

112a. Ribisl KM, Fernandez ME, Friedman DB, et al. Impact of the Cancer Prevention and Control Research Network: Accelerating the Translation of Research Into Practice. *Am J Prev Med.* Mar 2017;52(3S3):S233–S240.

113. Dworkin S, Pinto R, Hunter J, Rapkin B, Remien R. Keeping the spirit of community partnerships alive in the scale up of HIV/AIDS prevention: critical reflections on the roll out of DEBI (Diffusion of Effective Behavioral Interventions). *Am J Community Psychol.* 2008;42(1-2):51–59.

114. Norton W, Amico K, Cornman D, Fisher W, Fisher J. An agenda for advancing the science of implementation of evidence-based HIV prevention interventions. *AIDS Behav.* 2009;13(3):424–429.

115. Kilbourne A, Neumann M, Pincus H, Bauer M, Stall R. Implementing evidence-based interventions in health care: application of the replicating effective programs framework. *Implement Sci.* 2007;2:42.

116. Collins CB, Jr., Sapiano TN. Lessons Learned From Dissemination of Evidence-Based Interventions for HIV Prevention. *Am J Prev Med.* 2016;51(4 Suppl 2):S140–S147.

117. Norton WE, Larson RS, Dearing JW. Primary care and public health partnerships for implementing pre-exposure prophylaxis. *Am J Prev Med.* 2013;44(1 Suppl 2):S77–S79.

118. Duffus WA, Weis K, Kettinger L, Stephens T, Albrecht H, Gibson JJ. Risk-based HIV testing in South Carolina health care settings failed to identify the majority of infected individuals. *AIDS Patient Care STDS.* 2009;23(5):339–345.

119. Stallworth J, Andía J, Burgess R, Alvarez M, Collins C. Diffusion of Effective Behavioral Interventions and Hispanic/Latino populations. *AIDS Educ Prev.* 2009;21(5 Suppl):152–163.

120. Mays V, Cochran S, Zamudio A. HIV Prevention research: are we meeting the needs of African American men who have sex with men? *J Black Psychol.* 2004;30(1):78–105.

121. Ford C, Whetten K, Hall S, Kaufman J, Thrasher A. Black sexuality, social construction, and research targeting "The Down Low" ("The DL"). *Ann Epidemiol.* 2007;17(3):209–216.

122. Goldbaum G, Perdue T, Wolitski R, Rietmeijer C, Hedrich A, Wood R, Fishbein M, Project ACD. Differences in risk behavior and sources of AIDS information among gay, bisexual, and straight-identified men who have sex with men. *AIDS Behav.* 1998;2(1):13–21.

123. Wingood GM, Diclemente RJ, Mikhail I, McCree DH, Davies SL, Hardin JW, Harris Peterson S, Hook EW, Saag M. HIV discrimination and the health of women living with HIV. *Women Health.* 2007;46(2/3):99–112.

124. Prather C, Fuller TR, King W, Brown M, Moering M, Little S, Phillips K. Diffusing an HIV prevention intervention for African American women: integrating Afrocentric components into the SISTA diffusion strategy. *AIDS Educ Prevent.* 2006;18(Supp A):149–160.

125. Freed G, Bordley W, DeFriese G. Childhood immunization programs: an analysis of policy issues. *Milbank Q.* 1993;71(1):65–96.

126. Hill HA, Elam-Evans LD, Yankey D, Singleton JA, Kolasa M. National, state, and selected local area vaccination coverage among children aged 19-35 months—United States, 2014. *MMWR Morb Mortal Wkly Rep.* 2015;64(33):889–896.

127. Hutchins S, Jiles R, Bernier R. Elimination of measles and of disparities in measles childhood vaccine coverage among racial and ethnic minority populations in the United States. *J Infect Dis.* 2004;189 Suppl 1:S146–S152.

128. Galea S, Sisco S, Vlahov D. Reducing disparities in vaccination rates between different racial/ethnic and socioeconomic groups: the potential of community-based multilevel interventions. *J Ambul Care Manage*. 2005;28(1):49–59.

129. Centers for Disease Control and Prevention. Influenza vaccination coverage among children and adults—United States, 2008-09 influenza season. *MMWR Morb Mortal Wkly Rep*. 2009;58(39):1091–1095.

130. Sabnis SS, Conway JH. Overcoming challenges to childhood immunizations status. *Pediatr Clin North Am*. 2015;62(5):1093–1109.

131. Varan AK, Rodriguez-Lainz A, Hill HA, Elam-Evans LD, Yankey D, Li Q. Vaccination coverage disparities between foreign-born and U.S.-born children aged 19-35 months, United States, 2010-2012. *J Immigr Minor Health*. 2016.

132. Hoekstra E, LeBaron C, Megaloeconomou Y, Guerrero H, Byers C, Johnson-Partlow T, Lyons B, Mihalek E, Devier J, Mize J. Impact of a large-scale immunization initiative in the Special Supplemental Nutrition Program for Women, Infants, and Children (WIC). *JAMA*. 1998;280(13):1143–1147.

133. Birkhead G, LeBaron C, Parsons P, Grabau J, Maes E, Barr-Gale L, Fuhrman J, Brooks S, Rosenthal J, Hadler S. The immunization of children enrolled in the Special Supplemental Food Program for Women, Infants, and Children (WIC). The impact of different strategies. *JAMA*. 1995;274(4):312–316.

134. Community Preventive Services Task Force. Vaccination 2016. Available from: https://www.thecommunityguide.org/topic/vaccination.

135. Dougherty D, Chen X, Gray DT, Simon AE. Child and adolescent health care quality and disparities: are we making progress? *Acad Pediatr*. 2014;14(2):137–148.

136. Suryadevara M, Bonville CA, Ferraioli F, Domachowske JB. Community-centered education improves vaccination rates in children from low-income households. *Pediatrics*. 2013;132(2):319–325.

137. Crocker-Buque T, Edelstein M, Mounier-Jack S. Interventions to reduce inequalities in vaccine uptake in children and adolescents aged <19 years: a systematic review. *J Epidemiol Community Health*. 2017;71(1):87–97.

138. Brabin L, Greenberg D, Hessel L, Hyer R, Ivanoff B, Van Damme P. Current issues in adolescent immunization. *Vaccine*. 2008;26(33):4120–4134.

139. Centers for Disease Control and Prevention. Vaccination coverage among adolescents aged 13-17 years--United States, 2008. *MMWR Morb Mortal Wkly Rep*. 2009;38(36):997–1001.

140. Dempsey AF, Zimet GD. Interventions to improve adolescent vaccination: what may work and what still needs to be tested. *Am J Prev Med*. 2015;49(6 Suppl 4):S445–S454.

141. Reagan-Steiner S, Yankey D, Jeyarajah J, Elam-Evans LD, Curtis CR, MacNeil J, Markowitz LE, Singleton JA. National, regional, state, and selected local area vaccination coverage among adolescents aged 13-17 years—United States, 2015. *MMWR Morb Mortal Wkly Rep*. 2016;65(33):850–858.

142. Ompad D, Galea S, Vlahov D. Distribution of influenza vaccine to high-risk groups. *Epidemiol Rev*. 2006;28:54–70.

143. Lu P, Bridges C, Euler G, Singleton J. Influenza vaccination of recommended adult populations, U.S., 1989-2005. *Vaccine*. 2008;26(14):1786–1793.

144. Fiscella K. Tackling disparities in influenza vaccination in primary care: it takes a team. *J Gen Intern Med*. 2014;29(12):1579–1581.

145. Lau D, Hu J, Majumdar SR, Storie DA, Rees SE, Johnson JA. Interventions to improve influenza and pneumococcal vaccination rates among community-dwelling adults: a systematic review and meta-analysis. *Ann Fam Med*. 2012;10(6):538–546.

146. Institute of Medicine (US) Committee on Lesbian Gay, Bisexual, and Transgender Health Issues and Research Gaps and Opportunities. *The health of lesbian, gay, bisexual, and transgender people: Building a foundation for better understanding*. Washington, DC: National Academy of Sciences, 2011.

147. Rudolph AE, Standish K, Amesty S, Crawford ND, Stern RJ, Badillo WE, Boyer A, Brown D, Ranger N, Orduna JM, Lasenburg L, Lippek S, Fuller CM. A community-based approach to linking injection drug users with needed services through pharmacies: an evaluation of a pilot intervention in New York City. *AIDS Educ Prev*. 2010;22(3):238–251.

148. Friedman SR, Cooper HL, Osborne AH. Structural and social contexts of HIV risk Among African Americans. *Am J Public Health*. 2009;99(6):1002–1008.

149. Reich AD, Hansen HB, Link BG. Fundamental interventions: how clinicians can address the fundamental causes of disease. *J Bioeth Inq*. 2016;13(2):185–192.

150. Walsh B, Doherty E, O'Neill C. Since the start of the vaccines for children program, uptake has increased, and most disparities have decreased. *Health Aff (Millwood)*. 2016;35(2):356–364.

151. Broder KR, Cohn AC, Schwartz B, Klein JD, Fisher MM, Fishbein DB, Mijalski C, Burstein GR, Vernon-Smiley ME, McCauley MM, Wibbelsman CJ; Working Group on Adolescent Prevention Priorities. Adolescent immunizations and other clinical preventive services: a needle and a hook? *Pediatrics.* 2008;121 Suppl 1:S25–S34.

152. Centers for Disease Control and Prevention. Vaccines for Children Program. 2016; Available from: https://www.cdc.gov/vaccines/programs/vfc/about/.

153. Immunize Action Coalition. State mandates on immunization and vaccine-preventable diseases. 2016.

154. National Committee for Quality Assurance. HEDIS & Performance Measurement. 2016; Available from: http://www.ncqa.org/hedis-quality-measurement.

155. National Committee for Quality Assurance. Proposed Changes to Existing Measures for HEDIS 2017: Immunization for Adolescents and Human Papillomavirus Vaccine for Female Adolescents. 2016.

156. Dzewaltowski D, Estabrooks P, Glasgow R. The future of physical activity behavior change research: what is needed to improve translation of research into health promotion practice? *Exerc Sport Sci Rev.* 2004;32(2):57–63.

28

Dissemination and Implementation Research in a Global Context

REBECCA LOBB, SHOBA RAMANADHAN, AND LAURA MURRAY

INTRODUCTION

Low- and middle-income countries (LMICs) account for over 80% of the world's population, so it is impossible to overstate the need for global dissemination and implementation (D&I) research for health in lower resource countries.[1] The burden and mortality from infectious and noncommunicable disease is greater for LMICs than for higher income countries.[2] Furthermore, the dissemination and implementation gap between research and practice is wider for LMICs compared with higher income countries.[2] Even relatively simple interventions such as vaccination coverage to prevent death in children under age 5 lag behind goals established by the World Health Organization (WHO). Regional rates show that the LMIC regions of Africa and Southeast Asia have the poorest vaccination coverage on the globe, 75% and 77% respectively, substantially under the WHO's goal of 90%. However, it is the variation in coverage within LMIC regions that reflects the true need for D&I research. Within the continent of Africa vaccination coverage varies from 11.4% in Chad to 90.3% in Rwanda.[3]

Noncommunicable disease has become a greater concern than communicable disease in LMICs, including mental and neurological disorders, which contribute to 28% of the burden of disease attributed to noncommunicable causes.[1,4] Cost is often cited as a deterrent to translating effective interventions to practice in LMICs. Yet, many evidence-based interventions (EBPs) would be affordable for LMICs if scaled to a population level. As an example, scaling-up a package of cost-effective treatment for schizophrenia, depression, bipolar affective disorder, and hazardous alcohol use would cost about $2 per person per year in low-income countries and $3 to $4 per person per year in lower middle-income countries.[1]

Other translational challenges to moving research into practice within LMICs include the relevance of the research to local settings. Decision-makers may fail to see the value of interventions that were developed with populations or settings that are not representative of LMICs. They may also have insufficient primary data to be able to act.[5] Also, interventions developed using randomized-controlled trials may not provide sufficient information about the acceptability, feasibility or effectiveness of the intervention when used in real world conditions in LMICs. An example is the randomized trials that provide overwhelming evidence in support of insecticide-treated mosquito nets to reduce individual risk of malaria-related morbidity and mortality.[6] Worldwide donations were made to mitigate cost as a barrier to use of mosquito nets in LMIC regions. However, one estimate found that only 33% of owners in LMICs used the mosquito netting.[6] Barriers to use included complaints of discomfort due to heat and confusion over the purpose of the nets. Some owners thought the purpose was to minimize sleep disturbance from mosquitos rather than prevent malaria transmission.[6] These factors, combined with the ingenuity of the owners and scarcity of food, contributed to use of nets for fishing.[6,7] The lack of information on implementation factors to complement data from the randomized trials led to the threat of overfishing and insecticide toxicity to fish and humans.[7] This extreme example of a global health innovation highlights the acute need for dissemination and implementation research in conjunction with effectiveness trials to improve the acceptability, feasibility, and effectiveness of EBPs to accelerate the translation of research to practice within LMIC regions of the globe.

The authors have adapted the WHO framework for the implementation research cycle to

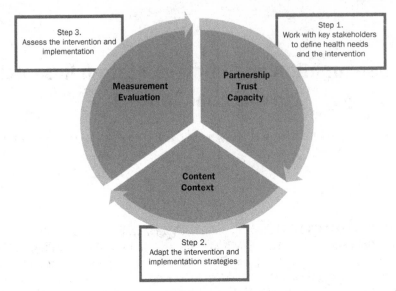

FIGURE 28.1 Implementation research cycle.

(Adapted from the World Health Organization.)

describe the nuances of D&I research for health in LMICs.[8] D&I research is a stepwise, cyclical process that involves: (1) working with key stakeholders to define health needs and appropriate interventions; (2) adapting the intervention and implementation strategies; and (3) assessing the intervention and implementation (Figure 28.1).[8] In-depth discussion of each step is provided in this chapter.

STEP 1. WORK WITH KEY STAKEHOLDERS

A participatory research approach (chapter 11) is necessary for D&I research in LMICs to assure attention to local health needs, the relevance of interventions, and feasibility to implement the interventions.[9] However, some considerations for building partnerships with stakeholders are uniquely emphasized for D&I research in LMICs, including partnership composition, building trust, and building capacity for future research and implementation.

Partnership Composition

To compensate for poorer infrastructure and lower resources in LMICs, partnership composition may need to be broader than required for participatory research conducted in higher income countries. Key stakeholders may include foreign governments, nongovernmental organizations, pharmaceutical and biotechnology companies in addition to the stakeholders usually engaged in D&I research in high-income countries (HICs; e.g., local organizations and residents). Ideally, ethnographic work would be an initial step to better understand the local context, problems, existing solutions, and challenges without relying just on "hearsay" of any one partner or "voice." However, D&I researchers should be aware that partnership composition will be strongly influenced by the initial partners identified to help champion the study in the local context because people tend to connect with people from similar disciplines.[10,11] To maximize the representativeness of key stakeholders, the research team can continuously monitor the impact of partnership composition on defining the problem and potential solutions to successfully implement the study.[10] Nabyonga-Orem et al. recommend "mapping the relevant stakeholders and devising the mechanism for their engagement and for how to resolve conflicts of interest and disagreements."[12] Connecting with the appropriate cross-section of local stakeholders for international collaborations for D&I research is critical to the project's success.

Building Trust

The weight of historical references and geographic distance between the Principal Investigator and LMIC can present barriers to the traditional methods for building trust with research stakeholders (e.g., communication, joint decision-making, time in the community).[13,14] D&I researchers should develop an understanding of the political and economic history of the LMIC and a sensitivity toward the power position of initial partners who may not be well connected with grassroots groups or end-users.[10] Trust can also be a function of concerns about research or a deeper concern related to historical interactions between outside researchers and stakeholders from the LMIC.[15] For example, a community-based participatory research study focused on "cervical health" among Black South African women found that partner communities were suspicious of research activities, having been subjected to a series of research activities in which White researchers collected data and left, without any improvement of the lives of the study participants or communities. The research team had to demonstrate that the work conducted would not be exploitative and would concretely benefit the community.[16] Ongoing engagement with stakeholders and investments in human capital (e.g., capacity-building), social capital (e.g., network development within and outside the community), and resource sharing (e.g., stipends and in-kind contributions) will contribute toward building trust with communities over time.[17] Time spent in the community building relationships and understanding culture and context is an important investment, particularly given issues of mistrust outlined, but also poses a challenge when members of the team live in different regions or parts of the world. As the penetration of new media technologies such as video calling increases, these innovations can be used to promote face-to-face interactions between stakeholders and the primary research team. Building trust may be accelerated by encouraging stakeholders from LMICs to have the researchers answer their questions before a project can be considered in that community.[18]

Building Capacity

D&I research in LMICs can have ripple effects to improve population health and build capacity for future research. Focusing on and testing implementation strategies in the local context will maximize the likelihood that D&I research will build capacity for health programs that can be sustained. The ripple effects of D&I research can begin as improvements in organizations or regions. For example, HIV prevention researchers have highlighted the important overlaps between capacity built for implementation research and capacity required for monitoring and evaluation efforts, management science, and continuous quality improvement.[19,20] The ripple effects can also have a direct positive impact on the local stakeholders who are invited to implement the EBPs. Training can elevate a persons' professional status in the community and have lasting effects on job opportunities and income.[21] However, D&I researchers should be cognizant of potential adverse consequences to the study if change in the implementer's social status means that participants in the study no longer view the stakeholder as "one of them." Hiring of local data collectors and project managers to leverage their language, cultural knowledge, and relationships to the community also builds capacity for future research. D&I researchers should engage fieldworkers to design study tools and research procedures to maximize the relevance and feasibility for implementation. Training in research methods and human subjects should be a priority and may include reading short excerpts from academic papers, critiquing interview strategies, or role playing.[22] The exchange of lay and scientific knowledge through training for in-country research support will build trust between researchers and local stakeholders and potentially generate ideas for future research collaborations.

STEP 2. ADAPT THE INTERVENTION AND IMPLEMENTATION STRATEGIES

The bulk of the evidence-based practices and implementation strategies come from HICs and cannot be directly transferred to LMICs that generally have fewer human, structural and financial resources to support implementation.[5,23,24] For this reason, D&I researchers will need to consider adapting both the intervention and implementation strategy for LMICs.[24] Regardless of the type of adaptations, a key feature of adaptation is that it must be systematic and strategic to balance flexibility with fidelity. Flexibility in program offerings not only supports adaptation from HICs to a given LMIC, but also within country translations of evidence to practice. Building flexibility into the design of EBPs allows decision-makers and practitioners to accommodate the range of populations and contexts, and combinations of these, in which an EBP might be used and facilitates scaling-up interventions found to be effective in LMICs.[25-27] The Stirman system provides a useful framework for classifying adaptations to EBPs, guiding the D&I researcher to consider how modifications are being made to the content or context and the nature of those modifications.[28]

Content Adaptations

Stirman describes content adaptations as modifications made to the EBPs or that impact how aspects of the EBP are delivered (e.g., shortening, adding elements, tailoring).[28] Common content adaptations to EBPs for implementation in LMICs include modifying language, adjusting for cultural relevance, or integration with another approach.[28] Modifications to language may include simplifying the language, reducing jargon, and adjusting activities for populations that may not be literate or with limited material resources.[29-31] For example, Kaysen and colleagues altered a worksheet used to challenge beliefs in an evidence-based cognitive process therapy intervention to make it pictorial and shortened the homework to maximize participation for the study population.[29] In a study of implementation of trauma-focused cognitive behavior therapy, Murray and colleagues adapted the implementation from a provider questioning approach to a provider storytelling approach to fit within the culture of Zambia.[32] The sessions were also extended up to 2-hours (from about 45–60 minutes) so providers had time to add analogies to the stories.[32] In global mental health research there has been an increase in transdiagnostic or common elements treatments to facilitate integration of different EBPs. These are models that teach a set of common practice elements that can be delivered in varying combinations to address a range of problems.[33-35]

Context Adaptations

Stirman refers to context adaptations as modifications made to the overall way treatment is delivered, which may include changes to the format and personnel who implement the EBP.[28] For example, the format of an HIV prevention program developed in the United States as a parent-focused intervention was modified to a family-focused intervention to account for the family structures in rural Kenya that emphasized a range of family members responsible for child-rearing.[28,36] Another strength of that program was that it leveraged the expertise of local staff and community members in the adaptation process, increasing the likelihood that the resulting program was context-appropriate.[28,36]

Context adaptations to personnel for implementation of EBPs in LMICs is common because of the shortage of human resources for health service delivery, and is referred to as "task-shifting." Task-shifting enables readily available workers with minimal or no professional clinical training to deliver EBPs that are usually delivered by specialists in HICs.[8] A series of studies in LMICs have used the task-shifting model to deliver mental health EBPs, demonstrating that it is feasible for providers with little or no prior mental health training, and often with little formal education at all, to assess mental health needs using locally validated measures and deliver EBPs effectively with positive clinical outcomes.[37-42] Adaptations that rely on task-shifting will also likely require changes to practitioner training. For example, an EBP for autism spectrum disorder was adapted from the United Kingdom to a site in India and a site in Pakistan. The use of nonspecialists to deliver the program required a change from a 2-day training for therapists to a 4-week training for nonspecialists, and clear referral patterns as well as newly developed measures for nonclinician competencies.[43] The change in provider type for this program also necessitated a change in delivery setting, with implications for available infrastructure and resources that must then be accounted for in the adapted version.

STEP 3. ASSESS THE INTERVENTION AND IMPLEMENTATION

Both measurement and evaluation methods are required to assess the intervention and implementation outcomes.

Measurement

Given the wide gap in use of EBPs, increasing reach is a priority outcome for D&I research in LMIC settings. Furthermore, acceptability of the EBP and implementation strategies in the local context and sustainability of the intervention effect after the funding period for research ends are key implementation outcome measures for D&I research in LMICs because of the need to build local capacity in low resources settings. The limited availability of existing instruments with sound psychometric properties for D&I research means that D&I researchers will need to consider the development of new measurement instruments for specific contexts and populations.[22] The Design, Implementation, Monitoring and Evaluation (DIME) process is a standardized approach to develop, test, and utilize context relevant measures for D&I research and for ongoing assessment of implementation constructs.[44] DIME has been successfully used to develop instruments with strong psychometric properties for administration in LMICs.[30,31] Another measurement consideration is that limited resources in LMICs may hinder ongoing measurement of implementation.[45] For this reason, D&I researchers should make efficient use of the resources that are available. The Apprenticeship Model is an example of efficient use of resources to ensure rigor in measurement and ongoing training of implementers.[33] The Model uses a staggered training approach that begins with an active in-person training, followed by practice and supervision by local supervisors who themselves are closely supervised by trainers. The implementers, local supervisor and trainer are independently responsible for using a checklist to assess the implementer's fidelity to completion of steps in a counseling protocol. Triangulation of the data sources inform the study about fidelity to the protocol, while discrepancies in fidelity ratings by the raters identifies opportunities for ongoing training to improve fidelity. Supervisors or the trainers can ensure that the implementers return to complete any missed component steps of the counseling session with the study participant.[33]

Evaluation

The limited studies of effective interventions in LMICs requires that D&I research examine not only what works to improve health outcomes but for whom the intervention works and in what conditions.[8,46] Careful selection of study designs will facilitate rigorous and informative evaluations of D&I research in LMICs. Useful study designs include hybrid trials, pragmatic designs, use of mixed methods, and use of repeat measures over time. Hybrid designs feature both evaluations of health impacts of the EBP and implementation success to address the limited research on EBPs in LMICs.[46] Pragmatic trials give greater consideration to the generalizability of findings across patients, implementers, outcomes, etc. while balancing the need for internal validity.[47] Mixed methods designs provide in-depth information about the implementation context, why an intervention worked (qualitative), the scope of problems or resources, and intervention effects (quantitative). Use of qualitative methods is essential for research conducted in LMICs because of the limited options for valid survey instruments to assess D&I constructs and the need to gain in-depth insights for intervention planning, implementation and evaluation from the local perspective. Relying only on quantitative methods for LMIC research would miss information that is important to studying D&I strategies and to understanding why an intervention worked or not. Quantitative and qualitative methods each contribute unique information and the methods can be integrated to provide additional insights beyond what either method contributes on its own.[48]

Furthermore, planning for dissemination and scale-up of effective interventions to LMICs is critical to realizing both the social and scientific value of D&I research. Plans for how the knowledge gained from the research will be translated and exchanged effectively for the LMIC, and resources needed to mobilize scale-up should begin early in the project.[8] WHO suggests working with in-country teams to develop scale-up strategies.[8] The following case study highlights many of the key features of evaluation that are most relevant to D&I research conducted in LMICs.

CASE STUDY

Background

South Africa carries a high burden of tuberculosis. High levels of poverty undermine adherence to tuberculosis treatment. Lutge et al. hypothesized that general economic support would increase adherence to treatment for tuberculosis. Their study was conducted in KwaZulu-Natal, one of South Africa's poorest and most populous provinces. KwaZulu-Natal has the highest incidence of tuberculosis in South Africa.[49]

D&I Study Design Features Relevant to LMICs

The trial was designed as a Hybrid III pragmatic cluster, randomized controlled trial of an implementation intervention strategy. Twenty clinics participated (10 intervention and 10 usual care) and all patients diagnosed with pulmonary drug-sensitive tuberculosis who initiated treatment were eligible to participate.[50] Another feature of this research was use of an explanatory mixed method design that involved quantitative data collection and analysis followed by a qualitative phase of research.[51] The implementation strategy consisted of a monthly voucher, redeemable for food, hypothetically freeing money for use elsewhere, such as for transport to the clinic for treatment. The Lutge intervention was pragmatic based on the PRECIS domain (chapter 19) practitioner expertise because nurses from the clinics distributed the vouchers to eligible patients instead of research staff, as well as the PRECIS domains practitioner adherence to the protocol and participant adherence to treatment because the follow-up intensity with the practitioners and patients was minimal.[47]

The quantitative evaluation was an intention-to-treat analysis that showed a small but nonsignificant improvement in treatment success rates in the intervention clinics compared with the control clinics. The collection of data on adherence, over time, enabled the research team to identify a strong dose–response effect. The quantitative implementation evaluation found that intervention reach was low, 36.2% of eligible patients did not receive the voucher at all. A subsequent qualitative evaluation of implementation outcomes (e.g., fidelity, acceptance) included interviews with practitioners and patients. The interviews revealed that among the most influential barriers to delivering the voucher was that practitioners made judgements about who they deemed financially worthy and patients felt guilty taking the vouchers because they knew people more financially disadvantaged than themselves.[50] These factors informed researchers why intervention reach was low and clarified quantitative findings.

Lessons Learned

By utilizing clinic staff to deliver the vouchers to patients and minimizing the intensity of follow-up, the investigators identified barriers to implementation that they did not anticipate. The pragmatic study design placed the overall small effect of the intervention and strong dose response within the context of the beliefs and behaviors of local practitioners and patients to identify opportunities to improve use of the vouchers in the field. These study design features are of critical importance to D&I research in LMICs, especially when the Principal Investigator is from another country and is unfamiliar with the local context. Had the investigators been able to use a comparative intervention in the comparison group, for example voucher plus education program for practitioners, they may have gleaned even more information from the trial, thus accelerating the translation of research to practice.

ETHICAL CONSIDERATIONS FOR D&I RESEARCH WITH LMICS

There are a wide range of ethical considerations for all research including research conducted within low-resource countries [52,53] (see chapter 4). However, D&I studies in LMICs prompt additional considerations, which are briefly highlighted here.

- **Local relevance:** Adoption of the strategy under study will likely require directing a portion of finite and limited resources away from other health activities. Thus, it is vital to ensure that the programs, policies, or practices under study have clinically or behaviorally meaningful impact and have not reached the implementation science phase simply because a researcher was able to publish a demonstration of impact and secure additional funding. In the same way, the program, practice, or policy, should be sustainable within the local context.[54]

- **Unintended consequences**: Researchers must consider the potential to create or increase disparities. Given the systems orientation of D&I research, the benefits and risks of the study must be considered at multiple levels of influence (e.g., individual, organizational, relational, and community).[22,55] Interventions designed to improve population health can widen health disparities when the population distribution of disease is associated with social or economic factors.[56] Multilevel evaluation frameworks such as RE-AIM (chapter 19) can draw attention to measures at multiple levels of influence that are relevant to translating research to practice. One must keep in mind that there are socioeconomic gradients within LMICs and the "inverse care law" applies: those with the most resources or power at hand will be the first to derive maximum benefits from population approaches intervenions.[56]

SUMMARY

The value and challenges associated with participatory research[57] are intensified for LMICs because of the geographic distance between the primary research team and research setting, the limited resources and infrastructure for health in

LMICs, and the linguistic and cultural diversity of the residents. D&I research is ideally suited to improve health for populations in LMICs because the emphasis on local context contributes to building trust between local stakeholders and researchers, and leverages emergent ideas for solutions to local problems. Moreover, the products of D&I research include practical information to improve use of EBPs in local settings and generalizable knowledge to advance science. The recent advances in frameworks (e.g., Stirman's, D.I.M.E, WHO) to guide adaptations of interventions for local context and the development of locally relevant measures can maximize the potential for D&I research to sustain intervention effects and facilitate scale-up of effective interventions.

SUGGESTED READINGS AND WEBSITES

Readings

Winer, M. and Ray, K. *Collaboration handbook: Creating, sustaining, and enjoying the journey.* Saint Paul, MN: Amherst H. Wilder Foundation; 2003.
This handbook provides activities and examples to enhance learning about creating, sustaining, and enjoying new ways of working with diverse stakeholders.

ESSENCE on Health Research. Seven Principles for Strengthening Research Capacity in low- and middle-income countries: simple ideas in a complex world. Good Practice Document Series. World Health Organization Reference Number: TDR/ESSENCE/2.14. 2014.
This report provides a pragmatic approach to conducting participatory research in LMICs to build capacity for future research.

Stirman SW, Miller CJ, Toder K, Calloway A. Development of a framework and coding system for modifications and adaptations of evidence-based interventions. *Implement Sci.* 2013;8(65.10):1186.
This manuscript describes a framework for classifying adaptations to EBPs that is useful for conducting systematic modifications to the content or context of interventions to enable scale-up of effective interventions.

Murray, L.K, Dorsey, S. Lewandowski, E. Global dissemination and implementation of child evidence-based practices in low resources countries. In: Beidas RS, Kendall PC, eds. *Dissemination and implementation of evidence-based practices in child and adolescent mental*

health. New York, NY: Oxford Univesity Press; 2014: 179–203.
This book chapter describes dissemination and implementation strategies that have been successfully used in LMICs including task-sharing and the apprenticeship model of trainging and supervision.

Selected Websites

Global Implementation Society. https://gis.globalimplementation.org/
The Global Implementation Society seeks to develop implementation practice and research as a as a professional discipline and to promote knowledge, skills, and service values of implementation to improve services and peoples' lives.

Alliance for Health Policy and Systems Research is an international collaboration hosted by the World Health Organization. http://www.who.int/alliance-hpsr/en/
The Alliance for Health Policy and Systems Research is an international collaboration hosted by the World Health Organization. The Alliance's mission has been to promote the generation and use of health policy and systems research as a means to strengthen the health systems of low- and middle-income countries. A list of courses and training on opportunities is available on the website.

The DIME Program Research Model: Design, Implementation, Monitoring and Evaluation. http://www.jhsph.edu/research/centers-and-institutes/center-for-refugee-and-disaster-response/response_service/AMHR/dime/index.html
The DIME model is a series of activities that combines evidence-based programming with rigorous monitoring and impact evaluation. The purpose is to provide a rational basis and approach for local programming while also generating information and lessons learned that can inform future services.

World Health Organization Implementation Research Toolkit. http://www.who.int/tdr/publications/year/2014/9789241506960_workbook_eng.pdf
The toolkit was developed by the Special Programme for Research and Training in Tropical Diseases to strengthen implementation research capacities of individuals and institutions in low-and middle-income countries where the greatest need exists.

World Health Organization. A Guide to Implementation Research in the Prevention and Control of Noncommunicable Diseases. http://apps.who.int/iris/bitstream/10665/252626/1/9789241511803-eng.pdf
This guide explores the way in which the interplay between a policy or intervention and its local context can affect implementation.

REFERENCES

1. Challenges and priorities for global mental health research in low- and middle-income countries. Symposium report. *Acad Med Sci.* 2008. https://acmedsci.ac.uk/file-download/34569-122838595851.pdf

2. Beaglehole R, Epping-Jordan J, Patel V, et al. Improving the prevention and management of chronic disease in low-income and middle-income countries: a priority for primary health care. *Lancet.* 2008;372(9642):940–949.

3. Restrepo-Mendex MC, Barros AJD, Wong KLM, et al. Inequalitites in full immunization coverage: trends in low- and middle-income countries. *Bull WHO.* 2016;94:794-805B. http://www.who.int/bulletin/volumes/94/11/15-162172/en/.

4. Maher D, Ford N, Unwin N. Priorities for developing countries in the global response to non-communicable diseases. *Global Health.* 2012;8:14.

5. McMichael C, Waters E, Volmink J. Evidence-based public health: what does it offer developing countries? *J Public Health.* 2005;27(2):215–221.

6. Pulford J, Hetzel MW, Bryant M, Siba PM, Mueller I. Reported reasons for not using a mosquito net when one is available: a review of the published literature. *Malaria J.* 2011;10:83.

7. Gettleman J. Meant to Keep Malaria Out, Mosquito Nets Are Used to Haul Fish. In: *New York Times* January 24, 2015. https://www.nytimes.com/2015/01/25/world/africa/mosquito-nets-for-malaria-spawn-new-epidemic-overfishing.html. Accessed November 11, 2016.

8. A guide to implementation research in the prevention and control of noncommunicable diseases. *Geneva: WHO Licence: CC BY-NC-SA 30 IGO.* 2016.

9. Lobb R, Colditz GA. Implementation science and its application to population health. *Annu Rev Public Health.* 2013;34:235–251.

10. Winer M, Ray K. *Collaboration handbook: Creating, sustaining, and enjoying the journey.* Saint Paul, MN: Amherst H. Wilder Foundation; 2003.

11. Lofters A, Virani T, Grewal G, Lobb R. Using knowledge exchange to build and sustain community support to reduce cancer screening inequities. *Prog Community Health Partnersh.* 2015;9(3):379–387.

12. Nabyonga-Orem J, Nanyunja M, Marchal B, Criel B, Ssengooba F. The roles and influence of actors in the uptake of evidence: the case of malaria treatment policy change in Uganda. *Implement Sci.* 2014;9:150.

13. Minkler M, Wallerstein N, eds. *Community based participatory research in health.* 2nd ed. San Francisco: Jossey-Bass; 2008.

14. Israel BA, Eng E, Schulz AJ, Parker EA, eds. *Methods for community-based participatory research for health.* 2nd ed. San Francisco: John Wiley & Sons; 2013.

15. Jao I, Kombe F, Mwalukore S, et al. Research stakeholders' views on benefits and challenges for public health research data sharing in Kenya: the importance of trust and social relations. *PloS One.* 2015;10(9):e0135545.

16. Mosavel M, Simon C, Van Stade D, Buchbinder M. Community-based participatory research (CBPR) in South Africa: engaging multiple constituents to shape the research question. *Soc Sci Med.* 2005;61(12):2577–2587.

17. Ramanadhan S, Viswanath K. Engaging Communities to Improve Health: Models, Evidence, and the Participatory Knowledge Translation (PaKT) Framework. In EB Fisher, L Cameron, AJ Christensen, U Ehlert, BF Oldenburg, F Snoek & Y Guo (Eds.), *Principles and Concepts of Behavioral Medicine: A Global Handbook*: Springer Science & Business Media. In press.

18. Silka L, Cleghorn GD, Grullon M, Tellez T. Creating community-based participatory research in a diverse community: a case study. *J Empir Res Hum Res Ethics.* 2008;3(2):5–16.

19. Schackman BR. Implementation science for the prevention and treatment of HIV/AIDS. *J Acquir Immune Defic Syndr.* 2010;55(Suppl 1):S27.

20. Norton WE, Amico KR, Cornman DH, Fisher WA, Fisher JD. An agenda for advancing the science of implementation of evidence-based HIV prevention interventions. *AIDS Behav.* 2009;13(3):424–429.

21. Pinto RM, da Silva SB, Penido C, Spector AY. International Participatory Research Framework: triangulating procedures to build health research capacity in Brazil. *Health Promot Int.* 2012;27(4):435–444.

22. Molyneux C, Goudge J, Russell S, Chuma J, Gumede T, Gilson L. Conducting health-related social science research in low income settings: ethical dilemmas faced in Kenya and South Africa. *J Int Dev.* 2009;21(2):309–326.

23. Cuijpers P, De Graaf I, Bohlmeijer E. Adapting and disseminating effective public health interventions in another country: towards a systematic approach. *Eur J Public Health.* 2005;15(2):166–169.

24. Wang Z, Norris SL, Bero L. Implementation plans included in World Health Organisation guidelines. *Implement Sci.* 2016;11(1).

25. Trickett EJ, Beehler S, Deutsch C, et al. Advancing the science of community-level interventions. *Am J Public Health.* 2011;101(8):1410–1419.

26. Mejia A, Calam R, Sanders MR. A review of parenting programs in developing countries: opportunities and challenges for preventing emotional and behavioral difficulties in children. *Clin Child Fam Psychol Rev.* 2012;15(2):163–175.

27. Michie S, Fixsen D, Grimshaw JM, Eccles MP. Specifying and reporting complex behaviour change interventions: the need for a scientific method. *Implement Sci.* 2009;4(1):1.

28. Stirman SW, Miller CJ, Toder K, Calloway A. Development of a framework and coding system for modifications and adaptations of evidence-based interventions. *Implement Sci.* 2013;8(65.10):1186.

29. Kaysen D, Lindgren K, Zangana GAS, Murray L, Bass J, Bolton P. Adaptation of cognitive processing therapy for treatment of torture victims: experience in Kurdistan, Iraq. *Psychol Trauma Theory Res Pract Policy.* 2013;5(2):184.

30. Murray LK, Beidas RS, Dorsey S, Skavenski S, Kasoma M, Mayeya J. Implementation research in low-resource settings. Seattle Implementation Research Conference; 2013; Seattle, Washington.

31. Verdeli H, Clougherty K, Onyango G, et al. Group interpersonal psychotherapy for depressed youth in IDP camps in Northern Uganda: adaptation and training. *Child Adolesc Psychiatr Clin North Am.* 2008;17(3):605–624.

32. Murray LK, Dorsey S, Skavenski S, et al. Identification, modification, and implementation of an evidence-based psychotherapy for children in a low-income country: the use of TF-CBT in Zambia. *Int J Ment Health Syst.* 2013;7(1):24.

33. Murray LK, Dorsey S, Haroz E, et al. A common elements treatment approach for adult mental health problems in low-and middle-income countries. *Cogn Behav Pract.* 2014;21(2):111–123.

34. Chorpita BF, Daleiden EL, Weisz JR. Identifying and selecting the common elements of evidence based interventions: a distillation and matching model. *Ment Health Serv Res.* 2005;7(1):5–20.

35. Mansell W, Harvey A, Watkins ER, Shafran R. Cognitive behavioral processes across psychological disorders: a review of the utility and validity of the transdiagnostic approach. *Int J Cogn Therapy.* 2008;1(3):181–191.

36. Poulsen MN, Vandenhoudt H, Wyckoff SC, et al. Cultural adaptation of a U.S. evidence-based parenting intervention for rural Western Kenya: from parents matter! To families matter! *AIDS Educ Prevent.* 2010;22(4):273–285.

37. Rahman A, Malik A, Sikander S, Roberts C, Creed F. Cognitive behaviour therapy-based intervention by community health workers for mothers with depression and their infants in rural Pakistan: a cluster-randomised controlled trial. *Lancet.* 2008;372(9642):902–909.

38. Bass JK, Annan J, McIvor Murray S, et al. Controlled trial of psychotherapy for Congolese survivors of sexual violence. *N Engl J Med.* 2013;368(23):2182–2191.

39. Bolton P, Bass J, Betancourt T, et al. Interventions for depression symptoms among adolescent survivors of war and displacement in northern Uganda: a randomized controlled trial. *JAMA.* 2007;298(5):519–527.

40. Bolton P, Lee C, Haroz EE, et al. A transdiagnostic community-based mental health treatment for comorbid disorders: development and outcomes of a randomized controlled trial among Burmese refugees in Thailand. *PLoS Med.* 2014;11(11):e1001757.

41. Murray LK, Skavenski S, Kane JC, et al. Effectiveness of trauma-focused cognitive behavioral therapy among trauma-affected children in Lusaka, Zambia: a randomized clinical trial. *JAMA Pediatr.* 2015;169(8):761–769.

42. Patel V, Weiss HA, Chowdhary N, et al. Effectiveness of an intervention led by lay health counsellors for depressive and anxiety disorders in primary care in Goa, India (MANAS): a cluster randomised controlled trial. *Lancet.* 2010;376(9758):2086–2095.

43. Divan G, Hamdani SU, Vajartkar V, et al. Adapting an evidence-based intervention for autism spectrum disorder for scaling up in resource-constrained settings: the development of the PASS intervention in South Asia. *Glob Health Act.* 2015;8.

44. Center for Refugee and Disaster Response. The DIME Program Research Model: Design, Implementation, Monitoring and Evaluation. http://www.jhsph.edu/research/centers-and-institutes/center-for-refugee-and-disaster-response/response_service/AMHR/dime/index.html. Accessed January 16, 2017.

45. Chambers DA, Glasgow RE, Stange KC. The dynamic sustainability framework: addressing the paradox of sustainment amid ongoing change. *Implement Sci.* 2013;8:117.

46. Curran GM, Bauer M, Mittman B, Pyne JM, Stetler C. Effectiveness-implementation hybrid designs: combining elements of clinical effectiveness and implementation research to enhance public health impact. *Med Care.* 2012;50(3):217–226.

47. Thorpe KE, Zwarenstein M, Oxman AD, et al. A pragmatic-explanatory continuum indicator summary (PRECIS): a tool to help trial designers. *J Clin Epidemiol.* 2009;62(5):464–475.

48. Fetters MD, Curry LA, Creswell JW. Achieving integration in mixed methods designs-principles

and practices. *Health Serv Res.* 2013;48(6 Pt 2):2134–2156.

49. Lutge E, Lewin S, Volmink J, Friedman I, Lombard C. Economic support to improve tuberculosis treatment outcomes in South Africa: a pragmatic cluster-randomized controlled trial. *Trials.* 2013;14:154.

50. Lutge E, Lewin S, Volmink J. Economic support to improve tuberculosis treatment outcomes in South Africa: a qualitative process evaluation of a cluster randomized controlled trial. *Trials.* 2014;15:236.

51. Creswell JW, Klassen AC, Plano Clark VL, Smith KC. Best practices for mixed methods research in the health sciences. *Bethesda (Maryland): National Institutes of Health.* 2011:2094–2103.

52. Benatar SR. Reflections and recommendations on research ethics in developing countries. *Soc Sci Med.* 2002;54(7):1131–1141.

53. Emanuel EJ, Wendler D, Killen J, Grady C. What makes clinical research in developing countries ethical? The benchmarks of ethical research. *J Infect Dis.* 2004;189(5):930–937.

54. Lomas J. Diffusion, dissemination, and implementation: who should do what? *Ann N Y Acad Sci* 1993;703:226–235

55. Guta A, Wilson MG, Flicker S, et al. Are we asking the right questions? A review of Canadian REB practices in relation to community-based participatory research. *J Empir Res Hum Res Ethics.* 2010;5(2):35–46.

56. Frohlich KL, Potvin L. Transcending the known in public health practice: the inequality paradox: the population approach and vulnerable populations. *Am J Public Health.* 2008;98(2):216–221.

57. Cargo M, Mercer SL. The value and challenges of participatory research: strengthening its practice. *Annu Rev Public Health.* 2008;29:325–350.

29

Future Issues in Dissemination and Implementation Research

ROSS C. BROWNSON, GRAHAM A. COLDITZ, AND ENOLA K. PROCTOR

INTRODUCTION

Two converging bodies of knowledge hold promise for bridging the gap between discovery of new research findings and application in public health and health care settings. First, the concept of evidence-based practice (in medicine, public health, and other related disciplines) is growing in prominence, due in part to a larger body of intervention research on what works to improve patient care or population health (e.g., the Clinical Guide[1] or Community Guide[2] recommendations on effective interventions).[3,4] Second, effective methods of dissemination and implementation (D&I) are needed to put evidence to work in "real world" settings.

Particularly related to this second point, this book provides a foundation in and strives to catalyze further knowledge development in the science of D&I research. While we continue to accumulate an evidence base on how to improve population health and patient care, knowledge about how to apply and evaluate the evidence is lacking for many settings and populations. This large gap can be filled by a growing investment in and lessons learned from D&I research, which elucidates the processes and factors that lead to widespread use of an evidence-based intervention by a particular population (e.g., youth, ethnic minorities, rural and underresourced communities, lower and middle income countries) or within a certain setting (e.g., worksite, school).[5] This research has begun to identify a number of important factors that enhance the uptake of evidence-based interventions in both practice (e.g., a primary care clinic) and policy (e.g., a state legislature) settings.

This chapter highlights several research topics that the authors believe are the most pressing areas for future inquiry. In part, the list was developed from the recommendations contained within the previous 28 chapters (see each chapter for details). The issues covered are not meant to be exhaustive; the intention is to identify the most promising areas that will move D&I science forward most quickly given the current state of the research and funding opportunities.

TERMINOLOGY AND THEORY

Developing the Terminology

For any field of scientific inquiry to thrive, consistent terminology is needed. Because D&I research in the health field has emerged from research traditions in diverse disciplines ranging from agriculture to education, there are numerous inconsistencies in the use and meaning of terms and main concepts.[5] While chapter 2 presents what we believe is a reasonable current snapshot of terminology for D&I research, further work is needed to standardize the terminology and to include more concepts from outside of health (e.g., D&I terms from business or organizational psychology). A particular concern is that the term "translation" is now being used for everything from cellular and molecular research to global health.[6]

Making Use of Theory and Frameworks

Theories and models explain behavior and suggest ways to achieve behavior change. A theory is a set of interrelated concepts that present a systematic view of events by specifying relations among variables in order to explain and predict events.[7] As illustrated in this book, D&I research can be enhanced by the use of theory, systematic planning frameworks, and logic models. Future research is needed to better understand which theories are best suited for various settings (schools, worksites, communities) and levels (policy, organizational change) and how theories might need to be adapted for D&I research on health disparities.

New models and frameworks have emerged, and are receiving increased attention (chapter 5). An area deserving more research involves recent attempts to apply D&I frameworks to population-level interventions such as policy dissemination and environmental change research.[8] Individual chapters should spark the testing of frameworks and models, as needed to lay out the complex array of factors required for successful dissemination of information and implementation of evidence-based programs in specific health care and public health settings. Given there are over 60 D&I models,[9] the emphasis should be on adapting and testing existing models rather than developing new ones.

METHODS AND MEASUREMENT

Developing New and Improved Measures

A public health and quality improvement adage is "what gets measured, gets done."[10] Successful progress of D&I science will require the development of practical measures of outcomes that are both reliable and valid. These enable empirical testing of the success of D&I efforts. While we have built many excellent surveillance systems for measuring long-term change (e.g., behavioral risk factors, mortality, cancer incidence), most of these are only partially helpful for D&I research, where a greater focus is needed on "midstream" and "upstream" factors.[11,12] Currently, there are very few measures designed to focus on D&I research at the population level; most are relevant for interventions addressing acute patient care. Moreover, most existing measures focus on ultimate outcomes, such as change in health status. Proximal measures of dissemination and implementation processes and outcomes are sorely needed. As new measures are developed (or existing metrics adapted), some key considerations include: which outcomes should be tracked and how long it will take to show progress; how implementation fidelity and adaptation can best be measured across a broad range of D&I studies; how to best determine criterion validity (how a measures compares with some "gold standard"); how to best measure moderating factors across a range of settings (e.g., schools, worksites); and

how common, practical, measures can be developed and shared so researchers are not constantly re-inventing measures.

Understanding How to Address Mis-implementation

Much of the current literature focuses on underuse of effective programs and interventions, a continuing public health need and a continued and important priority in implementation science. More than a decade ago in a landmark study, McGlynn and colleagues reported that adults in the United States received only about half of recommended health care services.[13] In the first comprehensive re-examination of that situation, Levine and colleagues recently reported improvement in some composite quality indicators: receipt of recommended medical treatment increased from 36% to 42% and recommended counseling increased from 43% to 50%[14] However two indicators worsened: avoidance of inappropriate medical treatment and avoidance of inappropriate antibiotics.

Of growing concern, and essential to provision of effective and appropriate health and public health care, is correction of the misuse of interventions. Mis-implementation is a process where effective interventions are ended or ineffective interventions are continued in public health settings (i.e., evidence-based decision-making is not occurring).[15,16] Various other terms can be used in describing programs ending prematurely such as de-adoption, de-implementation, termination, and discontinuation.[16] As part of the cultural shift needed toward the acceptance of de-adoption within medicine,[17] many medical practices are deemed ineffective or unsafe.[18] And the Institute of Medicine estimates that 30% of health care spending in the United States—about $750 billion per year—is unnecessary.[19] There is sparse literature on mis-implementation in public health practice. The Choosing Wisely Campaign, launched in 2012 by the American Board of Internal Medicine Foundation, strives to reduce low-value care through public education campaigns directed at both health care consumers and providers. Reducing use of familiar interventions runs into oftenly staunchly held assumptions that "more is better."[20] A richer understanding of mis-implementation will help us better allocate already limited resources to be used more efficiently. This knowledge will also allow researchers and practitioners to prevent the continuation of ineffective programs or discontinuation of effective programs.

Moving from Theory to Evidence-Based D&I Strategies

Our knowledge base about *how to* disseminate or how to implement lags far behind our knowledge base of *what to* disseminate or what to implement. That is, we have a growing repertoire of evidence-based interventions, programs, and policies, but few dissemination or implementation strategies that have been tested and shown to be effective. Therefore, as noted in chapter 13, we need well-designed studies to develop and test D&I strategies.

Understanding Fidelity, Adaptation, and Their Connections to D&I Research

Fidelity, defined in chapter 16 as the "extent to which the intervention was delivered as planned,"[21] is currently not well understood within the realm of D&I research. Key to the concept of fidelity is also the concept of adaptability, or the ability of the target audience to adapt the intervention to their own population. Striking a balance between adaptability and fidelity is challenging, but there are several models currently in place that have been able to strike this balance. The challenge in the future is to develop a means of evaluating these models in a way that helps determine their utility across myriad settings, populations, and health outcomes. Another key need is for more transparent reporting of program implementation and consistency of implementation across settings, staff, target groups, and time.

Several important topics can help inform our knowledge on fidelity and D&I research. Researchers can collaborate to design interventions and develop measures that assess and maximize the fidelity of the intervention. Practitioners are well suited to identify the evidence-based interventions that would be best suited for their populations and settings and assess how successfully the interventions are delivered. By doing this, practice-based evidence can be developed. Policymakers play key roles in creating the infrastructure needed to open up the lines of communication between researchers, practitioners, and intervention developers. Finally, the reviewers and editors of professional journals can make a greater effort to increase (and not punish) transparent reporting of issues around program implementation and adaptation. For example, the recently establish Standards for Reporting Implementation Studies (StaRI) support transparent and accurate reporting in D&I science.[22]

Building the Evidence on External Validity

As described in this book, there are numerous forms of evidence. Some types of evidence inform our knowledge about the etiology of disease.[23] Other evidence demonstrates the relative effectiveness of specific interventions to address a particular health condition. However, what is fundamental to D&I research and is often missing is a body of evidence that can help to determine the generalizability of an intervention from one population and/or setting to another, that is, the core concepts of external validity (see chapter 18).[24] There are many remaining research questions related to external validity—for example: Which factors need to be taken into account when an internally valid program or policy is implemented in a different setting or with a different population subgroup? How does one balance the concepts of fidelity and adaptation (reinvention)? If the adaptation process changes the original intervention to such an extent that the original efficacy data may no longer apply, then the program may be viewed as a new intervention under very different contextual conditions. How might we efficiently and effectively measure external validity across a wide range of intervention studies? How can systematic reviews more fully incorporate concepts of external validity? Green has recommended that the implementation of evidence-based approaches requires careful consideration of the "best processes" needed when generalizing research to alternate populations, places, and times.[25] This greater attention to external validity has many benefits including greater relevance and enhanced credibility of findings from D&I research for practitioners and policymakers and a better understanding of what constitutes an "effective" intervention (i.e., based solely on whether it worked in a narrowly defined population or a broader understanding of the key factors needed for replication or "scaling-up"[26]). At the earliest stages, D&I research could benefit from more consistent application of what is being called "exploratory evaluation" or "evaluability assessment." (i.e., a pre-evaluation activity designed to maximize the chances that any subsequent evaluation will result in useful information).[27,28]

Understanding the Contributions of Economic Evaluation

As noted in chapter 6, economic evaluation is an important tool for D&I research. It can provide information to help assess the relative value of alternative expenditures on health services and public health programs. For example, cost-effectiveness analysis (CEA) can suggest the relative value of alternative interventions (i.e., health return on dollars invested) and can play key roles in a whole range of D&I studies. It may also help inform strategies for de-implementation of ineffective strategies and guidelines. While CEA has been increasingly applied to medical and public health interventions, it is seldom used in a systematic manner for D&I research.

Improving the Knowledge Base on Sustainability

Sustainability describes the extent to which an evidence-based intervention can deliver its intended benefits over an extended period of time after external support from the donor agency is terminated.[29] Rarely do studies assess long-term sustainability of practice changes, even when implementation of effective practices is successful. This is a priority area for research, as the inability to overcome barriers to sustainability and scalability prevents population-wide benefit of new health care and public health discoveries.[30] Most implementation practice and research focuses on initial uptake, by early adopters, of one health intervention at a time. It is important that D&I research begin to tackle later-stage challenges of scaling up and sustaining evidence-supported interventions in complex community settings that serve vulnerable populations.

Improvement Science and Implementation Science: Defining Boundaries and Increasing the Interface

The fields of quality improvement and implementation science have complementary goals and as of yet distinct foci and stakeholders. Quality improvement in health service delivery is a major initiative in high-income countries, while implementation science focuses increasingly on increasing the adoption, scale-up, and spread of effective programs and interventions in low-resourced settings, domestically and globally. Quality improvement typically focuses on the "here and now"—quickly addressing adverse clinical events through locally generated and applied approaches and monitoring change through iterative cycles of improvement focused solutions. While also concerned with local clinical issues, the focus of implementation science is broader. Implementation science looks not toward local solutions but rather published research findings and evidence-based prevention programs or interventions, and works toward their adoption and sustained use by engagement of stakeholders and systems and through use of implementation strategies, which are increasingly evidence based themselves. Work at the interface of quality improvement and implementation science has two complementary priorities. First, the field will be informed by clearer delineation of the boundaries and potential interface of these two approaches, which have a common goal of improving health services and patient outcomes. Second, synergy could be advanced by exploring paths toward leveraging the local energy, commitment, and resources that characterize quality improvement while extending the generalizability of results through the application of systematic and theory-driven implementation science methods.

Documenting the Public Health Impact of D&I Research

It is critical that D&I researchers document the incremental advances in improved health care that result from dissemination and implementation. In many studies, the success of the implementation is assumed and evaluated from data on clinical outcomes alone. This may obscure D&I's unique value added to the quality of health care and public health. Woolf asserts that later stage translation research can do more to decrease morbidity and mortality than a new imaging device or class of drugs.[31] Indeed some studies show that health care can be improved as much as 68% through educational outreach and social marketing, and by 250% through clinician performance feedback.[32-34] Dissemination and implementation researchers should find the confidence to propose and strive toward these kinds of measureable impacts. We need methods and data to demonstrate the potential of D&I research to ultimately reduce the burden of disease and improve the quality of lives.

STRATEGIES AND POPULATIONS

Conducting Research in High-Risk Populations and Low-Resource Health Systems

As noted in chapter 27, despite enormous gains in health over the past century, several populations lag behind in realizing these gains in life years and quality of life (ethnic minorities, low-income and low-literacy populations). Moreover, under-resourced settings lag behind in the capacity to implement and sustain good care. This leads to a great urgency for D&I approaches among high-risk populations and low-resource systems where health disparities exist. There are several priorities for research. Perhaps most fundamental, we need to better understand how evidence-based interventions can be adapted and replicated successfully in low-income, minority, low-health literacy, and disadvantaged groups. Second, more inquiry is needed to understand how to maintain cultural appropriateness as a means of increasing "buy-in" from the target population. As was discussed in chapter 17, there are several key strategies for improving the cultural adaptation of interventions, including tailoring the intervention to the target audience. This emphasizes a need for delivery of interventions in the native language of the population and targeting specific cultural groups rather than trying to implement an intervention across several cultural backgrounds. Third, following on the principles of participatory research,[35] we need to balance "top-down" (researcher-driven) approaches with "bottom-up" approaches that closely involve the populations suffering from health disparities in the research process. Finally, we need cost-efficient methods to disseminate, train, implement, and monitor quality in underresourced health settings.

Learning from Global Efforts

Nearly every D&I issue has a global footprint, since diseases do not know borders and shared solutions are needed. This can readily be seen if one lines up goals of the World Health Organization with national health plans. While it is important to acknowledge that public health challenges in less-developed countries are compounded by poverty and hunger, diminished public infrastructure, and the epidemiologic transition to behaviors that pose risks more typically found in higher income countries, many of the D&I research issues described in this book still have applicability (see chapter 28). There is, however, little data available on the reach of evidence-based practices across developed and less-developed regions of the world.

As this work develops, there are many areas that are likely to lead to advances in D&I research. These could include: (1) adapting methods of surveillance from one country to another;[36] (2) understanding how to adapt an effective intervention in one geographic region to the context of another geographic region;[37,38] (3) implementing innovative methods for building capacity in evidence-based decision-making;[39] and (4) identifying effective methods for delivery of health care services in one country that could be applied to another.

Understanding How to Start Early: Designing for Dissemination and Implementation

The failure to address, during an intervention's intial design and testing, factors associated with its eventual adoption is a significant contributor to the often cited 17-year gap between discovery and delivery in routine care. While an assumed linear, stepwise progression from discovery to implementation has intutitive appeal, D&I science's inherent ability to span boundaries positions it for the kinds of partnerships and scientific synergy that could speed and improve uptake.[40] Ultimately, we need to better understand how to design interventions with the elements most critical for external validity in mind, addressing these issues during early developmental phases— not near the end of a project.

Designing for dissemination is defined as: "an active process that helps to ensure that public health interventions, often evaluated by researchers, are developed in ways that match well with adopters' needs, assets, and time frames."[41] A study of public health researchers in the United States found considerable room for improvement in designing for dissemination.[41] About half of respondents (53%) had a person or team in their unit dedicated to dissemination. Seventeen percent of all respondents used a model to plan their dissemination activities. One third of respondents (34%) always or usually involved stakeholders in the research process.

The difficulty in designing for dissemination is due in part to differing priorities between researchers and practitioners.[42] For researchers, partly because of funding, recognition, and other issues, priority is often on discovery (not application) of new knowledge; whereas for practitioners and policymakers, the focus often is on practical ways to apply these discoveries for their settings, often with some adaptation for local relevance.[43] The chasm between researchers and practitioners was illustrated in a "Designing for Dissemination" workshop sponsored by the US National Cancer Institute.[44] In this workshop, all participants acknowledged the importance of dissemination. Researchers reported that their role was to identify effective interventions but were not responsible for dissemination of research findings. Similarly, practitioners did not believe they were responsible for dissemination. Unfortunately, when no one believes it is their job to disseminate, the activity often falls through the cracks or sinks to low priority in already overstressed organizations.

Many areas are ripe for improvements in how we design for D&I. Through its establishment of six IGNITE (genomic medicine demonstration sites), the NIH has prioritized bringing implementation science to genomic medicine. Implementation science should be leveraged to help shape delivery of precision medicine by helping inform the fit between new genomically informed interventions and such contextual factors as stakeholder attitudes and decision patterns, required practice infrastructure supports, and health policy and financing. Moreover, implementation strategies offer promise to support genomics implementation in a wide range of health care systems.[45]

Based on a growing body of literature,[41,46,47] specific actions could improve designing for dissemination across levels of system, process, and production. It is important to place a greater emphasis on building strategic partnerships early in the D&I process; to develop new and more rapid methods for determining when a new program or policy is ready for adoption in a nonresearch setting (e.g., exploratory evaluation[27]); and to understand new ways of ensuring that the intervention is developed in ways that match well with adopters' needs, assets, and time frame. The D&I science toolkit offers several aids to designing for dissemination and implementation, including models for early planning,[48] design innovations (e.g., hybrid designs and pragmatic trials), and assessment of D&I outcomes pertinent to early phases of implementation research such as acceptability and feasiblity (chapter 14).

PARTNERSHIPS

Applying Transdisciplinary Approaches

Transdisciplinary research provides valuable opportunities to collaborate on interventions to improve the health and well-being of both individuals and communities.[42,49-51] For example,

tobacco research and control efforts and, more recently, physical activity projects have been successful in facilitating cooperation among disciplines such as advertising, policy, business, economics, medical science, and behavioral science. Research activities within multidisciplinary tobacco networks try to fill the gaps between scientific discovery and research translation by engaging a wide range of stakeholders.[52-54] Progress in D&I research will depend not only on fields like medicine or public health, but importantly on other disciplines such as law, business, economics, agriculture, marketing, transportation, urban planning, and education. Moreover, unlike tobacco control, disseminating and implementing interventions to address other public health problems (e.g., obesity) will necessarily involve partnerships among government, nongovernmental organizations, academic and the private sectors. We have begun to identify factors that facilitate transdisciplinary research in basic sciences, etiologic research, and intervention trials, including the breadths of disciplines involved, prior work together among researchers, spatial proximity of researchers, face-to-face interaction, and support from leadership.[55,56] There is sparse understanding of how best to facilitate transdisciplinary D&I research as "best practice," making this a research priority.

Building Knowledge on Participatory Approaches

As noted in chapter 11, participatory research methods have the potential to improve D&I research by involving community members and stakeholders in the decision-making processes, thus enhancing the relevance and overall quality of research. Within community and public health settings, participatory research builds trust, respect, capacity, empowerment, accountability, and sustainability,[57,58] all of which is critical to enhancing the success of D&I efforts further on. This has tremendous potential for the successful dissemination of research findings and also for conducting D&I research. Community engagement and participation can play roles in D&I research across a wide spectrum, ranging from engaging consumers, patients, or practitioners as advisors, to hiring research staff from communities being targeted, to full participation from community members in all research activities. An important future D&I research area is to understand how to best link the needs of community members or practitioners participation with the objectives of researchers.

TRAINING AND SUPPORT

Developing Training Programs

As the field of D&I research advances, increasing opportunities for training becomes essential to meeting the full potential of the discipline to improve population health in an efficient and timely manner.[59] In the United States, the Implementation Research Institute (supported by the National Institute on Mental Health)[60-62] and the Mentored Training in Dissemination and Implementation Research for Cancer (supported by the National Cancer Institute)[63-65] support training among researchers. More broadly, the structure of this training institute may serve as a model and catalyst for other NIH and CDC areas of focus to initiate parallel training programs. For example, the NIH Training Institute for Dissemination and Implementation Research in Health was launched in August 2011.[66] In Canada, initiatives include the Knowledge Translation training workshops and a Canadian Institutes of Health Research Strategic Training Initiative in Health Research, which funds a knowledge utilization studies program at the University of Alberta. This new training program aims to provide advanced training in the science of knowledge translation research, link trainees and mentors, and partner with national and international research groups to promote knowledge translation training and research. From funded initiatives such as these, we hope to see shared curriculum developed. The scope of material offered in these chapters should advance methods for design, improve standards for reporting, and provide examples of applications of D&I research methods. One remaining question is how to incorporate D&I methods into standard, ongoing public health training across disciplines such as environmental health sciences, behavioral sciences, and so forth—this raises issues of curriculum coordaintion and rigor in methods across applications.

Developing Resources and Academic Incentives

To further advance the field, the growing emphasis on funding D&I research must withstand competitive pressures for funding resources within numerous federal agencies (e.g., NIH, CDC, AHRQ, VA) and at the same time we need foundations and other funding agencies to embrace the principles of D&I research to make this area a top priority. Given the lean budget years ahead, creative approaches to funding are needed, including cofunding between federal agencies and foundations. Importantly as we move along the discovery to application pipeline, there is a need to include an emphasis on many issues covered in these chapters (e.g., funding to better understand the role of fidelity, support for more research on organizational factors). More generally, additional funding resources for methods research that can grow out of the applications of D&I research projects will broaden the science base on which we build a sustainable field of scientific research. Increasing emphasis is needed on how to develop resources and sustain implementation after the research funding has ended. This can be particularly challenging in settings with limited resources.

As noted in chapter 1, in parallel with funding for research studies, our institutions must develop more career paths for promotion and tenure of faculty who engage in D&I research. Simply put, systems changes are needed in our academic institutions so that D&I research and the time commitments needed to build relationships and knowledge users are recognized and more highly valued and rewarded. As we look forward to the future of D&I research, each health sector and government research and practice funding agency will need to evaluate priorities and determine its interest in funding collaborative initiatives. Since the field of D&I research often involves projects with long time horizons and numerous disciplines, junior investigators will need to be afforded adequate support and time to show progress and ways to provide credit and incentives within the many disciplinary "silos."

SUMMARY

There is enormous potential to advance the health of patients and the community through greater focus on implementing what we already know, and through greater application of the methods outlined in this book—D&I research. More simply put, taking what we know about improving health and putting it into practice must be our highest priority.[42]

This chapter has highlighted just a sample of the many rich areas for D&I research that will assist us in shortening the gap between discovery and practice, thus beginning to realize the benefits of research for patients, families, and communities. Greater emphasis on implementation in challenging settings, including lower and middle income countries and underresourced communities in higher income countries will add to the lessons we must learn to fully reap the benefit of our advances in D&I research methods. Moreover, collaboration and multidisciplinary approaches to D&I research will help to make efforts more consistent and more effective moving forward. Thus, we will be better able to identify knowledge gaps that need to be addressed in future D&I research, ultimately informing the practice and policies of clinical care and public health services.

ACKNOWLEDGMENTS

The authors are grateful for helpful input on this chapter from Drs. David Chambers, Mariah Dreisinger, Russ Glasgow, and Jon Kerner.

REFERENCES

1. US Preventive Services Task Force. Guide to Clinical Preventive Services. http://www.ahrq.gov/sites/default/files/wysiwyg/professionals/clinicians-providers/guidelines-recommendations/guide/cpsguide.pdf. Accessed February 12, 2017.

2. Task Force on Community Preventive Services. Guide to Community Preventive Services. www.thecommunityguide.org. Accessed February 12, 2017.

3. Satterfield JM, Spring B, Brownson RC, et al. Toward a transdisciplinary model of evidence-based practice. Milbank Q. 2009;87(2):368–390.

4. Brownson R, Baker E, Deshpande A, Gillespie K. Evidence-based public health. 3rd ed. New York: Oxford University Press; 2017.

5. Rabin B, Brownson R. Developing the terminology for dissemination and implementation research. In: Brownson R, Colditz G, Proctor E, eds. Dissemination and implementation research in health: translating science to practice. New York: Oxford University Press; 2012: 23–51.

6. Kerner JF. Integrating research, practice, and policy: what we see depends on where we stand. J Public Health Manag Pract. 2008;14(2):193–198.

7. Glanz K, Bishop DB. The role of behavioral science theory in development and implementation of public health interventions. Annu Rev Public Health. 2010;31:399–418.

8. Jilcott S, Ammerman A, Sommers J, Glasgow RE. Applying the RE-AIM framework to assess the public health impact of policy change. Ann Behav Med. 2007;34(2):105–114.

9. Tabak RG, Khoong EC, Chambers DA, Brownson RC. Bridging research and practice: models for dissemination and implementation research. Am J Prev Med. 2012;43(3):337–350.

10. Thacker SB. Public health surveillance and the prevention of injuries in sports: what gets measured gets done. J Athl Train. 2007;42(2):171–172.

11. Brownson RC, Jones E. Bridging the gap: translating research into policy and practice. Prev Med. 2009;49(4):313–315.

12. McKinlay JB. Paradigmatic obstacles to improving the health of populations--implications for health policy. Salud Publica Mex. 1998;40(4):369–379.

13. McGlynn EA, Asch SM, Adams J, et al. The quality of health care delivered to adults in the United States. N Engl J Med. 2003;348(26):2635–2645.

14. Levine DM, Linder JA, Landon BE. The quality of outpatient care delivered to adults in the United States, 2002 to 2013. JAMA Intern Med. 2016;176(12):1778–1790.

15. Brownson RC, Allen P, Jacob RR, et al. Understanding mis-implementation in public health practice. Am J Prev Med. 2015;48(5):543–551.

16. Gnjidic D, Elshaug AG. De-adoption and its 43 related terms: harmonizing low-value care terminology. BMC Med. 2015;13:273.

17. Gunderman RB, Seidenwurm DJ. De-Adoption and Un-Diffusion. J Am Coll Radiol. 2015;12(11):1162–1163.

18. Prasad V, Ioannidis JP. Evidence-based de-implementation for contradicted, unproven, and aspiring healthcare practices. Implement Sci. 2014;9:1.

19. Yong P, Saunders R, Olsen L, eds. The healthcare imperative: lowering costs and improving outcomes: Workshop series summary. Washington, DC: Institute of Medicine. National Academies Press; 2010.

20. Schlesinger M, Grob R. Treating, fast and slow: Americans' understanding of and responses to low-value care. Milbank Q. 2017;95(1):70–116.

21. Linnan L, Steckler A. Process evaluation and public health interventions: An overview. In: Steckler A, Linnan L, eds. Process evaluation in public health interventions and research. San Francisco: Jossey-Bass; 2002:1–23.

22. Pinnock H, Barwick M, Carpenter CR, et al. Standards for Reporting Implementation Studies (StaRI) Statement. BMJ. 2017;356:i6795.

23. Brownson RC, Baker EA, Leet TL, Gillespie KN, True WR. Evidence-based public health. 2nd ed. New York: Oxford University Press; 2011.

24. Green LW, Glasgow RE. Evaluating the relevance, generalization, and applicability of research: issues in external validation and translation methodology. Eval Health Prof. 2006;29(1):126–153.

25. Green LW. From research to "best practices" in other settings and populations. *Am J Health Behav.* 2001;25(3):165–178.

26. Norton W, Mittman B. *Scaling up health promotion/disease prevention programs in community settings: Barriers, facilitators, and initial recommendations.* Hartford, CT: Patrick and Catherine Weldon Donaghue Medical Research Foundation; 2010.

27. Leviton LC, Khan LK, Rog D, Dawkins N, Cotton D. Evaluability assessment to improve public health policies, programs, and practices. *Annu Rev Public Health.* 2010;31:213–233.

28. Dunet DO, Losby JL, Tucker-Brown A. Using evaluability assessment to support the development of practice-based evidence in public health. *J Public Health Manag Pract.* 2013;19(5):479–482.

29. Shediac-Rizkallah MC, Bone LR. Planning for the sustainability of community-based health programs: conceptual frameworks and future directions for research, practice and policy. *Health Educ Res.* 1998;13(1):87–108.

30. Proctor E, Luke D, Calhoun A, et al. Sustainability of evidence-based healthcare: research agenda, methodological advances, and infrastructure support. *Implement Sci.* 2015;10:88.

31. Woolf SH. The meaning of translational research and why it matters. *JAMA.* 2008;299(2):211–213.

32. Bennett JW, Glasziou PP. Computerised reminders and feedback in medication management: a systematic review of randomised controlled trials. *Med J Aust.* 2003;178(5):217–222.

33. Thomson O'Brien MA, Oxman AD, Davis DA, Haynes RB, Freemantle N, Harvey EL. Educational outreach visits: effects on professional practice and health care outcomes. *Cochrane Database Syst Rev.* 2000(2):CD000409.

34. Woolf SH, Johnson RE. The break-even point: when medical advances are less important than improving the fidelity with which they are delivered. *Ann Fam Med.* 2005;3(6):545–552.

35. Minkler M, Wallerstein N. *Community-based participatory research for health: From process to outcomes.* 2nd ed. San Francisco: Jossey-Bass; 2008.

36. Schmid T, Zabina H, McQueen D, Glasunov I, Potemkina R. The first telephone-based health survey in Moscow: building a model for behavioral risk factor surveillance in Russia. *Soz Praventivmed.* 2005;50(1):60–62.

37. Cambon L, Minary L, Ridde V, Alla F. Transferability of interventions in health education: a review. *BMC Public Health.* 2012;12:497.

38. Cuijpers P, de Graaf I, Bohlmeijer E. Adapting and disseminating effective public health interventions in another country: towards a systematic approach. *Eur J Public Health.* 2005;15(2):166–169.

39. Diem G, Brownson RC, Grabauskas V, Shatchkute A, Stachenko S. Prevention and control of noncommunicable diseases through evidence-based public health: implementing the NCD 2020 action plan. *Glob Health Promot.* 2016;23(3):5–13.

40. Ramsey AT. More Than Just the Endgame: The Role of Implementation Science For Early-Stage Innovations In Behavioral Health. https://publichealth.wustl.edu/just-endgame-role-implementation-science-early-stage-innovations-behavioral-health-sciences/. Accessed April 3, 2017.

41. Brownson RC, Jacobs JA, Tabak RG, Hoehner CM, Stamatakis KA. Designing for dissemination among public health researchers: findings from a national survey in the United States. *Am J Public Health.* 2013;103(9):1693–1699.

42. Colditz GA, Emmons KM, Vishwanath K, Kerner JF. Translating science to practice: community and academic perspectives. *J Public Health Manag Pract.* 2008;14(2):144–149.

43. Kreuter MW, Bernhardt JM. Reframing the dissemination challenge: a marketing and distribution perspective. *Am J Public Health.* 2009;99(12):2123–2127.

44. National Cancer Institute. *Designing for dissemination: Conference summary report.* Washington, DC: National Cancer Institute; 2002.

45. Chambers DA, Feero WG, Khoury MJ. Convergence of implementation science, precision medicine, and the learning health care system: a new model for biomedical research. *JAMA.* 2016;315(18):1941–1942.

46. Glasgow RE, Emmons KM. How can we increase translation of research into practice? Types of evidence needed. *Annu Rev Public Health.* 2007;28:413–433.

47. Owen N, Goode A, Fjeldsoe B, Sugiyama T, Eakin E. Designing for the dissemination of environmental and policy initiatives and programs for high-risk groups. In: Brownson R, Colditz G, Proctor E, eds. *Dissemination and implementation research in health: Translating science to practice.* New York: Oxford University Press; 2012: 114–127.

48. Marshall M, de Silva D, Cruickshank L, Shand J, Wei L, Anderson J. What we know about designing an effective improvement intervention (but too often fail to put into practice). *BMJ Qual Saf.* 2017;26(7):578–582.

49. Harper GW, Neubauer LC, Bangi AK, Francisco VT. Transdisciplinary research and evaluation for community health initiatives. *Health Promot Pract.* 2008;9(4):328–337.

50. Stokols D. Toward a science of transdisciplinary action research. *Am J Community Psychol.* 2006;38(1-2):63–77.

51. Ciesielski TH, Aldrich MC, Marsit CJ, Hiatt RA, Williams SM. Transdisciplinary approaches enhance the production of translational knowledge. *Transl Res.* 2017;182:113–134.

52. Kobus K, Mermelstein R. Bridging basic and clinical science with policy studies: The Partners with Transdisciplinary Tobacco Use Research Centers experience. *Nicotine Tob Res.* 2009;11(5):467–474.

53. Kobus K, Mermelstein R, Ponkshe P. Communications strategies to broaden the reach of tobacco use research: examples from the Transdisciplinary Tobacco Use Research Centers. *Nicotine Tob Res.* 2007;9 Suppl 4:S571–S582.

54. Morgan GD, Kobus K, Gerlach KK, et al. Facilitating transdisciplinary research: the experience of the transdisciplinary tobacco use research centers. *Nicotine Tob Res.* 2003;5 Suppl 1:S11–S19.

55. Stokols D, Harvey R, Gress J, Fuqua J, Phillips K. In vivo studies of transdisciplinary scientific collaboration: lessons learned and implications for active living research. *Am J Prev Med.* 2005;28(2 Suppl 2):202–213.

56. Emmons KM, Viswanath K, Colditz GA. The role of transdisciplinary collaboration in translating and disseminating health research: lessons learned and exemplars of success. *Am J Prev Med.* 2008;35(2 Suppl):S204–S210.

57. Cargo M, Mercer SL. The value and challenges of participatory research: strengthening its practice. *Annu Rev Public Health.* 2008;29:325–350.

58. Miller AL, Krusky AM, Franzen S, Cochran S, Zimmerman MA. Partnering to translate evidence-based programs to community settings: bridging the gap between research and practice. *Health Promot Pract.* 2012;13(4):559–566.

59. Chambers DA, Proctor EK, Brownson RC, Straus SE. Mapping training needs for dissemination and implementation research: lessons from a synthesis of existing D&I research training programs. *Transl Behav Med.* 2016 Mar 30 [Epub ahead of print].

60. Luke DA, Baumann AA, Carothers BJ, Landsverk J, Proctor EK. Forging a link between mentoring and collaboration: a new training model for implementation science. *Implement Sci.* 2016;11(1):137.

61. Proctor EK, Landsverk J, Baumann AA, et al. The implementation research institute: training mental health implementation researchers in the United States. *Implement Sci.* 2013;8:105.

62. Washington University in St. Louis. Implementation Research Institute. http://iristl.org/. Accessed February 12, 2017.

63. Brownson RC, Colditz GA, Dobbins M, et al. Concocting that magic elixir: successful grant application writing in dissemination and implementation research. *Clin Transl Sci.* 2015;8(6):710–716.

64. Padek M, Colditz G, Dobbins M, et al. Developing educational competencies for dissemination and implementation research training programs: an exploratory analysis using card sorts. *Implement Sci.* 2015;10:114.

65. Washington University in St. Louis. Mentored Training for Dissemination & Implementation Research in Cancer. http://mtdirc.org/. Accessed February 12, 2017.

66. Meissner HI, Glasgow RE, Vinson CA, et al. The U.S. training institute for dissemination and implementation research in health. *Implement Sci.* 2013;8:12.

INDEX

Note: Page numbers in **bold** indicate chapter subjects and authors. Page numbers in *italics* indicate tables and charts.